PHTLS

Prehospital Trauma Life Support

TRAUMA FIRST RESPONSE

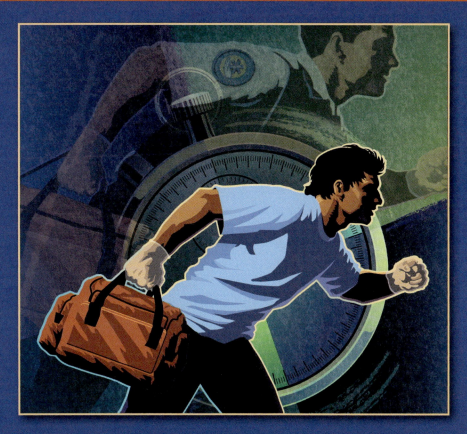

"The fate of the wounded rest in the hands of the one who applies the first dressing."

—Nicholas Senn, MD (1844–1908)
American Surgeon (Chicago, Illinois)
Founder, Association of Military Surgeons
of the United States

PHTLS
Prehospital Trauma Life Support

TRAUMA FIRST RESPONSE

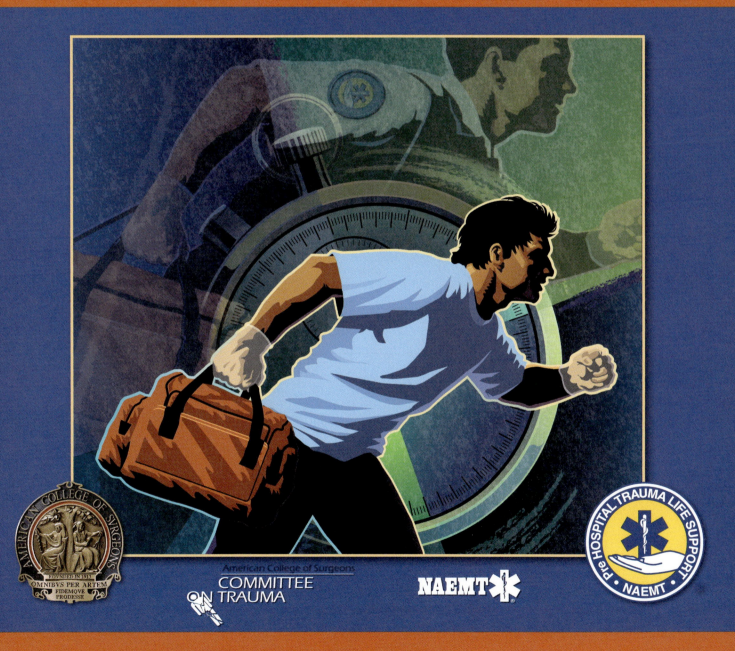

American College of Surgeons
COMMITTEE ON TRAUMA

NAEMT

ELSEVIER
MOSBY JEMS

Prehospital Trauma Life Support Committee of The National Association of Emergency Medical Technicians in Cooperation with The Committee on Trauma of The American College of Surgeons

MOSBY JEMS
ELSEVIER

3251 Riverport Lane
St. Louis, MO 63043

Notices

Knowledge and best practice in this field are constantly changing. As new research and experience broaden our understanding, changes in research methods, professional practices, or medical treatment may become necessary.

Practitioners and researchers must always rely on their own experience and knowledge in evaluating and using any information, methods, compounds, or experiments described herein. In using such information or methods they should be mindful of their own safety and the safety of others, including parties for whom they have a professional responsibility.

With respect to any drug or pharmaceutical products identified, readers are advised to check the most current information provided (i) on procedures featured or (ii) by the manufacturer of each product to be administered, to verify the recommended dose or formula, the method and duration of administration, and contraindications. It is the responsibility of practitioners, relying on their own experience and knowledge of their patients, to make diagnoses, to determine dosages and the best treatment for each individual patient, and to take all appropriate safety precautions.

To the fullest extent of the law, neither the Publisher nor the authors, contributors, or editors, assume any liability for any injury and/or damage to persons or property as a matter of products liability, negligence or otherwise, or from any use or operation of any methods, products, instructions, or ideas contained in the material herein.

Publisher: Andrew Allen
Managing Editor: Laura Bayless
Publishing Services Manager: Catherine Jackson
Design Direction: Jessica Williams

Printed in Canada

CONTRIBUTORS

EDITOR

Peter T. Pons, MD, FACEP
Associate Medical Director, PHTLS
Emergency Medicine
Denver, Colorado

EDITOR-IN-CHIEF

Norman E. McSwain, Jr., MD, FACS, NREMT-P
Professor of Surgery
Medical Director, PHTLS
Tulane University Department of Surgery
New Orleans, Louisiana

ASSOCIATE EDITORS

Will Chapleau, EMT-P, RN, TNS, CEN
Chairman, PHTLS Executive Council
Manager, ATLS Program
American College of Surgeons
Chicago, Illinois

Gregory Chapman, EMT-P, RRT
Vice Chairman, PHTLS Executive Council
Center for Prehospital Medicine
Department of Emergency Medicine
Carolinas Medical Center
Charlotte, North Carolina

Jeffrey S. Guy, MD, MSc, MMHC, FACS, EMT-P
Associate Medical Director, PHTLS
Associate Professor of Surgery
Director, Regional Burn Center
Vanderbilt University School of Medicine
Nashville, Tennessee

Jeffrey P. Salomone, MD, FACS, NREMT-P
Associate Medical Director, PHTLS
Associate Professor of Surgery
Emory University School of Medicine
Atlanta, Georgia

CONTRIBUTORS

Brad L. Bennett, PhD, NREMT-P, FAWM
CAPT, USN (Ret)
Adjunct Asst Professor, Military and Emergency
  Medicine Department
Uniformed Services University of the Health Sciences
Bethesda, Maryland

Matthew Bitner, MD
Division of Emergency Medicine
Department of Surgery
Duke University, School of Medicine
Durham, North Carolina

Frank K. Butler, Jr., MD
CAPT, MC, USN (Ret)
Chairman
Committee on Tactical Combat Casualty Care
Defense Health Board

Howard Champion, MD, FRCS, FACS
Senior Advisory in Trauma
Professor of Surgery and Military and Emergency Medicine
Uniformed Services University of the Health Sciences
Washington, DC

Will Chapleau, EMT-P, RN, TNS, CEN
Chairman, PHTLS Executive Council
Manager, ATLS Program
American College of Surgeons
Chicago, Illinois

Gregory Chapman, EMT-P, RRT
Vice Chairman, PHTLS Executive Council
Center for Prehospital Medicine
Department of Emergency Medicine
Carolinas Medical Center
Charlotte, North Carolina

Jeffrey S. Guy, MD, MSc, MMHC, FACS, EMT-P
Associate Medical Director, PHTLS
Associate Professor of Surgery
Director, Regional Burn Center
Vanderbilt University School of Medicine
Nashville, Tennessee

Norman E. McSwain, Jr., MD, FACS, NREMT-P
Professor of Surgery
Medical Director, PHTLS
Tulane University Department of Surgery
New Orleans, Louisiana

Peter T. Pons, MD, FACEP
Associate Medical Director, PHTLS
Emergency Medicine
Denver, Colorado

Jeffrey P. Salomone, MD, FACS, NREMT-P
Senior Associate Medical Director, PHTLS
Associate Professor of Surgery
Emory University School of Medicine
Atlanta, Georgia

Joseph A. Salomone, III, MD
Associate Professor of Emergency Medicine
University of Missouri, Kansas City
Kansas City, Missouri

INTERNATIONAL CONTRIBUTORS

Dr. Alberto Adduci, Italy

Dhary Al Rasheed, Saudi Arabia

Dr. Saud Al Turki, Saudi Arabia

Shaikha M. Al-Alawi, Oman

Stuart Alves, United Kingdom

Dr. Paul Barbevil, Uruguay

Dr. Jaime A. Cortés-Ojeda, Costa Rica

Kenneth D'Alessandro, Saudi Arabia

Jan Filippo, Netherlands

Dr. Subash Gautam, United Arab Emirates

Bernhard Gliwitzky, Germany

Steve Griesch, Luxemburg

Dr. Thorsten Hauer, Germany

Konstantin Karavasilis, Georgia

Fabrice Lamarche, Belgium

Dr. Salvijus Milasius, Lithuania

Dr. Ana Maria Montanez, Peru

Philip Nel, South Africa

Dr. Fernando Novo, Brazil

Dr. Gonzalo Ostria, Bolivia

Christoph Redelsteiner, Austria

John Richardsen, Norway

Dr. Osvaldo Rois, Argentina

Michal Soczynski, Poland

Dr. Javier Gonzales Uriarte, Spain

Lisbeth Wick, France

Patrick Wick, France

REVIEWERS

Jeffrey Asher, NREMT-P
Chief Paramedic Instructor
Chippewa Valley Technical College
Eau Claire, Wisconsin

Kevin Thomas Collopy, BA, CCEMT-P, NREMT-P, WEMT
Flight Paramedic, Spirit Ministry Medical Transportation
Lead Instructor, Wilderness Medical Associates
Ministry Health Care
Marshfield, Wisconsin

Steven Dralle, MBA, LP
San Antonio, Texas

Mark Goldstein, RN, MSN, EMT-P I/C
Emergency Services Operations Manager
Memorial Health System
Colorado Springs, Colorado

Marguerite X. Haaga, BA, EMSI, Paramedic
Center for Public Safety Education
East Berlin, Connecticut

Deborah L. Petty, BS, CICP, EMT-P I/C
Paramedic Training Officer
St. Charles County Ambulance District
St. Peters, Missouri

William E. Rich, EMT-P, AAS-EMT, CEM
Emergency Management Specialist
Centers for Disease Control
Atlanta, Georgia

Adriana Laura Torrez, LP, AAS
EMS Education Coordinator
Methodist Health System
Dallas, Texas

Our continued thanks go out to the reviewers of PHTLS
Prehospital Trauma Life Support, Seventh Edition:

P. David Adelson, MD
Director, Children's Neuroscience Institute
Chief of Pediatric Neurosurgery
Phoenix Children's Hospital
Phoenix, Arizona

Kristen D. Borchelt, RN, NREMT-P
Cincinnati Children's Hospital
Cincinnati, Ohio

Timothy Scott Brisbin, RN, BSN, NREMT-P
Director
The Center for Prehospital Medicine
Department of Emergency Medicine
Carolinas Medical Center
Charlotte, North Carolina

Jeffrey S. Cain, MD
US Army Institute of Surgical Research
Fort Sam Houston, Texas

David W. Callaway, MD
Beth Israel Deaconess Medical Center
Boston, Massachusetts

Erik Carlsen, NREMT-P
Lead Instructor/Coordinator
EMS Education MAST Ambulance Inc./Kansas City Missouri
    Tactical Medic Team
Kansas City, Missouri

Greg Clarkes, EMT-P
Canadian College of EMS
Edmonton, Alberta, Canada

Jo Ann Cobble, EdD, Paramedic, RN
Dean, Division of Health Professions
Oklahoma City Community College
Oklahoma City, Oklahoma

Arthur Cooper, MD, MS, FACS, FAAP, FCCM, FAHA
Professor of Surgery
Director of Trauma and Pediatric Surgical Services Columbia
University Medical Center
Affiliation at Harlem Hospital
New York, New York

Phil Currance, EMT-P, RHSP
Deputy Commander Colorado-2 DMAT
National Medical Response Team—Central
National Disaster Medical System/St. Anthony Central
Hospital
Denver, Colorado

Fidel O. Garcia, EMT-P
President
Professional EMS Education, LLC
Grand Junction, Colorado

Rudy Garrett, AS, NREMT-P, CCEMT-P
Flight Paramedic
Airmethods Kentucky
Somerset, Kentucky

J. Scott Hartley, NREMTP, EMSI, PHTLS Affiliate Faculty
ALS Affiliates Inc.
Omaha, Nebraska

Gary Hoertz, Paramedic
EMS Division Chief
Kootenai Fire & Rescue
Post Falls, Idaho

Debra Houry, MD, MPH
Associate Professor
Vice Chair for Research, Department of Emergency Medicine
Director, Center for Injury Control
Emory University
Atlanta, Georgia

John M. Kirtley, BA, NREMT-P
EMS Program Coordinator
J. Sargeant Reynolds Community College
Richmond, Virginia

Glen Larson, CD, REMTP, RN, ASEMS, AS(n), BGS
EMT & Paramedic Instructor
Canadian College of EMS
Edmonton, Alberta, Canada

Douglas W. Lundy, MD, FACS
Orthopaedic Trauma Surgeon
Resurgens Orthopaedics
Marietta, Georgia

William T. McGovern, BS, EMT-P, EMS I, FSI
Quality Assurance Coordinator–Field Services/Assistant
    Fire Chief
Hunter's Ambulance Service/Yalesville Volunteer Fire
    Department
Meriden, Connecticut/Wallingford, Connecticut

Chad E. McIntyre, AAS, NREMT-P, FP-C
Shands Jacksonville Trauma & Flight Services
Jacksonville, Florida

Reylon Meeks, RN, PhDc
Clinical Nurse Specialist
Blank Children's Hospital
Des Moines, Iowa

Jeff J. Messerole, Paramedic
Clinical Instructor
Spencer Hospital
Spencer, Iowa

Gregory S. Neiman, BA, NREMT-P
BLS Training Specialist
Virginia Office of EMS
Richmond, Virginia

Dennis Parker, MA, EMT-P, I/C
EMS Program Coordinator
Tennessee Tech University
Cookeville, Tennessee

David Pecora, EMT-P, PA
Morgantown, West Virginia

Timothy Penic, NREMT-P, CCP
Field Operations Supervisor
Medstar EMS
Fort Worth, Texas

Deborah L. Petty, BS, CICP, EMT-P I/C
Paramedic Training Officer
St. Charles County Ambulance District
St. Peters, Missouri

Jean-Cyrille Pitteloud, MD, DEAA
Hôpital du Valais
Sion, Switzerland

Larry Richmond, AS, NREMT-P, CCEMT-P
EMS Coordinator
Rapid City Indian Health Service Hospital
Rapid City, South Dakota

David Stamey, CCEMT-P
EMS Training Administrator
District of Columbia Fire & EMS Department
Washington, DC

Nerina Stepanovsky, PhD, RH, EMT-P
Emergency Medical Services Program
St. Petersburg College
St. Petersburg, Florida

Kevin M. Sullivan, MS, NREMT-P
Grady EMS
Atlanta, Georgia

David M. Tauber, NREMT-P, CCEMT-P, FP-C, I/C
Education Coordinator/Executive Director
New Haven Sponsor Hospital Program/Advanced Life
  Support Institute
New Haven, Connecticut/Conway, New Hampshire

Javier Uriarte, MD
Leioa, Bizkaia, Spain

Jason J. Zigmont, PhD, NREMT-P
Yale New Haven Health System
New Haven, Connecticut

PUBLISHER ACKNOWLEDGMENTS

The publisher would also like to thank the following agencies for assisting us with the photos and videos created for this book:

Dixie Blatt and the staff at St. John's Mercy Medical Center

Creve Coeur Fire Protection District

Cabin John Park Volunteer Fire Department

Montgomery County Fire Rescue Service

Montgomery County Volunteer Fire Rescue Association

Annapolis Fire Department

Prince Georges County Fire Department

NATIONAL ASSOCIATION OF EMTS BOARD OF DIRECTORS

Connie Meyer
President

Don Lundy
President Elect

Charlene Donahue
Secretary

Richard Ellis, NREMT-P
Treasurer

Patrick F. Moore
Immediate Past President

DIRECTORS

Rod Barrett	James (Jim) A. Judge, III
Aimee Binning	Chuck Kearns
Jennifer Frenette	Dennis Rowe
Paul Hinchey	Jules Scadden
Sue Jacobus	James M. Slattery
KC Jones	

PHTLS EXECUTIVE COUNCIL

Will Chapleau, EMT-P, RN, TNS, CEN
Chairman, PHTLS Executive Council
Manager, ATLS Program
American College of Surgeons
Chicago, Illinois

Gregory Chapman, EMT-P, RRT
Vice Chairman, PHTLS Executive Council
Center for Prehospital Medicine
Department of Emergency Medicine
Carolinas Medical Center
Charlotte, North Carolina

Augie Bamonti, EMT-P
AFB Consulting
Chicago Heights Fire Department (Ret)
Chicago Heights, Illinois

Frank K. Butler, Jr., MD
CAPT, MC, USN (Ret)
Chairman
Committee on Tactical Combat Casualty Care
Defense Health Board

Corine Curd
PHTLS International Office Director
NAEMT Headquarters
Clinton, Mississippi

Jeffrey S. Guy, MD, MSc, MMHC, FACS, EMT-P
Associate Medical Director, PHTLS
Associate Professor of Surgery
Director, Regional Burn Center
Vanderbilt University School of Medicine
Nashville, Tennessee

Michael J. Hunter
Deputy Chief Worcester EMS
UMass Memorial Medical Center—University Campus
Worcester, Massachusetts

Craig H. Jacobus, EMT-P, BA/BS, DC
EMS Faculty Metro Community College
Fremont, Nebraska

Norman E. McSwain, Jr., MD, FACS, NREMT-P
Medical Director, PHTLS
Professor of Surgery
Tulane University School of Medicine
New Orleans, Louisiana

Peter T. Pons, MD, FACEP
Associate Medical Director, PHTLS
Emergency Medicine
Denver, Colorado

Dennis Rowe, EMT-P
Director, Rural/Metro EMS
Lenoir City, Tennessee

Lance Stuke, MD, MPH
Assistant Professor of Surgery
LSU Department of Surgery
New Orleans, Louisiana

PHTLS HONOR ROLL

PHTLS continues to prosper and promote high standards of trauma care all over the world. It would not be able to do this without the contributions of many dedicated and inspired individuals over the past three decades. Some of those mentioned below were instrumental in the development of our first textbook. Others were constantly "on the road" spreading the word. Still others "put out fires" and otherwise problem-solved to keep PHTLS growing. The PHTLS Executive Council, along with the editors and contributors of this, our first edition, would like to express our thanks to all of those listed below. PHTLS lives, breathes, and grows because of the efforts of those who volunteer their time to what they believe in.

Gregory H. Adkisson
Melissa Alexander
Jameel Ali
Augie Bamonti
J.M. Barnes
Morris L. Beard
Ann Bellows
Ernest Block
Chip Boehm
Don E. Boyle
Susan Brown
Susan Briggs
Jonathan Busko
Alexander Butman
H. Jeannie Butman
Christain E. Callsen, Jr.
Steve Carden
Edward A. Casker
Bud Caukin
Hank Christen
David Ciraulo
Victoria Cleary
Philip Coco
Frederick J. Cole
Keith Conover
Arthur Cooper
Jel Coward
Alice "Twink" Dalton
Michael D'Auito

Judith Demarest
Joseph P. Dineen
Leon Dontigney
Joan Drake-Olsen
Mark Elcock
Blaine L. Endersen
Betsy Ewing
Mary E. Fallat
Milton R. Fields, III
Scott B. Frame†
Sheryl G.A. Gabram
Bret Gilliam
Jack Grandey
Vincent A. Greco
Nita J. Ham
Larry Hatfield
Mark C. Hodges
Walter Idol
Alex Isakov
Len Jacobs
Craig Jacobus
Lou Jordan
Richard Judd
Jon A. King
Jon R. Krohmer
Peter LeTarte
Robert W. Letton, Jr.
Dawn Loehn
Mark Lockhart

Robert Loftus
Greg C. Lord
Fernando Magallenes-Negrete
Paul M. Maniscalco
Scott W. Martin
Don Mauger
William McConnell
Merry McSwain
John Mechtel
Claire Merrick
Bill Metcalf
George Moerkirk
Stephen Murphy
Lawrence D. Newell
Jeanne O'Brien
Dawn Orgeron
Eric Ossmann
James Paturas
Joseph Pearce
Thomas Petrich
Valerie J. Phillips
James Pierce
Brian Plaisier
Mark Reading
Brian Reiselbara
Lou Romig
Donald Scelza
John Sigafoos

Paul Silverston
David Skinner
Dale C. Smith
Richard Sobieray
Sheila Spaid
Michael Spain
Don Stamper
Kenneth G. Swan
Kenneth G. Swan, Jr.
David M. Tauber
Joseph J. Tepas, III
Brian M. Tibbs
Josh Vayer
Richard Vomacka†
Robert K. Waddell, II
Michael Werdmann
Carl Werntz
Elizabeth Wertz
Keith Wesley
David E. Wesson
Roger D. White
Kenneth J. Wright
David Wuertz
Al Yellin
Steven Yevich
Doug York
Alida Zamboni

Again, thanks to all of you, and thanks to everyone around the world for making PHTLS work.
PHTLS Executive Council
Editors and Contributors of PHTLS

†Deceased.

ACKNOWLEDGMENTS

In 1624 John Donne wrote that "No man is an island, entire of itself." This describes in many ways the process of the publication of a book. Certainly, no editor is an island. Textbooks, such as the PHTLS Trauma First Response (TFR) book; courses, especially those that involve audiovisual material; and instructor manuals cannot be published by editors in isolation. As a matter of fact, much, if not most, of the work involved in publishing a textbook is done not by the editors and the authors whose names appear on the cover and on the inside of the book, but by the publisher's staff. This first edition of PHTLS TFR is certainly no exception.

From the American College of Surgeons Committee on Trauma, Carol Williams, Executive Secretary of the Committee on Trauma; John Fildes, MD, FACS, the current Chairman of the Committee on Trauma; and Wayne Meredith, MD, FACS, the ACS Medical Director of Trauma, have provided outstanding support for this edition as well as for PHTLS.

Within Mosby, Linda Honeycutt led the effort to bring this edition out on time, Laura Bayless has been an outstanding editor, Megan Greiner at Graphic World Inc. has brought this project to fruition, and Joy Knobbe has worked hard on the public relations for this book.

The editors and authors whose wives, children, and significant others have tolerated the long hours in the preparation of the material are obviously the backbone of any publication.

Peter T. Pons, MD, FACEP
Norman McSwain, MD, FACS, NREMT-P

FOREWORD

In Argentina, in Latin America, and around the world, trauma is a major cause of morbidity as a result of vehicle crashes, violence, and work-related accidents, among other causes.

A response to this issue began in Argentina in 1954 through the local chapter of the American College of Surgeons. It would take 35 more years for the first ATLS course to be conducted in 1989.

During the following years, trauma patient care became vital due to the growing number of victims and the poor training of people in prehospital care.

The thousands of people killed or permanently disabled in Argentina paid a heavy price, both socially and economically for the country. Thus, in 1996, the PHTLS program in Argentina was started by the international faculty of Norman McSwain, Will Chapleau, and Greg Chapman. Seventy instructors were trained, and Argentina was divided into eight regions comprising 23 provinces. Since its inception, the course has expanded throughout the country, becoming a golden milestone in the creation of integrated prehospital and hospital responses in the public and the private sphere.

From then until now, this course has trained physicians, nurses, firefighters, rescue groups, military personnel, and industrial brigades, from Argentina to neighboring Latin American countries. To date, the PHTLS program in our country has conducted international conferences and trauma update workshops for successive editions.

With the support of the PHTLS international office, managed by Will Chapleau and Corine Curd, and with the generous collaboration of other Latin American coordinators from Mexico, Colombia, Brazil, Bolivia, as well as different faculty from the United States, we accomplish these activities. Also, the PHTLS Program in Argentina has contributed to and coordinated the implementation of the program in countries such as Bolivia, Uruguay, Chile, Peru, and now Ecuador.

Personally, as an emergency doctor with more than 30 years of medical and scientific experience in academic societies related to the critically ill, I have to highlight the ongoing development of the program that, with its narrow sense based on scientific evidence, makes the PHTLS course universally adopted in over 40 countries in both the civilian and military worldwide.

It's been 15 years since the first course in our country. We have trained more than 7,500 students. Worldwide we have educated more than half a million providers. All this would not have been possible without the daily efforts of people like Norman McSwain, Will Chapleau, Jeff Salomone, and other greats, such as Scott Frame, who are no longer with us, and hundreds of managers and trainers in the other 50 countries that work day after day teaching and applying the concepts and skills of the program to their patients.

Today in Argentina, the initial management of trauma patient has a single protocol, "the PHTLS kind."

It is an honor shared by all of us who work on the scene, to feel part of this work philosophy and a sense of belonging. One takes great pride when a firefighter, a doctor, a soldier, or a brigade says, "I'm PHTLS," and when we work among the victims of an accident, I feel that these 15 years of training have borne fruit and I understand "they are making a difference."

I will always remember a phrase from Norman McSwain in Argentina: "If one of us can once again save a victim, you can change the world." Thus, overcoming any geopolitical barrier, PHTLS is a bridge of knowledge over the world.

Oswaldo Rois, MD
President, Fundación EMME
Director, PHTLS Argentina

PREFACE

The assessment and management of traumatic injury victims is a team effort. This team starts with those who first encounter the patient in the prehospital setting. In fact, much of how a patient is ultimately managed throughout his or her health care course depends on the assessment and care provided in the field. This process begins with the very first person who evaluates and treats the trauma victim. It is to these individuals that this text and program are dedicated.

Prehospital care providers should accept the responsibility to provide patient care that is as close to absolutely perfect as possible. This cannot be achieved with insufficient knowledge of the subject. We must remember that the patient did not choose to be involved in a traumatic situation. The provider, on the other hand, has chosen to be there to take care of the patient. The prehospital care provider is obligated to give 100% of his or her effort during contact with every patient. The patient has had a bad day; the provider cannot also have a bad day. The prehospital care provider must be sharp and capable in the competition between the patient and death and disease.

The patient is the most important person at the scene of an emergency. There is no time to think about the order in which the patient assessment is performed or what treatments should take priority over others. There is no time to practice a skill before using it on a particular patient. There is no time to think about where equipment or supplies are housed within the jump kit. There is no time to think about where to transport the injured patient. All of this information and more must be stored in the mind, and all supplies and equipment must be present in the jump kit when the provider arrives on the scene. Without the proper knowledge or equipment, the provider may neglect to do things that could potentially increase the patient's chance of survival. The responsibilities of a provider are too great to make such mistakes.

Those who deliver care in the prehospital setting are integral members of the trauma patient care team, as are the nurses or physicians in the emergency department, operating room, intensive care unit, ward, and rehabilitation unit. Prehospital care providers must be practiced in their skills so that they can move the patient quickly and efficiently out of the environment of the emergency and transport the patient quickly to the closest appropriate hospital.

WHY PHTLS?

Course Education Philosophy

Prehospital Trauma Life Support (PHTLS) focuses on principles, not preferences. By focusing on principles of good trauma care, PHTLS promotes critical thinking. The Executive Committee of the PHTLS Division of the National Association of Emergency Medical Technicians (NAEMT) believes that, given a good fund of knowledge, prehospital care providers are capable of making reasoned decisions regarding patient care. Rote memorization of mnemonics is discouraged. Furthermore, there is no one "PHTLS way" of performing a specific skill. The principle of the skill is taught, and then one acceptable method of performing the skill that meets the principle is presented. The authors realize that no one method can apply to the myriad unique situations encountered in the prehospital setting.

Up-to-Date Information

Development of the PHTLS Trauma First Response program began in 2009, immediately on the heels of the revision for the seventh edition of the PHTLS program. PHTLS Trauma First Response is specifically designed for the unique requirements of those individuals who are first to arrive to care for trauma patients in the prehospital setting. Included is a CD-ROM with video clips of skills. Note throughout the book the 💿 symbol references indicating that more information can be found on the CD-ROM.

Scientific Base

The authors and editors have adopted an "evidence-based" approach that includes references from the medical literature supporting the key principles, and additional position papers published by the national organizations are cited when applicable. Many references have been added, allowing those providers with an inquisitive mind to read the scientific data supporting our recommendations.

Support for NAEMT

The NAEMT provides the administrative structure for the PHTLS program. No proceeds from the PHTLS TFR program (surcharges or royalties from the text and audiovisuals) go to the editors or authors of this work or to the American College of Surgeons Committee on Trauma or any other physician-oriented organization. All profits from the PHTLS program are channelled back into NAEMT to provide funding for issues and programs that are of prime importance to EMS professionals, such as educational conferences and the lobbying of legislators on behalf of prehospital care providers.

PHTLS Is a World Leader

Because of the unprecedented success of PHTLS, the program has continued to grow by leaps and bounds and we now offer the Trauma First Response text and program to those who can benefit from this knowledge. PHTLS courses continue to proliferate across the United States, and the US military has adopted it, teaching the program to US Armed Forces personnel at over 100 training sites worldwide. PHTLS has been exported to more than 50 nations, and many others are expressing interest in bringing PHTLS to their countries in efforts to improve prehospital trauma care levels.

Prehospital care providers have the responsibility to assimilate this knowledge and these skills in order to use them for the benefit of the patients for whom the providers are responsible. The editors and authors of this material and the Executive Committee of the PHTLS Division of the NAEMT hope that you will incorporate this information into your

practice and daily rededicate yourself to the care of those persons who cannot care for themselves—the trauma patients.

Peter T. Pons, MD, FACEP
Editor
Norman E. McSwain, Jr., MD, FACS, NREMT-P
Editor-in-Chief, PHTLS
Will Chapleau, EMT-P, RN, TNS, CEN
Gregory Chapman, EMT-P, RRT
Jeffrey S. Guy, MD, MSc, MMHC, FACS, EMT-P
Jeffrey P. Salomone, MD, FACS, NREMT-P
Associate Editors

CONTENTS

SPECIFIC SKILLS

ATLS

As happens so often in life, a personal experience brought about the changes in emergency care that resulted in the birth of the Advanced Trauma Life Support ATLS course for physicians (and eventually the PHTLS program). ATLS started in 1978, 2 years after a private plane crash in a rural area of Nebraska. The ATLS course was born out of that mangled mass of metal, the injured, and the dead.

The pilot, an orthopaedic surgeon, his wife, and family of four children were flying in their twin-engine airplane when it crashed. His wife was killed instantly. The children were critically injured. They waited for what seemed like an eternity for help to arrive, but it never did. After approximately 8 hours, he walked ⅝ of a mile along a dirt road to a highway and flagged down a car after two trucks didn't stop. They drove to the accident site and loaded the children in the car and drove to the closest hospital, a few miles south of the crash site.

When they approached the emergency room door of this rural hospital, they found it was locked and had to knock to get in. A little later the two general practitioners in this small farming community arrived. One of the doctors picked up one of the injured children by the shoulders and the knees and took him into the x-ray room. Later, he returned and announced there was no skull fracture. The cervical spine had not been considered. He then began suturing the laceration. Finally, the pilot called his physician partner and told him what had happened and that they would get to Lincoln as soon as they could.

The doctors and staff in this little hospital had little or no preparation for this type of situation. There was an obvious lack of training for triage and proper treatment.

Folks got tired of the criticism of the treatment received in the rural setting of the crash. The complaint was not about the care at any particular facility, but about the general lack of a delivery system to treat the acute trauma patient in the rural setting. They decided they wanted to educate rural physicians in a systematic way to treat trauma patients and chose to use a similar format to ACLS and call it ATLS.

A syllabus was created and organized into a logical approach to manage trauma. The "treat as you go" methodology was developed. The ABCs of trauma were developed to prioritize the order of assessment and treatment. The prototype was field tested in Auburn, Nebraska, in 1978 with the help of many. The course was presented to the University of Nebraska and, eventually, to the American College of Surgeons Committee on Trauma.

Since that first course in Auburn, Nebraska, three decades have passed and ATLS keeps spreading and growing. What was originally intended as a course for rural Nebraska became a course for the whole world in all types of trauma settings and served as the basis for PHTLS.

PHTLS

As Richard H. Carmona, MD, former United States Surgeon General, stated in his foreword to the sixth edition of this book, "It has been said that we stand on the shoulders of giants in many apparent successes, and PHTLS is no different. With great vision and passion, as well as challenges, a small group of leaders persevered and developed PHTLS over a quarter of a century ago."

Often referred to as "The Father of EMS," Joseph D. "Deke" Farrington, MD, FACS (1909–1982), penned the article "Death in a Ditch," which many believe signalled the turning point in modern EMS in the United States. In 1958, he convinced the Chicago Fire Department that firefighters should be trained to manage emergency patients. Working with Dr. Sam Banks, Deke started the Trauma Training Program in Chicago. Millions have been trained following the guidelines developed in this landmark program. Deke continued to work at every level 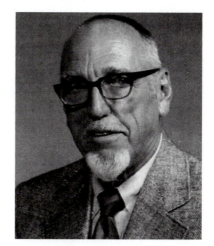 of EMS from the field to education to legislation, ensuring that EMS would grow into the profession in which we work today. The principles set forth by Deke's work form a part of the nucleus of PHTLS, and his are among the shoulders on which we all stand.

The first chairman of the ATLS ad hoc committee for the American College of Surgeons and Chairman of the Prehospital Care Subcommittee on Trauma for the American College of Surgeons, Dr. Norman E. McSwain, Jr., FACS, knew that what they had begun with ATLS would have a profound effect on the outcome of trauma patients. Moreover, he had a strong sense that an even greater effect could come from bringing this type of critical training to prehospital care providers.

Dr. McSwain, a founding member of the board of directors of the National Association of Emergency Medical Technicians (NAEMT), gained the support of the Association's president, Gary Labeau, and began to lay plans for a prehospital version of ATLS. President Labeau directed Dr. McSwain and Robert Nelson, NREMT-P, to determine the feasibility of an ATLS-type program for prehospital care providers.

As a professor of surgery at Tulane University School of Medicine in New Orleans, Louisiana, Dr. McSwain gained the university's support in putting together the draft curriculum of what was to become Prehospital Trauma Life Support (PHTLS). With this draft in place, a PHTLS committee was established in 1983. This committee continued to refine the curriculum, and later that same year, pilot courses were conducted in Lafayette and New Orleans, Louisiana, and at Marian Health Center in Sioux City, Iowa; Yale University School of Medicine in New Haven, Connecticut; and Norwalk Hospital in Norwalk, Connecticut.

Richard W. "Rick" Vomacka (1946–2001) was a part of the task force that developed the PHTLS course based on the Advanced Trauma Life Support program of the American College of Surgeons. PHTLS became his passion as the course came together, and he traveled around the country in the early 1980s conducting pilot courses and regional faculty workshops and worked with Dr. McSwain and the other original task force members to fine-tune the program. Rick was the key to the close relationship that developed between PHTLS and the US military, and he also worked on the first international PHTLS course sites. Rick was a big part of PHTLS's beginnings and will always be remembered with gratitude for his hard work and dedication to the cause of improving care for trauma patients.

National dissemination began with three intensive workshops taught in Denver, Colorado; Bethesda, Maryland; and Orlando, Florida, between September 1984 and February 1985. The graduates of these early courses formed what would be the "Barnstormers," PHTLS national and regional faculty members who traveled the country training additional faculty members, spreading the word that PHTLS had arrived.

Alex Butman along with Rick Vomacka worked diligently, and frequently used money out of their own pockets, to bring the first two editions of the PHTLS program to fruition. Without their help and work, PHTLS would never have begun.

Early courses focused on advanced life support (ALS). In 1986, a course that encompassed basic life support (BLS) was developed. The course grew exponentially. Beginning with those first few enthusiastic faculty members, first dozens, then hundreds, and now thousands of providers annually participate in PHTLS courses all over the world.

As the course grew, the PHTLS committee became a division of the NAEMT. Course demand and the need to maintain course continuity and quality necessitated the building of networks of affiliate state, regional, and national faculty members. There are national coordinators for every country, and in each country, there are regional and state coordinators along with affiliate faculty members to make sure that information is disseminated and courses are consistent whether a provider participates in a program in Chicago Heights, Illinois, or Buenos Aires, Argentina.

Throughout the growth process, medical oversight has been provided through the American College of Surgeons Committee on Trauma. For nearly 20 years, the partnership between the American College of Surgeons and the NAEMT has ensured that course participants receive the opportunity to give trauma patients everywhere their best chance at survival.

Now, PHTLS is pleased to offer the Trauma First Response program, which furthers the goal of providing knowledge and education to those involved in trauma care. PHTLS recognized that, in many cases, trauma patient assessment and management begin even before the arrival of public safety agencies and EMS ambulances. In fact, care begins with those individuals who respond to the call for help and who, in many instances, are responsible for activating the formal medical response system. It is for these individuals that the Trauma First Response program was developed under the leadership of Dr. Norman McSwain, Will Chapleau, and Dr. Peter Pons.

It is on the shoulders of these, and many more individuals too numerous to mention, that PHTLS stands and continues to grow.

PHTLS in the Military

Beginning in 1988, the US military aggressively set out to train its medics in PHTLS. Coordinated by DMRTI, the Defense Medical Readiness Training Institute at Fort Sam Houston in Texas, PHTLS is taught all over the United States, Europe, and Asia, and anywhere the flags of the US military fly. In 2001, the Army's 91WB program standardized the training of over 58,000 Army medics to include PHTLS. A military chapter was added in the fourth edition. After the fifth edition was initially published, a strong relationship was forged between the PHTLS organization and the newly established Committee on Tactical Combat Casualty Care. The initial fruit born of this relationship was an extensively revised military chapter in the fifth edition (revised), and a military version of the book was published in 2004. This collaboration has led to the creation of multiple military chapters for the sixth edition military PHTLS text. PHTLS has been taught numerous times "in theater" during the Afghanistan and Iraq wars and has contributed to the lowest mortality rate from any armed conflict in US history.

International PHTLS

The sound principles of prehospital trauma management emphasized in the PHTLS course have led prehospital care providers and physicians outside the United States to request the importation of the program to their various countries. ATLS faculty members presenting ATLS courses worldwide have assisted in this. This network provides medical direction and course continuity.

As PHTLS has moved across the United States and around the globe, we have been struck by the differences in our cultures and climates and also by the similarities of the people who devote their lives to caring for the sick and injured. All of us who have been blessed with the opportunity to teach overseas have experienced the fellowship with our international partners and know that we are all one people in pursuit of caring for those who need care the most.

The PHTLS family continues to grow with nearly a million students trained in 50 countries. Annually, we are running over 2,600 courses, with 34,000 students.

The nations in the ever-growing PHTLS family (as of the publication of this edition) include Argentina, Australia, Austria, Barbados, Belgium, Bolivia, Brazil, Canada, Chile, China and Hong Kong, Colombia, Costa Rica, Cyprus, Denmark, France, Georgia, Germany, Greece, Grenada, Ireland, Israel, Italy, Lithuania, Luxembourg, Mexico, Netherlands, New Zealand, Norway, Oman, Panama, Peru, Philippines, Poland, Portugal, Saudi Arabia, Scotland, Spain, Sweden, Switzerland, Trinidad and Tobago, United Arab Emirates, the United Kingdom, the United States, Uruguay, and Venezuela. Demonstration courses have been run in Bulgaria, Macedonia, and soon, Croatia, with hopes to establish faculty members there. Japan, Korea, South Africa, Ecuador, Paraguay, and Nigeria all hope to join the family in the near future.

Translations

Our growing international family has spawned translations of the text. The text is currently available in English, Spanish, Greek, Portuguese, French, Dutch, Georgian, Chinese, and Italian. Negotiations are ongoing to have the text published in a number of additional languages. Toward that end, there are subtitles in several languages on the CD-ROM that accompanies this book.

Vision for the Future

The vision for the future of PHTLS is family. The father of PHTLS, Dr. McSwain, remains the foundation for the growing family that provides vital training and contributes knowledge and experience to the world. The inaugural international PHTLS Trauma Symposium was held near Chicago, Illinois, in the year 2000. In 2010, the first European PHTLS meeting was held. These programs bring the work of practitioners and researchers around the globe together to determine the standards of trauma care for the new millennium.

Now, with the publication of the PHTLS Trauma First Response book and the development and implementation of the PHTLS TFR course, the principles of, knowledge, and education about trauma patient management are being extended to those who are first to assess and treat the trauma patient.

The support of the PHTLS family worldwide, all volunteering countless hours of their lives, allows the PHTLS leadership to keep PHTLS growing. This leadership consists of the following:

PHTLS Executive Council

International PHTLS Chairs

Will Chapleau, EMT-P, RN, TNS	1996–present
Elizabeth M. Wertz, RN, BSN, MPM	1992–1996
James L. Paturas	1991–1992
John Sinclair, EMT-P	1990–1991
David Wuertz, EMT-P	1988–1990
James L. Paturas	1985–1988
Richard Vomacka, REMT-P	1983–1985

Medical Director of PHTLS International

Norman E. McSwain, Jr., MD, FACS, NREMT-P	1983–present

Associate PHTLS Medical Directors

Jeffrey S. Guy, MD, FACS, EMT-P	2001–present
Peter T. Pons, MD, FACEP	2000–present
Lance Stuke, MD, MPH	2010–present

As we continue to pursue the potential of the PHTLS course and the worldwide community of prehospital care providers, we must remember our commitment to the following:

- Rapid and accurate assessment
- Identification of shock and hypoxemia
- Initiation of the right interventions at the right time
- Timely transport to the right place

It is also fitting to reprise our mission statement, which was written in a marathon session at the NAEMT conference in 1997. The PHTLS mission continues to be to provide the highest quality prehospital trauma education to all who wish to avail themselves of this opportunity. The PHTLS mission also enhances the achievement of the NAEMT mission. The PHTLS program is committed to quality and performance improvement. As such, PHTLS is always attentive to changes in technology and methods of delivering prehospital trauma care that may be used to enhance the clinical and service quality of this program.

National Association of Emergency Medical Technicians

The NAEMT represents the interests of prehospital care providers all over the world.

NAEMT was founded with the help of the National Registry of EMTs (NREMT) in 1975. Since its inception, the association has worked to promote professional status for prehospital care providers from the first responder to the administrator. Its educational programs began as a way of providing meaningful continuing education to providers at every level and have become the standard of prehospital continuing education all over the world.

NAEMT has reciprocal relationships with dozens of United States and international federal and private agencies that influence every aspect of prehospital care. The NAEMT's participation ensures that the voice of prehospital care is heard in determining the future of our practice.

NAEMT MISSION

The mission of the National Association of Emergency Medical Technicians, Inc., is to be a professional representative organization that will receive and represent the views and opinions of prehospital care personnel and to influence the future advancement of EMS as an allied health profession. NAEMT will serve its professional membership through educational programs, liaison activity, development of national standards and reciprocity, and the development of programs to benefit prehospital care personnel.

With this mission clearly defined and passionately pursued, NAEMT will continue to provide leadership in this developing specialty of prehospital care into the future.

CHAPTER 1

Introduction to PHTLS and TFR

CHAPTER OBJECTIVES

At the completion of this chapter, the reader will be able to do the following:

✓ Recognize the magnitude of the problem both in human and financial terms caused by traumatic injury.

✓ Understand the history and evolution of prehospital trauma care.

✓ Identify and recognize the components and importance of prehospital research and literature.

Our patients did not choose us. We chose them. We could have chosen another profession, but we did not. We have accepted the responsibility for patient care in some of the worst situations: when we are tired or cold; when it is rainy and dark; when we cannot predict what conditions we will encounter. We must either accept this responsibility or surrender it. We must give our patients the very best care that we can—not while we are daydreaming, not with unchecked equipment, not with incomplete supplies, and not with yesterday's knowledge. We cannot know what medical information is current, we cannot claim to be ready to care for our patients if we do not read and learn each day. Prehospital Trauma Life Support (PHTLS) provides a part of that knowledge to the working trauma responder but, more important, it ultimately benefits the person who needs our all—the patient. At the end of each patient encounter, we should feel that the patient received nothing short of our very best.

The opportunity for a medical first responder to help another person is greater in the management of trauma patients than in any other patient encounter. The chance for survival of a trauma patient who receives excellent trauma care is probably greater than that of any other patient. The trauma first responder can lengthen the life span and productive years of the trauma patient and benefit society by virtue of the care provided.

The Problem

In the United States, about 60 million injuries occur each year; 40 million people will require emergency department (ED) care for their injuries, and 2.5 million will be hospitalized. Each year, 9 million of these injuries are disabling. Approximately 8.7 million trauma patients will be temporarily disabled, and 300,000 will be permanently disabled.[3,18]

Trauma is the leading cause of death in persons between 1 and 44 years of age.[1] About 80% of teenage deaths and 60% of

childhood deaths are secondary to trauma. Trauma continues to be the seventh leading cause of death in elderly persons. Almost three times more Americans die of trauma *each year* than died in the entire Vietnam War.[2] Every 10 years, more Americans die of trauma than have died in all U.S. military conflicts combined. Only in the fifth decade of life do cancer and heart disease compete with trauma as a leading cause of death. The cost for care of trauma patients is staggering. Billions of dollars are spent on the management of trauma patients, not including the dollars lost in wages, insurance administration costs, property damage, and employer costs. Lost productivity from disabled trauma patients is the equivalent of 5.1 million years at a cost of more than $65 billion annually. For patients who die, 5.3 million years of life are lost (34 years per person) at a cost of more than $50 billion. Comparatively, the costs (measured in dollars and in years lost) for cancer and heart disease are much less, as illustrated in Figure 1-1.

Prehospital care providers can do little to increase the survival of a cancer patient. However, for the trauma patient, prehospital care providers often make the difference between life and death; between temporary disablement and serious or permanent disability; or between a life of productivity and a life of destitution and welfare. For example, proper protection of a possible broken neck (fractured cervical spine) by a prehospital care provider may make the difference between lifelong paralysis and a productive, healthy life of unrestricted activity. Prehospital care providers encounter many more examples almost every day.

Trauma is a worldwide problem. Although the events that produce injuries and deaths may differ from country to country, the consequences are not. We who work to provide trauma care have an obligation not only to be able to treat injuries after they occur, but ideally to help prevent them from occurring in the first place.

Trauma care is divided into three phases: pre-event, event, and post-event. The trauma first responder has responsibilities in each phase.

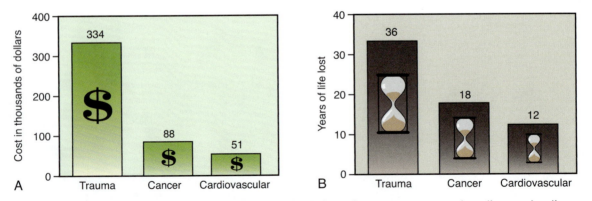

FIGURE 1-1   A, Comparative costs in thousands of dollars to U.S. victims of trauma, cancer, and cardiovascular disease each year. **B,** Comparative number of years lost as a result of trauma, cancer, and cardiovascular disease.

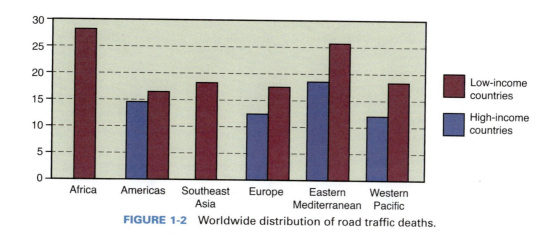

FIGURE 1-2 Worldwide distribution of road traffic deaths.

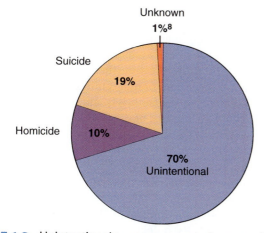

FIGURE 1-3 Unintentional trauma accounts for more deaths than all other causes of trauma death combined.
(Data from the National Center for Injury Prevention and Control: *WISQARS leading causes of death reports, 1999–2006.* Atlanta, Centers for Disease Control and Prevention.)

FIGURE 1-4 Motor vehicle trauma and firearms account for almost half the deaths that result from traumatic injury.
(Data from the National Center for Injury Prevention and Control: *WISQARS leading causes of death reports, 1999–2006,* Atlanta, Centers for Disease Control and Prevention.)

Pre-event Phase

Trauma is no accident, even though it is often referred to as such. An *accident* is defined as either "an event occurring by chance or arising from unknown causes" or "an unfortunate occurrence resulting from carelessness, unawareness, ignorance." Most trauma deaths and injuries fit the second definition but not the first. Most trauma deaths and injuries are preventable. Traumatic incidents fall into two categories: *intentional* and *unintentional.*

The pre-event phase of a trauma incident involves the circumstances leading up to an injury. Efforts to minimize the impact of injury in this phase are primarily focused on injury prevention. In working toward prevention of injuries, the public must be educated to utilize safe home and workplace practices, increase the use of vehicle occupant restraint systems, promote methods to reduce the use of weapons in criminal activities, and promote nonviolent conflict resolution. In addition to caring for the trauma patient, all members of the

health care delivery team have a responsibility to reduce the number of victims.

Currently, unintentional trauma and violence cause more deaths annually in the United States than all other diseases combined (Figures 1-2 and 1-3). Motor vehicles and firearms are involved in more than one half of all trauma deaths, most of which are preventable. Violence accounts for more than one third of these deaths (Figure 1-4).

Motorcycle helmet usage laws are one example of how legislation has affected injury prevention. In 1966 the U.S. Congress gave the Department of Transportation the authority to mandate that states pass legislation requiring the use of motorcycle helmets. The use of helmets subsequently increased to almost 100%, and the fatality rate from motorcycle crashes decreased dramatically. Congress removed this authority in 1975 and more than half the states repealed or modified the existing legislation, resulting in increased death rates in 2006 and 2007.[4] The increase in motorcycle deaths was 11% in 2006.[5] Only 20 states have universal helmet laws. In states with such laws, helmet usage is 74%, whereas in states without such laws the usage rate is 42%.[6] Another example of preventable trauma deaths involves the use of alcohol and driving.[7] As a result of pressure to change state laws for the level of intoxication while driving and through the educational activities of such organizations as Mothers Against Drunk Drivers (MADD), the number of drivers under the influence of alcohol involved in fatal crashes has been consistently decreasing since 1989.

Another way to prevent trauma is through the use of child safety seats. Many trauma centers, law enforcement organizations, and Emergency Medical Services (EMS) agencies conduct programs to educate parents in the correct installation and use of child safety seats.

The other component of the pre-event phase is the personal preparation of trauma care responders for events that are not prevented. Preparation includes proper and complete education with updated information. In addition, it is necessary to be familiar with the available equipment on the response unit at the beginning of every shift and to review your individual responsibilities and duties.

Event Phase

This phase is the moment of the actual trauma. Steps performed in the pre-event phase can influence the outcome of the event phase. This applies not only to our patients, but also to ourselves. Whether driving a personal vehicle or an emergency response vehicle or physically caring for a patient, trauma first responders need to protect themselves and teach others by example. It is important to always drive safely, follow traffic laws, and use the protective devices available, such as vehicle restraints and personal protective equipment such as gloves. Patient outcome will be optimized by assuring that the additional resources are requested, that the EMS system has been activated, and by appropriately prioritizing the interventions provided to the injured patient.

Post-event Phase

Obviously, the worst possible outcome after a traumatic event is death of the patient. Death after sustaining trauma generally occurs in one of three time periods.[8] The *first phase* of deaths occurs within the first few minutes and up to an hour after an incident. These deaths would likely occur even with prompt medical attention. The best way to combat these deaths is through injury prevention and safety strategies. The *second phase* of deaths occurs within the first few hours of an incident. These deaths can be prevented by good prehospital care and good hospital care. The *third phase* of deaths occurs several days to several weeks after the incident. These deaths are generally caused by multiple organ failure. Much more needs to be learned about managing and preventing multiple

organ failure; however, early and aggressive management of shock in the prehospital setting can prevent some of these deaths (Figure 1-5).

R Adams Cowley, MD, founder of the Maryland Institute of Emergency Medical Services (MIEMS), one of the first trauma centers in the United States, described and defined what he called the "Golden Hour."[9] Based on his research, Cowley believed that patients who received definitive care soon after an injury had a much higher survival rate than those whose care was delayed. We now refer to this concept as the Golden Period because it is not always 1 hour. Some patients have less time and others have more time; however, one cannot predict in advance how much time each patient actually has before their chance for survival disappears. Therefore, for the trauma first responder, this means ensuring that the patient is receiving adequate oxygen, controlling obvious external hemorrhage, and activating the EMS system to provide rapid transportation to a facility that is prepared to continue the process of resuscitation as quickly as possible.

An average urban EMS system in the United States has a *response time* (from notification that the incident occurred until arrival on the scene) of 6 to 8 minutes. A typical transport time to the receiving facility is another 8 to 10 minutes. Between 15 and 20 minutes of the Golden Period are already used just to arrive at the scene and transport the patient. If prehospital care at the scene is not efficient and well organized, an additional 30 to 40 minutes can be spent on the scene. With this time on the scene added to the transport time, the "Golden Hour" has already passed before the patient ever arrives at the hospital. This is where the trauma first responder can truly benefit the patient. By quickly evaluating the situation and the patient, performing needed treatment, and being ready to give a rapid, organized report to EMS responders, the trauma

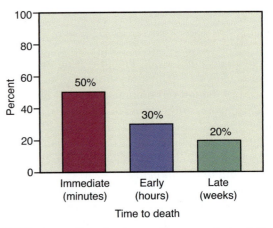

FIGURE 1-5 Immediate deaths can be prevented only by injury prevention education because some patients' only chance is for the incident not to have occurred. Early deaths can be prevented through timely, appropriate prehospital care to reduce mortality and morbidity. Late deaths can be prevented only through prompt transport to a hospital appropriately staffed for trauma care.

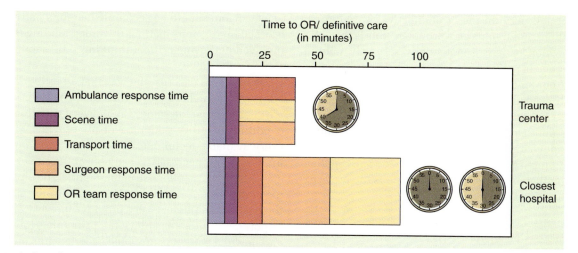

FIGURE 1-6 In locations where trauma centers are available, bypassing hospitals not committed to the care of trauma patients can significantly improve patient care. In severely injured trauma patients, definitive patient care generally occurs in the operating room (OR). An extra 10 to 20 minutes spent en route to a hospital with an in-house surgeon and in-house OR staff significantly reduces the time to definitive care in the OR. *Blue,* EMS response time. *Purple,* on-scene time. *Red,* EMS transport time. *Orange,* surgical response from out of hospital. *Yellow,* OR team response from out of hospital.

first responder can help minimize the amount of time spent on the scene with the patient once EMS arrives. EMS has the responsibility of actually transporting the patient to an appropriate facility. A trauma center that has a surgeon available either before or shortly after the arrival of the patient, a well-trained and trauma-experienced emergency medicine team, and an operating room (OR) team immediately available can often have a trauma patient with life-threatening hemorrhage in the OR within 10 to 15 minutes of the patient's arrival to the hospital. This can be the difference between life and death. On the other hand, a hospital without such in-house surgical capabilities must await the arrival of the surgeon and the surgical team before transporting the patient from the ED to the OR. Additional time may then elapse before the hemorrhage can be controlled, resulting in an associated increase in mortality rate (Figure 1-6). There is a significant increase in survival if non–trauma centers are bypassed and all severely injured patients are taken to a trauma center.[10–17]

The Art and Science of Medicine

It has been understood and accepted for many years that medicine is not an exact science and that there is much art in the practice of medicine. This includes all aspects of medicine and all practitioners, from allied health personnel to nurses and physicians. Medicine has changed a great deal since the early 1900s. At that time, there were no antibiotics and a minimal understanding of not only childhood illness, but all disease and illness; only rudimentary surgery was avail-

able; and medication was mostly herbal remedies. We have moved a long way toward the science side. In recent decades technology has advanced at a rapid rate as electronics have developed and as research has allowed us to better understand patient care. The practice of medicine has become more and more a science and less and less an art. However, the art remains and medicine is still a long way from the precise science of math or physics.

It was not until the 1950s that there was thought to be any benefit to training those who encountered the patient before arrival to the emergency room, and back then it was a "room," usually at the rear of the hospital and often locked until someone came to open it. The fund of knowledge provided to the prehospital provider has significantly advanced in the years since. With this growth comes the major responsibility that all prehospital providers ensure that they are up to date with the latest knowledge and that their skills are finely honed. This knowledge is gained from reading and continuing education, whereas the skills improve only with experience and critique, like those of a surgeon or an airplane pilot. Just as a pilot does not solo after one flight, so too does the trauma care provider not mature from using a skill once or in one situation.

The science of prehospital care, and the understanding to make fully correct decisions when dealing with a patient, includes a working knowledge of (1) anatomy—the organs, bones, muscles, arteries, nerves, and veins (perhaps not all the names but certainly where they are in the patient); (2) physiology of how the body works and responds to trauma; and (3) the appropriate interventions to perform in a given situation.

Yet, with all these advances, it is the art of medicine that continues to rely on healthcare providers to use their knowledge and critical thinking skills to make appropriate judgments and decisions to identify the immediate problem faced by the patient and perform the most effective procedures to benefit the patient. For trauma care providers, this is the determination of which patient is potentially seriously injured, which patient needs rapid transportation to the hospital; how much should be done and what techniques should be used to accomplish needed interventions; and what equipment is the best to use in what situation. This is all the art of medicine. Perhaps another word is preference. Which technique, procedure or device does the trauma care provider have in their scope of practice that will meet the needs of the patient in the situation that exists at the time? Which is the preferred method of managing the patient's problem?

Principles and Preferences

The science of medicine provides the *principles* of medical care. Simply stated, principles are those things that must be accomplished or ensured by the healthcare provider to optimize patient survival and outcome. How these principles are implemented by the individual provider to most efficiently manage the patient at the time of patient contact depends on his or her *preferences,* based on the situation that exists at the specific time, the clinical condition of the patient, the provider's own individual training and skills, and the equipment available. This is how the **science and art** of medicine come together for the good of patient care.

The preferences of how to accomplish the principles depend on four factors (Figure 1-7).

The philosophy of the PHTLS program is that no one situation is the same as any other situation. No one patient is the same as any other patient. PHTLS teaches the importance of having a strong understanding of the subject matter and the skills necessary to accomplish needed interventions. The judgments and decisions made on the scene should be individualized to the needs of this specific patient being dealt with at this specific time and in this specific situation. Protocols are not the final answer. Protocols are not flexible enough to meet the variability associated with every event. The provider must know the scene, the situation, the abilities of the providers involved, and the equipment available. Understanding

what can and should be accomplished for a particular patient is based on this information. By understanding the principles involved and using **critical thinking** skills, appropriate decisions can be made.

Preferences describe the way that an individual prehospital provider can best accomplish the principle. The principle will not be done the same way in every situation or for every condition of every patient. Not all providers have skill in every available technique. The tools to carry out these techniques are not necessarily available at the site of all emergencies. Just because one instructor, lecturer, or physician director prefers one particular technique does not mean that it is the best technique for every provider in every situation. The important point is to achieve the principle. How this is done and how the patient is provided care depends on the four factors listed in Figure 1-7 and described in more detail next.

Situation

Situation involves all the factors at a scene that can affect what care is provided to a patient. These include but are certainly not limited to the following: hazards on the scene, number of patients involved, location of the patient, position of the vehicle, contamination or hazardous materials concerns, fire (or chance of fire), weather, scene control and security by law enforcement, time and distance to medical care (including qualifications of the closest hospital and the trauma center if different), number of EMS providers and other possible helpers on the scene, bystanders, transportation available on the scene, other transportation available at a distance (e.g., helicopters, additional ambulances, etc.), and many more. All these conditions may be constantly changing. These factors and many others will change the way that you as a prehospital provider can respond to the needs of the patient.

The importance of and difference between principle and preference can be demonstrated using spinal immobilization in the following examples. The *principle* is that a potential spine injury must be considered in a patient with a significant mechanism of injury. The *preference* is in how spinal immobilization is to be carried out in a particular patient—in other words, What is the best way to ensure that the spine is immobilized given the circumstances involved? The art is how the prehospital provider carries this out to achieve the principle.

Situation 1:
- Automobile crash
- Bull's-eye fracture of the windshield
- Warm, sunny day
- No traffic on the road

Management:
- Patient examined in the car
- Cervical collar applied
- Patient secured to the short backboard

FIGURE 1-7   Principles versus Preferences

Principle is what is necessary for patient improvement or survival. *Preference* is how the principle is achieved in the time needed and by the provider available. The preference used to accomplish the principle depends on four factors:

- *Situation* that exists
- *Condition* of the patient
- *Fund of knowledge* of the provider
- *Equipment* available

- Rotated onto the long backboard
- Removed from the car
- Placed on the stretcher
- Physical assessment completed
- Patient transported to the hospital

Situation 2:
- Same as Situation 1, except gasoline is dripping from the gas tank
- Concern for fire

Management:
- Rapid extraction techniques used
- Patient moved significant distance from the vehicle
- Physical assessment completed
- Patient transported to the hospital

Situation 3:
- Vehicle is on fire
- Patient unable to move

Management:
- No assessment
- Patient dragged from the fire
- Placed on backboard
- Moved quickly at a distance from the fire
- Patient assessment completed
- Transported quickly to the hospital, depending on patient's condition

Condition of the Patient

For the component of the decision-making process that concerns the medical condition of the patient, the major question that affects decision making is, How injured is the patient? Some examples of issues that will help this determination include the cause of the medical condition, the age of the patient, physiologic factors (e.g., blood pressure, pulse, ventilatory rate, skin temperature, etc.), the etiology of the trauma, the patient's medical condition before the event, medication that the patient is using, illicit drug use, alcohol use, and many others.

Fund of Knowledge of the Provider

The **fund of knowledge** of the provider comes from several sources, including initial training, recent continuing education, experience in the field, experience with this specific condition, and skill with the available potential procedures that the patient might require.

Equipment Available

The trauma care provider will use the equipment or supplies they have been trained to use and have at hand.

The goal of patient care is to achieve the principle. How this is achieved and the decision made by the trauma care provider to manage the patient is the preference based on the situation, patient condition, fund of knowledge, and skill and equipment available at the time the patient presents. That action is determined by the provider's knowledge of all four components outlined earlier.

For example, when a non-breathing patient is encountered, the principle is that the airway must be opened and oxygen delivered to the lungs. The preference chosen depends on the four factors described earlier. Therefore, any of the following might occur:

- A bystander on the street with only cardiopulmonary resuscitation (CPR) training may perform mouth-to-mask ventilation
- An EMT may choose an oral airway and bag-mask ventilation
- A paramedic may choose to place an endotracheal (ET) tube or may decide that it is more advantageous to use the bag-mask device with rapid transportation
- A military corpsman in combat may chose a cricothyroidotomy or nothing at all if enemy fire is too intense
- A physician in the ED may chose paralytic drugs or fiber-optic-guided ET tube placement

None of the choices are wrong at a specific time for a given patient (situation, patient condition, fund of knowledge, experience/skill equipment available) and, in the same way, none are correct all the time for the same reasons.

Critical Thinking

In order to successfully accomplish the principle needed for a particular patient and to choose the best preference to implement the principle, critical thinking skills are as important as, and may be even more important than, the manual skills that will be used to perform an intervention. Critical thinking in medicine is a process whereby the medical care provider assesses the situation, the patient, and all the resources that are available. This information is then rapidly analyzed and integrated to provide the best care possible to the patient. This requires that the provider develop a plan of action, initiate this plan, reassess the plan as the process of caring for the patient moves forward, and make adjustments in the plan as the patient condition changes, until that phase of care is completed (Figure 1-8).

Critical thinking is a learned skill that improves with usage and experience, as do all skills.[19] If students are to function successfully as healthcare providers, they must be equipped with the lifelong learning and critical thinking skills necessary to acquire and process information in a rapidly changing world.[20]

For the prehospital provider, this process begins with the initial information provided at the time of the call for assis-

---

FIGURE 1-8 Steps in Critical Thinking

ASSESSMENT

What is going on? What needs to be done? What are the resources to achieve the goal? Analysis will involve: the scene survey, identification of any hazards to either the patient or to the provider, condition of the patient, rapidity required for resolution, location of the care (in the field, during transport, and after arrival to the hospital), number of patients on the scene, number of transport vehicles required, need for more rapid transportation (aeromedical), destination of the patient for the appropriate care.

ANALYSIS

Each of these described conditions needs to be individually and rapidly analyzed and cross-referenced with the provider's fund of knowledge and resources available, and then steps defined to provide the best care.

CONSTRUCTION OF A PLAN

The plan to achieve the best outcome for the patient is developed and critically reviewed. Is any step false? Are the planned steps all achievable? Are the resources available that will allow the plan to move forward? Will they, more likely than not, lead to a successful outcome?

ACTION

The plan is enacted and started in motion. This is done decisively and with strength of command so that there is no question or hesitation on the part of any of the individuals involved as to what needs to be accomplished, who is in command, and who is making the decisions. If the decisions are incorrect or incomplete or are causing difficulties or complications, the person in command must make appropriate changes. The input for change can come from observations of the commander or from other sources available.

REASSESSMENT

Is the process moving correctly? Has the situation on scene changed? What is the patient's condition? How has the treatment plan changed the patient condition? Does anything in the action plan need to be changed?

CHANGES ALONG THE WAY

Any changes identified by the commander are assessed and analyzed as described earlier and alterations made as appropriate so as to continue the best possible care to the patient. Decision making and reassessing the patient must be done without the worry that change is a sign of weakness or poor initial decision making. Such change based on patient need is not a weakness but rather a strength. Once a decision is made, as the process continues and the situation and patient respond, the provider reassesses and makes appropriate changes as required to provide the best possible care to the patient.

---

tance and continues until the handoff in the hospital to the next component in the chain of patient care. This critical thinking process first requires that the prehospital care provider assess and reassess the scene and situation in which the patient is encountered. Then the patient's condition must be frequently assessed and reassessed. Critical thinking is also involved in the selection of best or most appropriate facility for the patient, the resources available, and the transportation time to the various facilities in the vicinity. All these critical decisions are based on the situation, the patient condition, the fund of knowledge of the prehospital provider, and the equipment available.

By using, analyzing, and integrating all this information, the field care provider develops an initial plan for caring for the injured trauma victim and moves that plan forward. For each step along the way, providers must reassess exactly how the patient has responded to the process. Prehospital providers must either continue the treatment plan or take steps to change the process as additional information becomes available. All this depends on the critical thinking skills used by each provider to carry out his or her responsibilities.

In other words, critical thinking involves how to best provide the principles of patient care needed by the patient based on the current circumstances that the provider has noted. This uses the basis of appropriate medical care advocated by PHTLS "Judgment based on knowledge." Critical thinking has been described as being based on concepts and principles, not hard and fast rules or step-by-step procedures.[22] The emphasis throughout PHTLS education is that protocols involving robotic recall are not beneficial for patient management. Guidelines for patient care must be flexible. Critical thinking requires that flexibility. Protocols should simply serve as guidelines to assist providers in aligning their thought process and should be integrated with thoughtful, insightful analysis of the situation and application of appropriate steps to ensure the best possible patient care in this unique situation.

In addition, all medical providers have biases that can affect the critical thinking process and decision making about the patient. These biases must be recognized and not allowed to intrude during the patient care process. These biases usually arise from previous experiences that resulted in either a significant positive or negative impact. By being aware of and controlling biases, all conditions are taken into consideration and action is based on the guiding principles of "Assume the worst possible injury is present and prove that it is not" and "Do no further harm." The patient's management plan is designed regardless of the attitudes of the provider regarding the "apparent" conditions that might have lead to the current circumstances. For example, the initial impression that a driver is intoxicated may be correct, but other conditions may exist as well. Because a victim is found to smell of alcohol does not mean he or she is not injured too. Because the victim is intoxicated with impaired mental facilities does not mean that some of that impairment might not be due to brain injury or decreased cerebral perfusion because of shock.

Often the answers to these sorts of questions cannot be obtained until the patient arrives at the hospital (or maybe even several days thereafter); therefore, the critical thinking prehospital provider's response must be based on a worst case scenario. Judgments must be made based on the best information available at the time. The critical thinker is constantly looking for other information as it becomes available; being able to act on it is another sign of a good critical thinker. The assessment of the patient, the situation, and the conditions must continue throughout the critical thinking process. The critical thinker is always looking for new information, making and revising judgments, and planning two to three steps beyond the current activity.

Trauma care is a field of quick action and reliance on the innate ability of the provider to respond decisively to varying presentations and varying diseases. These quick actions require the skill of critical thinking and deciding, based on the current knowledge, which steps provide the best chance for patient survival.

Critical thinking at the site of an emergency must be swift, thorough, flexible, and objective. The emergency medical care provider at the site of an emergency may have only seconds to assess the situation, the condition of the patient, and the resources; make decisions; and commence patient care. This encompasses the processes of discernment, analysis, evaluation, judgment, reevaluation, and revised decision making, until the patient finally arrives at the hospital. In contrast, the critical care thinking process of an administrator may allow for several days, weeks, or even months. In EMS, a strong fund of knowledge possessed by the provider and the ability to communicate these judgments with strength and conviction to all involved in the response to the patient are the foundation for critical thinking.

As is taught in Chapter 3 on Assessment of the Scene and Patient, information is gathered using all the provider's senses—vision, smell, touch, hearing—and simultaneously fed into the "computer" inside the brain. The provider then analyzes the data obtained based on the predetermined priorities of the primary survey (airway, ventilation, and circula-

tion), resuscitation, and rapid transportation to the appropriate medical facility to then select the appropriate management steps for the individual needs of that particular patient. Typically, the process of evaluating a trauma patient begins with the ABCDE (Airway, Breathing, Circulation, Disability, and Exposure) priorities. However, if the patient is in shock because of severe ongoing external hemorrhage, then a pressure dressing (and tourniquet if that fails) over the site of severe hemorrhage is the appropriate initial step. Critical thinking is the recognition that following the standard ABCDE priority may lead to a patient who has an airway but who has now bled to death, so instead of addressing the airway, control of the bleeding was the appropriate first step. Critical thinking is the process of recognizing that if the pressure dressing is not working, something more needs to be done and application of a tourniquet is the next best step to stop the hemorrhage. How the brain of the provider functionally arrived at this decision is *critical thinking*. It is based on the assessment of the situation, the condition of the patient, the fund of knowledge of the prehospital provider, the skills of the provider, and the equipment available. "Critical thinking is a pervasive skill that involves scrutinizing, differentiating, and appraising information and reflecting on the information gained in order to make judgments and inform clinical decisions."[21]

The art and science of medicine, the knowledge of principles, and the appropriate application of preferences will lead to the anticipated outcome of the very best care possible given the circumstances in which the care is provided. There are essentially four steps in the process of caring for acute injuries: (1) the prehospital phase; (2) the initial (resuscitative) phase in the hospital; (3) the stabilization and definitive care phase; and (4) long-term resolution and rehabilitation to return the patient to a functional status. All these phases use the same principles of patient care in each step of the patient's care. All providers throughout the phases of the patient's care must use critical thinking. Critical thinking steps flow from the time of the injury until the time that the patient goes home. Each critical thinking step along the way varies according to the resources that are available to provide this care and the condition of the patient during each individual step. Therefore, understanding the principles of management, the options available, reassessment as the situation and the conditions change, and modification of the management plan throughout the entire patient's care requires use of the critical thinking process.

EMS personnel are directly involved in the initial (prehospital) phase of care but must use critical thinking and be aware of the entire process to produce seamless patient care as the patient moves through the system. The field care provider must think beyond the current situation to the definitive care needs and the patient's ultimate outcome. The goal is to manage the patient's injuries so that they heal and the patient can be discharged from the hospital in the best possible condition.

SUMMARY

- Principles or science
  - What the patient must have in order to optimize outcome and survival
- Preferences or art
  - Methods of achieving the principle
  - Considerations for choosing the method
- Situation that currently exists
- Condition of the patient
- Knowledge and experience
- Equipment available
- Critical thinking
  - Assess all concerns and components of the traumatic event at hand
- Use all senses to achieve assessment
- Review the need for additional information, equipment, personnel
- Identify hospitals in the vicinity and their capability
- Develop a plan of action and management
- Reassess the situation, patient, response to the action plan
- Mid-course correction(s) as necessary
- Goal is successful management
- Critical thinking is *not* following protocols
- Critical thinking *is* swift, flexible, objective

References

1. American College of Surgeons Committee on Trauma: *Advanced Trauma Life Support (ATLS) Manual,* ed 8, 2008, American College of Surgeons, Chicago, IL.
2. *US casualties in Iraq.* Available at www.globalsecurity.org/military/ops/iraq_casualties. Accessed February 23, 2009.
3. US Department of Transportation, National Highway Traffic Safety Administration: Not-in-traffic surveillance 2007—highlights. In NHTSA's National Center for Statistics and Analysis: *Traffic safety facts,* HS 811 085, Washington, DC, 2009.
4. US Department of Transportation, National Highway Traffic Safety Administration: Motorcycles. In NHTSA's National Center for Statistics and Analysis: *Traffic safety facts,* HS 810 990, Washington, DC, 2007.
5. Cars Blog: *Motorcycle death rates doubled; supersport bikes the most dangerous.* Available at blogs.consumerreports.org/cars/2007/09/motorcycle-deat. Accessed January 25, 2010.
6. Krisberg K: Motorcycle safety, helmets an issue as US deaths increase: more than 5,000 US deaths in 2007. *The Nations Health* 38(9), November 1, 2008.
7. Mothers Against Drunk Driving: Profile, Irving, TX, 2009, Center for Consumer Freedom. www.activistcash.com/organization_overview.cfm/oid/17. Accessed January 25, 2010.
8. Trunkey DD: Trauma. *Sci Am* 249(2):28, 1983.
9. R Adams Cowley Shock Trauma Center: *Tribute to R Adams Cowley, MD.* Available at www.umm.edu/shocktrauma/history.htm. Accessed March 27, 2008.
10. Trauma victims' survival may depend on which trauma center treats them. October 2005. http://news.bio-medicine.org/medicine-news-3/Trauma-victims-survival-depend-on-which-trauma-center-treats-them-8343-1/. Accessed January 25, 2010.
11. Peleg K, Aharonson-Daniel L, Stein M, et al: Increased survival among severe trauma patients: the impact of a national trauma system. *Arch Surg* 139(11):1231–1236, 2004.
12. Edwards W: Emergency medical systems significantly increase patient survival rates. Part 2. *Can Doct* 48(12):20–24, 1982.
13. Haas B, Jurkovich GJ, Wang J, et al: Survival advantage in trauma centers: expeditious intervention or experience? *J Am Coll Surg* 208(1):28–36, 2009.
14. Scheetz LJ: Differences in survival, length of stay, and discharge disposition of older trauma patients admitted to trauma centers and nontrauma center hospitals. *J Nurs Scholarsh* 37(4):361–366, 2005.
15. Norwood S, Fernandez L, England J: The early effects of implementing American College of Surgeons Level II criteria on transfer and survival rates at a rurally based community hospital. *J Trauma* 39(2):240–244; discussion 244–245, 1995.
16. Kane G, Wheeler NC, Cook S, et al: Impact of the Los Angeles County trauma system on the survival of seriously injured patients. *J Trauma* 32(5):576–583, 1992.
17. Hedges JR, Adams AL, Gunnels MD: ATLS practices and survival at rural level III trauma hospitals, 1995–1999. *Prehosp Emerg Care* 6(3):299–305, 2002.
18. Townsend CM Jr, Beauchamp RD, Evers BM, Mattox KL, editors: *Sabiston textbook of surgery,* ed 18, Philadelphia, PA, 2008, Saunders Elsevier.
19. Hendricson WD, Andrieu SC, Chadwick DG, et al: Educational strategies associated with development of problem-solving, critical thinking, and self-directed learning. *J Dent Educ* 70(9):925–36, 2006.
20. Cotter AJ: Developing critical thinking skills. *EMS Mag* 36(7):86, 2007.
21. Banning M: Measures that can be used to instill critical thinking skills in nurse prescribers. *Nurse Educ Pract* 6(2):98–105, 2006.
22. Caroll RT: *Becoming a Critical Thinker:* A Guide for the New Millenium, ed 2, 2005, Pearson Custom Publishing.

Suggested Reading

Callaham M: Quantifying the scanty science of prehospital emergency care. *Ann Emerg Med* 30:785, 1997.

Cone DC, Lewis RJ: Should this study change my practice? *Acad Emerg Med* 10:417, 2003.

Haynes RB, McKibbon KA, Fitzgerald D, et al: How to keep up with the medical literature. II. Deciding which journals to read regularly. *Ann Intern Med* 105:309, 1986.

Keim SM, Spaite DW, Maio RF, et al: Establishing the scope and methodological approach to out-of-hospital outcomes and effectiveness research. *Acad Emerg Med* 11:1067, 2004.

Lewis RJ, Bessen HA: Statistical concepts and methods for the reader of clinical studies in emergency medicine. *J Emerg Med* 9:221, 1991.

MacAvley D: Critical appraisal of medical literature: an aid to rational decision making. *Fam Pract* 12:98, 1995.

Reed JF III, Salen P, Bagher P: Methodological and statistical techniques: what do residents really need to know about statistics? *J Med Syst* 27:233, 2003.

Sackett DL: How to read clinical journals. V. To distinguish useful from useless or even harmful therapy. *Can Med Assoc J* 124:1156, 1981.

CHAPTER 2

Mechanisms of Injury and Kinematics of Trauma

CHAPTER OBJECTIVES

At the completion of this chapter, the reader will be able to do the following:

- ✓ Define energy in the context of causing injury.

- ✓ Describe the association among the laws of motion and energy and the kinematics of trauma.

- ✓ Describe the relationship of injury and energy exchange to speed.

- ✓ Discuss energy exchange and the production of cavitation.

- ✓ Given the description of a motor vehicle crash, use kinematics to predict the likely injury pattern for an unrestrained occupant.

- ✓ Associate the principles of energy exchange with the pathophysiology of injury to the head, spine, thorax, abdomen, and extremities resulting from that exchange.

- ✓ Describe the specific injuries and their causes as related to interior and exterior vehicle damage.

- ✓ Describe the function of restraint systems for vehicle occupants.

- ✓ Relate the laws of motion and energy to mechanisms other than motor vehicle crashes (e.g., blasts, falls).

- ✓ Describe the five phases of blast injury and the injuries produced in each phase.

- ✓ Describe the differences in the production of injury with low-, medium-, and high-energy weapons.

- ✓ Discuss the relationship of the frontal surface of an impacting object to energy exchange and injury production.

- ✓ Integrate principles of the kinematics of trauma into patient assessment.

SCENARIO

You and your partner are dispatched to a two-car collision. The day is warm and sunny. The scene is secured by law enforcement when you arrive.

On arrival you confirm that there are only two cars involved. The first car is in the ditch on the right side of the road and has impacted a tree at the passenger side door. There are bullet holes in the left front door. At least three holes are visible to you. There are two occupants in the vehicle.

The other car veered off the left side of the road and has hit a utility pole, centered between the two headlights. There are two people in that car. It is an old vehicle without air bags. There is a bent steering wheel and on the driver's side there is a bull's-eye fracture of the windshield. On the passenger side as you look into the car, you find an indentation in the lower part of the passenger-side dash. None of the passengers in either vehicle are wearing a safety belt. You are dealing with four injured patients, two in each car, and all have remained in the cars.

It is your responsibility to assess the patients and assign priority for transportation. Take the patients one at a time and describe them based on the kinematics.

Unexpected traumatic injuries are responsible for more than 169,000 deaths in the United States each year.[1] Vehicle collisions accounted for more than 37,000 deaths and more than 4 million injured persons in 2008.[2,3] This problem is not limited to the United States; other countries have an equal frequency of vehicular trauma, although the vehicles may be different. Penetrating trauma from guns is very high in the United States. In 2006, there were almost 31,000 deaths from firearms. Of these, more than 13,000 were homicides.[1] In 2008 there were more than 78,000 non-fatal firearm injuries reported.[2] Blast injuries are a major cause of injuries in many countries, whereas penetrating injuries from knives are prominent in others. Successful management of trauma patients depends on identification of injuries or potential injuries and the use of good assessment skills. It is often difficult to determine the exact injury produced, but understanding the potential for injury and the potential for significant blood loss will allow the provider to use the critical thinking process to recognize this likelihood and make appropriate triage, management, and transportation decisions.

The management of any patient begins (after initial resuscitation) with the history of the patient's injury. In trauma, the history is the story of the impact and the energy exchange that resulted from this impact.[4] An understanding of the energy exchange process will lead to suspicion of 95% of potential injuries.

When the provider, at any level of care, does not understand the principles of kinematics or the mechanisms involved, injuries may be missed. An understanding of these principles will increase the level of suspicion based on the pattern of injuries likely associated with the survey of the scene on arrival. This information and the suspected injuries can be used to properly assess the patient on the scene and be transmitted to the physicians and nurses in the emergency department (ED). At the scene and en route, these suspected injuries can be managed to provide the most appropriate patient care and "do no further harm."

Injuries that are not obvious but still severe can be fatal if they are not managed at the scene and en route to the trauma center or appropriate hospital. Knowing where to look and how to assess for injuries are as important as knowing what to do after finding injuries. A complete, accurate history of a traumatic incident and proper interpretation of this data will provide such information. Most of a patient's injuries can be predicted by a proper survey of the scene, even before examining the patient.

This chapter discusses the general principles and mechanical principles involved in the kinematics of trauma; the sections on the regional effects of blunt and penetrating trauma address local injury pathophysiology. The general principles are the laws of physics that govern energy exchange and the general effects of the energy exchange. Mechanical principles address the interaction of the human body with the components of the crash for blunt trauma (e.g., motor vehicles, three- and two-wheeled vehicles, and falls), penetrating trauma, and blasts.

A crash is the energy exchange that occurs when an object with energy, usually something solid, impacts the human body. It is not only the collision of a motor vehicle but also the crash of a falling body onto the pavement, the impact of a bullet on the external and internal tissues of the body, and the overpressure and debris of a blast. All these involve energy exchange, all result in injury, all involve potentially life-threatening conditions, and all require correct management by a knowledgeable and insightful prehospital care provider.

General Principles

A traumatic event is divided into three phases: precrash, crash, and post-crash. Again, the term *crash* does not necessarily mean a vehicular crash. The crash of a vehicle into a pedestrian, a missile (bullet) into the abdomen, and a construction worker striking the asphalt after a fall are all examples. In each case, energy is exchanged between a moving object and the tissue of the human body or between the moving human body and a stationary object.

The precrash phase includes all of the events that preceded the incident. Conditions that are present before the incident but important in the management of the patient's injuries are assessed as part of the precrash history. These include such things as a patient's acute or preexisting medical conditions (and medications to treat those conditions), ingestion of recreational substances (illegal and prescription drugs, alcohol, etc.), the use of safety devices such as seat belts or helmets, and a patient's state of mind. Typically, young trauma patients do not have chronic illnesses. With older patients, however, medical conditions that are present before the trauma event can cause serious complications in the prehospital assessment and management of the patient and can significantly influence the outcome. For example, the elderly driver of a vehicle that has struck a utility pole may have chest pain suggestive of a myocardial infarction (heart attack). Did the driver hit the utility pole and have a heart attack, or did he have a heart attack and then strike the utility pole? Does the patient take medication (e.g., beta blocker) that will prevent elevation of the pulse in shock? Most of these conditions directly influence the assessment and management strategies discussed in subsequent chapters but are important in overall patient care as well, even if they do not necessarily influence the kinematics of the crash.

The *crash phase* begins at the time of impact between one moving object and a second object. The second object can be moving or stationary and can be either an object or a person. Three impacts occur in most vehicular crashes: (1) the impact of the two objects involved, (2) the impact of the occupants into the vehicle, and (3) the impact of the vital organs inside the occupants. For example, when a vehicle strikes a tree, the first impact is the collision of the vehicle into the tree. The second impact is the occupant of the vehicle striking the steering wheel or windshield. If the patient is restrained, an impact occurs between the occupant and the seat belt. The third impact is between the patient's internal organs and his or her chest wall, abdominal wall, or skull. In a fall, only the second and third impacts are involved.

The direction in which the energy exchange occurs, the amount of energy that is exchanged, and the effect that these forces have on the patient are all important considerations as assessment begins.

During the *post-crash phase,* the information gathered about the crash and precrash phases is used to assess and manage a patient. This phase begins as soon as the energy from the crash is absorbed. The onset of the complications from life-threatening trauma can be slow or fast (or these complications can be prevented or significantly reduced), depending in part on the care provided at the scene and en route to the hospital. In the post-crash phase the understand-

ing of the kinematics of trauma, the index of suspicion regarding injuries, and strong assessment skills all become crucial to the patient outcome.

Simply stated, the **precrash** phase is where ***prevention*** can change the outcome. The **crash** phase is that portion of the traumatic event that involves the ***exchange of energy,*** or the kinematics (mechanics of energy). Lastly, the **post-crash** phase is the ***patient care*** phase.

To understand the effects of the forces that produce bodily injury, the prehospital care provider needs first to understand two components—energy exchange and human anatomy.

For example, in a motor vehicle crash (MVC), what does the scene look like? Who hit what and at what speed? How long was the stopping time? Were the victims using appropriate restraint devices such as seat belts? Did the air bag deploy? Were the children restrained properly in seats, or were they unrestrained and thrown about the vehicle? Were occupants thrown from the vehicle? Did they strike objects? If so, how many objects and what was the nature of those objects? These and many other questions must be answered if the prehospital care provider is to understand the exchange of forces that took place and translate this information into a prediction of injuries and appropriate patient care.

The process of surveying the scene to determine what forces and motion were involved and what injuries might have resulted from those forces is called *kinematics.* Because kinematics is based on fundamental principles of physics, an understanding of the pertinent laws of physics is necessary.

Energy

The initial component in obtaining a history is to evaluate the events that occurred at the time of the crash (Figure 2-1) and to estimate the energy that was exchanged with the human body and a gross approximation of the specific conditions that resulted.

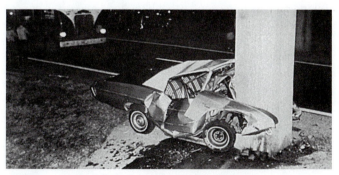

FIGURE 2-1 Evaluating the scene of an incident is critical. Such information as direction of impact, passenger compartment intrusion, and amount of energy exchanged provides insight into the possible injuries of the occupants. This photograph was in the first edition of the PHTLS text and, although an older-model vehicle, continues to show the concept of mechanism of injury.

Laws of Energy and Motion

Newton's first law of motion states that a body at rest will remain at rest and a body in motion will remain in motion unless acted on by an outside force. The skier in Figure 2-2 was stationary until the energy from gravity moved him down the slope. Once in motion, although he leaves the ground, he will remain in motion until he hits something or returns to the ground and comes to a stop.

As previously mentioned, in any collision, when the body of the potential patient is in motion, there are three collisions: (1) the vehicle hitting an object (moving or stationary); (2) the potential patient hitting the inside of the vehicle, crashing into an object, or being struck by energy in an explosion; and (3) the internal organs interacting with the walls of a compartment of the body or being torn loose from their supporting structures. An example is a person sitting in the front seat of a vehicle. When the vehicle hits a tree and stops, the unrestrained person continues in motion, and at the same rate of speed, until he or she hits the steering column, dashboard, and windshield. The impact with these objects stops the forward motion of the torso or head, but the internal organs of the person remain in motion until the organs hit the inside of the chest wall, abdominal wall, or skull, halting the forward motion.

The *law of conservation of energy combined with Newton's second law of motion* describes that energy cannot be created or destroyed but can be changed in form. The motion of the vehicle is a form of energy. To start the vehicle, gasoline explodes within the cylinder of the engine. This moves the pistons. The motion of the pistons is transferred by a set of gears to the wheels, which grasp the road as they turn and impart motion to the vehicle. To stop the vehicle, the energy of its motion must be changed to another form, such as the heat generated by the friction of applying the brakes or crashing into an object and bending the frame. When a driver brakes, the energy of motion is converted into the heat of friction (thermal energy) by the brake pads on the brake drums/disk and by the tires on the roadway. The vehicle decelerates.

Just as the mechanical energy of a vehicle that crashes into a wall is dissipated by the bending of the frame or other parts of the vehicle (Figure 2-3), the energy of motion of the organs and the structures inside the body must be dissipated as these organs stop their forward motion. The same concepts apply to the human body when it is stationary and comes into contact with an object in motion, such as a knife, a bullet, or a baseball bat.

Kinetic energy is a function of an object's mass and velocity. By knowing the approximate magnitude of the kinetic energy involved in a crash, the likelihood of injury can be predicted. Simply stated, the greater the kinetic energy involved, the greater the likelihood of serious or multiple injuries.

The mathematical formula to calculate kinetic energy is as follows:

Kinetic energy =

One half the mass times the velocity squared

$$KE = \tfrac{1}{2}mv^2$$

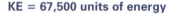

Although they are not exactly the same, a victim's weight is used to represent his or her mass. Likewise, speed is used to represent velocity (which really is speed and direction).

Thus the kinetic energy involved when a 150-pound (68-kg) person travels at 30 mph (48 km/hr) is calculated as follows:

$$KE = \frac{150}{2} \times 30^2$$

KE = 67,500 units of energy

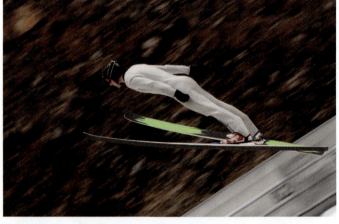

FIGURE 2-2 A skier was stationary until the energy from gravity moved him down the slope. Once in motion, although he leaves the ground, the momentum will keep him in motion until he hits something or returns to the ground and the transfer of energy (friction or a collision) causes him to come to a stop.

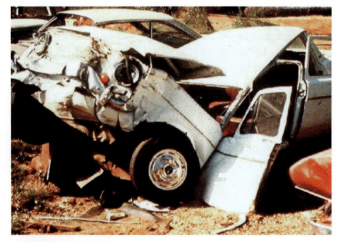

FIGURE 2-3 Vehicle stops suddenly against a dirt embankment.

As just shown, a 150-pound (68-kg) person traveling at 30 mph (48 km/hr) would have 67,500 units of energy that has to be converted to another form when he or she stops. This change takes the form of damage to the vehicle and injury to the person in it, unless the energy dissipation can take some less harmful form, such as on a seat belt or into an air bag.

Which factor in the formula, however, has the greatest effect on the amount of kinetic energy produced: mass or velocity? Consider adding 10 pounds to the 150-pound person traveling at 30 mph (48 km/hr) in the prior example, now making the mass equal to 160 pounds (72 kg):

$$KE = \frac{160}{2} \times 30^2$$

$$KE = 72,000 \text{ units}$$

As the mass has increased, so has the amount of kinetic energy.

Finally, returning to this same example of a 150-pound (68-kg) person, instead of increasing the mass by 10 pounds if the speed is increased by 10 mph (16 km/hr), the kinetic energy is as follows:

$$KE = \frac{150}{2} \times 40^2$$

$$KE = 120,000 \text{ units}$$

These calculations demonstrate that increasing the velocity (speed) increases the kinetic energy much more than increasing the mass. Much more energy exchange will occur (and therefore produce greater injury to either the occupant or the vehicle or both) in a high-speed crash than in a crash at a slower speed. The velocity is exponential and the mass is linear; this is critical even when there is a great mass disparity between two objects.

Mass × acceleration = force = mass × deceleration

Force (energy) is required to put an object into motion. This force (energy) is required to create a specific speed. The speed imparted is dependent on the weight (mass) of the structure. Once this energy is passed on to the object and it is placed in motion, the motion will remain until the energy is given up (Newton's first law of motion). This loss of energy will place other components in motion (tissue particles) or be lost as heat (dissipated into the brake disks on the wheels). An example of this process can be illustrated using a gun and a patient. In the chamber of a gun is a cartridge that contains gunpowder. If this gunpowder is ignited, it burns rapidly, creating energy that pushes the bullet out of the barrel at a great speed. This speed is equivalent to the weight of the bullet and the amount of energy produced by the burning of the gunpowder or force. To slow down (Newton's first law of motion), the bullet must give up its energy into the structure that it hits. This will produce an explosion in the tissue that is equal to the explosion

that occurred in the chamber of the gun when the initial speed was given to the bullet. The same phenomenon occurs in the moving automobile, the patient falling from a building, or the explosion of an improvised explosive device (IED).

Another important factor in any crash is the *stopping distance.* The shorter the stopping distance and the quicker the rate of that stop, the more energy that is transferred to the patient and the more damage or injury that is done to the patient. A vehicle that stops by hitting a brick wall and one that stops when the brakes are applied dissipate the same amount of energy, just in a different manner. The rate of energy exchange (into the vehicle body or into the brake disks) is different and occurs over a different distance. In the first instance, the energy is absorbed in a very short distance and amount of time by the bending of the frame of the vehicle. In the latter case, the energy is absorbed over a longer distance and period of time by the heat of the brakes. The forward motion of the occupant of the vehicle (energy) is absorbed in the first instance by damage to the soft tissue and bones of the occupant. In the latter case, the energy is dissipated, along with the energy of the vehicle, into the brakes.

This inverse relationship between stopping distance and injury also applies to falls. A person has a better chance of surviving a fall if he or she lands on a compressible surface, such as deep powder snow. The same fall terminating on a hard surface, such as concrete, can produce more severe injuries. The compressible material (i.e., the snow) increases the stopping distance and absorbs at least some of the energy rather than allowing all the energy to be absorbed by the body. The result is decreased injury and damage to the body. This principle also applies to other types of crashes. In addition, an unrestrained driver will be more severely injured than a restrained driver. The restraint system, rather than the body, will absorb a significant portion of the energy transfer.

Therefore, once an object is in motion and has energy in the form of motion, in order for it to come to a complete rest, the object must lose all its energy by converting the energy to another form or transferring it to another object. For example, if a vehicle strikes a pedestrian, the pedestrian is knocked away from the vehicle (Figure 2-4). Although the vehicle is somewhat slowed by the impact, the greater force of the vehicle imparts much more acceleration to the more lightweight pedestrian than it loses in speed because of the mass difference between the two. The softer body parts of the pedestrian versus the harder body parts of the vehicle also means more damage to the pedestrian than to the vehicle.

Energy Exchange between a Solid Object and the Human Body

When the human body collides with a solid object, or vice versa, the number of body tissue particles that are impacted by the solid object determines the amount of energy exchange that takes place. This transfer of energy produces the amount of damage (injury) that occurs to the patient. The number of

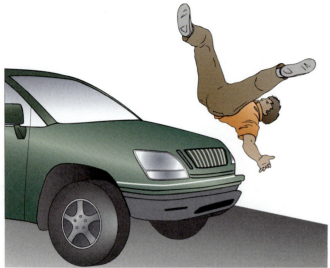

FIGURE 2-4 The energy exchange from a moving vehicle to a pedestrian crushes tissue and imparts speed and energy to the pedestrian to knock the victim away from the point of impact. Injury to the patient can occur at the point of impact as the pedestrian is hit by the vehicle and as the pedestrian is thrown to the ground or into another vehicle.

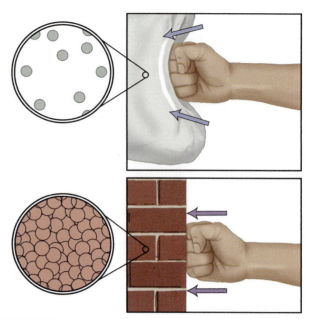

FIGURE 2-5 The fist absorbs more energy colliding with the dense brick wall than with the less dense feather pillow, which dissipates the force.

tissue particles affected is determined by (1) the density (particles per volume) of the tissue and (2) the size of the contact area of the impact.

Density

The denser a tissue is (measured in particles per volume), the greater the number of particles that will be hit by a moving object and therefore the greater the rate and the total amount of energy exchanged. Driving a fist into a feather pillow and driving a fist at the same speed into a brick wall will produce different effects on the hand. The fist absorbs more energy colliding with the dense brick wall than with the less dense feather pillow (Figure 2-5).

Simplistically, the body has three different types of tissue densities: *air density* (much of the lung and some portions of the intestine), *water density* (muscle and most solid organs, e.g., liver, spleen), and *solid density* (bone). Therefore, the amount of energy exchange (with resultant injury) will depend on which type of organ is impacted.

Contact Area

Wind exerts pressure on a hand when it is extended out of the window of a moving vehicle. When the palm of the hand is horizontal and parallel to the direction of the flow through the wind, some backward pressure is exerted on the front of the hand (fingers) as the particles of air strike the hand. Rotating the hand 90 degrees to a vertical position places a larger surface area into the wind; thus more air particles make contact with the hand, increasing the amount of force on it.

For trauma events, the impact surface area of the body can be modified by any change in the impact surface area of

the striking object. Examples of this effect include the front of an automobile, a baseball bat, a rifle bullet, or a shotgun. The automobile's front surface contacts a large portion of the victim. A baseball bat contacts a smaller area and a bullet a very small area. The amount of energy exchange that would produce damage to the patient depends then on the energy of the object and the density of the tissue in the pathway of the energy exchange.

If all the impact energy is in a small area and this force exceeds the resistance of the skin, the object is forced though the skin. This is the definition of **penetrating trauma.** If the force is spread out over a larger area and the skin is not penetrated, it is a **blunt trauma.** In either instance, a cavity in the patient is created by the force of the impacting object. Even with something like a bullet, the impact surface area can be different based on such factors as bullet size, its motion (tumble) within the body, deformation ("mushroom"), and fragmentation.

Cavitation

The basic mechanics of energy exchange are relatively simple. The impact on the tissue particles accelerates those tissue particles away from the point of impact. These tissues then become moving objects themselves and crash into other tissue particles, producing a "falling domino" effect. A common game that provides a visual effect of cavitation is pool.

The cue ball is driven down the length of a pool table by the force of the muscles in the arm. The cue ball crashes into the racked balls at the other end of the table. The energy from the arm into the cue ball is thus transferred onto each of the racked balls (Figure 2-6). The cue ball gives up its energy

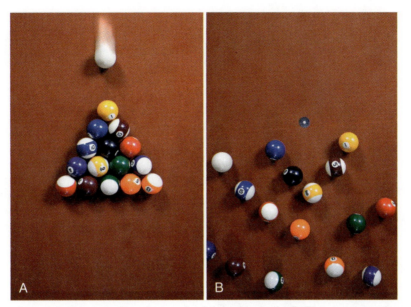

FIGURE 2-6 **A,** The energy of a cue ball is transferred to each of the other balls. **B,** The energy exchange pushes the balls apart, or creates a cavity.

to the other balls. The other balls began to move while the cue ball, which has lost its energy, slows or even stops. The other balls take on this energy as motion and move away from the impact point. A cavity has been created where the rack of balls once was. The same kind of energy exchange occurs when a bowling ball rolls down the alley, hitting the set of pins at the other end. The result of this energy exchange is a cavity. This sort of energy exchange occurs in both blunt and penetrating trauma.

Similarly, when a solid object strikes the human body or when the human body is in motion and strikes a stationary object, the tissue particles of the human body are knocked out of their normal position, creating a hole or cavity. Thus this process is called *cavitation.*

Two types of cavities are created[9]:

1. A temporary cavity is caused by stretching of the tissues that occurs at the time of impact. Because of the elastic properties of the body's tissues, some or all of the contents of the temporary cavity return to their previous position. The size, shape, and portions of the cavity that become part of the permanent damage depend on the tissue type, the elasticity of the tissue, and how much rebound of tissue occurs. The extent of this cavity is usually not visible when the prehospital or hospital provider examines the patient, even seconds after the impact.

2. A permanent cavity is left after the temporary cavity collapses and is the visible part of the tissue destruction. In addition, a crush cavity is produced by the direct impact of the object on the tissue. Both of these can be seen when the patient is examined (Figure 2-7).

The amount of the temporary cavity that remains as a permanent cavity is related to the elasticity (stretch ability) of the tissue involved. For example, forcefully swinging a baseball bat into a steel drum leaves a dent, or cavity, in its side.

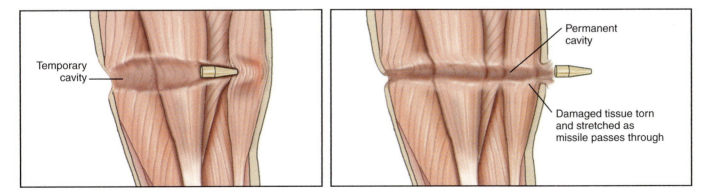

FIGURE 2-7 Damage to tissue is greater than the permanent cavity that remains from a missile injury. The faster or heavier the missile, the larger the temporary cavity and the greater the zone of tissue damage.

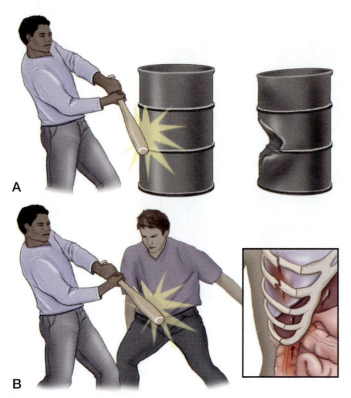

FIGURE 2-8   **A,** Swinging a baseball bat into a steel drum leaves a dent, or cavity, in its side. **B,** Swinging a baseball bat into a person usually leaves no visible cavity as the elasticity of the trunk returns the body back to its normal shape.

Swinging the same baseball bat with the same force into a similarly sized and shaped mass of foam rubber will leave no dent once the bat is removed (Figure 2-8). The difference is *elasticity;* the foam rubber is more elastic than the steel drum. The human body is more like the foam rubber than the steel drum. If a person punches a fist into another person's abdomen, he or she would feel the fist go in. However, when the person pulls the fist away, a dent is not left. Similarly, a baseball bat swung into the chest will leave no obvious cavity in the thoracic wall, but it would cause damage, both from direct contact and from the cavity created by the energy

exchange. The history of the incident and its interpretation provide the information needed to determine the potential size of the temporary cavity at the time of impact. The organs or the structures involved predict injuries.

When the trigger of a loaded gun is pulled, the firing pin strikes the cap and produces an explosion in the cartridge. The energy created by this explosion is exchanged onto the bullet, which speeds from the muzzle of the weapon. The bullet now has energy, or force (acceleration × mass = force). Once such force is imparted, the bullet cannot slow down until acted on by an outside force (Newton's first law of motion). In order for the bullet to stop inside the human body, an explosion must occur within the tissues that is equivalent to the explosion in the weapon (acceleration × mass = force = mass × deceleration) (Figure 2-9). This explosion is the result of energy exchange accelerating the tissue particles out of their normal position, creating a cavity.

Blunt and Penetrating Trauma

Trauma is generally classified as either blunt or penetrating. However, the energy exchange and the injury produced are similar in both types of trauma. Cavitation occurs in both. Only the type and direction are different. The only real difference is penetration of the skin. If an object's entire energy is concentrated on one small area of skin, the skin likely will tear, and the object will enter the body and create a more concentrated energy exchange along the pathway. This can result in greater destructive power to one area. A larger object whose energy is dispersed over a much larger area of skin may not penetrate the skin. The damage will be distributed over a larger area of the body, and the injury pattern will be less localized. An example would be the difference in a gunshot impact versus the impact of a large truck into a pedestrian (Figure 2-10).

The cavitation in blunt trauma is often only a temporary cavity and is directed away from the point of impact. Penetrating trauma creates both a permanent and a temporary cavity. The temporary cavity that is created will spread away from the pathway of this missile in both frontal and lateral directions.

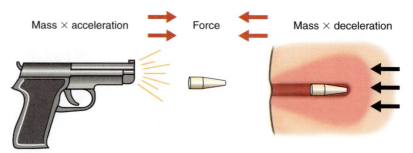

Mass × acceleration   Force   Mass × deceleration

FIGURE 2-9   As a bullet travels through tissue, its kinetic energy is transferred to the tissue that it comes in contact with, accelerating it away from the bullet.

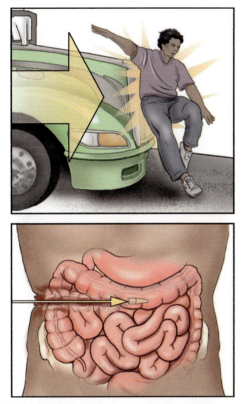

FIGURE 2-10 The force from a collision of a vehicle with a person is generally distributed over a large area, whereas the force of the collision between a bullet and person is localized to a very small area and results in penetration of the body and underlying organs.

Blunt Trauma

Mechanical Principles

This section is divided into two major parts. The mechanical and structural effects on the vehicle of a crash are discussed first and then the internal effects on the organs and body structures. Both are important and must be understood to properly assess the trauma patient and the potential injuries that exist after the crash.

The on-scene observations of the probable circumstances that led to a crash resulting in blunt trauma provide clues as to the severity of the injuries and the potential organs involved. The factors to assess are (1) direction of the impact, (2) external damage to the vehicle (type and severity), and (3) internal damage (e.g., occupant compartment intrusion, steering wheel/column bending, windshield bull's eye fractures, mirror damage, dashboard knee impacts).

In blunt trauma, two forces are involved in the impact: shear and compression, both of which may result in cavitation. *Shear* is the result of one organ or structure (or part of an organ or structure) changing speed faster than another organ or structure (or part of an organ or structure). This difference in acceleration (or deceleration) causes the parts to separate and tear. *Compression* is the result of an organ or structure (or part of an organ or structure) being directly squeezed between other organs or structures. Injury can result from any type of impact, such as MVCs (vehicle or motorcycle), pedestrian collisions with vehicles, falls, sports injuries, or blast injuries. All these mechanisms are discussed separately, followed by the results of this energy exchange on the specific anatomy in each of the body regions.

As discussed previously in this chapter, three collisions occur in blunt trauma. The first is the collision of the vehicle into another object. The second is the collision that occurs when the potential patient strikes the inside of the vehicular passenger compartment, strikes the ground at the end of a fall, or is stuck by the force created in an explosion. The third is when the internal structures within the various regions of the body (head, chest, abdomen, etc.) strike the wall of that region or are torn (shear force) from their attachment within this compartment. The first of these will be discussed as it relates to vehicle crashes, falls, and explosions. The latter two will be discussed in the specific regions involved.

Motor Vehicle Crashes

Many forms of blunt trauma occur, but MVCs (including motorcycle crashes) are the most common. In 2008, 86% of MVC fatalities were vehicle occupants. The remaining 14% were pedestrians, cyclists, and other non-occupants, as reported by the National Highway Traffic Safety Administration (NHTSA).[2]

MVCs can be divided into the following five types[6]:

1. Frontal impact
2. Rear impact
3. Lateral impact
4. Rotational impact
5. Rollover

Although each pattern has variations, accurate identification of the five patterns will provide insight into other, similar types of crashes.

In MVCs and other rapid-deceleration mechanisms, such as snowmobile, motorcycle, and boating crashes and falls from heights, three collisions occur: (1) the vehicle collides with an object or with another vehicle, (2) the unrestrained occupant collides with the inside of the vehicle, and (3) the occupant's internal organs collide with one another or with the wall of the compartment that contains them.

An example is a vehicle hitting a tree. The first collision occurs when the vehicle strikes the tree. The vehicle stops, but the unrestrained driver keeps moving forward. The second collision occurs when the driver hits the steering wheel, windshield, or some other part of the occupant compartment. Now the driver's torso stops moving forward, but many internal organs keep moving until they strike another organ or cavity wall or are suddenly stopped by a ligament, fascia, vessel, or muscle. This is the third collision.

One method to estimate the potential for injury to the occupant is to look at the vehicle and determine which of the five types of collisions occurred, the energy exchange involved, and the direction of the impact. The occupant receives the same type of force as the vehicle and from the same direction as did the vehicle. The amount of force exchanged with the occupant, however, may be somewhat reduced by absorption of energy by the vehicle.

Frontal Impact. In Figure 2-11, for example, the vehicle has hit a utility pole in the center of the car. The impact point stopped its forward motion, but the rest of the car continued forward until the energy was absorbed by the bending of the car. The same type of motion occurs to the driver, resulting in injury. The stable steering column is impacted by the chest, perhaps in the center of the sternum. Just as the car continued in forward motion, significantly deforming the front of the vehicle; so too will the driver's chest. As the sternum stops its forward motion against the dash, the posterior thoracic wall continues until the energy is absorbed by the bending and possible fracture of the ribs. This process will also crush the heart and the lungs between the sternum and the vertebral column and the posterior thoracic wall.

The amount of damage to the vehicle indicates the approximate speed of the vehicle at the time of impact. The greater the intrusion into the body of the vehicle, the greater the speed at the time of impact. The greater the vehicle speed, the greater the energy exchange and the more likely the occupants are to be injured.

Although the vehicle suddenly ceases to move forward in a frontal impact, the occupant continues to move and will follow one of two possible paths: either up-and-over or down-and-under.

The use of a seat belt and the deployment of an air bag or restraint system will absorb some or most of the energy, thus reducing the injury to the victim. For clarity and simplicity of discussion the occupant is these examples will be assumed to be without restraint.

Up-and-Over Path. In this sequence the body's forward motion carries it up and over the steering wheel (Figure 2-12). The head is usually the lead body portion striking the windshield or windshield frame or roof. The head then stops its forward motion. The torso continues in motion until its energy/force is absorbed along the spine. The cervical spine is the least

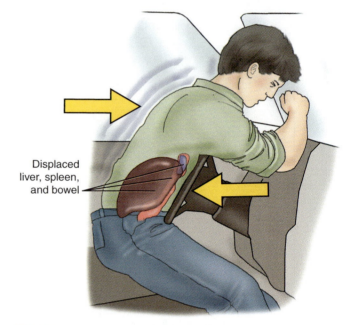

Displaced liver, spleen, and bowel

FIGURE 2-12 Configuration of the seat and position of the occupant can direct the initial force on the upper torso, with the head as the lead point.

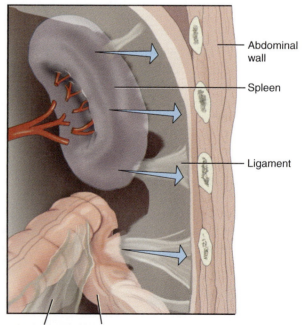

Abdominal wall

Spleen

Ligament

Mesentery   Large intestine

FIGURE 2-13 Organs can tear away from their point of attachment to the abdominal wall. The spleen, kidney, and small intestine are particularly susceptible to these types of shear forces.

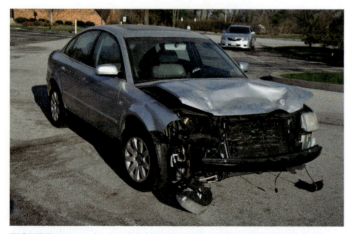

FIGURE 2-11 As a vehicle impacts a utility pole, the front of the car stops but the rear portion of the vehicle continues traveling forward, causing deformation of the vehicle.

protected segment of the spine. The chest or abdomen then collides with the steering column, depending on the position of the torso. Impact of the chest into the steering column produces thoracic cage, cardiac, lung, and aortic injuries (see Regional Effects of Blunt Trauma). Impact of the abdomen into the steering column can compress and crush the solid organs, produce overpressure injuries, especially to the diaphragm, and rupture of the hollow organs. The kidneys, spleen, and liver are also subject to shear injury as the abdomen strikes the steering wheel and abruptly stops. An organ may be torn from its normal anatomic restraints and supporting tissues. For example, the continued forward motion of the kidneys after the vertebral column has stopped moving pro-

duces shear along the attachment of the organs at their blood supply. The aorta and vena cava are tethered tightly to the posterior abdominal wall and vertebral column. The continued forward motion of the kidneys can stretch the renal vessels to the point of rupture (Figure 2-13). A similar action may tear the aorta in the chest as the unattached arch becomes the tightly adhered descending aorta (Figure 2-14).

Down-and-Under Path. In a down-and-under path the occupant moves forward, downward and out of the seat into the dashboard (Figure 2-15). The importance of understanding kinematics is illustrated by the injuries produced to the lower extremity in this pathway. Many of the injuries are difficult

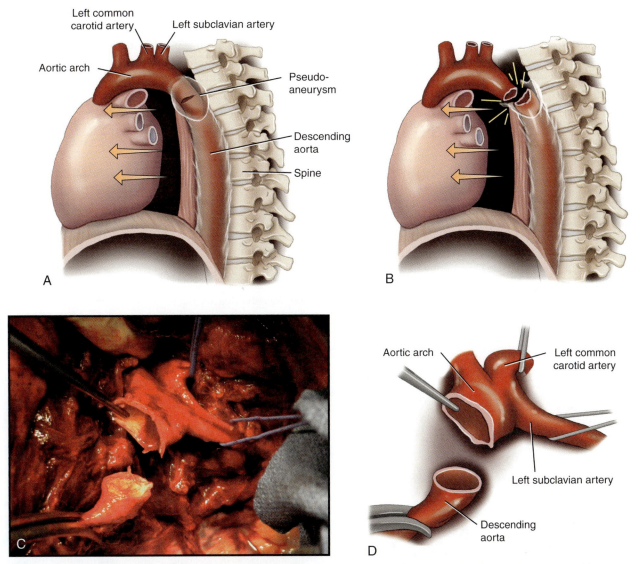

FIGURE 2-14 A, The descending aorta is a fixed structure that moves with the thoracic spine. The arch, aorta, and heart are freely movable. Acceleration of the torso in a lateral-impact collision or rapid deceleration of the torso in a frontal-impact collision produces a different rate of motion between the arch-heart complex and the descending aorta. This motion may result in a tear of the inner lining of the aorta that is contained within the outermost layer, producing a pseudoaneurysm. **B,** Tears at the junction of the arch and descending aorta may also result in a complete rupture, leading to immediate exsanguination in the chest. **C** and **D,** Operative photograph and drawing of a traumatic aortic tear.
(**A** from McSwain NE Jr, Paturas JL: *The basic EMT: comprehensive prehospital patient care,* ed 2, St Louis, 2001, Mosby.)

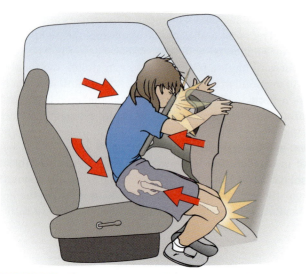

FIGURE 2-15 The occupant and the vehicle travel forward together. The vehicle stops, and the unrestrained occupant continues forward until something stops that motion.

to identify; therefore, an understanding of the mechanism of injury is very important.

The foot, if planted on the floor panel or on the brake pedal with a straight knee, can twist as the continued torso motion angulates and fractures the ankle joint. More often, however, the knees are already bent, and the force is not directed to the ankle. Therefore, the knees strike the dashboard.

The knee has two possible impact points against the dashboard: the tibia and the femur (Figure 2-16, *A*). If the tibia hits the dashboard and stops first, the femur remains in motion and overrides it. A dislocated knee, with torn ligaments, tendons, and other supporting structures, can result. Because the popliteal artery lies close to the knee joint, dislocation of the joint is often associated with injury to the vessel. The artery can be completely disrupted or the lining alone (intima) may be dam-

aged (Figure 2-16, *B*). In either case, a blood clot may form in the injured vessel, resulting in significantly decreased blood flow to the leg tissues below the knee. Early recognition of the knee injury and the potential for vascular injury will alert the physicians to the need for assessment of the vessel in this area.

Early identification and treatment of such a popliteal artery injury significantly decreases the complications of distal limb ischemia (lack of blood flow and oxygen). Perfusion (blood flow) to this tissue needs to be reestablished within about 6 hours or amputation will result. Delays could occur because the prehospital care provider failed to consider the kinematics of the injury or overlooked important clues during assessment of the patient.

Although most of these patients have evidence of injury to the knee, an imprint on the dashboard where the knee impacted is a key indicator that significant energy was focused on this joint and adjacent structures (Figure 2-17). Further investigation is needed in the hospital to better eliminate the possible injuries.

When the femur is the point of impact, the energy is absorbed on the bone shaft, which can then break (Figure 2-18). The continued forward motion of the pelvis onto the femur that remains intact can override the femoral head, resulting in a posterior dislocation of the acetabular joint (Figure 2-19).

After the knees and legs stop their forward motion, the upper body will bend forward into the steering column or dashboard. The unrestrained victim may then sustain many of the same injuries described previously for the up-and-over pathway.

Recognizing these potential injuries and relaying the information to the ED physicians can result in long-term benefits to the patient.

Rear Impact. Rear-impact collisions occur when a slower-moving or stationary vehicle is struck from behind by a vehicle moving at a faster rate of speed.[7] For ease of understanding, the more rapidly moving vehicle is called the "bullet

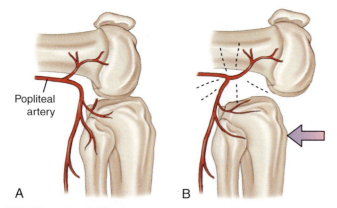

FIGURE 2-16 **A,** The knee has two possible impact points in a motor vehicle crash: the femur and the tibia. **B,** The popliteal artery lies close to the joint, tightly tied to the femur above and tibia below. Separation of these two bones stretches, kinks, and tears the artery.

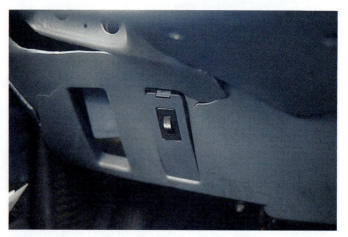

FIGURE 2-17 The impact point of the knee on the dashboard indicates both a down-and-under pathway and a significant absorption of energy along the lower extremity.

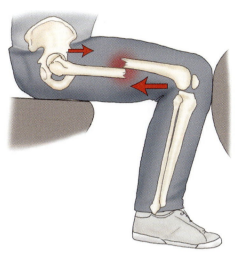

FIGURE 2-18 When the femur is the point of impact, the energy is absorbed on the bone shaft, which can then break.

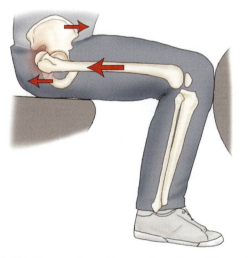

FIGURE 2-19 The continued forward motion of the pelvis onto the femur can override the femur's head, resulting in a posterior dislocation of the femur on the acetabular joint.

vehicle," and the slower or stopped object is called the "target vehicle." In such collisions the energy of the bullet vehicle at the moment of impact is converted to acceleration of the target vehicle and damage to both vehicles. The greater the difference in the momentum of the two vehicles, the greater the force of the initial impact and the more energy that is available to create damage and acceleration.

During a rear impact, the target vehicle in front is accelerated forward. Everything that is attached to the frame will also move forward and at the same rate of speed. This includes the seats in which the occupants are riding. The unattached objects in the vehicle, including the occupants, will begin forward motion only after something in contact with the frame begins to transmit the energy of the frame motion to these objects or occupants. As an example, the torso is accelerated by the back of the seat after some of the energy has been

absorbed by the springs in the seats. If the headrest is improperly positioned behind and below the occiput of the head, the head will begin its forward motion after the torso, resulting in hyperextension of the neck. Shear and stretching of the ligaments and other support structures, especially in the anterior part of the neck, can result in injury (Figure 2-20, *A*).

If the headrest is properly positioned, the head moves at approximately the same time as the torso without hyperextension (Figures 2-20, *B,* and 2-21). If the target vehicle is allowed to move forward without interference until it slows to a stop, the occupant will probably not suffer significant injury because most of the body's motion is supported by the seat, similar to an astronaut launching into orbit.

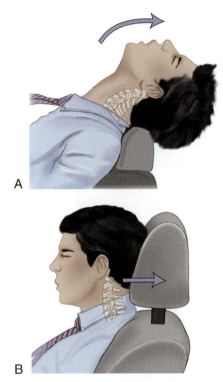

FIGURE 2-20   **A,** A rear-impact collision forces the torso forward. If the headrest is improperly positioned, the head is hyperextended over the top of the headrest. **B,** If the headrest is up, the head moves with the torso and neck injury is prevented.

FIGURE 2-21   Headrests
If it can be proved that the victim's headrest was not properly positioned when the neck injury occurred, some courts consider reducing the liability of the party at fault in the crash on the grounds that the victim's negligence contributed to the injuries *(contributory negligence).* Similar measures have been considered in cases of failure to use occupant restraints. Elderly patients have a high frequency of injury.[8]

However, if the vehicle strikes another vehicle or object or if the driver slams on the brakes and stops suddenly, the occupants will continue forward, following the characteristic pattern of a frontal-impact collision. The collision then involves two impacts, rear and frontal. The double impact increases the likelihood of injury.

Lateral Impact. Lateral-impact mechanisms come into play when the vehicle is involved in an intersection ("T-bone") collision or when the vehicle veers off the road and impacts a utility pole, tree, or other obstacle on the roadside sideways. If the collision is at an intersection, the target vehicle is accelerated from the impact in the direction away from the force created by the bullet vehicle. The side of the vehicle or the door that is struck is thrust against the side of the occupant. The occupants may then be injured as they are accelerated laterally (Figure 2-22) or as the passenger compartment is bent inward by the door's projection (Figure 2-23). Injury caused

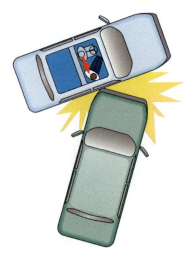

FIGURE 2-22 Lateral impact of the vehicle pushes the entire vehicle into the unrestrained passenger. A restrained passenger moves laterally with the vehicle.

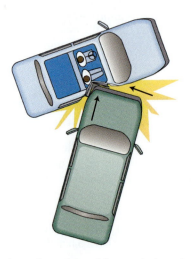

FIGURE 2-23 Intrusion of the side panels into the passenger compartment provides another source of injury.

by the vehicle's movement is less severe if the occupant is restrained and moves with the initial motion of the vehicle.[9]

Five body regions can sustain injury in a lateral impact:

1. *Clavicle.* The clavicle (collarbone) can be compressed and fractured if the force is against the shoulder (Figure 2-24, *A*).
2. *Chest.* Compression of the thoracic (chest) wall inward can result in fractured ribs, pulmonary contusion, or compression injury of the solid organs beneath the rib cage, as well as overpressure injuries (e.g., pneumothorax) (Figure 2-24, *B*). Shear injuries of the aorta can result from the lateral acceleration (25% of aortic shear injuries occur in lateral-impact collisions).[10–12]
3. *Abdomen and pelvis.* The intrusion compresses and fractures the pelvis and pushes the head of the femur through the acetabulum (Figure 2-24, *C*). Occupants on the driver's side are vulnerable to splenic injuries because the spleen is on the left side of the body, whereas those on the passenger side are more likely to receive an injury to the liver.
4. *Neck.* The torso can move out from under the head in lateral collisions, as well as in rear impacts. The attachment point of the head is posterior and inferior to the center of gravity of the head. Therefore, the motion of the head in relationship to the neck is lateral flexion and rotation.

    The contralateral side of the spine will be opened (distraction) and the ipsilateral side compressed. This can fracture the vertebrae or, more likely, produce jumped facets and possible dislocation, as well as spinal cord injury (Figure 2-25).
5. *Head.* The head can impact the frame of the door.

Near-side impacts produce more injuries than far-side impacts.

Rotational Impact. Rotational-impact collisions occur when one corner of a vehicle strikes an immovable object, the corner of another vehicle, or a vehicle moving slower or in the opposite direction of the first vehicle. Following Newton's first law of motion, this corner of the vehicle will stop while the rest of the vehicle continues its forward motion until all its energy is completely transformed.

Rotational-impact collisions result in injuries that are a combination of those seen in frontal impacts and lateral collisions. The victim continues to move forward and then is hit by the side of the vehicle (as in a lateral collision) as the vehicle rotates around the point of impact (Figure 2-26). *More severe injuries are seen in the victim closest to the point of impact.*

Rollover. During a rollover, a vehicle may undergo several impacts at many different angles, as may the unrestrained occupant's body and internal organs (Figure 2-27). Injury and damage can occur with each of these impacts. In rollover collisions a restrained patient often sustains shearing-type injuries because of the significant forces created by a rolling vehicle.

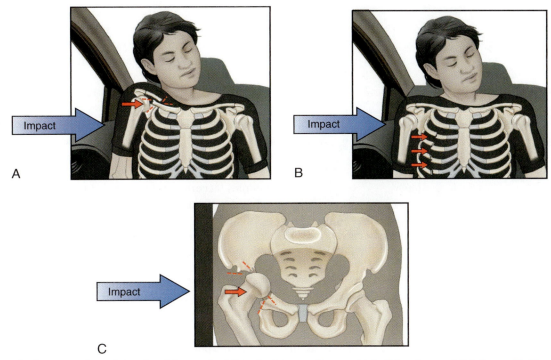

FIGURE 2-24   **A,** Compression of the shoulder against the clavicle produces midshaft fractures of this bone. **B,** Compression against the lateral chest and abdominal wall can fracture ribs and injure the underlying spleen, liver, and kidney. **C,** Lateral impact on the femur pushes the head through the acetabulum or fractures the pelvis.

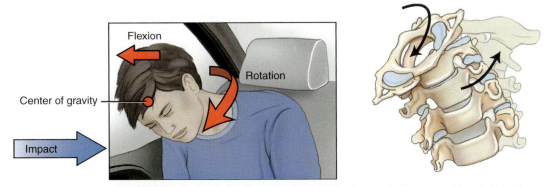

FIGURE 2-25   The center of gravity of the skull is anterior and superior to its pivot point between the skull and cervical spine. During a lateral impact, when the torso is rapidly accelerated out from under the head, the head turns toward the point of impact in both lateral and anterior-posterior angles. Such motion separates the vertebral bodies from the side of opposite impact and rotates them apart. Jumped facets, ligaments, tears, and lateral compression fractures result.

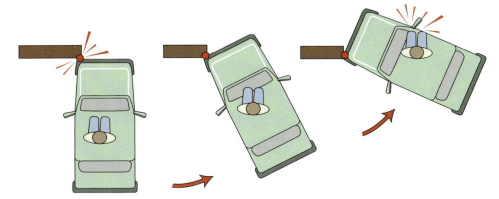

FIGURE 2-26   The victim in a rotational impact crash first moves forward and then laterally as the vehicle pivots around the impact point.

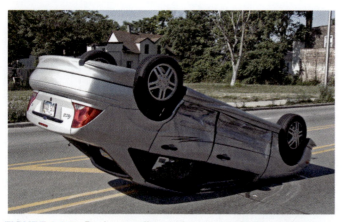

FIGURE 2-27 During a rollover, the unrestrained occupant can be wholly or partially ejected out of the vehicle or can bounce around inside the vehicle. This action produces multiple and somewhat unpredictable injuries that are usually severe.

The forces are similar to the forces of a spinning carnival ride. Although the occupants are held securely by restraints, the internal organs still move and can tear at the connecting tissue areas. More serious injuries result from being unrestrained. In many cases the occupants are ejected from the vehicle as it rolls and are either crushed as the vehicle rolls over them or sustain injuries from the impact with the ground. If the occupants are ejected onto the roadway, they can be struck by oncoming traffic. The NHTSA reports that in crashes involving fatalities in the year 2008, 77% of occupants who were totally ejected from a vehicle were killed.[13]

Vehicle Incompatibility. The type of vehicle involved in the crash plays a significant role in the potential for injury and death to the occupants. For example, in a lateral impact between two cars that lack air bags, the occupants of the car struck on its lateral aspect are almost six times more likely to die than the occupants in the vehicle striking that car. This can be largely explained by the relative lack of protection on the side of a car compared with the large amount of deformation that can occur to the front end of a vehicle before there is intrusion into the passenger compartment. However, when the vehicle that is struck in a lateral collision (by a car) is a sport utility vehicle (SUV), van, or pickup truck rather than a car, the risk of death to occupants is almost the same for all vehicles involved. Thus, SUVs, vans, and pickup trucks provide additional protection to their occupants because the passenger compartment sits higher off the ground than that of a car, and the occupants sustain less of a direct blow in a lateral impact.

More serious injuries and a greatly increased risk of death to vehicle occupants have been documented when a car is struck on its lateral aspect by a van, SUV, or pickup. In a lateral-impact collision between a van and a car, the occupants of the car struck broadside are 13 times more likely to die than those in the van. If the striking vehicle is a pickup truck or SUV, the occupants of the car struck broadside are 25 to 30 times more likely to die than those in the pickup truck or SUV. This tremendous disparity results from the

higher center of gravity and increased mass of the van, SUV, or pickup truck. Knowledge of vehicle types where occupants were located in a crash may lead the prehospital care provider to have a higher index of suspicion for serious injury.

Occupant Protective and Restraining Systems

Seat Belts. In the injury patterns described previously, the victims were assumed to be unrestrained. The NHTSA reported that in 2008 only 17% of occupants were unrestrained, compared with 67% in a 1999 NHTSA report.[13] Ejection from vehicles accounted for approximately 25% of the 44,000 vehicular deaths in 2002. About 77% of passenger vehicle occupants who were totally ejected were killed[13]; 1 in 13 ejection victims sustained a spine fracture. After ejection from a vehicle, the body is subjected to a second impact as the body strikes the ground (or another object) outside the vehicle. This second impact can result in injuries that are even more severe than the initial impact. The risk of death for ejected victims is six times greater than for those who are not ejected. Clearly, seat belts save lives.[6]

From 2004 through 2008, more than 75,000 lives were saved by the use of these restraining devices.[14] The NHTSA estimates that more than 255,000 lives have been saved in the United States alone since 1975. The NHTSA reports that more than 13,000 lives were saved by seat belts in the United States in 2008 and that if all occupants wore restraints, the total lives saved would have been more than 17,000.

What occurs when the victims are restrained? If a seat belt is positioned properly, the pressure of the impact is absorbed by the pelvis and the chest, resulting in few, if any, serious injuries (Figure 2-28). The proper use of restraints transfers

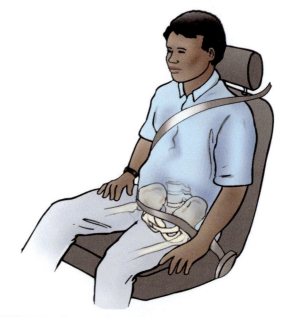

FIGURE 2-28 A properly positioned seat belt is located below the anterior superior iliac spine on each side, above the femur, and is tight enough to remain in this position. The bowl-shaped pelvis protects the soft intraabdominal organs.

the force of the impact from the patient's body to the restraint belts and restraint system. With restraints, the chance of receiving life-threatening injuries is greatly reduced.[6,15,16]

Seat belts must be worn properly to be effective. An improperly worn belt may not protect against injury in the event of a crash, and it may even cause injury. When lap belts are worn loosely or are strapped above the pelvis, compression injuries of the soft abdominal organs can occur. Injuries of the soft intraabdominal organs (spleen, liver, and pancreas) result from compression between the seat belt and the posterior abdominal wall (Figure 2-29). Increased intraabdominal pressure can cause diaphragmatic rupture and herniation of abdominal organs. Lap belts should also not be worn alone but in combination with a shoulder restraint. Anterior compression fractures of the lumbar spine can occur as the upper and lower parts of the torso pivot over the lap belt and the restrained twelfth thoracic (T12), first lumbar (L1), and second lumbar (L2) vertebrae. Many occupants of vehicles still place the diagonal strap under the arm and not over the shoulder.

As laws on mandatory seat belt use are passed and enforced, the overall severity of injuries decreases and the number of fatal crashes is significantly reduced.

Air Bags. Air bags (in addition to seat belts) provide supplemental protection to the occupant of a vehicle. Originally, front-seat driver and passenger air bag systems were designed to cushion the forward motion of only the front-seat occupants. The air bags absorb energy slowly by increasing the body's stopping distance. They are extremely effective in the first collision of frontal and near-frontal impacts (the 65%–70% of crashes that occur within 30 degrees of the headlights). However, air bags deflate immediately after the impact and therefore are not effective in multiple-impact or rear-impact collisions. An air bag deploys and deflates within 0.5 seconds. As the vehicle veers into the path of an

oncoming vehicle or off the road into a tree after the initial impact, no air bag protection is left. Side air bags add to the protection of occupants.

When air bags deploy, they can produce minor but noticeable injuries that the prehospital care provider needs to manage. These include abrasions of the arms, chest, and face (Figure 2-30); foreign bodies to the face and eyes; and injuries caused by the occupant's eyeglasses (Figure 2-31). Air bags

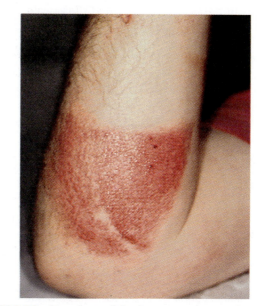

FIGURE 2-30 Abrasions of the forearm are secondary to rapid expansion of the air bag when the hands are tight against the steering wheel.
(From McSwain NE Jr, Paturas JL: *The basic EMT: comprehensive prehospital patient care*, ed 2, St Louis, 2001, Mosby.)

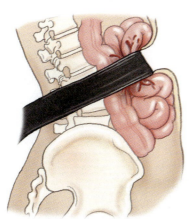

FIGURE 2-29 A seat belt that is incorrectly positioned above the brim of the pelvis allows the abdominal organs to be trapped between the moving posterior wall and the belt. Injuries to the pancreas and other retroperitoneal organs result, as well as blowout ruptures of the small intestine and colon.

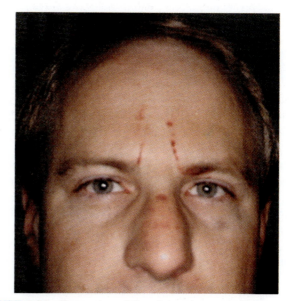

FIGURE 2-31 Expansion of the air bag into eyeglasses produces abrasions.
(From McSwain NE Jr, Paturas JL: *The basic EMT: comprehensive prehospital patient care*, ed 2, St Louis, 2001, Mosby.)

that do not deploy can still be dangerous to both the patient and the prehospital care provider (Figure 2-32). Air bags can be deactivated by an extrication specialist trained to do so properly and safely. Such deactivation should *not* delay patient care or extrication of the critical patient.

Air bags pose a significant hazard to infants and children if the child is either unrestrained or placed in a rear-facing child seat on the front passenger compartment. Of the more than 290 deaths from air bag deployments, almost 70% were passengers in the front seat and 90 of those were infants or children.

Motorcycle Crashes

Motorcycle crashes account for a significant number of the motor vehicle deaths each year. Although the laws of physics for motorcycle crashes are the same, the mechanism of injury varies from automobile and truck crashes. This variance occurs in each of the following types of impacts: head-on, angular, and ejection. An additional factor that leads to increased death, disability, and injury is the lack of structural framework around the biker that is present in other motor vehicles.

Head-on Impact. A head-on collision into a solid object stops the forward motion of a motorcycle (Figure 2-33). Because the motorcycle's center of gravity is above and behind the front axle, which is the pivot point in such a collision, the motorcycle will tip forward, and the rider will crash into the handlebars. The rider may receive injuries to the head, chest, abdomen, or pelvis depending on which part of the anatomy strikes the handlebars. If the rider's feet remain on the pegs of the motorcycle and the thighs hit the handlebars, the forward motion will be absorbed by the midshaft of the femur, usually resulting in bilateral femoral fractures (Figure 2-34). "Open-book" pelvic fractures are a common

result of the interaction between the biker's pelvis and the handlebars.

Angular Impact. In an angular-impact collision, the motorcycle hits an object at an angle. The motorcycle will then collapse onto the rider or cause the rider to be crushed between the motorcycle and the object struck. Injuries to the upper or lower extremities can occur, resulting in fractures and extensive soft tissue injury (Figure 2-35). Injuries can also occur to organs of the abdominal cavity as a result of energy exchange.

Ejection Impact. Because of the lack of restraint, the rider is susceptible to being ejected. The rider will continue in flight until the head, arms, chest, abdomen, or legs strike another object, such as a motor vehicle, a telephone pole, or the road. Injury will occur at the point of impact and will radiate to the rest of the body as the energy is absorbed.[6]

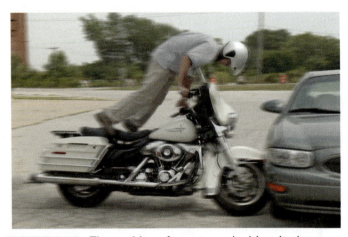

FIGURE 2-33 The position of a motorcycle driver is above the pivot point of the front wheel as the motorcycle impacts an object head-on.

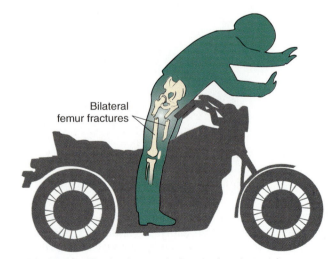

Bilateral femur fractures

FIGURE 2-34 The body travels forward and over the motorcycle, causing the thighs and the femurs to impact the handlebars. The driver can also be ejected.

FIGURE 2-32   Air Bags

Front-seat passenger air bags have been shown to be dangerous to children and small adults, especially when children are placed in incorrect positions in the front seat or with incorrectly installed child car seats. Children 12 years of age and younger should always be in the proper restraint device for their size and should be in the back seat. At least one study has demonstrated that almost 99% of parents checked did not know how to properly install child restraining systems.[17]

Drivers should always be at least 10 inches (25 cm) from the air bag cover, and front-seat passengers should be at least 18 inches (45 cm) away. In most cases, when the proper seating arrangements and distances are used, air bag injuries are limited to simple abrasions.

In many cars, air bags are now available in the sides and tops of doors.

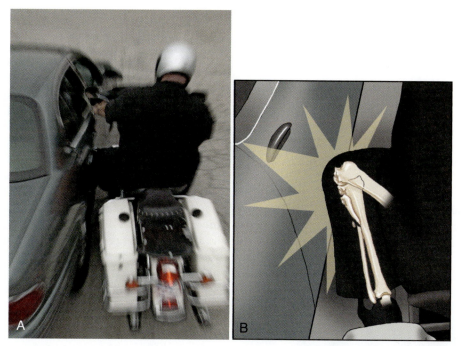

FIGURE 2-35   If the motorcycle does not hit an object head-on, it collapses like a pair of scissors, trapping the rider's lower extremity between the object impacted and the motorcycle.

Injury Prevention. Many riders do not use proper protection. Protection for motorcyclists includes boots, leather clothing, and helmets. Of the three, the *helmet* affords the best protection. It is built similar to the skull: strong and supportive externally and energy absorbent internally. The helmet's structure absorbs much of the impact, thereby decreasing injury to the face, skull, and brain. Failure to use helmets has been shown to increase head injuries by more than 300%. The helmet provides only minimal protection for the neck but does not itself cause neck injuries. Mandatory helmet laws work. For example, Louisiana had a 60% reduction in head injuries in the first 6 years after passing a helmet law. Most states that have passed mandatory helmet legislation have found an associated reduction in motorcycle incidents.

"Laying the bike down" is a protective maneuver used by bikers to separate them from the motorcycle in an impending crash (Figure 2-36). The rider turns the motorcycle sideways and drags the inside leg on the ground. This action slows the rider more than the motorcycle so that the motorcycle will move out from under the rider. The rider will then slide along on the pavement but will not be trapped between the motorcycle and any object it hits. These riders usually receive abrasions ("road rash") and minor fractures but generally avoid the severe injuries associated with the other types of impact, unless they directly strike another object (Figure 2-37).

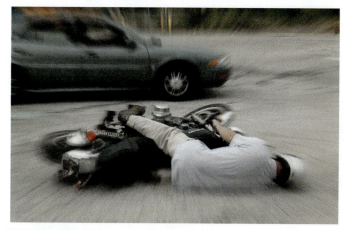

FIGURE 2-36   To prevent being trapped between two pieces of steel (motorcycle and vehicle), the rider "lays the bike down" to dissipate the injury. This often causes abrasions ("road rash") as the rider's speed is slowed on the asphalt.

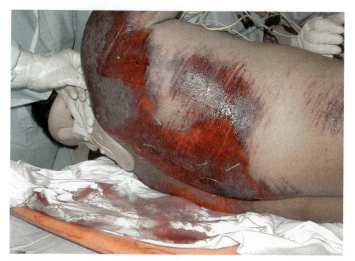

FIGURE 2-37   Road burns after a motorcycle crash without protective clothing.

Pedestrian Injuries

Pedestrian collisions with MVCs have three separate phases, each with its own injury pattern, as follows:

1. The initial impact is to the legs and sometimes the hips (Figure 2-38, *A*).
2. The torso rolls onto the hood of the vehicle (and may strike the windshield) (Figure 2-38, *B*).
3. The victim falls off the vehicle and onto the ground, usually headfirst, with possible cervical spine trauma (Figure 2-38, *C*).

The injuries produced in pedestrian crashes vary according to the height of the victim and the height of the vehicle (Figure 2-39). The impact points on a child and an adult standing in front of a car present different anatomical structures to the vehicles. Because they are shorter, children are initially struck higher on the body than adults (Figure 2-40, *A*). The first impact generally occurs when the bumper strikes the child's legs (above the knees) or pelvis, damaging the femur or pelvic girdle. The second impact occurs almost instantly afterward as the front of the vehicle's hood continues forward and strikes the child's thorax. Then the head and face strike the front or top of the vehicle's hood (Figure 2-40, *B*). Because of the child's smaller size and weight, the child may not be thrown clear of the vehicle, as usually occurs with an adult. Instead, the child may be dragged by the vehicle while partially under the vehicle's front end (Figure 2-40, *C*). If the child falls to the side, the lower limbs may also be run over by a front wheel. If the child falls backward, ending up completely under the vehicle, almost any injury can occur (e.g., being dragged, struck by projections, or run over by a wheel).

If the foot is planted on the ground at the time of impact, the child will receive energy exchange at the upper leg, hip,

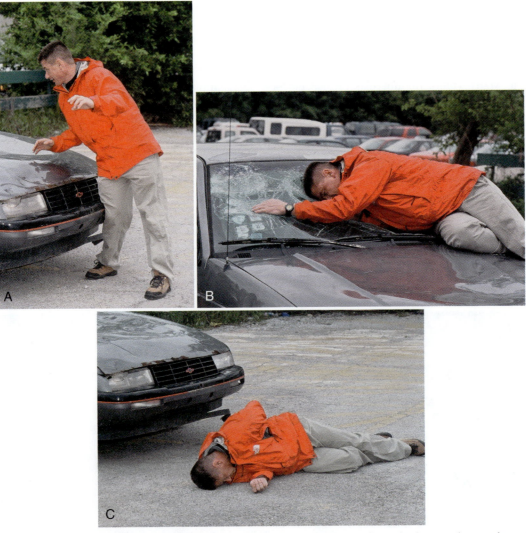

FIGURE 2-38   A, *Phase 1.* When a pedestrian is struck by a vehicle, the initial impact is to the legs and sometimes to the hips. **B,** *Phase 2.* The torso of the pedestrian rolls onto the hood of the vehicle. **C,** *Phase 3.* The pedestrian falls off the vehicle and hits the ground.

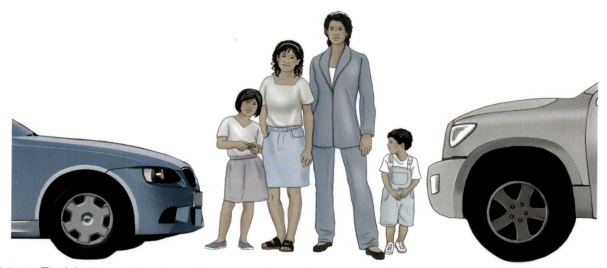

FIGURE 2-39   The injuries resulting from vehicle-pedestrian crashes vary according to the height of the victim and the height of the vehicle.

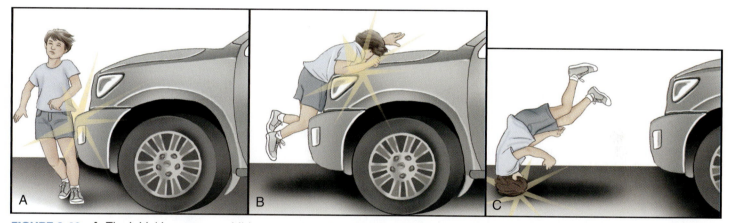

FIGURE 2-40   **A,** The initial impact on a child occurs when the vehicle strikes the child's upper leg or pelvis. **B,** The second impact occurs when the child's head and face strike the front or top of the vehicle's hood. **C,** A child may not be thrown clear of a vehicle but may be trapped and dragged by the vehicle.

and abdomen. This will force the hips and abdomen away from the impact. The upper part of the torso will come along later, as will the planted foot. The energy exchange moving the torso but not the feet will fracture the pelvis and shear the femur, producing severe angulation at the point of impact and possible spine injury as well.

To complicate these injuries further, a child will likely turn toward the car out of curiosity, exposing the anterior body and face to injuries, whereas an adult will attempt to escape and will be hit in the back or the side.

Adults are usually struck first by the vehicle's bumper in the lower legs, fracturing the tibia and fibula. The collision continues into the pelvis and chest as the victim is impacted. As the victim is impacted by the front of the vehicle's hood, depending on the height of the hood, the abdomen and thorax are struck by the top of the hood and the windshield. This substantial second strike can result in fractures of the upper femur, pelvis, ribs, and spine, producing intraabdominal or intrathoracic crush and shear. If the victim's head strikes the hood or if the victim continues to move up the hood so that the head strikes the windshield, injury to the face, head, and cervical and thoracic spine can occur. If the vehicle has a large frontal area (e.g., trucks and SUVs), the potential patient's entire body is hit simultaneously.

The third impact occurs as the victim is thrown off the vehicle and strikes the pavement. The victim can receive a significant blow on one side of the body, injuring the hip, shoulder, and head. Head injury often occurs when the victim strikes either the vehicle or the pavement. Similarly, because all three impacts produce sudden, violent movement of the torso, neck, and head, an unstable spine fracture may result. After falling, the victim may be struck by a second vehicle traveling next to or behind the first.

As with an adult, any child struck by a vehicle can receive some type of head injury. Because of the sudden, violent forces acting on the head, neck, and torso, cervical spine injuries are high on the suspicion list.

Knowing the specific sequence of multiple impacts in pedestrian versus motor vehicle crashes and understanding the multiple underlying injuries that they can produce are key to making an initial assessment and determining the appropriate management of a patient.

Falls

Victims of falls can also sustain injury from multiple impacts. An estimation of the height of the fall, the surface on which the victim landed, and the part of the body struck first are important factors to determine as these are indications of the energy involved and thus the energy exchange that occurred. Victims who fall from greater heights have a higher incidence of injury because their velocity increases as they fall. Falls from greater than three times the height of the victim are often severe. The type of surface on which the victim lands, and particularly its degree of *compressibility* (ability to be deformed by the transfer of energy), also has an effect on stopping distance.

The pattern of injury in falls occurring feet first is called *Don Juan syndrome*. Only in the movies can the character Don Juan jump from a high balcony, land on his feet, and painlessly walk away. In real life, bilateral fractures of the calcaneus (heel bone), compression or shear fractures of the ankles, and distal tibial or fibular fractures are often associated with this syndrome. After the feet land and stop moving, the legs are the next body part to absorb energy. Tibial plateau fractures of the knee, long-bone fractures, and hip fractures can result. The body is compressed by the weight of the head and torso, which are still moving, and can cause compression fractures of the spinal column in the thoracic and lumbar areas. Hyperflexion occurs at each concave bend of the S-shaped spine, producing compression injuries on the concave side and distraction injuries on the convex side. This victim is often described as breaking his or her "S."

If a victim falls forward onto the outstretched hands, the result can be bilateral compression and flexion fractures (Colles fractures) of the wrists. If the victim did not land on the feet, the prehospital care provider will assess the part of the body that struck first, evaluate the pathway of energy displacement, and determine the injury pattern.

If the falling victim lands on the head with the body almost in line, as often occurs in shallow-water diving injuries, the entire weight and force of the moving torso, pelvis, and legs compress the head and cervical spine. A fracture of the cervical spine is a common result, as with the up-and-over pathway of frontal-impact collisions.

Sports Injuries

Severe injury can occur during many sports or recreational activities, such as skiing, diving, baseball, and football. These injuries can be caused by sudden deceleration forces or by excessive compression, twisting, hyperextension, or hyperflexion. In recent years, various sports activities have become available to a wide spectrum of occasional, recreational participants who often lack the necessary training and conditioning or the proper protective equipment. Recreational sports and activities include participants of all ages. Sports such as downhill skiing, water-skiing, bicycling, and skateboarding, are all potentially high-velocity activities. Other sports, such as trail biking, all-terrain vehicle (ATV) riding, and snowmobiling, can produce velocity deceleration, collisions, and impacts similar to motorcycle crashes or MVCs.

The potential injuries of a victim who is in a high-speed collision and then ejected from a skateboard, snowmobile, or bicycle are similar to those sustained when a person is ejected from an automobile at the same speed because the amount of energy is the same. The specific mechanisms of MVCs and motorcycle crashes were described earlier.

The potential mechanisms associated with each sport are too numerous to list in detail. However, the general principles are the same as for MVCs. While assessing the mechanism of injury, the prehospital care provider considers the following questions to assist in the identification of injuries:

- What forces acted on the victim, and how?
- What are the apparent injuries?
- To what object or part of the body was the energy transmitted?
- What other injuries are likely to have been produced by this energy transfer?
- Was protective gear being worn?
- Was there sudden compression, deceleration, or acceleration?

What injury-producing movements occurred (e.g., hyperflexion, hyperextension, compression, excessive lateral bending)?

When the mechanism of injury involves a high-speed collision between two participants, as in a crash between two skiers, reconstruction of the exact sequence of events from eyewitness accounts is often difficult. In such crashes the injuries sustained by one skier are often clues for examination of the other. In general, which part of one victim struck what part of the other victim and what injury resulted from the energy transfer are important. For example, if one victim sustains an impact fracture of the hip, a part of the other skier's body must have been struck with substantial force and therefore must have sustained a similar high-impact injury. If the second skier's head struck the first skier's hip, the trauma first responder will suspect potentially serious head injury and an unstable spine for the second skier.

Broken or damaged equipment is also an important indicator of injury and must be included in the evaluation of the mechanism of injury. A broken sports helmet is evidence of the magnitude of the force with which it struck. Because skis are made of highly durable material, a broken ski indicates that extreme localized force came to bear, even when the mechanism of injury may appear unimpressive. A snowmobile with a severely dented front end indicates the force with which it struck a tree. The presence of a broken stick after an ice hockey skirmish raises the question of whose body broke it, how, and specifically what part of the victim's body was struck by the stick or fell on it.

Victims of significant crashes who complain of no apparent injuries must be assessed as if severe injuries exist. The steps are as follows:

1. Evaluate the patient for life-threatening injury.
2. Evaluate the patient for mechanism of injury. (What happened and exactly how?)
3. Determine how the forces that produced injury in one victim may have affected any other person.
4. Determine whether any protective gear was worn (it may have already been removed).
5. Assess damage to the protective equipment. (What are the implications of this damage relative to the patient's body?)
6. Assess the patient for possible associated injuries.

High-speed falls, collisions, and falls from heights without serious injury are common in many contact sports. The ability of athletes to experience incredible collisions and falls while sustaining only minor injury, largely as a result of impact-absorbing equipment, may be confusing. The potential for injury in sports participants may be overlooked. The principles of kinematics and careful consideration of the exact sequence and mechanism of injury will provide insight into sports collisions in which greater forces than usual came to bear. Kinematics is an essential tool in identifying possible underlying injuries and determining which patients require further evaluation and treatment at a medical facility.

Regional Effects of Blunt Trauma

The body can be divided into six regions: head, neck, thorax, abdomen, pelvis, and extremities. Each body region is subdivided into (1) the external part of the body, usually comprised of skin, bone, soft tissue, vessels, and nerves; and (2) the internal part of the body, usually vital internal organs. The injuries produced as a result of shear, cavitation, and compression forces are used to provide an overview in each component and region for potential injuries.

Head

The only indication that compression and shear injuries have occurred to the patient's head may be a soft tissue injury to

the scalp, a contusion of the scalp, or a bull's-eye fracture of the windshield (Figure 2-41).

Compression. When the body is traveling forward with the head leading the way, as in a frontal vehicular crash or a headfirst fall, the head is the first structure to receive the impact and the energy exchange. The continued momentum of the torso then compresses the head. The initial energy exchange occurs on the scalp and the skull. The skull can be compressed and fractured, pushing the broken bony segments of the skull into the brain (Figure 2-42).

Shear. After the skull stops its forward motion, the brain continues to move forward, becoming compressed against the intact or fractured skull, with resultant concussion, contusions, or lacerations. The brain is soft and compressible; therefore, its length is shortened. The posterior part of the brain can continue forward, pulling away from the skull, which has already stopped moving. As the brain separates from the skull, stretching or breaking (shearing) of brain tissue itself or any blood vessels in the area occur (Figure 2-43). Hemorrhage into

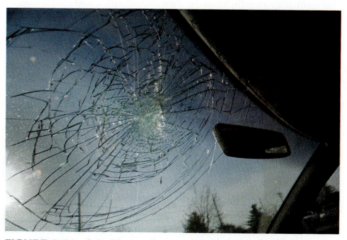

FIGURE 2-41 A bull's-eye fracture of the windshield is a major indication of skull impact and energy exchange to both the skull and the cervical spine.

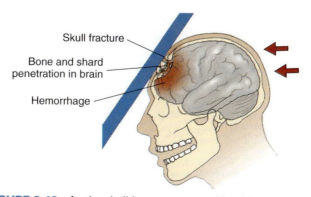

Skull fracture

Bone and shard penetration in brain

Hemorrhage

FIGURE 2-42 As the skull impacts a movable object, pieces of bone are fractured and are pushed into the brain substance.

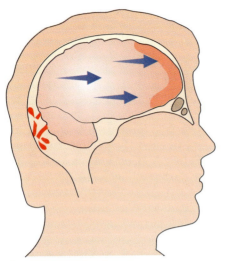

FIGURE 2-43   As the skull stops its forward motion, the brain continues to move forward. The part of the brain nearest the impact is compressed, bruised, and perhaps even lacerated. The portion farthest from the impact is separated from the skull, with tearing and lacerations of the vessels involved.

the epidural, subdural, or subarachnoid space can then result, as well as stretching and shearing of brain tissue itself (diffuse axonal injury of the brain). If the brain separates from the spinal cord, it will most likely occur at the brainstem.

Neck

Compression. The dome of the skull is fairly strong and can absorb the impact of a collision; however, the cervical spine is much more flexible. The continued pressure from the momentum of the torso toward the now stationary skull produces angulation or compression of the spine (Figure 2-44). Hyperextension or hyperflexion of the neck often results in fracture or dislocation of one or more vertebra and injury to the spinal cord. The result can be jumped (dislocated) facets, potential fractures, spinal cord compression, or unstable neck fractures (Figure 2-45). Direct in-line compression crushes the

bony vertebral bodies. Both angulation and in-line compression can result in an unstable spine.

Shear. The skull's center of gravity is anterior and cephalad to the point at which the skull attaches to the bony spine. Therefore, a lateral impact on the torso when the neck is unrestrained will produce lateral flexion and rotation of the neck (see Figure 2-25). Extreme flexion or hyperextension may also cause stretching injuries to the soft tissues of the neck.

Thorax

Compression. If the impact of a collision is centered on the anterior part of the chest, the sternum will receive the initial energy exchange. When the sternum stops moving, the posterior thoracic wall (muscles and thoracic spine) and the organs in the thoracic cavity continue to move forward until the organs strike and are compressed against the sternum.

The continued forward motion of the posterior thorax bends the ribs. If the tensile strength of the ribs is exceeded, fractured ribs and flail chest can develop (Figure 2-46). This is similar to what happens when a vehicle stops suddenly against a dirt embankment (see Figure 2-3). The frame of the vehicle bends, which absorbs some of the energy. The rear of the vehicle continues to move forward until the bending of the frame absorbs all the energy. In the same way, the posterior thoracic wall continues to move until the ribs absorb all the energy. Compression of the chest wall is common with frontal and lateral impacts and produces an interesting phe-

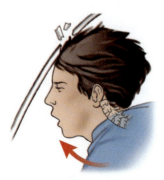

FIGURE 2-44   The skull often stops its forward motion, but the torso does not. Just as the brain compresses within the skull, the torso continues its forward motion until its energy is absorbed. The weakest point of this forward motion is the cervical spine.

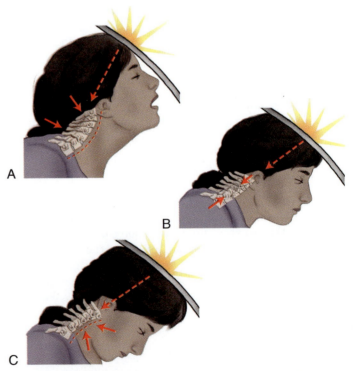

FIGURE 2-45   The spine can be compressed directly along its own axis or angled in hyperextension or hyperflexion.

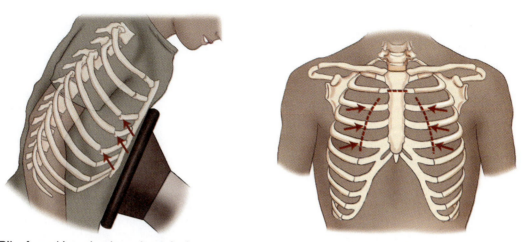

FIGURE 2-46   Ribs forced into the thoracic cavity by external compression usually fracture in multiple places, producing the clinical condition known as *flail chest.*

nomenon called the *paper bag effect,* which may result in a pneumothorax (collapsed lung). A victim instinctively takes a deep breath and holds it just before impact. This closes the glottis, effectively sealing off the lungs. With a significant energy exchange on impact and compression of the chest wall, the lungs may then burst like a paper bag full of air that is popped (Figure 2-47). The lungs can also become compressed and contused, compromising ventilation.

Compression injuries of the internal structures of the thorax may also include cardiac contusion, which occurs as the heart is compressed between the sternum and the spine and can result in significant dysrhythmias (heart rhythm abnormalities). Perhaps a more common injury is compression of the lungs leading to pulmonary contusion (bruising

and hemorrhage of the lung tissue). Although the clinical consequences may develop over time, immediate loss of the ability of the patient to properly ventilate may occur. Pulmonary contusion can have consequences in the field for the prehospital provider and for the physicians during resuscitation after arrival in the hospital. In situations where long transportation times are required, this condition can play a role en route.

Shear.   The heart, ascending aorta, and aortic arch are relatively unrestrained within the thorax. The descending aorta, however, is tightly adherent to the posterior thoracic wall and the vertebral column. The resultant motion of the aorta is similar to holding the flexible tubes of a stethoscope just below where

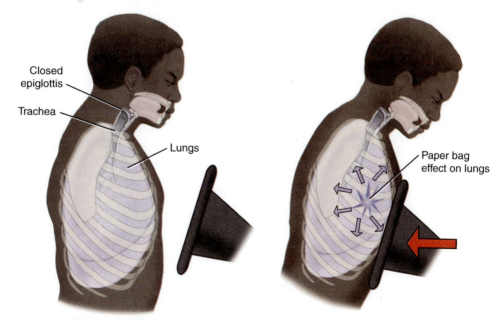

Closed epiglottis

Trachea

Lungs

Paper bag effect on lungs

FIGURE 2-47   Compression of the lung against a closed glottis, by impact on either the anterior or the lateral chest wall, produces an effect similar to compressing a paper bag when the opening is closed tightly by the hands. The paper bag ruptures, as does the lung.

the rigid tubes from the earpiece end and swinging the acoustic head of the stethoscope from side to side. As the skeletal frame stops abruptly in a collision, the heart and the initial segment of the aorta continue their forward motion. The shear forces produced can tear the aorta at the junction of the portion that moves freely with the tightly bound portion (see Figure 2-14).

An aortic tear may result in an immediate, complete transection of the aorta followed by rapid exsanguination. Some aortic tears are only partial, and one or more layers of tissue remain intact. However, the remaining layers are under great pressure, and a traumatic aneurysm often develops, similar to the bubble that can form on a weak part of a tire. The aneurysm can eventually rupture minutes, hours, or days after the original injury. Approximately 80% of these patients die on the scene at the time of the initial impact. Of the remaining 20%, one third will die within 6 hours, one third will die within 24 hours, and one third will live 3 days or longer. It is important that the prehospital care provider recognize the potential for such injuries and relay this information to the hospital personnel.

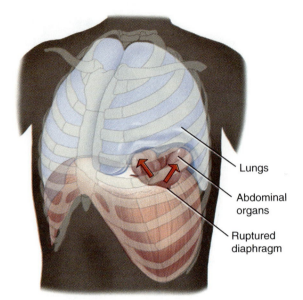

FIGURE 2-48 With increased pressure inside the abdomen, the diaphragm can rupture.

Abdomen

Compression. Internal organs pressed by the vertebral column into the steering wheel or dashboard during a frontal collision may rupture. The effect of this sudden increase in pressure is similar to the effect of placing the internal organ on an anvil and striking it with a hammer. Solid organs commonly injured in this manner include the pancreas, spleen, liver, and kidneys.

Injury may also result from overpressure in the abdomen. The *diaphragm* is a ¼-inch thick (5-mm) muscle located across the top of the abdomen and separates the abdominal cavity from the thoracic cavity. Its contraction causes the pleural cavity to expand for breathing. The anterior abdominal wall comprises two layers of fascia and one very strong muscle. Laterally there are three muscle layers with associated fascia, and the lumbar spine and its associated muscles provide strength to the posterior abdominal wall. The diaphragm is the weakest of all the walls and structures surrounding the abdominal cavity. It may be torn or ruptured as intraabdominal pressure increases (Figure 2-48). This injury has four common consequences:

1. The "bellows" effect that is usually created by the diaphragm is lost and breathing is affected.
2. The abdominal organs can enter the thoracic cavity and reduce the space available for lung expansion.
3. The displaced organs can become ischemic from compression of their blood supply.
4. If intraabdominal hemorrhage is present, the blood can also cause a hemothorax.

Shear. Injury to the abdominal organs occurs at their points of attachment to the mesentery. During a collision, the forward motion of the body stops but the organs continue to move forward, causing tears at the points of attachment of organs to the abdominal wall. If the organ is attached by a pedicle (a stalk of tissue), the tear can occur where the pedicle attaches to the organ, where it attaches to the abdominal wall, or anywhere along the length of the pedicle (see Figures 2-13 and 2-14). Organs that can shear this way are the kidneys, small intestine, large intestine, and spleen.

Another type of injury that often occurs during deceleration is laceration of the liver caused by its impact with the ligamentum teres. The liver is suspended from the diaphragm but is only minimally attached to the posterior abdomen near the lumbar vertebrae. The ligamentum teres attaches to the anterior abdominal wall at the umbilicus and to the left lobe of the liver in the midline of the body. (The liver is not a midline structure; it lies more on the right than on the left.) A down-and-under pathway in a frontal impact or a feet first fall causes the liver to bring the diaphragm with it as it descends into the ligamentum teres (Figure 2-49). The ligamentum teres will fracture or transect the liver, analogous to a cheese slicer cutting cheese.

Pelvic fractures are the result of damage to the external abdomen and may cause injury to the bladder or lacerations of the blood vessels in the pelvic cavity. Approximately 10% of patients with pelvic fractures also have a genitourinary injury.

Pelvic fractures resulting from compression from the side, usually caused by a lateral-impact collision, have two components. One is the compression of the proximal femur into the pelvis, which pushes the head of the femur through the acetabulum itself. This often produces radiating fractures that involve the entire joint. Further compression of the femur or the lateral walls of the pelvis produce compression fractures

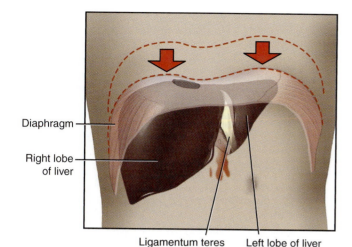

Diaphragm

Right lobe
of liver

Ligamentum teres   Left lobe of liver

FIGURE 2-49   The liver is not supported by any fixed
structure. Its major support is by the diaphragm, which is
freely movable. As the body travels in the down-and-under
pathway, so does the liver. When the torso stops but the liver
does not, the liver continues downward onto the ligamentum
teres, tearing the liver. This is much like pushing a cheese-
cutting wire into a block of cheese.

of the pelvic bones or the ring of the pelvis. Because a ring
generally cannot be fractured in only one place, this usually
means two fractures to the ring, although some of the fractures may involve the acetabulum.

Shear fractures usually involve the ilium and the sacral
area. This shearing force tears the joint open. Because the
joints in a ring such as the pelvis generally must be fractured
in two places, this often produces a fracture somewhere else
along the pelvic ring.

The other type of compression fracture occurs anteriorly
when the compression is over the symphysis pubis. This will
either break the symphysis by pushing in on both sides or
break one side and push it back toward the sacroiliac joint.
This opens the joint, producing the so-called open-book
fracture.

Penetrating Trauma

Physics of Penetrating Trauma

The principles of physics discussed earlier are equally important when dealing with penetrating injuries.

Energy cannot be created or destroyed, but it can be
changed in form. This principle is important in understanding penetrating trauma. For example, although a lead bullet is
in the brass cartridge casing that is filled with explosive powder, the bullet itself has no force. However, when the primer
explodes, the powder burns, producing rapidly expanding
gases that are transformed into force. The bullet then moves
out of the gun and toward its target.

After this force has acted on the missile, the bullet will
remain at that speed and force until it is acted on by an outside force. When the bullet hits something, such as a human
body, it strikes the individual tissue cells. The energy (speed
and mass) of the bullet's motion is exchanged for the energy
that crushes these cells and moves them away (cavitation)
from the path of the bullet.

Factors That Affect the Size of the Frontal Area

The larger the frontal area of the moving missile, the greater
the number of particles that will be hit; therefore, the greater
the energy exchange that occurs and the larger the cavity that
is created. The size of the frontal surface area of a projectile
is influenced by three factors: profile, tumble, and fragmentation. Energy exchange or potential energy exchange can be
analyzed based on these factors.

Profile.   *Profile* describes an object's initial size and whether
that size changes at the time of impact. The profile, or frontal
area, of an ice pick is much smaller than that of a baseball bat,
which in turn is much smaller than that of a truck. A hollow-
point bullet flattens and spreads on impact (Figure 2-50). This
change enlarges the frontal area so that it hits more tissue particles and produces greater energy exchange. As a result, a
larger cavity forms and more injury results.

In general, a bullet should remain very aerodynamic as it
travels through the air en route to the target. Low resistance
while passing through the air (hitting as few air particles as
possible) to travel is a good thing. This will allow it to maintain most of its speed. To achieve this, the frontal area is kept
small in a conical shape. A lot of drag (resistance to travel) is
a bad thing. A good bullet design would have very little drag
while passing through the air but much more drag when passing through the body's tissues. If that missile strikes the skin
and becomes deformed, covering a larger area, creating much
more drag, then a much greater energy exchange will occur.
Therefore, the ideal bullet is designed to keep its shape while
in the air and only deform on impact.

FIGURE 2-50   Expanding Bullets

A munitions factory in Dum Dum, India, manufactured a
bullet that expanded when it hit the skin. Ballistic experts
recognized this design as one that would cause more damage
than is necessary in war; therefore, these bullets were
prohibited in military conflicts. The Petersburg Declaration
of 1868 and the Hague Convention of 1899 affirmed this
principle, denouncing these "dum-dum" projectiles and
other expanding missiles, such as silver tips, hollow-points,
scored-lead cartridges or jackets, and partially jacketed
bullets, and outlawing their use in war.

Tumble. *Tumble* describes whether the object turns over and over and assumes a different angle inside the body than the angle assumed as it entered the body, thus creating more drag inside the body than in the air. A wedge-shaped bullet's center of gravity is located nearer to the base than to the nose of the bullet. When the nose of the bullet strikes something, it slows rapidly. Momentum continues to carry the base of the bullet forward, with the center of gravity seeking to become the leading point of the bullet. A slightly asymmetrical shape causes an end-over-end motion, or tumble. As the bullet tumbles, the normally horizontal sides of the bullet become its leading edges, thus striking far more particles than when bullet was in the air (Figure 2-51). More energy exchange is produced, and therefore greater tissue damage occurs.

Fragmentation. *Fragmentation* describes whether the object breaks up to produce multiple parts or rubble and therefore more drag and more energy exchange. There are two types of fragmentation rounds: (1) fragmentation on leaving the weapon (e.g., shotgun pellets) (Figure 2-52) and (2) fragmentation after entering the body. This can be active or passive fragmentation. Active fragmentation involves a bullet that has an explosive inside it that detonates inside the skin. Bullets with soft noses or vertical cuts in the nose and safety slugs that contain many small fragments to increase body damage by breaking apart on impact are examples of passive fragmentation. The resulting mass of fragments creates a larger frontal area than a single solid bullet, and energy is dispersed rapidly into the tissue. If the missile shatters, it will spread out over a wider area, with two results: (1) more tissue particles will be struck by the larger frontal projection, and (2) the injuries will be distributed over a larger portion of the body because more organs will be struck (Figure 2-53). The multiple pieces of shot from a shotgun blast produce similar results. Shotgun wounds are an excellent example of the fragmentation injury pattern.

Damage and Energy Levels
The damage caused in a penetrating injury can be estimated by classifying penetrating objects into three categories according to their energy capacity: low-, medium-, and high-energy weapons.

Low-Energy Weapons. Low-energy weapons include hand-driven weapons such as a knife or ice pick. These missiles

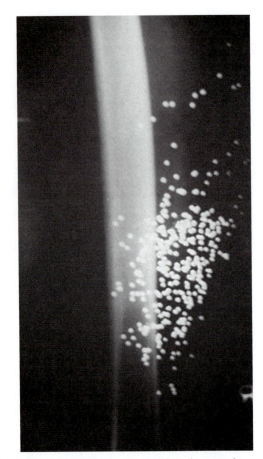

FIGURE 2-52   Maximum fragmentation damage is caused by a shotgun.

produce damage only with their sharp points or cutting edges. Because these are low-velocity injuries, they are usually associated with less secondary trauma (i.e., less cavitation will occur). Injury in these victims can be predicted by tracing the path of the weapon into the body. If the weapon has been

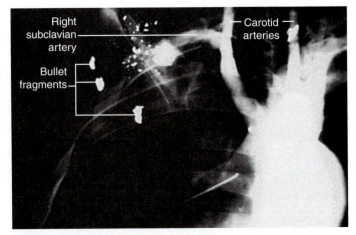

FIGURE 2-53   When the missile breaks up into smaller particles, this fragmentation increases its frontal area and increases the energy distribution.
(McSwain NE Jr: Pulmonary chest trauma. In Moylan JA, editor: *Principles of trauma,* New York, 1992, Gower.)

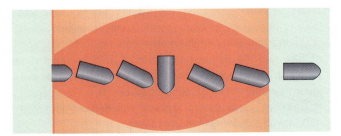

FIGURE 2-51   Tumble motion of a missile maximizes its damage at 90 degrees.

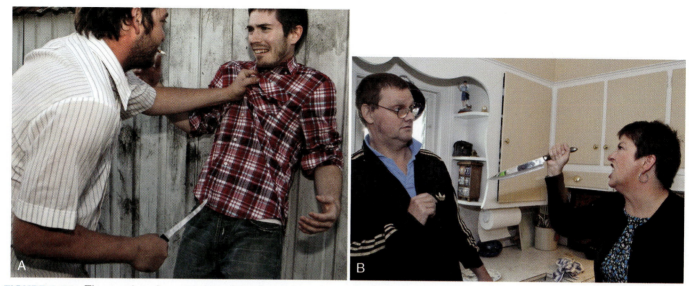

FIGURE 2-54   The gender of an attacker often determines the trajectory of the wound in stabbing incidents. Male attackers tend to stand upward, whereas female attackers tend to stand downward.

removed, the prehospital care provider should try to identify the type of weapon used.

The gender of the attacker is an important factor in determining the trajectory of a knife. Men tend to thrust with the blade on the thumb side of the hand and with an upward or inward motion, whereas women tend to hold the blade on the little finger side and stab downward (Figure 2-54).

An attacker may stab a victim and then move the knife around inside the body. A simple entrance wound may produce a false sense of security. The entrance wound may be small, but the damage inside may be extensive. The potential scope of the movement of the inserted blade is an area of possible damage (Figure 2-55).

Evaluation of the patient for associated injury is important. For example, the diaphragm can reach as high as the nipple line on deep expiration. A stab wound to the lower chest can injure intraabdominal as well as intrathoracic structures and a wound of the upper abdomen may also involve the lower chest.

Penetrating trauma can result from impaled objects such as fence posts and street signs in vehicle crashes and falls, ski poles in snow sports, and handlebar injuries in bicycling.

Medium-Energy and High-Energy Weapons. Firearms fall into two groups: medium energy and high energy. Medium-energy weapons include handguns and some rifles whose muzzle velocity is 1000 feet per second. The temporary cavity created by this weapon is three to five times the caliber of the bullet. High-energy weapons have muzzle velocity in excess of 2000 feet per second and significantly greater muzzle energy. They create a temporary cavity 25 times or more than the caliber of the bullet. It is obvious that as the amount of gunpowder in the cartridge increases and the size of the bullet increases, the speed and mass of the bullet and therefore its kinetic energy increase (Figure 2-56, *A* and *B*). The mass of the bullet is an important but smaller component (KE = $\frac{1}{2}$ mv^2). The bullet mass is not to be discounted, however. In the Civil War, a Kentucky long rifle firing a 0.55-caliber Minie ball had almost the same muzzle energy as the current M16 used in Iraq. The mass of the missile becomes more important when considering the damage produced by a 12-gauge shotgun at close range or an improvised explosive device (IED). In general, medium-energy and high-energy weapons damage not only the tissue directly in the path of the missile but also the tissue involved in the temporary cavity on each side of the missile's path. The variables of missile profile, tumble, and fragmentation influence the rapidity of the energy exchange and therefore the extent and direction of the injury. The force of the tissue particles being moved out of the direct path of the missile compresses and stretches the surrounding tissue (Figure 2-57).

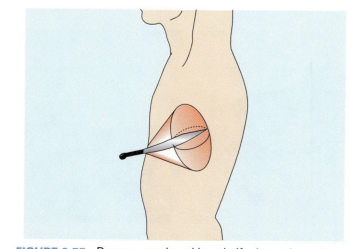

FIGURE 2-55   Damage produced by a knife depends on the movement of the blade inside the victim.

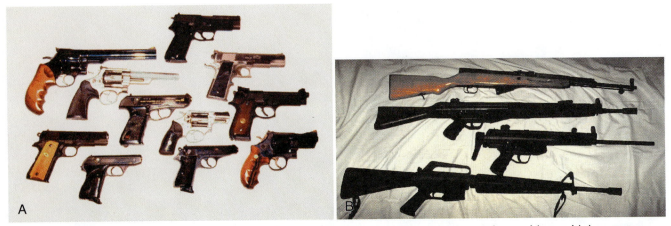

FIGURE 2-56   **A,** Medium-energy weapons are usually guns that have short barrels and contain cartridges with less power.
B, High-energy weapons.
(From McSwain NE Jr, Paturas JL: *The basic EMT: comprehensive prehospital patient care,* ed 2, St Louis, 2001, Mosby.)

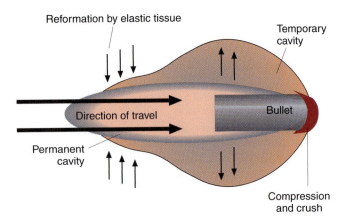

FIGURE 2-57   A bullet crushes tissues directly in its path. A cavity is created in the wake of the bullet. The crushed part is permanent. The temporary expansion can also produce injury.

High-energy weapons discharge high-energy missiles (Figure 2-58). Tissue damage is much more extensive with a high-energy penetrating object than with one of medium energy. The vacuum created in the cavity created by this high-speed missile can pull clothing, bacteria, and other debris from the surface into the wound.

A consideration in predicting the damage from a gunshot wound is the range or *distance* from which the gun (either medium or high energy) is fired. Air resistance slows the bullet; therefore, increasing the distance will decrease the energy at the time of impact and will result in less injury. Most shootings are done at close range with handguns, so the probability of serious injury is related to both the anatomy involved and the energy of the weapon rather than loss of kinetic energy.

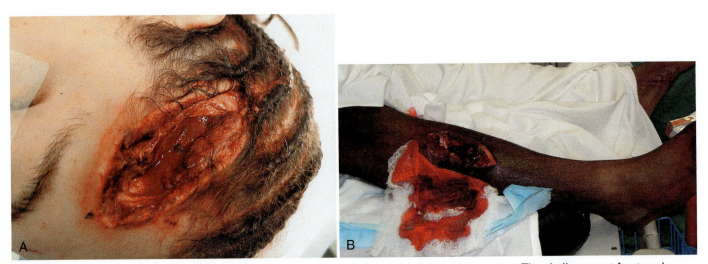

FIGURE 2-58   **A,** Graze wound to the scalp created by a projectile from a high-velocity weapon. The skull was not fractured.
B, High-velocity gunshot wound to the leg demonstrating the large, permanent cavity.

Anatomy

Entrance and Exit Wounds

Tissue damage will occur at the site of missile entry into the body, along the path of the penetrating object, and on exit from the body. Knowledge of the victim's position, the attacker's position, and the weapon used is helpful in determining the path of injury. If the entrance wound and the exit wound can be related, the anatomical structures that would likely be in this pathway can be approximated.

Evaluating wound sites provides valuable information to direct the management of the patient and to relay to the receiving facility. Do two holes in the victim's abdomen indicate that a single missile entered and exited, or that two missiles entered and are both still inside the patient? Did the missile cross the midline (usually causing more severe injury) or remain on the same side? In what direction did the missile travel? What internal organs are likely to have been in its path?

Entrance and exit wounds usually, but not always, produce identifiable injury patterns to soft tissue. Evaluation of the apparent trajectory of a penetrating object is very helpful to the clinician. This information should be given to the physicians in the hospital. On the other hand, prehospital providers (and most physicians) do not have the experience or the expertise of a forensic pathologist; therefore, the assessment of which wound is an entrance and which is an exit is fraught with uncertainty. Such information is solely for patient care to try to gauge the trajectory of the missile and not for legal purposes to determine specifics about the incident. These two issues should not be confused. The provider must have as much information as possible to determine the potential injuries sustained by the patient and to best decide how the patient is to be managed. The legal issues related to the specifics of entrance and exit are best left to others. An entrance wound from a gunshot lies against the underlying tissue, but an exit wound has no support. The former is typically a round or oval wound, depending on the entry path, and the latter is usually a *stellate* (starburst) wound (Figure 2-59). Because the missile is spinning as it enters the skin, it leaves a small area of abrasion (1–2 mm) that is pink (Figure 2-60). Abrasion is not present on the exit side. If the muzzle was placed directly against the skin at the time of discharge, the expanding gases will enter the tissue and produce crepitus on examination (Figure 2-61). If the muzzle is within 2 to 3 inches (5–7 cm), the hot gases that exit will burn the skin; at 2 to 6 inches (5–15 cm) the smoke will adhere to the skin; and inside 10 inches (25 cm) the burning cordite particles will tattoo the skin with small (1–2 mm) burned areas (Figure 2-62).

Regional Effects of Penetrating Trauma

This section discusses the injuries sustained by various parts of the body during penetrating trauma.

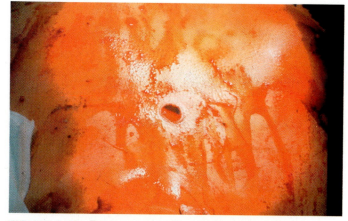

FIGURE 2-59 Entrance wound is usually round or oval in shape, and exit wound is often stellate or linear.

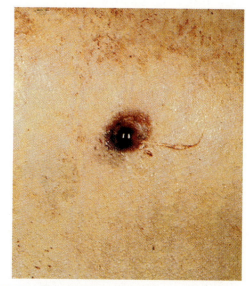

FIGURE 2-60 The abraded edge indicates that the bullet traveled from top right to bottom left.

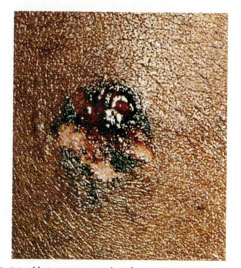

FIGURE 2-61 Hot gases coming from the end of a muzzle held in proximity to the skin produce partial-thickness and full-thickness burns on the skin.

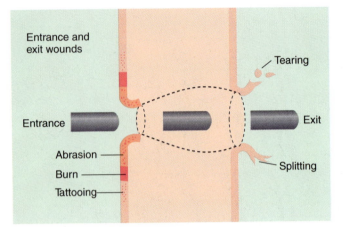

FIGURE 2-62   On entrance, spin and compression of the bullet produce round or oval holes. On exit, the wound is pressed open.

Head. After a missile penetrates the skull, its energy is distributed within a closed space. Particles accelerating away from the missile are forced against the unyielding skull, which cannot expand as can skin, muscle, or even the abdomen. Thus the brain tissue is compressed against the inside of the skull, producing more injury than would otherwise occur if it could expand freely. It is like putting a firecracker in an apple and then placing the apple in a metal can. When the firecracker explodes, the apple will be destroyed against the

wall of the can. If the forces are strong enough, the skull may explode from the inside out (Figure 2-63).

A bullet may follow the curvature of the interior of the skull if it enters at an angle and has insufficient force to exit the skull. This path can produce significant damage (Figure 2-64). Because of this characteristic, small-caliber, medium-velocity weapons, such as the 0.22-caliber or 0.25-caliber pistol, have been called "assassin's weapons." They go in and exchange all their energy into the brain.

Thorax. Three major groups of structures are inside the thoracic cavity: the pulmonary system, vascular system, and gastrointestinal tract. This does not include the bone and muscle of the chest wall. One or more of the anatomical structures of these systems may be injured by a penetrating object.

Pulmonary System. Lung tissue is less dense than blood, solid organs, or bone; therefore, a penetrating object will hit fewer particles, exchange less energy, and do less damage to lung tissue. Damage to the lungs can be clinically significant (Figure 2-65), but fewer than 15% of patients will require surgical exploration.[18]

Vascular System. Smaller vessels that are not attached to the chest wall may be pushed aside without significant damage. However, larger vessels, such as the aorta and vena cava, are less mobile because they are tethered to the spine or the heart. They cannot move aside easily and are more susceptible to damage.

The myocardium (almost totally muscle) stretches as the bullet passes through and then contracts, leaving a smaller

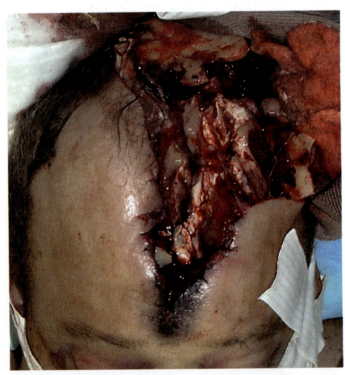

FIGURE 2-63   After a missile penetrates the skull, its energy is distributed within a closed space. It is like putting a firecracker in a closed container. If the forces are strong enough, the container (the skull) may explode from the inside out.

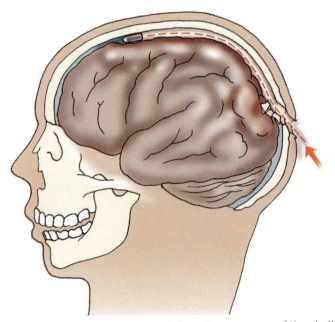

FIGURE 2-64   The bullet may follow the curvature of the skull. (From McSwain NE Jr, Paturas JL: *The basic EMT: Comprehensive prehospital patient care*, ed 2, St Louis, 2001, Mosby.)

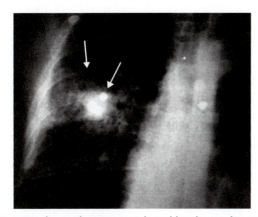

FIGURE 2-65   Lung damage produced by the cavity at a distance from the point of impact.

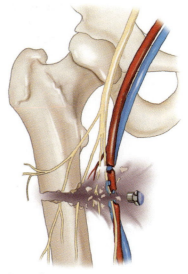

FIGURE 2-66   Bone fragments become secondary missiles themselves, producing damage by the same mechanism as the original penetrating object.

defect. The thickness of the muscle may control a low-energy penetration, such as by a knife or even a small medium-energy 0.22-caliber bullet. This closure can prevent immediate exsanguination and allow time to transport the victim to an appropriate facility.

Gastrointestinal Tract. The esophagus, the part of the gastrointestinal tract that traverses the thoracic cavity, can be penetrated and can leak its contents into the thoracic cavity. The signs and symptoms of such an injury may be delayed for several hours or several days.

Abdomen. The abdomen contains structures of three types: air filled, solid, and bony. Penetration by a low-energy missile may not cause significant damage; only 30% of knife wounds penetrating the abdominal cavity require surgical exploration to repair damage. A medium-energy injury (e.g., handgun wound) is more damaging; 85% to 95% require surgical repair. However, in injuries caused by medium-energy missiles, the damage to solid and vascular structures often does not produce immediate exsanguination. This enables prehospital care providers to transport the patient to an appropriate facility in time for effective surgical intervention.

Extremities. Penetrating injuries to the extremities can include damage to bones, muscles, nerves, or vessels. When bones are hit, bony fragments become secondary missiles, lacerating surrounding tissue (Figure 2-66). Muscles often expand away from the path of the missile, causing hemorrhage. The missile may penetrate blood vessels, or a near-miss may damage the lining of a blood vessel, causing clotting and obstruction of the vessel within minutes or hours.

Shotgun Wounds

Although shotguns are not high-velocity weapons, they are high-energy weapons; at close range they can be more lethal than some of the most high-energy rifles. Handguns and rifles predominantly use *rifling* (grooves) on the inside of the barrel to spin a single missile in a flight pattern toward the target.

In contrast, most shotguns possess a smooth, cylindrical tube barrel that directs a load of missiles in the direction of the target. Devices known as *chokes* and *diverters* can be attached to the end of a shotgun barrel to shape and form the column of missiles into specific patterns (e.g., cylindrical or rectangular). Regardless, when a shotgun is fired, a large number of missiles are ejected in a *spread,* or *spray,* pattern. The barrels may be shortened ("sawed off") to prematurely widen the trajectory of the missiles.

Although shotguns may use various types of ammunition, the structure of most shotgun shells is similar. A typical shotgun shell contains gunpowder, wadding, and projectiles. When discharged, all these individual components are propelled from the muzzle and can inflict injury on the victim. Certain types of gunpowder can *stipple* ("tattoo") the skin in close-range injuries. Wadding, which is usually lubricated paper, fibers, or plastic used to separate the shot (missiles) from the charge of gunpowder, can provide another source of infection into the wound if not removed. The missiles can vary in size, weight, and composition. A wide variety of missiles are available, from compressed metal powders to *birdshot* (small metal pellets), *buckshot* (larger metal pellets), *slugs* (a single metal missile), and more recently, plastic and rubber alternatives. The average shell is loaded with 1 to $1\frac{1}{2}$ ounces of shot. Fillers that are placed with the shot (polyethylene or polypropylene granules) can become embedded in the superficial layers of the skin.

An average birdshot shell may contain 200 to 2000 pellets, whereas a buckshot shell may contain only 6 to 20 pellets (Figure 2-67). It is important to note that as the size of the buckshot pellets increases, they approach the wounding characteristics of 0.22-caliber missiles in regard to effective range and energy transfer characteristics. Larger "magnum"

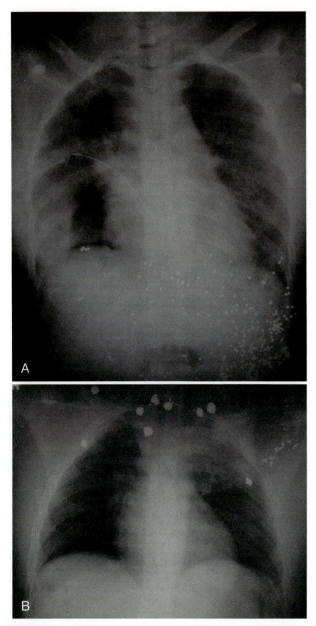

FIGURE 2-67 An average birdshot shell may contain 200 to 2000 pellets (**A**), whereas a buckshot shell may contain only 6 to 20 pellets (**B**).

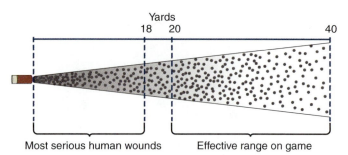

FIGURE 2-68   The diameter of the spread of a shot column expands as range increases.
(From DeMuth WE: The mechanism of gunshot wounds. *J Trauma* 11:219, 1971.)

shells are also available. These shells may contain more shot and a larger charge of gunpowder, or only the larger powder charge, to boost the muzzle velocity of the shot.

The type of ammunition used is important in gauging injuries, but the *range* (distance) at which the patient was shot provides the most important variable when evaluating the shotgun injury victim. Shotguns eject a large number of missiles, most of which are spherical. These projectiles are especially susceptible to the effects of air resistance, thereby quickly slowing once they exit the muzzle (Figure 2-68). The effect of air resistance on the projectiles decreases the effective range of the weapon and changes the basic charac-

teristics of wounds that it generates. Consequently, shotgun wounds have been classified into four major categories: contact, close-range, intermediate-range, and long-range wounds (Figure 2-69).

Contact wounds occur when the muzzle is touching the patient at the time the weapon is discharged. This typically results in circular entrance wounds, which may or may not have soot or an imprint of the muzzle (see Figure 2-61). Searing or burning of the wound edges is common, secondary to the high temperatures and the expansion of hot gases as the missiles exit the muzzle. Some contact wounds may be more stellate (star shaped) in appearance, caused by the superheated gases from the barrel escaping from the tissue. Contact wounds usually result in widespread tissue damage and are associated with high mortality. The length of a standard shotgun barrel makes it difficult to commit suicide with this weapon, because it is difficult to reach and pull the trigger. Such attempts usually result in a split face without the shot reaching the brain.

Close-range wounds (less than 6 feet), although still typically characterized by circular entrance wounds, will likely have more evidence of soot, gunpowder, or filler stippling around the wound margins than contact wounds. Additionally, abrasions and markings from the impact of the wadding that coincide with the wounds from the missiles may be found. Close-range wounds also create significant damage in the patient; missiles fired from this range still retain sufficient energy to penetrate deep structures and exhibit a slightly wider spread pattern. This increases the extent of injury as missiles travel through soft tissue.

Intermediate-range wounds are characterized by the appearance of satellite pellet holes emerging from the border around a central entrance wound. This pattern is a result of individual pellets spreading from the main column of shot and generally occurs at a range of 6 to 18 feet. These injuries are a mixture of deep penetrating wounds and superficial wounds and abrasions. Because of the deep penetrating components of this injury, however, victims may still have a relatively high mortality rate.

Long-range wounds are rarely lethal. These wounds are typically characterized by the classic spread of scattered pellet wounds and result from a range of greater than 18 feet.

FIGURE 2-69   **Patterns of Shotgun Injury**

Type	Wound Appearance	Injury	Mortality
Contact		Widespread tissue damage	85%–90%
Close		Penetrates beyond deep fascia	15%–20%
Intermediate		Penetrates subcutaneous tissue and deep fascia	0%–5%
Long range		Superficial skin penetration	0%

Modified from Sherman RT, Parrish RA: Management of shotgun injuries: a review of 152 cases. *J Trauma* 18:236, 1978.

However, even at these slower velocities, the pellets can cause significant damage to certain sensitive tissues (e.g., eyes). In addition, larger buckshot pellets can retain sufficient velocity to inflict damage to deep structures, even at long range. The prehospital care provider also needs to consider the cumulative effects of many small missile wounds and their locations, focusing on sensitive tissues. *Adequate exposure* is essential when examining all patients involved in trauma, and shotgun injuries are no exception.

These varying characteristics need to be taken into account when evaluating injury patterns in patients with shotgun injuries. For example, a single circular shotgun wound could represent a contact or close-range injury with birdshot or buckshot in which the missiles have retained a tight column or grouping. Conversely, this may also represent an intermediate-range to long-range injury with a slug or solitary missile. Only detailed examination of the wound will allow differentiation of these injuries that will likely involve significant damage to internal structures despite strikingly different missile characteristics.

Contact and close-range wounds to the chest may result in a large, visually impressive wound causing an open pneumothorax, and bowel may eviscerate from such wounds to the abdomen. On occasion, a single pellet from an intermediate-range wound may penetrate deep enough to perforate the bowel, leading eventually to peritonitis, or may damage a major artery, resulting in vascular compromise to an extremity. Alternatively, a patient who presents with multiple small wounds in a spread pattern may have dozens of entrance wounds. However, none of the missiles may have retained enough energy to penetrate through fascia, let alone produce significant damage to internal structures.

Although immediate patient care must always remain the priority, any information (shell type, suspected range of the patient from the weapon, number of shots fired) that prehospital care providers can gather from the scene and relay to the receiving facility can assist with appropriate diagnostic eval-

uation and treatment of the shotgun-injured patient. Furthermore, recognition of various wound types can aid providers in maintaining a high index of suspicion for internal injury regardless of the initial impression of the injury.

Blast Injuries

Injury from Explosions

Explosive devices are the most commonly used weapons in combat and by terrorists. Explosive devices cause human injury by multiple mechanisms, some of which are exceedingly complex. The greatest challenges for clinicians at all levels of care in the aftermath of an explosion are the large numbers of casualties and multiple penetrating injuries (Figure 2-70).[19]

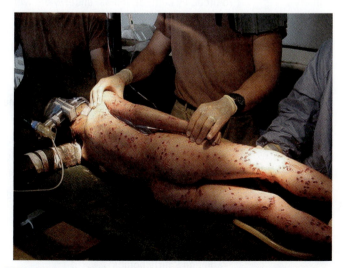

FIGURE 2-70   Patient with multiple fragment wounds from a bomb blast.

Physics of Blast

Explosions are physical, chemical, or nuclear reactions that result in the almost instantaneous release of large amounts of energy in the form of heat and rapidly expanding, highly compressed gas, capable of propelling fragments at extremely high velocities. The energy associated with an explosion can take multiple forms: kinetic and heat energy in the "blast wave," kinetic energy of fragments formed by the breakup of the weapon casing and surrounding debris, and electromagnetic energy.

Blast waves can travel at more than 16,400 feet (5000 meters) per second. When a blast occurs, a sudden increase in pressure surrounds objects close to the explosion, compressing them on all sides with a rise in pressure, called the shock front or shock wave, up to a peak overpressure value. Following the shock front, the overpressure drops down to ambient pressure, and then a partial vacuum is often formed as a result of air being sucked back (Figure 2-71). There is also a blast "wind." The primary significance of the blast wind is that it propels fragments at speeds in excess of several thousand meters per second (faster than standard ballistic weapons such as bullets and shells).[20] Whereas the effective range of the pressure effect is measured in tens of feet, the fragments accelerated by the dynamic pressure will quickly outpace the blast wave to become the dominant cause of injury out to ranges of thousands of feet.

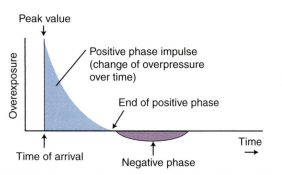

FIGURE 2-71 Pressure-Time History of a Blast Wave. This graph shows the sudden massive increase in pressure (blast overpressure) after the decrease in pressure and negative pressure phase.
(Source: Blast injuries. Idealized graph of a blast pressure wave over time. Courtesy Bowen TE, Bellamy RF, editors: *Emergency war surgery*, Washington, DC, United States Government Printing Office, 1988.)

Interaction of Blast Waves with the Body

Blast waves interact with the body and other structures by transmitting energy from the blast wave into the structure. This energy causes the structure to deform in a manner that depends on the strength and elasticity of the structure being loaded. The differences in density of components within a structure cause complex re-formations, convergences, and couplings of the transmitted blast waves. This occurs particularly with large-density interfaces such as solid tissue to air or liquid (e.g., lung, heart, liver, and bowel).

Explosion-Related Injuries

Injuries from explosions are generally classified as primary, secondary, tertiary, quaternary, and quinary after the injury taxonomy described in Department of Defense Directive 6025.21E[20] (Figures 2-72 and 2-73). Detonation of an explo-

FIGURE 2-72   Blast Injury Categories

Category	Definition	Typical Injuries
Primary	Produced by contact of blast shockwave with body Stress and shear waves occur in tissues Waves reinforced/reflected at tissue density interfaces Gas-filled organs (lungs, ears, etc.) at particular risk	Tympanic membrane rupture Blast lung Eye injuries Concussion

Secondary	Ballistic wounds produced by:
	    Primary fragments (pieces of exploding weapon)
	    Secondary fragments (environmental fragments, e.g., glass)
	Threat of fragment injury extends further than that from blast wave
		Penetrating injuries
		Traumatic amputations
		Lacerations

Tertiary	Blast wave propels individuals onto surfaces/objects or objects onto individuals, causing whole body translocation Crush injuries caused by structural damage and building collapse	Blunt injuries Crush syndrome Compartment syndrome
Quaternary	Other explosion-related injuries, illnesses, or disease	Burns Toxic gas and other inhalation injury Injury from environmental contamination
Quinary	Injuries resulting from specific additives such as bacteria and radiation ("dirty bombs")	

Centers for Disease Control and Prevention: *Explosions and blast injuries: a primer for clinicians.* Available at www.bt.cdc.gov/masscasualties/explosions.asp. Accessed July 21, 2010.

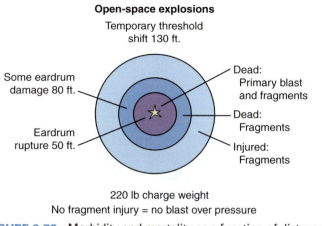

Open-space explosions

Temporary threshold
shift 130 ft.

Some eardrum
damage 80 ft.

Dead:
Primary blast
and fragments

Dead:
Fragments

Injured:
Fragments

Eardrum
rupture 50 ft.

220 lb charge weight
No fragment injury = no blast over pressure

FIGURE 2-73 Morbidity and mortality as a function of distance from open-space detonation of a 22-pound (approximately 100-kg) charge.

sive device sets off a chain of interactions in the objects and people in its path.[19] If an individual is close enough, the initial blast wave increases pressure in the body, causing stress and shear, particularly in gas-filled organs such as the ears, lungs, and (rarely) bowels. These primary blast injuries are more common when the explosion occurs in an enclosed space because the blast wave bounces off surfaces, thus enhancing the destructive potential of the pressure waves.[21] Immediate death from pulmonary barotrauma (blast lung) occurs more often in enclosed-space than in open-air bombings.[22–24] The most common form of primary blast injury is tympanic membrane (eardrum) rupture.[25,26] Tympanic membrane rupture, which may occur at pressures as low as 5 psi,[27,28] is often the only significant overpressure injury experienced. The next major injury occurs at less than 40 psi, a threshold known to be associated with pulmonary injuries, including pneumo-thorax, air embolism, interstitial and subcutaneous emphy-sema, and pneuomediastinum.[29]

The shock front of the blast wave quickly dissipates and is followed by the blast wind, which propels fragments to create multiple penetrating injuries. Although these are termed sec-ondary injuries, they are usually the predominant wounding agent.[19] The blast wind also propels large objects into people or people onto hard surfaces (whole or partial body transloca-tion), creating blunt (tertiary blast) injuries; this category of injury also includes crush injuries caused by structural col-lapse.[29] Heat, flames, gas, and smoke generated during explo-sions cause quaternary injuries that include burns, inhalation injury, and asphyxiation.[15] Quinary injuries are produced when bacteria, chemicals, or radioactive materials are added to the explosive device and released upon detonation.

Injury from Fragments

Conventional explosive weapons are designed to maximize damage caused by fragments. With initial velocities of many thousands of feet per second, the distance that fragments may be thrown for a 50-pound (23-kg) bomb will be well over 1000 feet (0.3 km), whereas the lethal radius of the blast over-

pressure is approximately 50 feet (about 15 meters). Both military and terrorist weapons developers, therefore, design weapons to maximize fragmentation injury so as to signifi-cantly increase the damage radius of a free-field explosive.

Very few explosive devices cause injury solely by blast overpressure, and serious primary blast injury is relatively rare compared with the large numbers of secondary and ter-tiary injuries. Thus, few patients have injuries dominated by primary blast effects. Because energy from the blast wave dissipates rapidly, most explosive devices are constructed to cause damage primarily from fragments. These may be pri-mary fragments, generated through the breakup of the casing surrounding the explosive, or secondary fragments, created from debris in the surrounding environment. Regardless of whether the fragments are created from shattered munitions casing, flying debris, or embedded objects that terrorists often pack into homemade bombs, they exponentially increase the range and lethality of explosives and are the primary cause of explosion-related injury.

Multi-Etiology Injury

In addition to the direct effects of an explosion, health care providers must be mindful of the other causes of injury from attacks with explosions. For instance, an IED that targets a vehicle may result in minimal initial damage to the vehicle occupants. However, the vehicle itself may be displaced ver-tically or vectored off course, resulting in occupant blunt trauma from collision, from flipping upside down as part of the vertical displacement process, or from rollover, such as down an embankment or culvert. In these circumstances, occupants sustain injury based on the mechanisms previ-ously described for blunt trauma. In the military setting, a vehicle's occupants may be afforded some protection from blunt injury by virtue of their body armor. Furthermore, the occupants of a vehicle disabled after an IED attack may be attacked with gunfire as they exit the vehicle and are subject to ambush, thus potentially becoming victims of penetrating injury.

Using Kinematics in Assessment

The assessment of a trauma patient must involve knowledge of kinematics. For example, a driver who hits the steering wheel (blunt trauma) will have a large cavity in the anterior chest at the time of impact; however, the chest rapidly returns to, or near to, its original shape as the driver rebounds from the steering wheel. If two trauma care providers examine the patient separately—one who understands kinematics and another who does not—the one without knowledge of kine-matics will be concerned only with the bruise visible on the outside of the patient's chest. The trauma care provider who understands kinematics will recognize that a large cavity was present at the time of impact; that the ribs had to bend in for the cavity to form; and that the heart, lungs, and great vessels were compressed by the formation of the cavity. Therefore, the knowledgeable responder will suspect injury to the heart, lungs, great vessels, and chest wall. The other prehospital care provider will not even be aware of these possibilities.

The knowledgeable trauma care provider suspecting serious intrathoracic injuries will assess for these potential injuries, manage the patient, and initiate transport more aggressively, rather than react to what otherwise appears to be only a minor closed, soft-tissue injury. Early identification, adequate understanding, and appropriate treatment of underlying injury will significantly influence whether a patient lives or dies.

SUMMARY

- Integrating the principles of the kinematics of trauma into the assessment of the trauma patient is key to discovering the potential for severe or life-threatening injuries.
- Up to 95% of the injuries can be anticipated by understanding the injury exchange that occurs with the human body at the time of a collision. Knowledge of kinematics allows for injuries that are not immediately apparent to be identified and treated as appropriate. Left unsuspected, undetected, and therefore untreated, these injuries contribute significantly to morbidity and mortality resulting from trauma.
- Energy cannot be created or destroyed, only changed in form. The kinetic energy of an object, expressed as a function of both velocity (speed) and mass (weight), is transferred to another object on contact.
- Damage to the object or body tissue impacted is not only a function of the amount of kinetic energy applied to it but also a function of the tissue's ability to tolerate the forces applied to it.

Blunt Trauma

- The direction of the impact determines the pattern of and potential for injury: frontal, lateral, rear, rotational, rollover, or angular.
- Ejection from a car reduces the protection on impact.
- Energy-absorbing protective devices are very important. These include seat belts, air bags, drop-down engines, and energy-absorbing auto parts, such as bumpers, collapsible steering wheels, dashboards, and helmets. On arrival, the damage to the vehicles and the direction of the impact will indicate which victims are most likely to have been more severely injured.
- Pedestrian injures vary according to the height of the victim and which part of the body had direct contact with the vehicle.

Falls

- The distance traveled before impact affects the severity of the injury sustained.
- The energy-absorbing capability of the target at the end of the fall (i.e., concrete vs. soft snow) affects the severity of the injury sustained.
- Identify the victim body parts that hit the target and progression of the energy exchange through the victim's body.

Blasts

- There are five types of injury in a blast:
  1. Primary—overpressure and underpressure
  2. Secondary—projectiles (most common source of injury from blasts)
  3. Tertiary—propulsion of the body into another object
  4. Quaternary—heat and flames
  5. Quinary—radiation, chemicals, bacteria

Penetrating Trauma

- The energy varies depending on the primary injuring agent:
  - Low energy—handheld cutting devices
  - Medium energy—handguns, some rifles
  - High energy—high-powered rifles
- The distance of the victim to the perpetrator and the objects that the bullet might have struck will affect the amount of energy at the time of impact with the body and therefore the available energy to be dissipated into the patient to produce damage to the body parts.
- Organs in proximity of the pathway of the penetrating object determine the potential life-threatening conditions.
- The pathway of the penetrating trauma is determined by the wound of entrance and the wound of exit.

SCENARIO SOLUTION

Patient 1: Driver of the vehicle with side impact. Two bullets traversed the door of the car. The patient has two left-side bullet wounds, one below the ribs and one above the ribs. The patient's blood pressure was low; therefore, the likely injuries in the chest include pneumothorax, hemothorax, and penetration of the heart and possibly major vessels. Below the ribs, penetration into the abdominal cavity could involve any of the abdominal organs with associated hemorrhage.

Patient 2: Passenger in vehicle with side impact of car. Because of the energy exchanged between the door and the occupant, you should suspect injury in all four side-impact areas—that is, the shoulder (clavicle), chest wall and thoracic cavity, abdominal cavity, and pelvis. Potential injuries in these areas include the following:

1. Fractured clavicle
2. Fractured ribs (potential flail chest)
3. Pulmonary contusions
4. Sheering related to the aorta
5. Pneumothorax
6. Abdomen (fractured liver or spleen)
7. Deceleration injury to the kidney
8. Fractured pelvis
9. Rotational injury of the cervical spine

Patient 3: Driver of the vehicle. With the bent steering wheel, you suspect an up-and-over pathway at the time of the collision into the pole, causing a frontal chest impact into the steering wheel and head impact into the windshield. Potential injuries include the following:

1. Myocardial contusion
2. Pneumothorax
3. Flail chest
4. Pulmonary contusion
5. Overpressure injury in the abdomen
6. Fractured liver and spleen
7. Cervical spine facture
8. Brain injury

Patient 4: Passenger in second vehicle. You suspect down-and-under pathway. Potential injuries include the following:

1. Fracture of the lower extremities (ankle, shaft of the femur)
2. Hip dislocation
3. Facial injuries
4. Cervical spine injury

One other additional important assessment to consider: How did the bullet holes get in the first car? Did you search the occupants for weapons? ■

References

1. National Center for Injury Prevention and Control: *WISQARS injury mortality reports, 1999– 2007*. Available at http://webappa.cdc.gov/sasweb/ncipc/mortrate10_sy.html. Accessed December 4, 2009.
2. National Highway Traffic Safety Administration. *National statistics*. Available at www.fars.nhtsa.dot.gov/Main/index.aspx. Accessed December 4, 2009.
3. National Center for Injury Prevention and Control: *WISQARS nonfatal injury reports*. Available at http://webappa.cdc.gov/sasweb/ncipc/nfirates2001.html. Accessed December 4, 2009.
4. Rogers CD, Pagliarello G, McLellan BA, Nelson WR: Mechanism of injury influences the pattern of injuries sustained by patients involved in vehicular trauma. *Can J Surg* 34(3):283–286, 1991.
5. Hollerman JJ, Fackler ML, Coldwell DM, Ben-Menachem Y: Gunshot wounds: 1. Bullets, ballistics, and mechanisms of injury. *AJR Am J Roentgenol* 155(4):685–690, 1990.
6. Simon BJ, Legere P, Emhoff T, et al: Vehicular trauma triage by mechanism: avoidance of the unproductive evaluation. *J Trauma* 37(4):645–649, 1994.
7. Hernandez IA, Fyfe KR, Heo G, Major PW: Kinematics of head movement in simulated low velocity rear-end impacts. *Clin Biomech* 20(10):1011–1018, 2005.
8. Parenteau C: Far-side occupant kinematics in low speed lateral sled. *Traffic Inj Prev* 7(2):164–170, 2006.
9. Kumaresan S, Sances A, Carlin F, et al: Biomechanics of side impact injuries: evaluation of seat belt restraint system, occupant kinematics and injury potential. *Conf Proc IEEE Eng Med Biol Soc* 1:87–90, 2006.
10. Siegel JH, Yang KH, Smith JA, et al: Computer simulation and validation of the Archimedes Lever hypothesis as a mechanism for aortic isthmus disruption in a case of lateral impact motor vehicle crash: a Crash Injury Research Engineering Network (CIREN) study. *J Trauma* 60(5):1072–1082, 2006.
11. Horton TG, Cohn SM, Heid MP, et al: Identification of trauma patients at risk of thoracic aortic tear by mechanism of injury. *J Trauma* 48(6):1008–1013; discussion 1013–1014, 2000.
12. Dyer DS, Moore EE, Ilke DN, et al: Thoracic aortic injury: how predictive is mechanism and is chest computed tomography a

reliable screening tool? A prospective study of 1,561 patients. *J Trauma* 48(4):673–682; discussion 682–683, 2000.

13. National Highway Traffic Safety Administration: *Traffic safety facts 2008.* Available at www.nrd.nhtsa.dot.gov/Pubs/811160. PDF. Accessed December 4, 2009.

14. National Highway Traffic Safety Administration: *Traffic safety facts crash stats.* Available at www-nrd.nhtsa.dot.gov/Pubs/811153.PDF. Accessed December 5, 2009.

15. Lindquist MO, Hall AR, Bjornstig UL: Kinematics of belted fatalities in frontal collisions: a new approach in deep studies of injury mechanism. *J Trauma* 61(6):1506–1516, 2006.

16. Siegel AW: Automobile collisions, kinematics and related injury patterns. *Calif Med* 116(2):16–22, 1972.

17. Fackler ML: Ballistic injury. *Ann Emerg Med* 15(12):1451–1455, 1986.

18. American College of Surgeons (ACS) Committee on Trauma: *Advanced trauma life support course,* Chicago, 2002, ACS.

19. Wade CE, Ritenour AE, Eastridge BJ, et al: Explosion injuries treated at combat support hospitals in the Global War on Terrorism. In Elsayed N, Atkins J, eds: *Explosion and blast-related injuries,* Philadelphia, Elsevier, 2008.

20. Champion HR, Baskin T, Holcomb JB: Injuries from explosives. In McSwain NE et al, editors: *National Association of Emergency Medical Technicians: PHTLS basic and advanced prehospital trauma life support: military edition,* ed 2, St Louis, 2006, Mosby.

21. Department of Defense Directive: *Medical research for prevention, mitigation, and treatment of blast injuries,* Number 6025.21E, July 5, 2006. Available at www.dtic.mil/whs/directives/corres/html/602521.htm. Accessed April 15, 2008.

22. Gutierrez de Ceballos JP, Turégano-Fuentes F, Perez-Diaz D, et al: 11 March 2004: The terrorist bomb explosions in Madrid, Spain—an analysis of the logistics, injuries sustained and clinical management of casualties treated at the closest hospital. *Crit Care* 9:104–111, 2005.

23. Gutierrez de Ceballos JP, Turégano Fuentes F, et al: Casualties treated at the closest hospital in the Madrid, March 11, terrorist bombings. *Crit Care Med* 2005;33(1 Suppl):S107–112.

24. Avidan V, Hersch M, Armon Y, et al: Blast lung injury: clinical manifestations, treatment, and outcome. *Am J Surg* 2005;190:927–931.

25. Leibovici D, Gofrit ON, Stein M, et al: Blast injuries: bus versus open-air bombings—a comparative study of injuries in survivors of open-air versus confined-space explosions. *J Trauma* 1996;41:1030-1035.

26. Ritenour AE, Wickley A, Ritenour JS, et al: Tympanic membrane perforation and hearing loss from blast overpressure in Operation Enduring Freedom and Operation Iraqi Freedom wounded. *J Trauma* 64:S174–178, 2008.

27. Zalewski T: Experimentelle Untersuchungen uber die Resistenz-fahigkeit des Trommelfells. *Z Ohrenheilkd* 52:109, 1906.

28. Helling ER: Otologic blast injuries due to the Kenya embassy bombing. *Mil Med* 169:872–876, 2004.

29. Nixon RG, Stewart C: *When things go boom: blast injuries. Fire engineering,* May 1, 2004. Available at www.fireengineering.com/articles/article_ display.html?id=204602. Accessed April 15, 2008.

Suggested Reading

Alderman B, Anderson A: Possible effect of airbag inflation on a standing child. In *Proceedings of 18th American Association of Automotive Medicine,* September 1974.

American College of Surgeons (ACS) Committee on Trauma: *Advanced trauma life support course,* Chicago, 2002, ACS.

Anderson PA, Henley MB, Rivara P, Maier RV: Flexion distraction and chance injuries to the thoracolumbar spine. *J Orthop Trauma* 5(2):153, 1991.

Anderson PA, Rivara FP, Maier RV, Drake C: The epidemiology of seatbelt-associated injuries. *J Trauma* 31(1):60, 1991.

Bartlett CS: Gunshot wound ballistics. *Clin Orthop* 408:28, 2003.

DePalma RG, Burris DG, Champion HR, Hodgson MJ: Current concepts: blast injuries, *N Engl J Med* 352:1335, 2005.

Di Maio VJM: *Gunshot wounds: practical aspects of firearms, ballistics and forensic techniques,* Boca Raton, Fla, 1999, CRC Press.

Fackler ML, Surinchak JS, Malinowski JA, Bowen RE: Bullet fragmentation: a major cause of tissue disruption. *J Trauma* 24:35, 1984.

Fackler ML, Surinchak JS, Malinowski JA, Bowen RE: Wounding potential of the Russian AK-47 assault rife. *J Trauma* 24:263, 1984.

Garrett JW, Braunstein PW: The seat belt syndrome, *J Trauma* 2:220, 1962.

Huelke DF, Mackay GM, Morris A: Vertebral column injuries and lap-shoulder belts. *J Trauma* 38:547, 1995.

Huelke DF, Moore JL, Ostrom M: Air bag injuries and occupant protection. *J Trauma* 33(6):894, 1992.

Joksch H, Massie D, Pichler R: *Vehicle aggressivity: fleet characterization using traffic collision data,* Washington, DC, 1998, NHTSA/Department of Transportation.

McSwain NE Jr: Kinematics. In Mattox KL, Feliciano DV, Moore EE, editors: *Trauma,* ed 4, New York, 1999, McGraw-Hill.

McSwain NE Jr, Brent CR: Trauma rounds: lipstick sign. *Emerg Med* 21:46, 1898.

National Safety Council (NSC): *Accident facts 1994,* Chicago, 1994, NSC.

Ordog GJ, Wasserberger JN, Balasubramaniam S: Shotgun wound ballistics. *J Trauma* 28:624, 1988.

Oreskovich MR, Howard JD, Compass MK, et al: Geriatric trauma: injury patterns and outcome. *J Trauma* 24:565, 1984.

Rutledge R, Thomason M, Oller D, et al: The spectrum of abdominal injuries associated with the use of seat belts. *J Trauma* 31(6):820, 1991.

States JD, Annechiarico RP, Good RG, et al: A time comparison study of the New York State Safety Belt Use Law utilizing hospital admission and police accident report information. *Accid Anal Prev* 22(6):509, 1990.

Swierzewski MJ, Feliciano DV, Lillis RP, et al: Deaths from motor vehicle crashes: patterns of injury in restrained and unrestrained victims. *J Trauma* 37(3):404, 1994.

Sykes LN, Champion HR, Fouty WJ: Dum dums, hollowpoints, and devastators: techniques designed to increase wounding potential of bullets. *J Trauma* 28:618, 1988.

CHAPTER 3

Assessment of the Scene and Patient

CHAPTER OBJECTIVES

At the completion of this chapter, the reader will be able to do the following:

✓ Identify potential threats to the safety of the patient, bystanders, and emergency personnel that are common to all emergency scenes.

✓ Identify potential threats that are unique to a given scenario, such as a motor vehicle crash (MVC).

✓ Integrate analysis of scene safety, scene situation, and kinematics into assessment of the trauma patient to make patient care decisions.

✓ Describe appropriate steps to take to recognize and remove potential threats to safety.

✓ Given a mass-casualty incident (MCI) scenario (hazardous material incident, weapon of mass destruction), integrate the use of a triage system into the management of the scene and make triage decisions based on assessment findings.

✓ Describe the significance of patient assessment in the context of overall management of the trauma patient.

✓ Demonstrate the discrete steps involved in assessing and managing the trauma patient.

✓ Given a scenario, adapt the 15-second global survey and primary survey to the particulars of the situation.

✓ Demonstrate the critical questioning needed to associate the physical examination and scene findings with their likely causes and consequences.

SCENARIO 1

You are dispatched to the scene of a tanker truck crash. As you begin to respond, you notice that it has just begun to snow. Dispatch provides the additional information that the driver of the truck is reported to be unconscious and bleeding from a large scalp laceration. In addition, a witness states that liquid from the vehicle is leaking onto the street.

As you arrive on the scene, what considerations are important before you contact the patient?

What are your concerns about the scene?

SCENARIO 2

You are awakened at 0400 on a Saturday to respond to the scene of a person who fell from a third floor balcony. As you go to the ambulance, you notice the temperature is 50 °F (10 °C). According to dispatch, bystanders report that the patient lost consciousness but now is awake. On arrival, you detect no threats to safety in your scene assessment. Bystanders state that he was partying in the apartment above and had been drinking some alcohol. They report that he seemed to land feet first onto the ground below and confirm that they witnessed the patient's loss of consciousness for a period of "several minutes." Approaching the patient, a young adult male, you kneel at his head, observing that he is conscious. You position your hands to provide cervical spine stabilization. In response to your questioning, you discover that the patient's chief complaint is foot and back pain. Your questioning serves the dual purpose of obtaining the patient's complaint and assessing his ventilatory effort. Detecting no shortness of breath, you proceed with further questioning as your partner obtains the patient's vital signs. The patient answers your questions appropriately to establish that he is oriented to person, place, and event.

Based on kinematics as they relate to this incident, what potential injuries do you anticipate finding during your assessment?

What are your next priorities?

How will you proceed with this patient?

The trauma care provider has the following three priorities on arrival to a scene:

1. The first priority for everyone involved at a trauma incident is assessment of the scene. *Scene assessment* involves establishing that the scene is safe and carefully considering the exact nature of the situation. In addition to patient and responder safety, the determination needs to be made as to what alteration in patient care is indicated by the current conditions. Assessment of scene safety and the situation is initiated while en route to the scene based on information from the dispatcher. It continues as the emergency medical services (EMS) unit and responders arrive on the scene, and as the providers approach

the patient. The issues identified in this evaluation must be addressed before beginning assessment of individual patients. In some situations, such as combat or tactical situations, this becomes even more critical and can alter the methods of how the principles of patient care are accomplished.

2. After performing the scene assessment, attention is turned to evaluating individual patients. Scene assessment includes an initial abbreviated form of triage so that the most severely injured patients are assessed first. The emphasis in order of priority is (a) conditions that may result in the loss of life, (b) conditions that may result in the loss of limb, and (c) all other conditions that do not threaten life or limb.

3. If the scene involves more than one patient, the situation is classified as either a multiple-patient incident or a mass-casualty incident (MCI). In an MCI the priority shifts from focusing all resources on the most injured patient to saving the maximum number of patients—that is, providing the greatest good to the greatest number. Triage is discussed in the final section of this chapter.

Scene Assessment

Scene and patient assessment starts long before the prehospital care provider arrives at the patient's side. Dispatch begins the process by providing the initial information about the incident and the patient, based on bystander reports or information provided by other public safety or prehospital care units first on the scene. The on-scene information-gathering process begins immediately upon arrival at the incident. Before making contact with the patient, the scene is evaluated by (1) obtaining a general impression of the situation for scene safety, (2) looking at the cause and results of the incident, and (3) observing family members or bystanders. A majority of patient injuries can be predicted based on an understanding of the kinematics and the effects on the patients.

Taking the time to prepare mentally for a call and practicing basic communication between partners may be the difference between a well-managed scene and a hostile confrontation (or a physical assault). Good observation, perception, and communication skills are the best tools.

The scene's appearance creates an impression that influences the entire assessment; therefore, correct evaluation of the scene is crucial. A wealth of information is gathered by simply looking, watching, listening, and cataloguing as much information as possible, including the mechanisms of injury, the present situation, and the overall degree of safety.

Just as the patient's condition can improve or deteriorate, so can the condition of the scene. Evaluating the scene initially, then failing to reassess how the scene may be changing can result in serious consequences to the care providers and the patient.

Scene assessment includes the following two major components:

1. *Safety.* The primary consideration when approaching any scene is the safety of the medical and rescue personnel. Rescue attempts should not be made by those untrained in the techniques required. When medical personnel become victims, they will no longer be able to assist other injured people and will add to the number of patients and decrease the number of care providers. Patient care needs to wait until the scene is secured.

    Scene safety involves not only rescuer safety but also patient safety. In general, patients in a hazardous situation should be moved to a safe area before assessment and treatment begin. Threatening conditions to patient or rescuer safety include fire, downed electrical lines, explosives, hazardous materials, including blood or body fluid, traffic, floodwater, weapons (e.g., guns, knives), and environmental conditions. Also, an assailant may still be on the scene and may intervene to harm the patient, rescuers, or others.

    The preferences employed for patient care can be drastically altered by the conditions on the scene. For example, an industrial explosion or chemical spill can produce dangerous conditions for the prehospital care provider that take precedent and alter the methods by which patient care is provided. (For more information on principle versus preference, see Chapter 1.)

    A final safety consideration involves bystanders and the public who may be present on a scene. While the responder's first priorities are to personal, partner, and patient safety, the safety of those who gather at emergency scenes must also be maintained. Police and fire responders can be extremely helpful in assuring that the public do not place themselves at risk at emergency scenes.

2. *Situation.* Assessment of the situation follows the safety assessment. Many issues must be assessed based upon the individual situation.

    - What really happened at the scene?
    - Why was help summoned?
    - What was the mechanism of injury (kinematics), and what forces and energies led to the victims' injuries? (See Chapter 2.)
    - How many people are involved, and what are their ages?
    - Are additional EMS units needed for treatment or transport?
    - Is mutual aid needed? Are any other personnel or resources needed (e.g., law enforcement, fire department, power company)?
    - Is special extrication or rescue equipment needed?
    - Is helicopter transport necessary?
    - Is a physician needed to assist with triage or on-scene medical care issues?
    - Could a medical problem be the instigating factor that led to the trauma (e.g., a vehicle crash that resulted from the driver's heart attack)?

Issues related to both safety and situation have significant overlap; many safety topics are also specific to certain situations, and certain situations pose serious safety hazards. These issues are discussed in further detail in the following sections.

Safety Issues

Traffic Safety

The majority of EMS responders who are killed or injured each year are involved in motor vehicle-related incidents.[1] Although most of these are related to direct ambulance collisions during the response phase, a subset of these fatalities and injuries occurs while working on the scene of a motor vehicle crash (MVC). In the United States, MVCs resulted in more than 1.9 million EMS responses in 2003.[2] Many factors can result in prehospital care providers being injured or killed on the scene of an MVC (Figure 3-1). Some factors, such as weather conditions (e.g., snow, ice, rain, fog) and road design (e.g., limited-access or rural roads), cannot be changed; however, the responder can be aware that these conditions exist and can act appropriately to mitigate these situations.[3]

Weather/Light Conditions

Many prehospital care responses to MVCs take place in adverse weather conditions and at night. These weather conditions vary by geographic location and time of the year. Providers in many areas need to deal with ice and snow during the winter months, whereas those in coastal and mountainous areas often confront fog. Rainstorms are common in most geographic areas, and sandstorms affect other regions. Incoming traffic may not see or be able to stop in time to avoid emergency vehicles or personnel parked on the scene.

Highway Design

High-speed, limited-access highways have made moving large amounts of traffic efficient, but when a crash occurs, the resulting traffic backup and "rubber necking" by drivers create dangerous situations for responders. Law enforcement is usually reluctant to shut down a limited-access highway and strives to keep the flow of traffic moving. Although this may seem to produce further danger to responders, it may prevent additional rear-end collisions caused by the backup of vehicles.

Rural roads present other problems. Although the volume of traffic is much less than on urban roadways, the windy, narrow, and hilly nature of these roads creates short sight distances for drivers as they approach the scene of an MVC. Rural roads may not be as well maintained as those in urban areas, resulting in slippery conditions long after a storm has passed and catching unsuspecting drivers off guard. Isolated

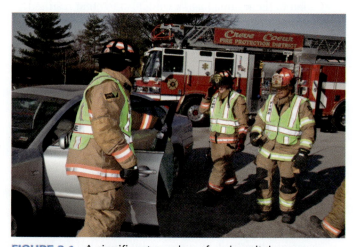

FIGURE 3-1 A significant number of prehospital care providers who are injured or killed are working at the scene of a motor vehicle crash.

areas of snow, ice, or fog that caused the original MVC may still be present, hinder EMS arrival, and may result in suboptimal conditions for oncoming drivers.

Prevention Strategies

It would be safest to respond to MVCs only during daylight hours on clear days; unfortunately, prehospital care providers need to respond at all times of day and in any weather condition. However, steps can be taken to reduce the risks of becoming a victim while working at an MVC. The best way is to not be there, particularly on limited-access highways. The number of people on the scene at any given time should be the number needed to accomplish the tasks at hand; for example, having three ambulances and a supervisor's vehicle at a scene that has only one patient dramatically increases the risk of a provider being hit by a passing vehicle. Although many dispatch protocols require multiple-ambulance response to limited-access highways, all but the initial ambulance should be staged at an on ramp nearby unless immediately needed.

The location of equipment on the ambulance also plays a role in safety. Equipment should be placed so that it can be gathered without stepping into the traffic flow. The passenger's side of the ambulance is usually toward the guardrails, and placing the equipment most often used at MVCs in these compartments will keep responders out of the traffic flow.

Reflective Clothing. In most cases of prehospital care responders being hit by oncoming vehicles, the drivers stated that they did not see the responder in the road. Both the National Fire Protection Association and the Occupational Safety and Health Administration (OSHA) have standards for reflective warning garments used on highways. OSHA has three levels of protection for workers on highways, with the highest level (level 3) being used at night on a high-speed roadway. The Federal Highway Administration has mandated that all workers, including public safety and first responders wear American National Standards Institute (ANSI) class 2 or class 3 reflective vests when responding to an incident on a highway funded with federal aid. Common sense indicates that prehospital care providers should wear reflective clothing at all motor vehicle–related crashes as a safety measure. The ANSI standards can be met either by affixing reflective material to the outer jacket or by wearing an approved reflective vest.

Vehicle Positioning and Warning Devices. Vehicle positioning at the scene of an MVC is of the utmost importance. The incident commander or the safety officer should ensure that responding vehicles are placed in the best positions to protect prehospital care providers. It is important for the first arriving emergency vehicles to "take the lane" of the accident (Figure 3-2). Although placement of the ambulance behind the scene will not facilitate loading of the patient, it will protect the responders and patients from oncoming traffic. As additional emergency vehicles arrive, they should generally be placed on the same side of the road as the incident. These vehicles should be placed farther away from the incident to give increased warning time to oncoming drivers.

Headlights, especially high beams, should be turned off so as not to blind oncoming drivers, except if the beams are being used to illuminate the scene. The number of warning lights at the scene should be evaluated; too many lights will only serve to confuse oncoming drivers. Many departments use warning signs stating "accident ahead" to give ample warning time for drivers. Flares may be arranged to warn and direct traffic flow; however, care should be used in dry conditions so as not to start grass fires. Reflective cones serve as good devices to direct traffic flow away from the lane taken up by the emergency (Figure 3-3).

If traffic needs to be directed, this should be done by law enforcement or those with special training in traffic control. Confusing or contradicting instructions given to drivers only create additional safety risks. The best situations are created when traffic is not impeded and normal flow can be maintained around the emergency. Construction sites provide an example of traffic flow around obstructions. Traffic issues at crash scenes can be handled in much the same way; prehospital care providers can observe construction sites to gain insight into how traffic flow may work better at an MVC.

Violence

Each call has the potential to take the EMS provider into an emotionally charged environment. Some EMS agencies have a policy that requires the presence of law enforcement before providers enter a scene of violence or potential violence. Even a benign-appearing scene has the potential to deteriorate into violence; therefore providers must always be alert to subtle clues suggesting a change in situation. The patient, family, or bystanders on the scene may not be able to perceive the situation rationally. These individuals may think that the response time was too long, may be oversensitive to words or actions, and may misunderstand the "usual" approach to patient assessment. Maintaining a confident and professional manner while demonstrating respect and concern is important to gain the patient's trust and achieve control of the scene.

It is important that EMS personnel train themselves to "observe" the scene and not just "look" at it. Learn to notice numbers and locations of individuals when arriving on the scene, movement of bystanders into or out of the scene, indicators of stress or tension, unexpected or unusual reactions to EMS presence, or other "gut" feelings that may be developing. Watch the hands; look for unusual bulges in waistbands, clothing that is "out of season" such as wearing an overcoat in warm weather, or oversized clothing that could easily hide a weapon.

If a developing threat is perceived, immediately begin preparing to leave the scene. An assessment or a procedure may need to be finished in the ambulance. The safety of the prehospital care providers takes priority.

Consider the following situation: You and your partner are in the living room of your patient's home. While your partner is checking the patient's blood pressure, an apparently intoxicated individual enters the room from the back of the house. He looks angry, and you notice what appears to be the butt of a gun sticking out of the waistband of his pants. Your partner does not see or hear this person enter the room because he is focused on the patient. The suspicious person begins to question your presence and is extremely agitated about your uniform and your badge. His hands repeatedly move toward, then away from, his waist. He begins to pace and mumble. How can you and your partner prepare for this sort of situation?

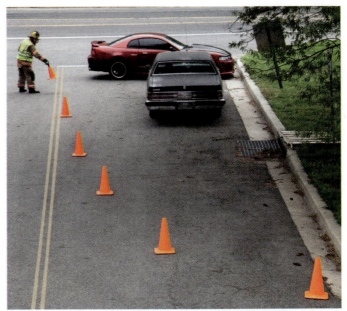

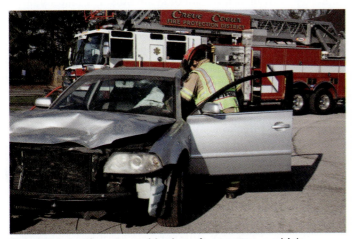

FIGURE 3-2 Correct positioning of emergency vehicle. (From McSwain N, Paturas J: *The basic EMT,* ed 2, St Louis, 2003, Mosby.)

FIGURE 3-3 Placement of traffic delineation devices. (From Henry M, Stapleton E: *EMT prehospital care,* ed 3, St Louis, 2004, Mosby.)

Managing the Violent Scene

Prior to the beginning of the day's EMS calls, partners need to discuss and agree on methods to handle the violent or disruptive patient. Attempting to develop a process when the event in ongoing is not the correct approach. Partners can use a hands-on/hands-off approach, as well as predetermined code words and hand signals, for emergencies. If both providers have all their attention focused on the patient, the scene can quickly become threatening, and early clues (as well as opportunities to retreat) may be missed.

- The role of the *hands-on* prehospital care provider is to take charge of the patient assessment, giving necessary attention to the patient. The *hands-off provider* stands back (until needed) to observe the scene, interact with family or bystanders, collect necessary information, and create better access and egress. In essence, the hands-off provider is monitoring the scene and "covering" his or her partner's back.
- A predetermined *code word* and *hand signals* allow partners to communicate a threat without alerting others of their concerns. In many situations, tension and anxiety are immediately reduced when an attentive prehospital care provider begins interacting with and assessing the patient.

There are various methods for dealing with a scene that has become dangerous, such as the following:

1. **Don't be there.** When responding to a known violent scene, stage at a safe location until the scene has been rendered safe by law enforcement and clearance to respond has been given.
2. **Retreat.** If threats are presented when approaching the scene, tactfully retreat to the vehicle and leave the scene. Stage at a safe location and notify appropriate personnel.
3. **Diffuse.** If a scene becomes threatening during patient care, use verbal diffusion skills to reduce tension and aggression (while preparing to leave the scene).
4. **Defend.** *As a last resort,* the prehospital care provider may find it necessary to defend himself or herself. It is important that such efforts are to "disengage and get away." Do not attempt to chase or subdue an aggressive party. Ensure that law enforcement personnel have been notified and are en route. Again, the safety of the providers is the priority.

Bloodborne Pathogens

Before the recognition of acquired immunodeficiency syndrome (AIDS) in the early 1980s, health care workers (HCWs) showed little concern over exposure to blood and body fluids. Despite knowledge that blood was known to transmit certain hepatitis viruses, prehospital care providers and others involved in emergency medical care often viewed contact with a patient's blood as an annoyance rather than an occupational hazard. Because of the high mortality rate associated with contracting AIDS, and the recognition that human immunodeficiency virus (HIV), the causative agent of AIDS, could be transmitted in blood, HCWs became much more concerned about the patient as a vector of disease. Federal agencies, such as the Centers for Disease Control and Prevention (CDC) and OSHA, developed guidelines and mandates for HCWs to minimize exposure to bloodborne illness, including HIV and hepatitis. The primary infections transmitted through blood include both hepatitis B (HBV) and hepatitis C (HCV) viruses and HIV. Although this issue became a concern because of HIV, it is important to note that infection by hepatitis is much easier than infection with HIV and requires much fewer virus organisms than HIV to become infected. It also carries a high mortality rate and is without specific treatment.

Epidemiologic data demonstrate that HCWs are much more likely to contract bloodborne illness from their patients than their patients are to contract disease from health professionals. Exposures to blood are typically characterized as either percutaneous or mucocutaneous. Percutaneous exposures occur when an individual sustains a puncture wound through intact skin from a contaminated sharp object, such as a needle or scalpel, with the risk of transmission being directly related to both the contaminating agent and the volume of infected blood introduced by the injury. Mucocutaneous exposures typically are less likely to result in transmission and include exposure of blood to nonintact skin, such as a soft tissue wound (e.g., abrasion, superficial laceration) or a skin condition (e.g., acne), or to mucous membranes (e.g., conjunctiva of eye).

Viral Hepatitis

Hepatitis can be transmitted to HCWs through needlesticks and mucocutaneous exposures on nonintact skin.

Although a number of hepatitis viruses have been identified, HBV and HCV are of most concern to HCWs experiencing a blood exposure. Viral hepatitis causes acute inflammation of the liver (Figure 3-4). The incubation period, from exposure until manifestation of symptoms, is generally 60 to 90 days. Up to 30% of those infected with HBV may have an asymptomatic course.

A vaccine derived from the hepatitis B surface antigen (HBsAg) can immunize individuals against HBV.[4] Before the development of this vaccine, more than 10,000 HCWs became infected with HBV annually, and several hundred would die each year from either severe hepatitis or complications of chronic HBV infection. OSHA now requires employers to offer the HBV vaccine to those workers in high-risk environments. All prehospital care providers should be immunized against HBV. Almost all those who complete the series of three vaccines will develop antibody (Ab) to HBsAg, and immunity can be determined by testing blood for the presence of HBsAb. If a HCW is exposed to blood from a patient who is potentially infected with HBV before the HCW has developed immunity (i.e., before completing the vaccine series), passive

FIGURE 3-4	Hepatitis

The clinical manifestations of viral hepatitis are right upper quadrant pain, fatigue, loss of appetite, nausea, vomiting, and alteration in liver function. Jaundice, a yellowish coloration of the skin, results from an increased level of bilirubin in the bloodstream. Although most individuals with hepatitis recover without serious problems, a small percentage of patients develop *acute fulminant hepatic failure* and may die. A significant number of those who recover will develop a carrier state, in which their blood can transmit the virus.

As in HBV, infection with HCV can range from a mild, asymptomatic course to liver failure and death. The incubation period for HCV is somewhat shorter than for HBV, typically 6 to 9 weeks. Chronic infections with HCV are much more common than with HBV, and about 80% to 85% of those who contract HCV will develop persistently abnormal liver function, predisposing them to *hepatocellular carcinoma.* Hepatitis C is primarily transmitted through blood, whereas hepatitis B can be transmitted through blood or sexual contact. About two thirds of intravenous drug abusers have been infected with HCV. Before routine testing of donated blood for presence of HBV and HCV, blood transfusion was the primary reason patients contracted hepatitis.

FIGURE 3-5	Human Immunodeficiency Virus

Two serotypes of HIV have been identified. HIV-1 accounts for virtually all AIDS in the United States and equatorial Africa, and HIV-2 is found almost exclusively in Western Africa. Although early victims of HIV were male homosexuals, intravenous drug users, or hemophiliacs, HIV disease is now found in many teenage and adult heterosexual populations, with the fastest-growing numbers in minority communities. The screening test for HIV is very sensitive, and false-positive tests occasionally occur. All positive screening tests should be confirmed with a more specific technique (e.g., Western blot electrophoresis).

After infection with HIV, when patients develop one of the opportunistic infections or cancers, they transition from being *HIV positive* to having AIDS. In the last decade, significant advances have been made in the treatment of HIV disease, primarily in developing new drugs to combat its effects. This has resulted in many individuals with HIV infection being able to lead fairly normal lives because the progression of the disease is slowed dramatically.

Although HCWs typically are more concerned about contracting HIV because of its uniformly fatal prognosis, they are at greater risk of contracting HBV or HCV.

protection from HBV can be conferred to the HCW with the administration of hepatitis B immune globulin (HBIG).

At present, no immune globulin or vaccine is available to protect HCWs from exposure to HCV, emphasizing the need for using Standard Precautions.

Human Immunodeficiency Virus

After infection, HIV targets the immune system of its new host. Over time the number of certain types of white blood cells falls dramatically, leaving the individual prone to developing unusual infections or cancers (Figure 3-5).

Only about 0.3% (about 1 in 300) of needlestick exposures to HIV-positive blood lead to infection, compared with infection rates of 23% to 62% (1 in 4 to 1 in 2) with exposure to HBV-infected needles. Infection with HCV falls between these two rates (1.8%; 1 in 50). The probable explanation for the varying rates of infection is the relative concentration of virus particles found in infected blood. In general, HBV-positive blood contains 100 million to 1 billion virus particles/mL, whereas HCV-positive and HIV-positive blood contains 1 million and 100 to 10,000 particles/mL, respectively. The risk of infection appears higher with exposure to a larger quantity of blood, exposure to blood from a patient with a more advanced stage of disease, a deep percutaneous injury, or an injury from a hollow-bore, blood-filled needle. HIV is primarily transmit-

ted through infected blood or semen, but vaginal secretions and pericardial, peritoneal, pleural, amniotic, and cerebrospinal fluids are all considered potentially infected. Unless obvious blood is present, tears, urine, sweat, feces, and saliva are generally considered noninfectious.

Standard Precautions

Because clinical examination cannot reliably identify all patients who pose a potential threat to HCWs, Standard Precautions were developed to prevent HCWs from coming into direct contact with a patient's blood or body fluid (e.g., saliva, vomit). OSHA has developed regulations that mandate employers and their employees to follow Standard Precautions in the workplace. Standard Precautions consist of both physical barriers to blood and body fluid and exposure as well as safe handling practices for needles and other "sharps." Because trauma patients often have external hemorrhage and because blood is an extremely high-risk body fluid, protective devices should be worn while caring for patients.

Physical Barriers

Gloves. Gloves should be worn when touching nonintact skin, mucous membranes, or areas contaminated by gross blood or other body fluids. Because perforations may readily occur in gloves while caring for a patient, gloves should be examined regularly for defects and changed immediately if a problem is noted (Figure 3-6).

Masks and Face Shields. Masks serve to protect the HCW's oral and nasal mucous membranes from exposure to infectious agents, especially in situations in which airborne pathogens are known or suspected. Masks and face shields should be changed immediately if they become wet or soiled.

Eye Protection. Eye protection must be worn in circumstances where droplets of infected fluid may be splattered, such as while providing airway management to a patient with blood in the oropharynx. Standard eyeglasses are not considered adequate because they lack side shields.

Gowns. Disposable gowns with impervious plastic liners offer the best protection, but they may be extremely uncomfortable and impractical in the prehospital environment. Gowns or clothing should be changed immediately if significant soilage occurs.

Resuscitation Equipment. HCWs should have access to bag-mask devices or mouthpieces to protect them from direct contact with a patient's saliva, blood, and vomit.

Handwashing. Handwashing is a fundamental principle of infection control. Hands should be washed with soap and running water if gross contamination with blood or body fluid occurs. Alcohol-based hand antiseptics are useful at preventing transmission of many infectious agents but are not appropriate for situations where obvious soiling has occurred; however, they can provide some cleansing and protective effect in situations where running water and soap are not available. After removal of gloves, hands should be cleansed with either soap and water or an alcohol-based antiseptic.

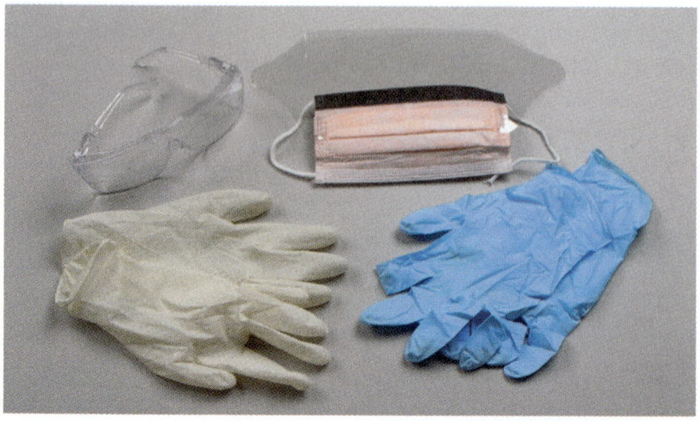

Preventing Sharps Injury. As noted earlier, percutaneous exposure to a patient's blood or body fluid constitutes a significant manner in which viral infections could be transmitted to HCWs. Many percutaneous exposures are caused by injuries from sticks with contaminated needles or other sharps used by the responder while caring for the patient. Eliminate unnecessary needles and sharps, never recap a used needle, and implement safety devices when possible (Figure 3-7).

Management of Occupational Exposure. In the United States, OSHA mandates that every organization providing health care have a control plan for managing occupational exposures of its employees to blood and body fluids. Each exposure should be thoroughly documented, including the type of injury and estimation of the volume of inoculate. If a HCW has a mucocutaneous or percutaneous exposure to blood or sustains an injury from a contaminated sharp, efforts are taken to prevent bacterial infection, including tetanus, and HBV and HIV infection. No prophylactic therapy to prevent HCV infection is currently approved or available. Figure 3-8 describes a typical blood and body fluid exposure protocol.

Hazardous Materials

Understanding the prehospital care provider's risk of exposure to hazardous materials is not as simple as recognizing environments that have obvious potential for hazardous material exposure. Hazardous materials are widespread in the modern world; vehicles, buildings, and even homes have hazardous material potential. For this reason, all prehospital

FIGURE 3-6 At a minimum, personal protective equipment for prehospital care providers should consist of gloves, mask, and eye protection.
(From Chapleau W: *Emergency first responder,* St Louis, 2004, Mosby.)

FIGURE 3-7 **Preventing Sharps Injury**

Prehospital care providers are at significant risk for injury from needles and other sharps. Strategies for reducing sharps injuries include the following:

- Use safety devices, such as shielded or retracting needles and scalpels and automatically retracting lancets.
- Use "needleless" systems that allow injection of medication at ports without needles.
- Refrain from recapping needles and other sharps.
- Immediately dispose of contaminated needles into rigid sharps containers rather than setting them down or handing them to someone else for disposal.
- Use prefilled medication syringes rather than drawing medication from an ampule.
- Provide a written exposure control plan, and ensure that all employees are aware of the plan.
- Maintain a sharps injury log.

FIGURE 3-8   Sample Exposure Protocol

After a percutaneous or mucocutaneous exposure to blood or other potentially infected body fluids, taking the appropriate actions and instituting appropriate post-exposure prophylaxis (PEP) can help minimize the potential for acquiring viral hepatitis or HIV infection. Appropriate steps include:

1. Prevention of bacterial infection.
   - Cleanse exposed skin thoroughly with germicidal soap and water; exposed mucous membranes (mouth, eyes) should be irrigated with copious amounts of water.
   - Administer tetanus toxoid booster, if not received in previous 5 years.
2. Baseline laboratory studies performed on both exposed health care worker (HCW) and source patient, if known.
   - *HCW:* Hepatitis B surface antibody (HBsAb), hepatitis C virus (HCV), and human immunodeficiency virus (HIV) tests.
   - *Source patient:* Hepatitis B and C serology and HIV test.
3. Prevention of hepatitis B virus (HBV) infection.
   - If the HCW has not been immunized against hepatitis B, the first dose of HBV vaccine is administered along with hepatitis B immune globulin (HBIG).

- If the HCW has begun but not yet completed the HBV vaccine series, or if the HCW has completed all HBV immunizations, HBIG is given if the HBsAb test fails to show the presence of protective antibodies and the source patient's tests demonstrate active infection with HBV. HBIG may be administered up to 7 days after an exposure and still be effective.
4. Prevention of HIV infection.
   - PEP depends upon the route of exposure (percutaneous vs. mucocutaneous) and the likelihood and severity of HIV infection in the source patient. If the source patient is known to be negative, PEP is not indicated, regardless of exposure route. In the past, when recommended, PEP has generally involved a two-drug regimen. With the development of numerous antiretroviral medications, the number of drug regimen combinations has increased. In addition, three-drug treatment is also warranted in specific cases involving high risk of transmission. It is therefore recommended that an exposed prehospital provider be evaluated by an expert to determine the most appropriate PEP regimen, given the circumstances of the particular exposure.

---

care providers require training to a minimum of the awareness level.

There are four levels of hazardous materials training.

- *Awareness:* This is the first of four levels of training available to responders and is designed to provide a basic level of knowledge.
- *Operations:* These responders are trained to set up perimeters and safety zones, limiting the spread of the event. Whereas awareness represents the minimum level of training, the operations level would be helpful for all responders, as well as providing the training to help control the event.
- *Technician:* Technicians are trained to work within the hazardous area and stop the release of hazardous materials.
- *Specialist:* This advanced level allows the responder to provide command and support skills to a hazardous materials (hazmat or HazMat) event.

Prehospital care providers accept that scene safety is the first part of the approach to every patient and every scene. An important part of determining the safety of the scene is to evaluate for the potential of hazmat exposure. Assessment of potential hazards should begin with dispatch. The information given by dispatch may establish a high index of suspicion. Additional information can be requested while en route

if prehospital care providers have any concerns or questions that could be relayed to the scene.

Once a scene has been determined to have hazmat involvement, the focus must shift to securing the scene and summoning help to safely isolate the involved area and remove and decontaminate the patients. The general simple rule is, "If the scene is not safe, make it safe." If the provider cannot make the scene safe, help should be summoned. The *Emergency Response Guidebook* (ERG), produced by the U.S. Department of Transportation, can be used to identify potential hazards (Figure 3-9). The book uses a simple system that allows identification of a material by its name or placard number. The text then refers the reader to a guide page that provides basic information about safe distances for rescuers, life and fire hazards, and the patient's likely complaints. Binoculars should be used to read labels; if labels can be read without the use of viewing devices, the provider is too close and likely to be exposed.

At a hazmat scene, security must be ensured: "Nobody in, nobody out." The staging area should be established upwind and uphill at a safe distance from the hazard. Entry into and exit from the scene should be denied until the arrival of hazmat specialists. In most cases, patient care will begin when the decontaminated patient is delivered to the prehospital care provider.

It is important for the prehospital care provider to understand the command system and structure of the work zones

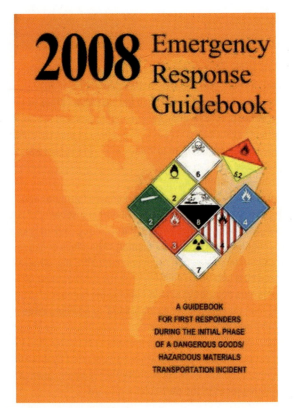

FIGURE 3-9 The *Emergency Response Guidebook* produced by the U.S. Department of Transportation provides critical information at the scene of a potential hazardous material ("hazmat") incident.

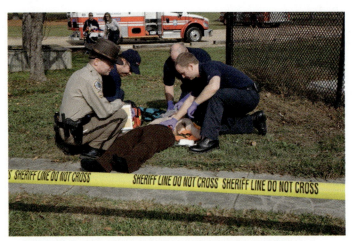

FIGURE 3-10 Prehospital care providers often have to manage patients at the scene of a crime and need to collaborate with law enforcement to preserve evidence. (From McSwain N, Paturas J: *The basic EMT,* ed 2, St Louis, 2003, Mosby.)

in a hazmat operation. Hazmat control operations are set up in zones.

- HOT: The "hot" zone is the area of highest contamination, and only specially trained and protected workers may enter this area. If patients are in this area, the hazmat team will bring them out.
- WARM: A contamination reduction corridor runs through the next zone, called the "warm" zone, where the patients will be decontaminated by the hazmat team. From here, they will move into the "cold" zone.
- COLD: The cold zone is an area that is free from contamination. Patient care activities generally occur outside the cold zone. The command post, treatment, and triage areas will be outside the cold zone. (See Weapons of Mass Destruction for further hazmat considerations.)

Situation Issues

Crime Scenes

Unfortunately, a sizable percentage of trauma patients encountered by many prehospital care providers, especially in urban settings, are intentionally injured. In addition to shootings and stabbings, patients may be victims of other types of violent crimes, including assaults with fists or blunt objects and attempted strangulation. In other cases, victims may have been intentionally struck by a vehicle or pushed from a structure, resulting in a significant fall. Even an MVC can be considered a crime scene if one of the drivers is thought to be under the influence of alcohol or other intoxicants, driving recklessly, or speeding (Figure 3-10).

When managing these types of patients, prehospital care personnel interact with law enforcement personnel. Although both EMS and law enforcement share the goal of preserving life, prehospital care providers and law enforcement personnel occasionally find that their duties at a crime scene come into conflict. EMS personnel focus on the need to assess a victim for signs of life and viability, whereas law enforcement personnel are concerned with preserving evidence at a crime scene or bringing a perpetrator to justice.

By being aware of the general approach taken by law enforcement personnel at a crime scene, prehospital care providers not only may aid their patient but also may better cooperate with law enforcement personnel, leading to the arrest of their patient's assailant.

At the scene of a major crime (homicide, suspicious death, rape, traffic death), most law enforcement agencies will collect and process evidence. Officers will typically perform the following duties:

- Initially canvass the scene to identify all evidence, including weapons and shell casings.
- Photograph the scene.
- Sketch the scene.
- Create a log of everyone who has entered the scene.
- Conduct a more thorough search of the entire scene, looking for all potential evidence.

- Look for and collect trace evidence, ranging from fingerprints to items that may contain DNA evidence (e.g., cigarette butts, strands of hair, fibers).

Police investigators believe that everyone who enters a crime scene brings some type of evidence to the scene and unknowingly removes some evidence from the scene. To solve the crime, a detective's goal is to identify the evidence deposited and removed by the perpetrator. To accomplish this, the investigators have to account for any evidence left or removed by other law enforcement officers, EMS personnel, and citizens who may have entered the scene. Careless behavior by prehospital care personnel at a crime scene may disrupt, destroy, or contaminate vital evidence, hampering a criminal investigation.

On occasion, prehospital care providers arrive at a potential crime scene before any law enforcement officers. If the victim is obviously dead, providers should carefully back out of the location without touching any items and await the arrival of officers. Although they would prefer that a crime scene not be disturbed, investigators realize that in some circumstances, prehospital care providers need to turn a body or move objects at a crime scene to access a victim and determine viability. If providers needed to transport a patient or move a body or other objects in the area before the arrival of law enforcement, investigators will typically ascertain the following:

- When were the alterations made to the scene?
- What was the purpose of the movement?
- Who made the alterations?
- At what time was the person's death identified by EMS personnel?

If trauma care providers entered a crime scene before law enforcement personnel, investigators may want to interview and formally take a statement from the providers regarding their actions or observations. Trauma care providers should never be alarmed or concerned about such a request. The purpose of the interview is not to critique the actions of the providers but to learn information that may prove helpful to the investigator in solving the case. Investigators may also request to take fingerprints of the prehospital care personnel if items in the crime scene were touched or handled by the crew without gloves.

Proper handling of a patient's clothing may preserve valuable evidence. If a patient's clothing needs to be removed, law enforcement officers and medical examiners prefer that prehospital care providers avoid cutting through bullet or knife holes in the clothing. If the clothing is cut, investigators may ask what alterations were made to the clothing, who made the alterations, and the reason for alterations. Any clothing that is removed should be placed in a paper (not plastic) bag and turned over to investigators.

One final important issue involving victims of violent crimes is the value of any statements made by the patient while under the care of prehospital care providers. Some patients, realizing the critical nature of their injuries, may tell providers who inflicted their injuries. This information should be documented and passed on to investigators. If possible, prehospital care personnel should inform officers of the critical nature of a patient's injuries so that a sworn officer can be present if the patient is capable of providing any information regarding the perpetrator: a "dying declaration."

Weapons of Mass Destruction

The response to a scene involving hazardous materials, as discussed earlier, includes similar safety and other concerns as the response to the scene involving a weapon of mass destruction (WMD).

Every scene that involves multiple victims or that was reported to have resulted from an explosion should trigger two questions:

1. Was a WMD was involved?
2. Could there be a secondary device intended to harm responders?

In particular, when many victims complain of similar symptoms or present with similar findings, a WMD should be considered. See Chapter 11, Disaster Management and Weapons of Mass Destruction, for greater detail.

The prehospital care provider needs to approach such scenes with extreme caution and resist the urge to rush in to care for the sickest victim.[5] This natural response of providers only serves to increase the victim count. Instead, the provider should approach the scene from an upwind position and take a moment to stop, look, and listen for clues that will alert the team to the possible presence of a WMD. Obvious spills of wet or dry material, visible vapors, and smoke should be avoided until the nature of the material has been ascertained. Enclosed or confined spaces should never be entered without appropriate personal protective equipment (PPE).

Once a WMD has been included as a possible cause, the prehospital care provider needs to take all appropriate steps for self-protection. These steps include the use of PPE appropriate to the function of the individual provider. Information that this may be a WMD incident should be relayed back to dispatch to alert incoming responders from all services. Staging areas for additional equipment, responders, and helicopters should be established upwind and at a safe distance from the site.

The scene should be secured and zones indicating hot, warm, and cold areas designated. Sites for decontamination should also be determined. Once the nature of the agent has been determined (chemical, biologic, or radiologic), specific requests for antidote or antibiotics can be made.

Scene Control Zones

As mentioned previously, to limit the spread of a hazardous material or WMD, the National Institute of Occupational Safety and Health (NIOSH) and the Environmental Protection Agency (EPA) have developed and advocated the use of control zones. The objective of this concept is to perform specific activities in specific zones. Adherence to such principles reduces the likelihood of spread of contamination and injury to rescue personnel and bystanders.

The zones are three concentric circles (Figure 3-11). The innermost zone, the *hot zone,* is the region immediately adjacent to the hazmat or WMD incident. The task of rescuers in this region is to evacuate the contaminated, injured patient, with no provision of patient care. In order to do so, generally the highest level of PPE must be utilized. The next zone, the *warm zone,* is where decontamination of victims, personnel, and equipment occurs. In this zone the only patient care administered is primary assessment and spinal immobilization, again by personnel using appropriate PPE. The outermost zone, the *cold zone,* is where equipment and personnel are staged. Once the patient is evacuated to the cold zone, providers can safely deliver definitive patient care. Figure 3-12 lists safe evacuation distances for bomb threats.

If a patient is delivered to the hospital or aid station from a hazmat or WMD scene, it is most prudent to reevaluate if that patient has been decontaminated and to mimic the concepts of these zones (see Figure 3-11).

Decontamination

Whether the incident involves a hazmat situation or a WMD, decontamination of an exposed individual often may be required. *Decontamination* is the reduction or removal of hazardous chemical, biologic, or radiologic agents. The provider's highest priority in the care of an exposed patient, as in any emergency, is personal and scene safety. If there is any question of a continued exposure hazard, assurance of personal safety is the first priority. Failure to do so will only produce an additional victim (the provider) and deprive those already injured of the provider's skills. Decontamination of the patient is the next priority. This will minimize the exposure risk to the provider during assessment and treatment of the patient and will prevent contamination of equipment, thereby avoiding the risk of exposure of other individuals from contaminated equipment and vehicles.

OSHA provides regulatory guidelines for PPE used by prehospital care providers during the emergency care of victims in a potentially hazardous environment. Individuals providing medical care in environments of an unknown hazard must have a minimum of appropriate training and be supplied and trained with level B protection. Level B protection consists of splash-protective, chemical-resistant clothing and self-contained breathing sources. Training in advance of the need to use this level of PPE is required.

If patients are conscious and able to assist, it is best to enlist their cooperation to have them perform as much of the decontamination as possible to reduce the likelihood of cross-

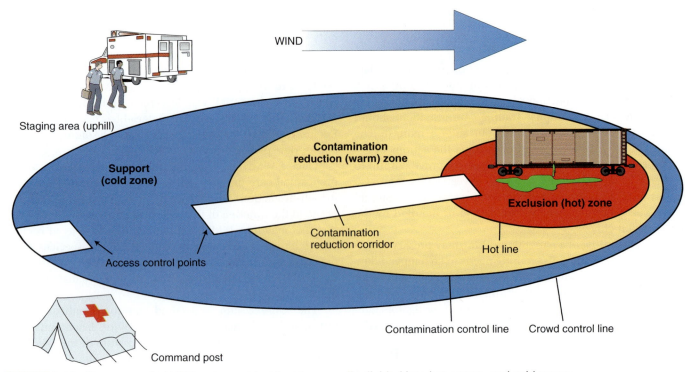

FIGURE 3-11 The scene of a WMD or hazmat incident is generally divided into hot, warm, and cold zones.
(From Chapleau W: *Emergency first responder,* St Louis, 2004, Mosby.)

FIGURE 3-12   **Bomb Threats: Safe Evacuation Distances**

Threat Description	Explosives Capacity (TNT Capacity) (pounds)	Building Evacuation Distance (feet)	Outdoor Evacuation Distance (feet)
Pipe bomb	5	70	850
Briefcase/suitcase bomb	50	150	1850
Compact sedan	500	320	1500
Full-size sedan	1000	400	1750
Passenger/cargo van	4000	650	2750
Small moving van, delivery truck	10,000	860	3750
Moving van, small tank truck	30,000	1240	6500
Semitrailer	60,000	1570	7000

(Modified from Messier DM: Explosive prospects: terrorist bombings present multifaceted response challenge. *Homeland response* 2(1), 2004.)

contamination to providers. Carefully remove the patient's clothes as well as jewelry and place these in plastic bags. Transfer the removed clothing carefully so as not to spread any particulate matter or splash any liquid onto noncontaminated personnel or surfaces. Brush any particulate matter off the patient, then irrigate copiously with water. Washing with water will dilute the concentration of the potentially hazardous material and remove any remaining agent. A common axiom is, "The solution to pollution is dilution." Successful decontamination requires large amounts of water. A common mistake made by the inexperienced prehospital care provider is to irrigate the patient with water only until the irrigant begins to spill onto the floor, which usually occurs after 1 or 2 L of irrigation. This practice has two problems: The area of body contamination is increased, and the offending agent is not diluted sufficiently to render the agent harmless. Failure to provide for adequate runoff and drainage of lavage fluid may cause injury to previously unexposed areas of the body as the contaminated lavage accumulates. Neutralizing agents for chemical burns are typically avoided. Often in the neutralizing process the agents give off heat in an exothermic reaction. Therefore, a well-meaning provider may create a thermal burn in addition to the chemical burn. Most commercially available decontamination solutions are made for the purpose of decontaminating equipment, not people.

Secondary Devices

Within months after the bombing at the 1996 Atlanta Summer Olympics, the metropolitan Atlanta area experienced two additional bombings. These bombings at an abortion clinic and a nightclub had secondary bombs planted and represented the first time in 17 years in the United States that secondary bombs had been planted, presumably to kill or injure rescuers responding to the scene of the first blast. Unfortunately, the secondary device at the abortion clinic was not detected prior to its detonation and it resulted in six casualties. Secondary devices have been used with regularity by terrorists in many countries. All prehospital care personnel need to be mindful of the potential presence of a secondary device. After these incidents, the Georgia Emergency Management Agency developed the following guidelines for rescuers and prehospital care personnel responding to the scene of a bombing where a secondary bomb might be planted[6]:

1. *Refrain from use of electronic devices.* Radio waves from cell phones and radios may cause a secondary device to detonate, especially if used close to the bomb. Equipment used by the news media may also trigger a detonation.
2. *Ensure sufficient boundaries for the scene.* The potential zone of danger (hot zone) should extend 1000 feet in all directions (including vertically) from the original blast site. As more powerful bombs are created, shrapnel may

travel further. The initial bomb blast may damage infrastructure, including gas lines and power lines, which may jeopardize the safety of rescuers. Access to and exit from the hot zone should be carefully controlled.

3. *Provide rapid evacuation of victims from the scene and hot zone.* Because the scene of a bomb blast is considered unsafe, triage of victims should not occur in the hot zone. An EMS command post (or triage area) should be established 2000 to 4000 feet from the scene of the initial bombing. Rescuers can rapidly evacuate victims from the bombing site, with minimal interventions, until victims and rescuers are out of the hot zone.

4. *Collaborate with law enforcement personnel on preserving and recovering evidence.* Bombing sites constitute a crime scene, and rescuers should disrupt the scene only as necessary to evacuate victims. Any potential evidence that is inadvertently removed from the scene with a victim should be documented and turned over to law enforcement personnel to ensure proper chain of custody. Prehospital care personnel can document exactly where they were in the scene and which items they touched.

Command Structure

An ambulance responding to a call will usually have one person in charge (the incident commander) and another person assisting in a rudimentary incident command structure. As an incident grows larger and more responders from various public safety and other agencies respond to the scene, the need for a formal system and structure to oversee and control the response becomes increasingly important.

Incident Command

The *incident command system* (ICS) has developed over the years as an outgrowth of planning systems used by firefighting services for multiple-service responses to major fire situations. The program gained acceptance particularly from the experience of wildland firefighters battling expansive firefronts, with deployment of dozens of diverse agencies.

Dealing with any incident, large or small, is enhanced by the precise command structure afforded by the ICS. At the core of ICS is the establishment of centralized command at the scene and the subsequent buildup of divisional responsibilities. The first arriving unit establishes the command center, and communications are established through command for the buildup of the response. The five key elements of incident command are as follows:

1. *Command* provides overall control of the event and the communications that will coordinate the movement of resources in and patients out of the incident scene.

2. *Operations* include divisions to handle the tactical needs of the event. Fire suppression, EMS, and rescue are examples of operational divisions.

3. *Planning* is a continuous process of evaluating immediate and potential needs of the incident and planning the

response. Throughout the event, this element will be used to evaluate the effectiveness of operations and to make suggested alterations in the response and tactical approach.

4. *Logistics* handles the task of acquiring resources and moving them where needed; these include personnel, shelter, vehicles, and equipment.

5. *Finance* tracks the money. Response personnel from all involved agencies as well as contractors, personnel, and vendors brought into service in the incident will be tracked so that the cost of the event can be determined and these groups can be paid for goods, supplies, equipment, and services.

National Incident Management System

On February 28, 2003, President George W. Bush directed the Secretary of Homeland Security through Presidential Directive HSPD-5 to produce a National Incident Management System (NIMS). This would establish a consistent, nationwide approach for federal, state, and local governments to work effectively together to prepare for, respond to, and recover from domestic incidents regardless of cause, size, or complexity.

NIMS focuses on the following incident management characteristics:

- Common terminology
- Modular organization
- Management by objectives
- Reliance on an incident action plan
- Manageable span of control
- Predesignated "incident mobilization center" locations and facilities
- Comprehensive resource management
- Integrated communications
- Establishment of transfer of command
- Chain of command and unity of command
- Unified command
- Accountability of resources and personnel
- Deployment
- Information and intelligence management

The key elements of NIMS are as follows:

1. ICS
2. Communications and information management
3. Preparedness
4. Joint information systems (consistent public information)
5. National Incident Management Integration Center (NIC)

Incident Action Plans

Incident action plans (IAPs) include overall incident objectives and strategies established by the IC or unified command. The planning section develops and documents the IAP. The IAP also addresses the tactical objectives and support activities for the operational period, which is generally 12 to 24 hours. The planning section also provides an ongoing critique, or "lessons learned" process, to ensure the response meets the needs of the event.

In very large incidents, multiple ICS organizations may be established. Area command may be established to manage multiple ICS organizations. Area command does not have operational responsibilities but will perform the following duties:

1. Set overall incident-related priorities for the agency
2. Allocate critical resources according to established priorities
3. Ensure that incidents are managed properly
4. Ensure effective communications
5. Ensure that incident management objectives are met and do not conflict with each other or with agency policies
6. Identify critical resource needs and report to the Emergency Operations Center(s)
7. Ensure that short-term emergency recovery is coordinated to assist in the transition to full recovery operations
8. Provide for personnel accountability and safe operating environments

Detailed information and training programs about the Incident Command System and the National Incident Management System can found on the Federal Emergency Management Agency's website (Figure 3-13).

FIGURE 3-13 Incident Command Training Resources

Federal Emergency Management Agency (FEMA): Incident command system (ICS) training:

ICS-100.a, Introduction to ICS (http://training.fema.gov/EMIWeb/IS/IS100A.asp)

ICS-200.a, Basic ICS (http://training.fema.gov/EMIWeb/IS/IS200A.asp)

ICS-700.a, NIMS, an Introduction (http://training.fema.gov/EMIWeb/IS/is700a.asp)

ICS-800.b, National Response Framework, an Introduction (http://training.fema.gov/EMIWeb/IS/IS800b.asp)

National Incident Management System (NIMS) and FEMA training: Contact your state Emergency Management Agency or Emergency Management Institute and National Fire Academy, Emmitsburg, Md. A variety of online correspondence and on-site courses are available (http://training.fema.gov/IS/crslist.asp).

For more information on NIMS, contact the NIMS Integrations Center: www.dhs.gov.

Patient Assessment and Triage

Once all of the preceding issues have been addressed, the actual process of assessing and treating patients can begin. The greatest challenge occurs when the prehospital care provider is faced with multiple victims.

Mass-casualty incidents (MCIs) occur in many sizes. Most rescuers have responded to incidents with more than one victim, but large-scale events with hundreds to thousands of victims are rarely encountered.

Triage is a French word meaning "to sort." Triage is a process that will be used to assign priority for treatment and transport. In the prehospital environment, triage is used in two different contexts, as follows:

1. **Sufficient resources are available to manage all patients.** In this triage situation, the most severely injured patients are treated and transported first, and those with lesser injuries are treated and transported later.
2. **The number of patients exceeds the immediate capacity of on-scene resources.** The objective in such triage is to ensure survival of the largest possible number of injured patients. Patients are sorted into categories for patient care. In an MCI, patient care must be rationed because the number of patients exceeds the available resources. Relatively few prehospital care providers ever experience an MCI with 50 to 100 or more simultaneously injured persons, but many will be involved in MCIs with 10 to 20 patients, and most prehospital veterans have managed an incident with 2 to 10 patients.

Incidents that involve sufficient rescuers and medical resources allow for treatment and transport of the most severely injured patients first. In a large-scale MCI, limited resources will require that patient treatment and transport be prioritized to salvage the victims with the greatest chance of survival (Figure 3-14). These victims are prioritized for treatment and transport.

The goal of patient management at the MCI scene is to do the most good for the most patients with the resources available. It is the responsibility of the prehospital care provider to make decisions about who is to be managed first. The usual rules about saving lives are different in MCIs. The decision is always to save the most lives; however, when the available resources are not sufficient for the needs of all of the injured patients present, these resources should be used for those patients who have the best chance of surviving. In a choice between a patient with a catastrophic injury such as severe brain trauma and a patient with acute intra-abdominal hemorrhage, the proper course of action in an MCI is to manage first the salvageable patient—the victim with the abdominal hemorrhage. Treating the patient with severe head trauma first will probably result in the loss of both patients; the head trauma patient may die because he or she may not be salvageable, and the abdominal hemorrhage patient may die because time, equipment, and personnel spent managing the unsalvageable patient kept this

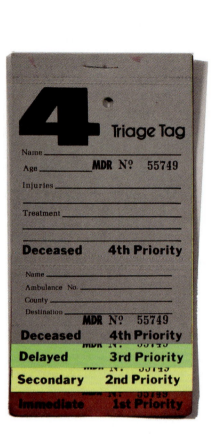
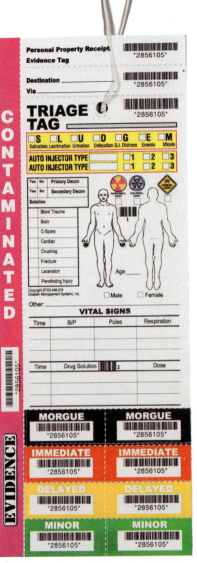
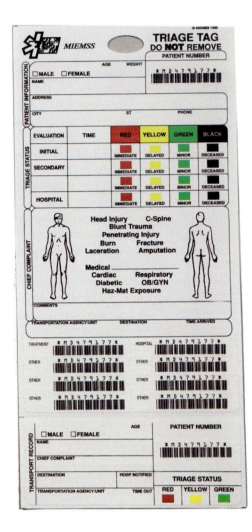

FIGURE 3-14 Example of a triage tag.
(From McSwain N, Paturas J: *The basic EMT,* ed 2, St Louis, 2003, Mosby.)

salvageable patient from receiving the simple care needed to survive until definitive surgical care was available.

In a triage MCI situation, the catastrophically injured patient may need to be considered "lower priority," with treatment delayed until more help and equipment become available. These are difficult decisions and circumstances, but a trauma care provider must respond quickly and properly. A medical care team should not attempt to resuscitate a traumatic cardiac arrest patient with little or no chance of survival while three other patients die because of airway compromise or external hemorrhage. The "sorting scheme" most often used divides patients into five categories based on need of care and chance of survival, as follows:

1. *Immediate.* Patients whose injuries are critical but who will require only minimal time or equipment to manage and who have a good prognosis for survival are classed as "immediate." An example is the patient with a compromised airway or massive external hemorrhage.

2. *Delayed.* Delayed patients are those whose injuries are serious but who do not require immediate management to salvage life or limb. An example is the patient with a long-bone fracture.

3. *Minor.* Patients, often called the "walking wounded," who have minor injuries that can wait for treatment or who may even assist in the interim by comforting other patients or helping as litter bearers.

4. *Expectant.* The category is for those patients whose injuries are so severe that they have only a minimal chance of survival. An example is the patient with a 90% full-thickness burn and thermal pulmonary injury.

FIGURE 3-15   START Triage

In 1983, medical personnel from Hoag Memorial Hospital and firefighter paramedics from the Newport Beach Fire Department created a triage process for first responders, *Simple Triage and Rapid Treatment* (START) (see Figure 3-16). This triage process was designed to identify critically injured patients easily and quickly. START does not establish a medical diagnosis but instead provides a rapid and simple sorting process. START uses three simple assessments to identify those victims most at risk to die from their injuries. Typically, the process takes 30 to 60 seconds per victim. START requires no tools, specialized medical equipment, or special knowledge.

HOW DOES START WORK?

The first step is to direct anyone who can walk to a designated safe area. If the victims can walk and follow commands, their condition is categorized as "minor," and they will be further triaged and tagged when more rescuers arrive. This now leads to a smaller group of presumably more seriously injured victims remaining for rescuers to triage. The mnemonic "30-2-can-do" is used as the START triage prompt (see Figure 3-17). The "30" refers to the patient's respiratory rate, the "2" refers to capillary refill, and the "can-do" refers to the ability of the patient to follow commands. Any victim with respirations

fewer than 30 per minute, capillary refill of less than 2 seconds, and the ability to follow verbal commands and who can walk is categorized as a "minor" patient. When victims meet these criteria but cannot walk, they are categorized as "delayed." Victims who are unconscious or have rapid breathing or who have delayed capillary refill or absent radial pulse are categorized as "immediate." While at the victim's side, two basic lifesaving measures can be performed: opening the airway and controlling external hemorrhage. For those victims who are not breathing, the rescuer should open the airway, and if breathing resumes, the victim is categorized as "immediate." No cardiopulmonary resuscitation (CPR) should be attempted. If the victim does not resume breathing, the victim is categorized as "dead." Bystanders or the "walking wounded" can be directed by the rescuer to help maintain the airway and hemorrhage control.

Retriage is also needed if lack of transportation prolongs the time the victims remain at the scene. Using START criteria, significantly injured victims may be categorized as "delayed." The longer they remain without treatment, the greater the chance their condition will deteriorate. Therefore, repeat evaluation and triage are appropriate over time.

---

5. *Dead.* Patients who are unresponsive, pulseless, and breathless are classified as "dead." In a disaster, resources rarely allow for attempted resuscitation of cardiac arrest patients.

Figures 3-15 to 3-17 describe a commonly used triage scheme known as START, which uses only four categories: immediate, delayed, minor, and dead (for more information, please see Chapter 11, Disaster Management and Weapons of Mass Destruction). Figures 3-18 and 3-19 describe the recently published SALT triage system.[7]

Trauma first responders should become aware of and knowledgeable about the triage system preferred and used by the emergency response system in their locale.

Patient Assessment

Assessment is the cornerstone of excellent patient care. For the trauma patient, as for other critically ill patients, assessment is the foundation on which all management and transportation decisions are based. The first goal in assessment is to determine a patient's current condition. In doing so an overall impression of a patient's status is developed and baseline values for the status of the patient's respiratory, circulatory, and neurologic systems established. Life-threatening conditions are rapidly

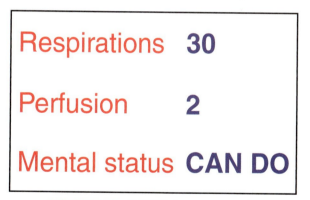

FIGURE 3-16 START triage mnemonic.

assessed and urgent interventions and resuscitation initiated. Any other conditions that require attention are identified and addressed before a patient is moved. If time allows, a secondary survey for non–life-or-limb-threatening injuries is conducted. Often this occurs during transportation of the patient.

All these steps are performed quickly and efficiently, with a goal of minimizing time spent on the scene. Critical patients should not remain in the field for care other than that needed to stabilize them for transport, unless they are trapped or other complications exist that prevent early transportation. By applying the principles learned in this course, on-scene

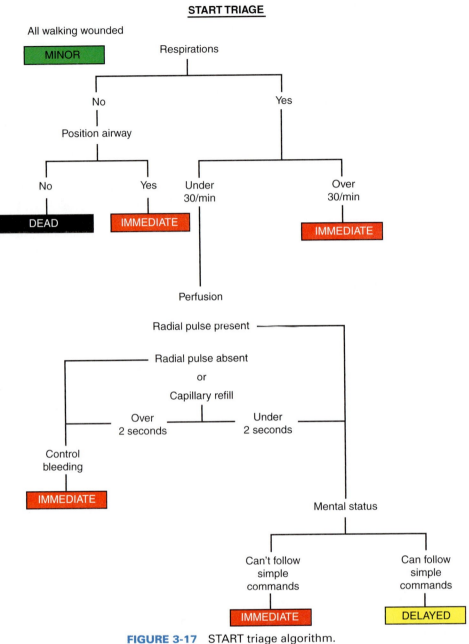

FIGURE 3-17 START triage algorithm.
(Courtesy Newport Beach Fire Department, Newport Beach, Calif.)

delay can be minimized and patients moved rapidly to an appropriate medical facility. Successful assessment and intervention require a strong knowledge base of trauma physiology and a well-thought-out plan of management that is carried out quickly and effectively.

The trauma management literature frequently mentions the need to transport the trauma patient to definitive surgical care within an absolute minimum amount of time after the onset of the injury. This is because a critical trauma patient who does not respond to initial therapy is most likely bleed-ing internally. This blood loss will continue until the bleeding is controlled. Except for the most basic external bleeding, this hemorrhage control can be accomplished only in the operating room (OR).

The primary concerns for assessment and management of the trauma patient, in order of importance, are (1) airway, (2) breathing and ventilation, (3) oxygenation, (4) hemorrhage control, (5) perfusion, and (6) neurologic function. This sequence protects the ability of the body to oxygenate and the ability of the red blood cells (RBCs) to deliver oxygen to

FIGURE 3-18 SALT Triage

This system uses a global sorting process, beginning by asking patients to walk or wave (follow commands). Those patients who do not respond are then assessed for life threats and subsequently categorized as immediate, delayed, minimal, or dead (See Figure 3-19).

the tissues. Hemorrhage control, which is only temporary in the field but permanent in the OR, depends on rapid transportation by the prehospital care providers and the presence of a trauma team that is immediately available on arrival at the medical facility.

R Adams Cowley, MD, developed the concept of the "Golden Hour" of trauma. He believed that the time between injury occurrence and definitive care was critical. During this period, when bleeding is uncontrolled and inadequate amounts of oxygen are being delivered to tissue because of decreased perfusion (circulation), damage occurs throughout the body. He stated that if bleeding is not controlled and tissue oxygenation is not restored within 1 hour of the injury, the patient's chances of survival plummet.

The Golden Hour is now referred to as the "Golden Period" because this critical time period is not necessarily 1 hour. Some patients have less than an hour in which to receive care, whereas others have more time. A trauma care provider is responsible for recognizing the urgency of a given situation and transporting a patient as quickly and as safely as possible to a facility where definitive care can be accomplished. To deliver the trauma patient to definitive care, the seriousness of the patient's life-threatening injuries must be quickly identified; only essential, lifesaving care at the scene provided; and rapid transportation to an appropriate medical facility undertaken. In many urban prehospital systems, the average time between injury and arrival of the ambulance to the scene is 8 to 9 minutes. Usually another 8 to 9 minutes are spent transporting the patient. If the providers spend only 10 minutes on the scene, 30 minutes of the Golden Period will have passed by the time a patient arrives at the receiving facility. Every additional minute spent on the scene is additional time that the patient is bleeding, and valuable time is ticking away from the Golden Period. To address this critical trauma management issue, quick, efficient evaluation and management of the patient is the ultimate objective.

SALT Mass Casualty Triage

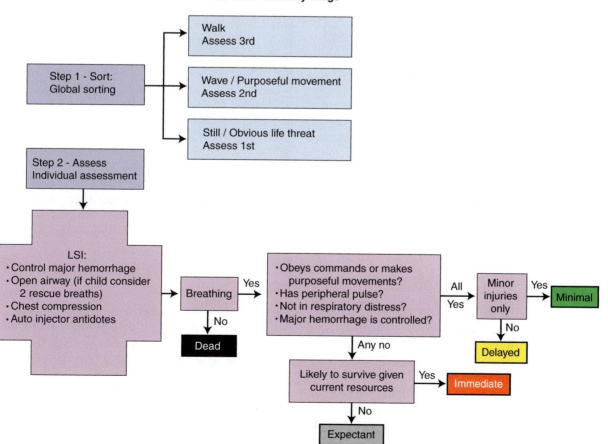

FIGURE 3-19 SALT triage algorithm.

Scene time should not exceed 10 minutes; the shorter the scene time, the better. The longer the patient is kept on scene, the greater the potential for blood loss and death. These time parameters change as delayed extrication, delayed transport, and other unexpected circumstances arise.

This chapter covers the essentials of patient assessment and initial management in the field and is based on the approach taught to physicians in the Advanced Trauma Life Support (ATLS) program.[8] The principles described are identical to those learned in initial basic or advanced provider training programs.

Establishing Priorities

There are three priorities on arrival to a scene, as follows:

1. The first priority for everyone involved at a trauma incident is assessment of the scene.
2. Recognition of the existence of multiple-patient incidents and MCIs. In an MCI the priority shifts from focusing all resources on the most injured patient to saving the maximum number of patients (providing the greatest good to the greatest number).
3. Once a brief scene assessment has been performed, attention can be turned to evaluating individual patients. The assessment and management process is begun by focusing on the patient or patients who have been identified as most critical, as resources allow. Emphasis is placed on the following, in this order: (a) conditions that may result in the loss of life, (b) conditions that may result in the loss of limb, and (c) all other conditions that do not threaten life or limb. Depending on the severity of the injury, the number of injured patients, and the proximity to the receiving facility, conditions that do not threaten life or limb may never be addressed.

Most of this chapter focuses on the *critical thinking* skills required to conduct a proper assessment, interpret the findings, and set priorities for proper patient care.

Primary Survey

Initial Assessment

In the critical multisystem trauma patient, the priority for care is the rapid identification and management of life-threatening conditions (Figure 3-20). More than 90% of trauma patients have simple injuries that involve only one system (e.g., an isolated limb fracture). For many of these single-system trauma patients, there is time to be thorough in both the primary and the secondary survey. For the critically injured patient, however, the provider may never conduct more than a primary survey. The emphasis is on rapid evaluation, initiation of resuscitation, and transportation to an appropriate medical

FIGURE 3-20   Multisystem versus Single-System Trauma Patient

- A *multisystem trauma patient* has injuries involving more than one body system, including the pulmonary, circulatory, neurologic, gastrointestinal, musculoskeletal, and integumentary systems. An example would be a patient involved in a motor vehicle crash who has a traumatic brain injury, pulmonary contusions, a splenic injury with shock, and a femur fracture.
- A *single-system trauma patient* has injury to only one body system. An example would be a patient with a simple ankle fracture and no evidence of blood loss or shock.

facility. This does not eliminate the need for prehospital management; it means that it needs to be *done faster, done more efficiently, and done en route to the receiving facility.*

Quick establishment of priorities and the initial evaluation of life-threatening injuries must be routine. Therefore, the components of the primary and secondary surveys need to be memorized and the logical progression of priority-based assessment and treatment understood. A prehospital care provider has to think about the pathophysiology of a patient's injuries and conditions; the provider cannot waste time trying to remember which priorities are the most important.

The most common basis of life-threatening injuries is lack of adequate tissue oxygenation, which leads to anaerobic (without oxygen) metabolism (energy production). Decreased energy production that occurs with anaerobic metabolism is termed *shock*. Three components are necessary for normal metabolism: (1) oxygenation of RBCs in the lungs, (2) delivery of RBCs to the cells throughout the body, and (3) off-loading of oxygen to these cells. The activities involved in the primary survey are aimed at identifying and correcting problems with the first two components.

General Impression

The primary survey begins with a simultaneous, or *global,* overview of the status of a patient's respiratory, circulatory, and neurologic systems to identify obvious, significant external problems with oxygenation, circulation, hemorrhage, or gross deformities. When initially approaching a patient, the prehospital care provider observes whether the patient appears to be moving air effectively, is awake or unresponsive, is holding himself or herself up, and is moving spontaneously. Once at the patient's side, a reasonable starting point is to ask the patient, "What happened to you?" If the patient answers with a coherent explanation in complete sentences, the prehospital care provider can conclude that the patient has an open airway, sufficient breathing to support speech, adequate blood supply to the brain, and reasonable neurologic functioning; that is, there are probably no immediate threats to this patient's life.

If a patient is unable to provide such an answer, a detailed primary survey to identify life-threatening problems is begun. While asking follow-up questions (e.g., "Where do you hurt?"), airway patency is further assessed and respiratory function is observed. A quick check of the radial pulse allows the prehospital care provider to evaluate the presence, quality, and rate (very fast, very slow, or generally normal) of circulatory activity. The provider can simultaneously feel the temperature and moistness of the skin while noting skin color and capillary refill. The patient's level of consciousness and mentation are determined by the appropriateness of the verbal responses. Then a rapid scan of the patient from head to foot, looking for signs of hemorrhage while gathering all the preliminary data for the primary survey, is performed. By doing these things, a quick, overall look at the patient has been accomplished, making the first few seconds with the patient a global survey of overall condition and an evaluation of life-threatening possibilities. The information obtained will help determine priorities, categorize the severity of the patient's injuries and conditions, and identify which injury or condition needs to be managed first. Within 15 to 30 seconds, a general impression of the patient's overall condition has been gained.

The general impression establishes whether the patient is presently or imminently in a critical state and rapidly evaluates the patient's overall systemic condition. The global overview and general impression often provide all of the information necessary to determine whether additional resources, such as advanced life support (ALS), are required. If helicopter transportation to a trauma facility is appropriate, this is often when the decision to request the helicopter is made. Delay in deciding that additional resources are necessary will only extend on-scene time. Early decision making will ultimately shorten scene time. Once a general impression of the patient's condition is obtained, the primary survey is performed unless a complication requires more care or evaluation.

The primary survey must proceed rapidly. The following discussion addresses the specific components of the primary survey and the order of priority for optimal patient management.

The following are the five steps involved in the primary survey, in order of priority:

A—Airway management and cervical spine stabilization
B—Breathing (ventilation)
C—Circulation and bleeding
D—Disability
E— Expose/Environment

Step A: Airway Management and Cervical Spine Stabilization

Airway

The patient's airway is quickly checked to ensure that it is *patent* (open and clear) and that no danger of obstruction exists. Common causes of airway obstruction include the tongue, damaged or broken teeth and dentures, vomit, blood, and other secretions. If the airway is compromised, it will have to be opened, initially using manual methods (trauma chin lift or trauma jaw thrust), and cleared of blood, body substances, and foreign bodies if necessary (Figure 3-21). Eventually, as equipment and time become available, airway management can advance to mechanical means (oral airway, nasal airway).

When evaluating most patients, breathing is normally a silent process that is really not noticeable. If the patient's breathing is, in fact, noticeable, then something is wrong with the patient's ability to ventilate. Patients who are making noise when they breathe often have airway obstruction. For example, snoring is a sound made during a patient's breathing that results from the tongue falling back and blocking the air passageways. This occurs commonly in patients who are supine on their backs and who have an alteration in their mental status. This obstruction can usually be easily relieved by performing the manual methods of a trauma jaw thrust or trauma chin lift.

Gurgling sounds when a patient is breathing indicate the accumulation of fluid (saliva, blood, vomit) in the airway. These need to be suctioned to clear the air passageway. A wheezing sort of sound heard when the patient is breathing in (inspiration) indicates the presence of a foreign body or other obstruction in the air passageway. Patients should be allowed to assume a position of comfort whenever possible. Attempts to remove the object may only force it deeper into the airways.

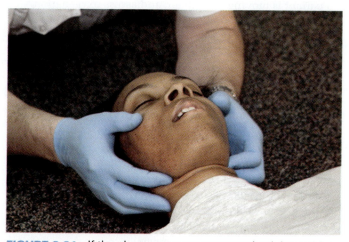

FIGURE 3-21 If the airway appears compromised, it must be opened while continuing to protect the spine.

Cervical Spine Stabilization

Every trauma patient with a significant mechanism of injury is suspected of spinal injury until spinal injury is conclusively ruled out. Therefore, when establishing an open airway, the possibility of cervical spine injury must always be considered. Excessive movement could either produce or aggravate spinal damage because bony compression of the spinal cord may occur in the presence of a fractured spine. The solution is to ensure that the patient's neck is manually maintained in the neutral position during the opening of the airway and when assisting breathing. This does not mean that the necessary airway maintenance procedures just described cannot or should not be applied. Instead, it means that the procedures will be performed while protecting the patient's spine from unnecessary movement. After initiating precautions for cervical injury, the patient's entire spine must be immobilized. Therefore, the patient's entire body must be in line and secured.

Step B: Breathing (Ventilation)

The first step is to effectively deliver oxygen to a patient's lungs to help maintain the aerobic metabolic process. Hypoxia (low oxygen levels in the blood) can result from inadequate ventilation of the lungs and leads to lack of oxygenation of the patient's tissues. Once the patient's airway is open, the quality and quantity of the patient's breathing (ventilation) can be evaluated, as follows:

1. Check to see if the patient is breathing.
2. If the patient is not breathing (apneic), immediately begin assisting ventilations with a bag-mask device with supplemental oxygen before continuing the assessment.
3. Ensure that the patient's airway is open and clear, continue assisted ventilation, and prepare to insert an oral or nasal airway.
4. If the patient is breathing, estimate the adequacy of the breathing rate and depth to determine whether the patient is moving enough air, and assess oxygenation. Provide supplemental oxygen using a face mask.
5. Quickly observe the patient's chest rise, and if the patient is conscious, listen to the patient talk to assess whether he or she can speak a full sentence without difficulty.

Although commonly referred to as the "respiratory rate," a more correct term is *ventilatory rate*. *Ventilation* refers to the process of inhalation and exhalation, whereas *respiration* best describes the physiologic process of gas exchange between the arteries and the alveoli. This text uses the term *ventilatory rate* rather than *respiratory rate*.

The ventilatory rate can be divided into the following five levels:

1. *Apneic.* The patient is not breathing.
2. *Slow.* A very slow ventilatory rate may indicate ischemia (decreased supply of oxygen) of the brain. If the ventilatory rate has dropped below 12 breaths/minute (*bradypnea*), it is usually necessary to either assist or completely take over the patient's breathing with a bag-mask device. Assisted or total ventilatory support with the bag-mask device should include supplemental oxygen (Figure 3-22).
3. *Normal.* If the ventilatory rate is between 12 and 20 breaths/minute (*eupnea*, a normal rate for an adult), the prehospital care provider watches the patient closely. Although the patient may appear stable, supplemental oxygen should be considered.
4. *Fast.* If the ventilatory rate is between 20 and 30 breaths/minute (*tachypnea*), the patient must be watched closely to see whether the patient is improving or deteriorating. The drive for increasing the ventilatory rate is accumulation of carbon dioxide (CO_2) in the blood or a decreased level of blood oxygen (O_2). When a patient displays an abnormal ventilatory rate, the reason must be investigated. A rapid rate indicates that not enough oxygen is reaching the body tissue. This lack of oxygen initiates anaerobic metabolism (see Chapter 5) and ultimately an increase in CO_2. The body's detection system recognizes an increased level of CO_2 and tells the ventilatory system to speed up to exhale this excess. Therefore, an increased ventilatory rate may indicate that the patient needs better perfusion or oxygenation, or both. Administration of supplemental oxygen is indicated for this patient, at least until the patient's overall status is determined. Concern must remain about the patient's ability to maintain adequate ventilation, and the prehospital care provider remains alert for any deterioration in overall condition.

FIGURE 3-22   Airway Management on Spontaneous Ventilation Rate

Ventilatory Rate (breaths/min)	Management
Slow (<12)	Assisted or total ventilation with ≥ 85% oxygen ($FiO_2 \geq 0.85$)
Normal (12–20)	Observation; consider supplemental oxygen
Too fast (20–30)	Administration of ≥ 85% oxygen ($FiO_2 \geq 0.85$)
Abnormally fast (>30)	Assisted ventilation ($FiO_2 \geq 0.85$)

FiO₂, Fraction of inspired oxygen concentration.

5. *Abnormally fast.* A ventilatory rate greater than 30 breaths/minute *(severe tachypnea)* usually indicates hypoxia, anaerobic metabolism, or both, with a resultant acidosis (buildup of acid). Ventilation with supplemental oxygen must be assisted immediately with a bag-mask device. A search for the cause of the rapid ventilatory rate should begin at once to ascertain if the cause is an oxygenation problem or an RBC delivery problem. Once the cause is identified, the intervention must occur immediately to correct the problem.

When assessing the trauma patient's ventilatory status, the ventilatory *depth* as well as the *rate* is assessed. A patient can be breathing at a normal ventilatory rate of 16 breaths/minute but have a greatly decreased ventilatory depth. Conversely, a patient can have a normal ventilatory depth but an increased or decreased ventilatory rate.

Step C: Circulation (Hemorrhage and Perfusion)

Assessing for possible bleeding, either externally or internally, and circulatory system compromise or failure is the next step in caring for the trauma patient. Oxygenation of the RBCs without delivery of the oxygen to the tissue cells is of no benefit to the patient. In the primary survey of a trauma patient, external hemorrhage must be identified and controlled. The provider can then obtain an adequate overall estimate of the patient's cardiac output and perfusion status.

Hemorrhage Control

External hemorrhage is identified and controlled in the primary survey. Hemorrhage control is included in the assessment of circulation because if gross bleeding is not controlled as soon as possible, the potential for the patient's death increases dramatically. The three types of external hemorrhage are as follows:

1. *Capillary bleeding* is caused by abrasions that have scraped open the tiny capillaries just below the skin's surface. Usually capillary bleeding will have slowed or even stopped before the arrival of prehospital care.
2. *Venous bleeding* is from deeper areas within the tissue and is usually controlled with a small amount of direct pressure. Venous bleeding is usually not life threatening unless the injury is severe or blood loss is not controlled.
3. *Arterial bleeding* is caused by an injury that has lacerated an artery. This is the most important and most difficult type of blood loss to control. It is characterized by spurting blood that is bright red. Even a small, deep arterial puncture wound can produce life-threatening arterial blood loss.

Hemorrhage control is a priority because every red blood cell counts. Rapid control of blood loss is one of the most important goals in the care of a trauma patient. The primary survey cannot advance unless hemorrhage is controlled.

In cases of external hemorrhage, application of direct pressure will control most major hemorrhage until the trauma care provider can transport the patient to a hospital where an OR and adequate equipment are available. Hemorrhage control is initiated during the primary survey and maintained throughout transport. The provider may require assistance to accomplish both ventilation and bleeding control in a critically injured patient.

Hemorrhage can be controlled in the following ways:

1. *Direct pressure.* Direct pressure is exactly what the name implies—applying pressure to the site of bleeding. This is accomplished by placing a dressing (e.g., 4-inch × 4-inch gauze) or abdominal pads directly over the site that is bleeding and applying pressure. The application and maintenance of direct pressure will require all of one provider's attention, preventing the provider from participating in other aspects of patient care. However, if assistance is limited, a pressure dressing can be fashioned out of gauze pads and an elastic bandage or a triangle bandage. If bleeding is not controlled, it will not matter how much oxygen or fluid the patient receives; circulation will not improve in the face of ongoing hemorrhage.

   It used to be taught that if the bandage became soaked with blood or if the wound bled through the bandage, one should apply additional dressings or gauze pads on top of the old ones and rebandage it. In fact, if the dressing becomes soaked with blood, it is not effectively controlling the bleeding. Therefore, the dressing should be removed, new gauze applied, and manual direct pressure with a hand pressing down on the wound performed in order to control the ongoing bleeding.
2. *Tourniquets.* Tourniquets have often been described as the technique of "last resort." Military experience in Afghanistan and Iraq, plus the routine and safe use of tourniquets by surgeons, has led to reconsideration of this approach.[9–11] The use of "elevation" and pressure on "pressure points" is no longer recommended because of insufficient data supporting their effectiveness.[12,13] Tourniquets, on the other hand, are very effective in controlling severe hemorrhage and should be used if direct pressure or a pressure dressing fails to control hemorrhage from an extremity.

   If internal hemorrhage is suspected, the thorax and abdomen are exposed to quickly inspect and palpate for signs of injury. The pelvis is also palpated because a pelvic fracture is a major source of intraabdominal bleeding. Most causes of internal hemorrhage are not controllable outside the hospital. The prehospital treatment is rapid delivery of the patient to a facility equipped and staffed for rapid control of hemorrhage in the OR (e.g., trauma center, if available).

Perfusion

The patient's overall circulatory status can be determined by checking the patient's mental status, pulse, skin color, temperature, and moisture; and capillary refilling time.

Mental Status. The patient's mental status provides an indication of the overall quality of the circulation. As the circulatory status worsens, the patient will often exhibit signs of confusion. Some patients will become combative and be uncooperative with efforts at treatment. As the blood loss progresses even further and circulation to the brain diminishes, the patient may lose consciousness completely.

Pulse. The pulse is evaluated for presence, quality, and regularity. The presence of a palpable peripheral pulse also provides an estimate of blood pressure. A quick check of the pulse reveals whether the patient has a fast heart rate (tachycardia), a slow heart rate (bradycardia), or an irregular rhythm. It can also reveal information about the systolic blood pressure. If a radial pulse cannot be felt in an uninjured extremity, the patient has a low blood pressure and likely has entered the *decompensated phase* of shock, a late sign of the patient's critical condition. In the primary survey, determination of an exact pulse rate is not necessary. Instead, a gross estimate is rapidly obtained, and assessment moves on to other gross evaluations. The actual pulse rate is obtained later in the process. If the patient lacks a palpable carotid or femoral pulse, he or she is in cardiopulmonary arrest (see later discussion).

Skin

Color. Adequate perfusion produces a pinkish hue to the skin. Skin becomes pale when blood is shunted away from an area. Pale coloration is associated with poor perfusion. Bluish coloration indicates a lack of adequate oxygen in the blood. Skin pigmentation can often make this determination difficult. Examination of the color of nail beds and mucous membranes serves to overcome this challenge because these changes in color usually first appear in the lips, gums, or fingertips.

Temperature. As with overall skin evaluation, skin temperature is influenced by environmental conditions. Cool skin indicates decreased perfusion, regardless of the cause. The prehospital care provider usually assesses skin temperature by touching the patient with the back of the hand; therefore, an accurate determination can be difficult with gloves donned. Normal skin temperature is warm to touch, neither cool nor hot. Normally the blood vessels are not dilated and do not bring the heat of the body to the surface of the skin.

Moisture. Dry skin indicates good perfusion. Moist skin is associated with shock and decreased perfusion. This decrease in perfusion is caused by blood being shunted to the main organs of the body as a result of vasoconstriction of peripheral vessels.

Capillary Refilling Time. The capillary refilling time is checked by pressing over the nail beds. This removes the blood from the visible capillary bed. The rate of return of blood to the nail beds (refilling time) is a tool for estimating blood flow through this most distant part of the circulation. A capillary refilling time of greater than 2 seconds indicates that the capillary beds are not receiving adequate perfusion. However, capillary refilling time by itself is a poor indicator of shock because it is influenced by so many other factors. For example, peripheral vascular disease (arteriosclerosis), cold temperatures, the use of pharmacologic vasodilators or constrictors, or the presence of neurogenic shock can skew the result. Refilling becomes a less useful check of cardiovascular function in these cases. Capillary refilling time has a place in the evaluation of circulatory adequacy, but it should always be used in conjunction with other physical examination findings, just as the prehospital care provider uses other indicators (e.g., blood pressure).

Step D: Disability

Having evaluated and corrected, to the extent possible, the factors involved in delivering oxygen to the lungs and circulating it throughout the body, the next step in the primary survey is the assessment of brain (cerebral) function, which is an indirect measurement of cerebral oxygenation. The goal is to determine the patient's level of consciousness (LOC) and ascertain the potential for hypoxia.

The trauma care provider can infer that a confused, belligerent, combative, or uncooperative patient is hypoxic until proved otherwise. Most patients want help when their lives are medically threatened. If a patient refuses help, the reason must be questioned. Does the patient feel threatened by the presence of a prehospital care provider on the scene? If so, further attempts to establish rapport will often help to gain the patient's trust. If nothing in the situation seems to be threatening, the source of the behavior should be assumed to be physiologic and reversible conditions identified and treated. During the assessment, the history can help determine whether the patient lost consciousness at any time since the injury occurred, what toxic substances might be involved, and whether the patient has any preexisting conditions that may produce a decreased LOC or aberrant behavior.

A decreased LOC alerts a prehospital care provider to the following four possibilities:

1. Decreased cerebral oxygenation (caused by hypoxia/hypoperfusion)
2. Central nervous system (CNS) injury
3. Drug or alcohol overdose
4. Metabolic derangement (diabetes, seizure, cardiac arrest)

The Glasgow Coma Scale (GCS) score is a tool used for determining LOC.[14] It is a quick, simple method for determining cerebral function and is predictive of patient outcome, especially the best motor response. It also provides a base-

Eye Opening	Points
Spontaneous eye opening	4
Eye opening on command	3
Eye opening to painful stimulus	2
No eye opening	1

Best Verbal Response	
Answers appropriately (oriented)	5
Gives confused answers	4
Inappropriate response	3
Makes unintelligible noises	2
Makes no verbal response	1

Best Motor Response	
Follows command	6
Localizes painful stimuli	5
Withdrawal to pain	4
Responds with abnormal flexion to painful stimuli (decorticate)	3
Responds with abnormal extension to pain (decerebrate)	2
Gives no motor response	1
Total	

FIGURE 3-23 Glasgow Coma Scale (GCS).

line of cerebral function for serial neurologic evaluations. The GCS score is divided into three sections: (1) *eye* opening, (2) best *verbal* response, and (3) best *motor* response (EVM). Each of the components should be reported and documented individually rather than as a total score.

The patient is assigned a score according to the *best* response to each component of the EVM (Figure 3-23). For example, if a patient's right eye is so severely swollen that the patient cannot open it, but the left eye opens spontaneously, the patient receives a "4" for the best eye movement. If a patient lacks spontaneous eye opening, the provider should use a verbal command ("Open your eyes"). If the patient does not respond to a verbal stimulus, a painful stimulus, such as nail bed pressure with a pen or squeezing of the axillary tissue, can be applied.

The patient's verbal response is determined by using a question such as, "What happened to you?" If fully oriented, the patient will supply a coherent answer. Otherwise, the patient's verbal response is scored as confused, inappropriate, unintelligible, or absent. If a patient has an airway in place, the GCS score contains only the eye and motor scales.

The third component of the GCS is the motor score. A simple, unambiguous command such as, "Hold up two fingers," or "Show me a hitchhiker's sign" is given to the patient. If the patient complies with the command, the highest score of "6" is given. If the patient fails to follow a command, a painful stimulus, as noted previously, should be used, and the patient's *best* motor response should be scored. A patient who attempts to push away a painful stimulus is considered to be "localizing." Other possible responses to pain include withdrawal from the stimulus, abnormal flexion (decorticate posturing) (Figure 2-24, *A*) or extension (decerebrate posturing) (Figure 2-24, *B*) of the upper extremities, or absence of motor function.

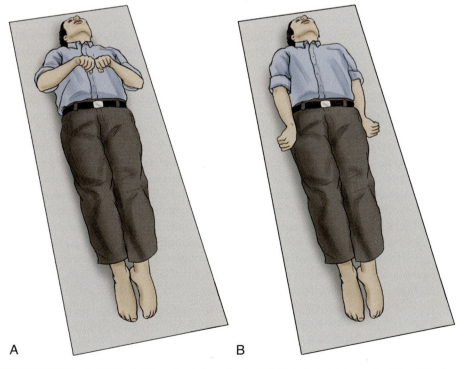

A   B

FIGURE 3-24 **A,** Flexion (decorticate) posturing. **B,** Extension (decerebrate) posturing.
(Aehlert B: *Paramedic practice today,* vol 1, St Louis, 2010, Mosby.)

The maximum GCS score is 15, indicating a patient with no disability, whereas the lowest score of 3 is generally an ominous sign. A score of less than 8 indicates a major injury, 9 to 12 a moderate injury, and 13 to 15 a minor injury. A GCS score of 8 is an indication for considering active airway management of the patient.

The prehospital care provider can easily calculate and relate the individual components of the score and will include them in the verbal report as well as in the patient care record.

If a patient is not awake, oriented, or able to follow commands, the prehospital care provider can assess the pupils quickly. Are the **p**upils **e**qual **a**nd **r**ound, **r**eactive to **l**ight (PEARRL)? Is each pupil of normal appearance, and does it react to light by constricting appropriately or is it unresponsive and dilated? A GCS score of less than 14 in combination with an abnormal pupil examination can indicate the presence of a life-threatening traumatic brain injury.

The acronym AVPU is often used to describe the patient's LOC. In this system, *A* stands for *alert, V* for responds to *verbal* stimulus, *P* for responds to *painful* stimulus, and *U* for *unresponsive.* This approach, although very simple, fails to properly provide information as to specifically *how* the patient responds to verbal or painful stimuli. In other words, if the patient responds to verbal questioning, is the patient oriented, confused, or mumbling incomprehensibly? Likewise, when the patient responds to painful stimulus, does the patient localize, withdraw, or demonstrate decorticate or decerebrate posturing? Because of its lack of precision, the use of AVPU has fallen into disfavor. Although the GCS is more complicated to remember than AVPU, repeated practice will make this crucial assessment second nature.

Step E: Expose/Environment

An early step in the assessment process is to remove a patient's clothes because exposure of the trauma patient is critical to finding all injuries (Figure 3-25). The saying, "The one part of the body that is not exposed will be the most severely injured part," may not always be true, but it is true often enough to warrant a total body examination. Also, blood can collect in and be absorbed by clothing and thereby go unnoticed. After seeing the patient's entire body, the prehospital care provider can then cover the patient again to conserve body heat. Although it is important to expose a trauma patient's body to complete an effective assessment, *hypothermia* is a serious problem in the management of a trauma patient. Only what is necessary should be exposed to the outside environment. Once the patient has been moved inside the warm emergency medical services (EMS) unit, the complete examination can be accomplished and the patient covered again as quickly as possible.

The amount of the patient's clothing that should be removed during an assessment varies depending on the conditions or injuries found. A general rule is to remove as much clothing as necessary to determine the presence

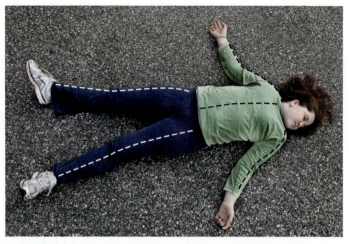

FIGURE 3-25 Clothing can be quickly removed by cutting, as indicated by the dotted lines.

or absence of a condition or injury. The prehospital care provider need not be afraid to remove clothing if it is the only way to complete the assessment and treatment properly. On occasion, patients can sustain multiple mechanisms of injury, such as experiencing a motor vehicle crash after being shot. Potentially life-threatening injuries may be missed if the patient is inadequately examined. Injuries cannot be treated if they are not first identified. Special care should be taken when cutting and removing clothing from a victim of a crime so as not to inadvertently destroy evidence (Figure 3-26).

Resuscitation

Resuscitation describes treatment steps taken to correct life-threatening problems as identified in the primary survey. PHTLS assessment is based on a "treat as you go" philosophy, in which treatment is initiated as each threat to life is identified, or at the earliest possible moment (Figure 3-27).

Limited Scene Intervention

Airway problems are managed as the top priority. If the airway is open but the patient is not breathing, ventilatory support is initiated. Ventilatory support includes administration of high supplemental oxygen as early as possible. If the patient is exhibiting signs of ventilatory distress and lowered levels of air exchange, ventilatory assistance is needed by way of a bag-mask device. Cardiac arrest is identified during the assessment of circulation and chest compressions begun, if appropriate. Exsanguinating hemorrhage is also controlled during this step. In a patient with adequate airway and breathing, hypoxia and shock (anaerobic metabolism), if present, can be rapidly corrected.

Transport

If life-threatening conditions are identified during the primary survey, the patient should be rapidly "packaged" after initiating limited field intervention. Transport of critically injured

Unfortunately, some trauma patients are victims of violent crimes. In these situations, it is important to do everything possible to preserve evidence for law enforcement personnel. When cutting clothing from a crime victim, care should be taken *not* to cut through holes in the clothing made by bullets (projectiles), knives, or other objects because this can compromise valuable forensic evidence. If clothing is removed from a victim of a potential crime, it should be placed in a paper (not plastic) bag and turned over to law enforcement personnel on scene before patient transport. Any weapons, drugs, or personal belongings found during patient assessment should also be turned over to law enforcement personnel, as well as thoroughly documented on the prehospital care report (PCR). If the patient's condition warrants transport before the arrival of law enforcement, these items are brought with the patient to the hospital, and the law enforcement agency is contacted and appraised of the destination facility.

In discussing the process of patient assessment, management, and decision making, the information must be presented in a sequential format (i.e., step A followed by step B followed by step C, etc.). Although presentation of information in this manner makes explanation easier and perhaps makes the concepts easier for a student to understand, that is not how the real world functions. In reality, these steps are accomplished virtually simultaneously. The prehospital care provider's brain is similar to a computer that can receive input from several sources at once (cerebral multitasking). The brain can assess data received simultaneously and is capable of prioritizing the information from all input sources, sorting them in such a way that orderly decision making follows.

The brain can gather most data in about 15 seconds. Simultaneous processing of these data and appropriate prioritization of the information by the prehospital care provider can identify the component that the provider must manage first. Although the ABCDE approach described in this chapter may not necessarily be the order in which the prehospital care provider collects or receives the information, it does serve to establish priorities for management.

The primary survey addresses life-threatening conditions. The secondary survey of the patient identifies possible limb-threatening injuries as well as other, less significant problems.

trauma patients to the closest appropriate facility should be initiated as soon as possible (Figure 3-28). Unless complicating circumstances exist, scene time should be as short as possible (limited to 10 minutes or less) for these patients. Limited scene time and initiation of rapid transport to the closest appropriate facility, preferably a trauma center, are fundamental aspects of prehospital trauma resuscitation. If transport time is prolonged, it may be appropriate to call for aid from a nearby ALS service that can intercept the basic unit en route. Helicopter evacuation to a trauma center is another option. Both the ALS service and the flight service will allow for advanced airway management, ventilatory management, and fluid replacement.

Secondary Survey (Detailed History and Physical Examination)

The secondary survey is a head-to-toe evaluation of a patient. The secondary survey is performed only after the primary survey is completed, all life-threatening injuries have been identified and treated, and resuscitation initiated. The objective of the secondary survey is to identify injuries or problems that were not identified during the primary survey. Because a well-performed primary survey will identify all life-threatening conditions, the secondary survey, by definition, deals with less serious problems. Therefore, a critical trauma patient is transported as soon as possible after conclusion of the primary survey and not held in the field in order to perform a secondary survey.

The secondary survey uses a "look, listen, and feel" approach to evaluate the skin and everything it contains. Rather than looking at the entire body at one time, returning to

listen to all areas, and finally returning to palpate all areas, the prehospital care provider "searches" the body. The provider identifies injuries and correlates physical findings region by region, beginning at the head and proceeding through the neck, chest, and abdomen to the extremities, concluding with a detailed neurologic examination. The following phrases capture the essence of the entire assessment process:

See, don't just look.
Hear, don't just listen.
Feel, don't just touch.

See
- Examine all of the skin of each region.
- Be attentive for external hemorrhage or signs of internal hemorrhage, such as distension of the abdomen, marked tenseness of an extremity or an expanding hematoma.
- Make note of soft tissue injuries, including abrasions, burns, contusions, hematomas, lacerations, and puncture wounds.
- Make note of any masses or swelling or deformation of bones.

FIGURE 3-28   Critical Trauma Patient

Limit scene time to 10 minutes or less when any of the following life-threatening conditions are present:

- Inadequate or threatened airway
- Impaired ventilation, as demonstrated by the following:
  - Abnormally fast or slow ventilatory rate
  - Hypoxia (SpO$_2$ < 95% even with supplemental oxygen)
  - Dyspnea
  - Open pneumothorax or flail chest
- Suspected pneumothorax
- Significant external hemorrhage or suspected internal hemorrhage
- Abnormal neurologic status
  - GCS score ≤ = 13
  - Seizure activity
  - Sensory or motor deficit
- Penetrating trauma to the head, neck, or torso, or proximal to elbow and knee in the extremities
- Amputation or near-amputation proximal to the fingers or toes
- Any trauma in the presence of the following:
  - History of serious medical conditions (e.g., coronary artery disease, chronic obstructive pulmonary disease, bleeding disorder)
  - Age > 55 years
  - Hypothermia
  - Burns
  - Pregnancy

- Make note of abnormal indentations on the skin and the skin's color.
- Make note of anything that does not "look right."

Hear

- Note any unusual sounds when the patient inhales or exhales.

Feel

- Carefully move each bone in the region. Note whether this produces crepitus, pain, or unusual movement.
- Firmly palpate all parts of the region. Note whether anything moves that should not, whether anything feels "squishy," if the patient complains of tenderness, where pulses are felt, whether pulsations are felt that should not be present, and whether all pulses are present.

Vital Signs

The quality of the pulse and ventilatory rates and the other components of the primary survey are continually reevaluated because significant changes can occur rapidly. Quantita-tive vital signs are measured and motor and sensory status evaluated in all four extremities as soon as possible, although this is normally not accomplished until the conclusion of the primary survey. Depending on the situation, a second provider may obtain vital signs while the first provider completes the primary survey, to avoid further delay. However, exact "numbers" for pulse rate, ventilatory rate, and blood pressure are not critical in the initial management of the patient with severe multisystem trauma. Therefore, the measurement of the exact numbers can be delayed until completion of the essential steps of resuscitation and stabilization.

A set of complete vital signs includes blood pressure, pulse rate and quality, ventilatory rate (including breath sounds), and skin color and temperature. A complete set of vital signs are evaluated and recorded every 3 to 5 minutes, as often as possible, or at the time of any change in condition or a medical problem. Even if an automated, noninvasive blood pressure device is available, the initial blood pressure should be taken manually. Automatic blood pressure devices may be inaccurate when the patient is significantly hypotensive.

SAMPLE History

A quick history is obtained on the patient, whenever possible. This information should be documented on the patient care report and passed on to the medical personnel at the receiving facility. The mnemonic SAMPLE serves as a reminder for the key components, as follows:

- *Symptoms:* What does the patient complain of? Pain? Trouble breathing? Numbness? Tingling? Burns? Bleeding?
- *Allergies:* Primarily to medications.
- *Medications:* Prescription and nonprescription drugs that the patient takes regularly.
- *Past medical and surgical history:* Significant medical problems for which the patient receives ongoing medical care; includes prior surgeries.
- *Last meal:* Many trauma patients will require surgery, and recent food intake increases the risk of aspiration during induction of anesthesia.
- *Events:* Leading up to the injury.

Head

Visual examination of the head and face will reveal contusions, abrasions, lacerations, bone asymmetry, hemorrhage, bony defects of the face and supportive skull, and abnormalities of the eye, eyelid, external ear, mouth, and mandible. The following are included during a head examination:

- Search thoroughly through the patient's hair for any soft tissue injuries
- Check pupil size for reactivity to light, equality, accommodation, roundness, and irregular shape
- Carefully palpate the bones of the face and skull to identify crepitus, deviation, depression, or abnormal mobil-

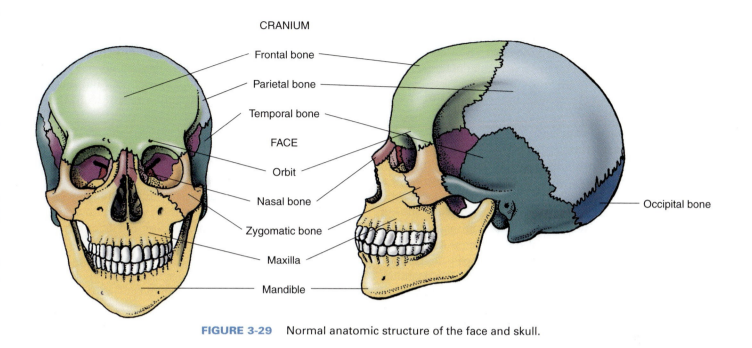

FIGURE 3-29   Normal anatomic structure of the face and skull.

ity (this is extremely important in the nonradiographic evaluation for head injury).

Figure 3-29 reviews the normal anatomic structure of the face and skull.

Neck

Visual examination of the neck for contusions, abrasions, lacerations, and deformities will alert the prehospital care provider to the possibility of underlying injuries. Palpation may reveal subcutaneous emphysema of a laryngeal, tracheal, or pulmonary origin. Crepitus of the larynx, hoarseness, and subcutaneous emphysema constitute a triad classically indicative of laryngeal fracture. Lack of tenderness of the cervical spine may help rule out cervical spine fractures (when combined with strict criteria), whereas tenderness may frequently indicate the presence of a fracture, dislocation, or ligamentous injury. Such palpation is performed carefully, ensuring that the cervical spine remains in a neutral, inline position.

Figure 3-30 reviews the normal anatomy of the neck.

Chest

Because the thorax is strong, resilient, and elastic, it can absorb a significant amount of trauma. Close visual examination of the chest for deformities, areas of paradoxical movement, contusions, and abrasions is necessary to identify underlying injuries. Other signs for which the prehospital care provider should watch closely include splinting and guarding; unequal bilateral chest excursion; and intercostal, suprasternal, or supraclavicular bulging or retraction.

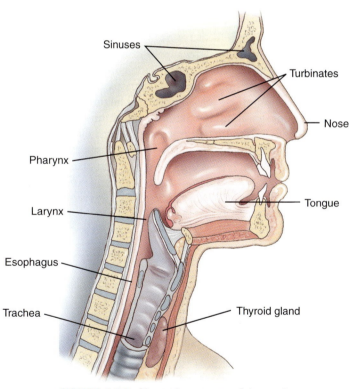

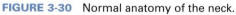

FIGURE 3-30   Normal anatomy of the neck.

For example, a contusion over the sternum may be the only indication of a cardiac injury. A stab wound near the sternum may indicate cardiac tamponade. A line traced from the fourth intercostal space anteriorly, to the sixth intercostal space laterally, and to the eighth intercostal space posteriorly defines the upward excursion of the diaphragm at full expiration (Figure 3-31). A penetrating injury that occurs below this line or with a path that may have taken it below this line should be considered to have traversed both the thoracic and abdominal cavities.

Abdomen

The abdominal examination begins, as with the other parts of the body, by visual evaluation. Abrasions and ecchymoses (bruises) indicate the possibility of underlying injury. The abdomen should be examined carefully, near the umbilicus, for a telltale transverse contusion, which suggests that an incorrectly worn seat belt has caused underlying injury. Almost 50% of patients with this sign will have an intestinal injury. Lumbar spine fractures may also be associated with the "seat belt sign."

Examination of the abdomen also includes palpation of each quadrant to evaluate tenderness, abdominal muscle guarding, and masses. When palpating, the trauma care provider notes whether the abdomen is soft or whether rigidity or guarding is present. There is no need to continue palpating after discovering abdominal tenderness or pain. Additional information will not alter prehospital management, and the only outcomes of a continued abdominal examination are further discomfort to the patient and delayed transportation to the receiving facility.

Pelvis

The pelvis is evaluated by observation and palpation. The pelvis is first visually examined for abrasions, contusions, lacerations, open fractures, and signs of distension. Pelvic fractures can produce massive internal hemorrhage, resulting in rapid deterioration of a patient's condition.

The pelvis is palpated only once for instability as part of the secondary survey. Because palpation can aggravate hem-

orrhage, this examination step should only be performed once and not repeated. Palpation is accomplished by gently first applying anterior-to-posterior pressure with the heels of the hands on the symphysis pubis and then medial pressure to the iliac crests bilaterally, evaluating for pain and abnormal movement. Any evidence of instability raises the likelihood of internal hemorrhage.

Back

The back of the torso should be examined for evidence of injury. This is best accomplished when logrolling the patient for placement onto the long backboard. Breath sounds can be auscultated over the posterior thorax at this time, and the spine should be palpated for tenderness and deformity.

Extremities

The examination of the extremities begins at the clavicle in the upper extremity and the pelvis in the lower extremity and then proceeds toward the most distal portion of each extremity. Each individual bone and joint is evaluated by visual examination for deformity, hematoma, or ecchymosis and by palpation to determine the presence of crepitus, pain, tenderness, or unusual movements. Any suspected fracture should be immobilized until x-ray confirmation of its presence or absence is possible. Circulation and motor and sensory nerve function at the distal end of each extremity are also checked. If an extremity is immobilized, pulses, movement, and sensation should be rechecked after splinting.

Neurologic Examination

As with the other regional examinations described, the neurologic examination in the secondary survey is conducted in much greater detail than in the primary survey. Calculation of the GCS score, evaluation of motor and sensory function, and observation of pupillary response are all included. When examining a patient's pupils, equality of response in addition to equality of size are evaluated. A small but significant portion of the population has pupils of differing sizes as a normal condition *(anisocoria)*. Even in these patients, however, the pupils should react to light in a similar manner. Pupils that react at differing speeds to the introduction of light are considered to be unequal. Unequal pupils in an unconscious trauma patient may indicate increased pressure inside the skull, caused by either swelling of the brain or a rapidly expanding intracranial hematoma (Figure 3-32). Direct eye injury can also cause unequal pupils.

A gross examination of sensory capability and response will determine the presence or absence of weakness or loss of sensation in the extremities and will identify areas that require further examination. The entire length of the spine, and thus the entire patient, need to be immobilized. Use of a long backboard, cervical collar, head pads, and straps is required. Immobilizing the head and neck only is inadequate to accomplish the necessary stabilization. If the body is not immobilized, a shift in the patient's body resulting from lift-

Lateral View of Diaphragm Position

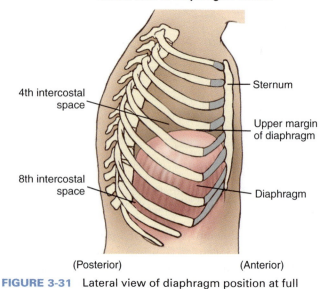

4th intercostal space

Sternum

Upper margin of diaphragm

8th intercostal space

Diaphragm

(Posterior)   (Anterior)

FIGURE 3-31 Lateral view of diaphragm position at full expiration.

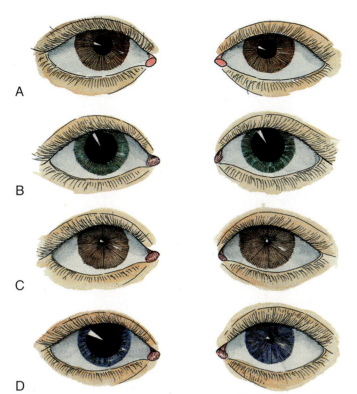

FIGURE 3-32   A, Normal pupils. **B,** Pupil dilation. **C,** Pupil constriction. **D,** Unequal pupils.

ing or ambulance movement will cause the body to move but not the head, which has been restrained, potentially causing further injury to the spinal cord. Protection of the entire spinal cord is required at all times.

Definitive Care in the Field

Included in assessment and management are the skills of packaging, transportation, and communication. Definitive care is the end phase of patient care. The following are examples of definitive care:

- For a patient with cardiac arrest, definitive care is defibrillation with resultant normal rhythm; cardiopulmonary resuscitation (CPR) is just a holding pattern until defibrillation can be accomplished.
- For a patient in a diabetic coma from low blood sugar, definitive care is intravenous glucose and a return to normal blood glucose levels.
- For a patient with an obstructed airway, definitive care is relief of the obstruction, which may be accomplished by jaw thrust and assisted ventilation.
- For the patient with severe bleeding, definitive care is hemorrhage control and resuscitation from shock.

In general, definitive care for many of the injuries sustained by the trauma patient can only be provided in the operating

room of a hospital. Anything that delays the administration of that definitive care will lessen the patient's chance for survival. The care given to the trauma patient in the field is similar to CPR for the cardiac arrest patient. It keeps the patient alive until something definitive can be done. For the trauma patient, the care given in the field is often only temporizing—buying the additional minutes needed to reach the OR.

Packaging

As discussed previously, spinal injury must be suspected in all trauma patients. Therefore, when indicated, stabilization of the spine should be an integral component of packaging the trauma patient. If time is available, the following are accomplished:

- Careful stabilization of extremity fractures using specific splints
- If the patient is in critical condition, immobilization of all fractures as the patient is stabilized on a long backboard ("trauma" board)
- Bandaging of wounds as necessary and appropriate

Transport

Transportation should begin as soon as the patient is loaded and stabilized. As discussed previously, delay at the scene to complete the secondary survey only extends the period before the receiving facility can administer blood and control hemorrhage. Continued evaluation and further resuscitation occur en route to the receiving facility. *For some critically injured trauma patients, initiation of transport is the single most important aspect of definitive care in the field.*

A patient whose condition is not critical can receive attention for individual injuries before transportation, but even this patient should be transported rapidly before a hidden condition becomes critical.

Field Triage Scheme

The Triage Decision Scheme, originally published by the American College of Surgeons (ACS) Committee on Trauma, is used to make prehospital patient triage decisions (Figure 3-33).[16] In some systems the Triage Decision Scheme is used in the process of determining the most appropriate receiving facility for a trauma patient. As with any algorithm, however, it should be used as a guideline and not as a replacement for good judgment. The Triage Decision Scheme divides triage into three prioritized steps that will assist in the decision as to when it is best to transport a patient to a trauma center, if available: (1) physiologic criteria, (2) anatomic criteria, and (3) mechanism of injury (kinematics). Following this scheme results in *over-triage* (more patients are taken to the trauma center than actually need a trauma center level of care), but this outcome is better than *undertriage* (patients needing a trauma center level of care are taken to nontrauma centers). Medical directors or local medical control boards should establish local protocols to familiarize prehospital field personnel with trauma centers.

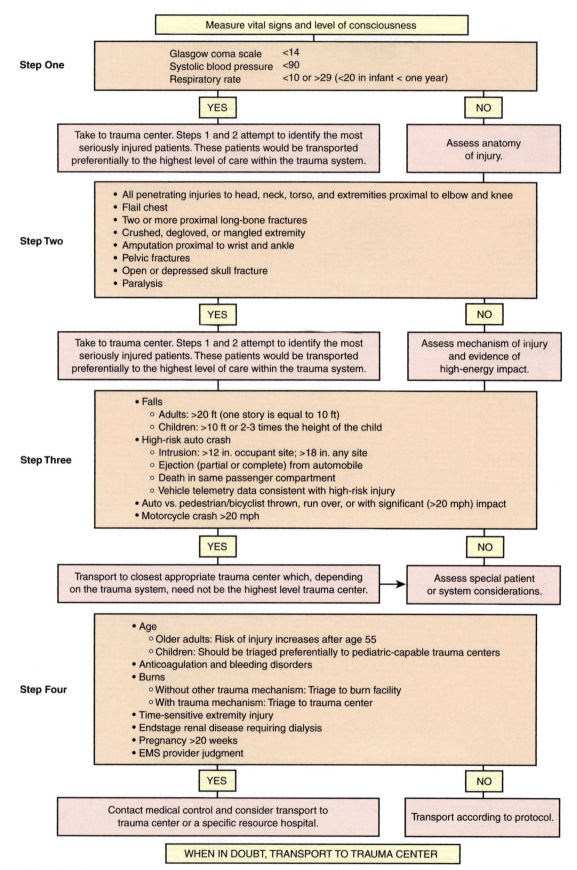

FIGURE 3-33 Deciding where to transport a patient is critical, with consideration of the type and location of available facilities. Situations that will most likely require an in-house trauma team are detailed in the Triage Decision Scheme.

Duration of Transport

The trauma care provider should choose a receiving facility according to the severity of the patient's injury. In simple terms, the patient should be transported to the closest appropriate facility (i.e., the closest facility most capable of managing the patient's problems). If the patient's injuries are severe or indicate the possibility of continuing hemorrhage, the provider should take the patient to a facility that will provide definitive care as quickly as possible (i.e., a trauma center, if available).

For example, if an ambulance responds to a call in 8 minutes and the prehospital team spends 6 minutes on the scene to package and load the patient into the transporting unit, 14 minutes of the Golden Period have passed. The closest hospital is 5 minutes away, and the trauma center is 14 minutes away. On arrival at the trauma center, the surgeon is in the emergency department (ED) with the emergency physician and the entire trauma team. The OR is staffed and ready. After 10 minutes in the ED for resuscitation and necessary radiographs and blood work, the patient is taken to the OR. The total time since the incident is now 38 minutes. In comparison, the closest hospital has an available emergency physician, but the surgeon and OR team are out of the hospital. In contrast to the patient's 10 minutes in the ED at the trauma center, the time in the ED at the nontrauma facility could stretch to 45 minutes until the surgeon arrives and examines the patient. Another 30 minutes could elapse while waiting for the OR team to arrive once the surgeon has examined the patient and decided to operate. The total time is 94 minutes, or 2½ times longer than the first scenario. The 9 minutes saved by the shorter ambulance ride actually cost 57 minutes, during which time operative management could have been started and hemorrhage control achieved.

In a rural community, the transport time to an awaiting trauma team may be 45 to 60 minutes or even longer. In this situation, the closest hospital with an on-call trauma team is the appropriate receiving facility.

Method of Transport

Another aspect in the transportation decision is the transportation method. Some systems offer an alternative option of air transportation. Air medical services may offer a higher level of care than ground units. Air transportation may also be quicker and smoother than ground transportation in some circumstances. As previously mentioned, if air transportation is available in a community and is appropriate for the specific situation, the earlier in the assessment process that the decision is made to call for air transport, the greater the likely benefit to the patient.

Monitoring and Reassessment

Ongoing Assessment

After the primary survey and initial care are complete, the patient must continuously be monitored, the vital signs reassessed, and the primary survey repeated several times while en route to the receiving facility or at the scene if transport is delayed. Continuous reassessment of the components of the primary survey will help ensure that unrecognized compromise of vital functions does not occur. Particular attention must be paid to any significant change in a patient's condition and management reevaluated if the patient's condition changes. Furthermore, the continued monitoring of a patient helps reveal conditions or problems that may have been overlooked or not apparent during the primary survey. Often the patient's condition will be obvious and looking at and listening to the patient provides much information. How the information is gathered is not as important as ensuring that *all* the information is gathered. Reassessment should be conducted as quickly and thoroughly as possible. Monitoring during a prolonged transport situation is described later.

Communication

Communication with the receiving facility should be undertaken as soon as possible. The information transmitted about a patient's condition, management, and the expected time of arrival will give the receiving facility time to prepare for the patient. Transmission of information about the mechanism of injury, the characteristics of the scene, the number of patients, and other pertinent facts allows the receiving facility staff to best coordinate its resources and meet each patient's needs.

Equally important is the written *prehospital care report* (PCR). A good PCR is valuable for the following two reasons:

1. It gives the receiving facility staff a thorough understanding of the events that occurred, the findings and treatment that were provided in the field, and the patient's condition should any questions arise after the prehospital care providers have left.
2. It helps ensure quality control throughout the prehospital system by making case review possible.

For these reasons, it is important that the trauma care provider fill out the PCR accurately and completely and provide it to the receiving facility. The report should stay with the patient; the report is of little use if it does not arrive until hours or days after the patient arrives.

The PCR becomes a part of the patient's medical record. It is a legal record of what was found and what was done and can be used as part of a legal action. The report is considered to be a complete record of the injuries found and the actions taken. A good adage to remember is, "If it is not on the report, it was not done." All that the prehospital care provider knows, has seen, and has done to the patient should be recorded in the report. Another important reason for providing a copy of the PCR to the receiving facility is that most trauma centers maintain a "trauma registry," a database of all trauma patients admitted to their facility. The prehospital information is an important aspect of this database and may aid in valuable research.

The prehospital care provider also verbally transfers responsibility for a patient ("sign off," "report off," or "transfer over") to the physician or nurse who takes over the patient's care at the receiving facility. This verbal report is typically more detailed than the radio report and less detailed than the written record, providing an overview of the significant history of the incident, the action taken by the prehospital care providers, and the patient's response to this action. The report must highlight any significant changes in the patient's condition that have taken place since transmitting the radio report. Transfer of important prehospital information further emphasizes the team concept of patient care.

Special Considerations

Abuse

A trauma care provider is often the first responder on the scene, allowing the provider to observe a potentially abusive situation. The provider inside a house can observe and relay the details about the scene to the receiving facility so that the appropriate social services in the area can be alerted. The prehospital care provider is usually the first, and sometimes the only, medically trained person to be in a position to observe, suspect and relay information about this silent danger.

Anyone at any age can be a potential abuser or victim of abuse. A pregnant woman, infant, toddler, child, adolescent, young adult, middle-aged adult, and older adult are all at risk for abuse. Several different types of abuse exist, including physical, psychological (emotional), and financial. Abuse may occur by *commission,* in which a purposeful act results in an injury (physical abuse or sexual abuse), or by *omission* (e.g., neglectful care of a dependent). This section does not discuss types of abuse and only introduces the reader to general characteristics and heightens a prehospital care provider's awareness and suspicion of abuse.

General characteristics of a potential abuser include dishonesty, the "story" not correlating with the injuries, a negative attitude, and abrasiveness with prehospital personnel. General characteristics of the abused patient include quietness, not wanting to elaborate on details of the incident, constant eye contact or lack of eye contact with someone at the scene, and minimization of personal injuries. Abuse, abusers, and the abused can take many different forms, and prehospital care providers need to keep suspicion high if the scene and the story do not correlate. The provider is required to relay suspicions and any information to the proper authorities.

Traumatic Cardiopulmonary Arrest

Cardiopulmonary arrest resulting from trauma differs from that caused by medical problems in three significant ways, as follows:

1. Most medical cardiac arrests are the result of either a respiratory problem, such as a foreign body airway obstruction, or a cardiac rhythm disturbance that prehospital care providers may be able to treat definitively in the field. Cardiac arrest resulting from injury most often results from exsan-

guination or, less often, a problem incompatible with life, such as a devastating brain or spinal cord injury, and the patient cannot be appropriately resuscitated in the field.

2. Medical arrests are best managed with attempts at stabilization at the scene (e.g., removal of airway foreign body, defibrillation). In contrast, traumatic cardiopulmonary arrest is best managed with immediate transport to a facility that offers immediate blood and emergent surgery.

3. Because of the differences in etiology and management, patients with traumatic cardiopulmonary arrest in the prehospital setting have an extremely low likelihood of survival. Less than 4% of trauma patients who require CPR in the prehospital setting survive to be discharged from the hospital, with most studies documenting that victims of penetrating trauma have a slightly better chance of survival over those of blunt trauma. Of the small percentage of patients who are discharged from the hospital alive, many sustain significant neurologic impairment.

In addition to the extremely low survival rate, resuscitation attempts in patients who are extremely unlikely to survive put prehospital care providers at risk from exposure to blood and body fluids as well as injuries sustained in motor vehicle crashes during emergent transport. Such unsuccessful attempts at resuscitation may divert resources away from other patients who are viable and have a greater likelihood of survival. For these reasons, good judgment needs to be exercised regarding the decision to initiate resuscitation attempts for victims of traumatic cardiopulmonary arrest.

The National Association of EMS Physicians collaborated with the ACS Committee on Trauma to develop guidelines for withholding or terminating CPR in the prehospital setting. Victims of drowning, lightning strike, or hypothermia and patients in whom the mechanism of injury does not correlate with the clinical situation (suggesting a nontraumatic cause) deserve special consideration before a decision is made to withhold or terminate resuscitation. A patient found in cardiopulmonary arrest at the scene of a traumatic event may have experienced the arrest because of a medical problem (e.g., myocardial infarction), especially if the patient is elderly and evidence of injury is minimal.

Withholding Cardiopulmonary Resuscitation

If, during the primary survey, patients are found to meet the following criteria, CPR may be withheld and the patient declared dead[17]:

- For victims of blunt trauma, resuscitation efforts may be withheld if the patient is pulseless and apneic on arrival of prehospital care providers.
- For victims of penetrating trauma, resuscitation efforts may be withheld if there are no signs of life (patients with no pupillary response to light, no spontaneous movement, no organized cardiac rhythm on electrocardiogram > 40 beats/minute).

- Resuscitation efforts are not indicated when the patient has sustained an obviously fatal injury (e.g., decapitation) or when evidence exists of dependent lividity, rigor mortis, and decomposition.

Basic Life Support

Guidelines for managing cardiopulmonary arrest have recently been revised and published by the American Heart Association.[18] After opening the airway with a trauma jaw thrust, ventilatory effort is assessed. If the patient is apneic, the prehospital care provider delivers two rescue breaths. These breaths are delivered slowly to prevent gastric inflation. Any obvious, exsanguinating hemorrhage should be controlled. If the patient remains unresponsive after these efforts, chest compressions are initiated. Cycles of compressions and ventilations are given. Compressions are delivered at 100. The individual delivering chest compressions is changed every 2 minutes to prevent fatigue. If an automated external defibrillator (AED) is available, the patient's cardiac rhythm is assessed and defibrillation performed if ventricular fibrillation is present.

Terminating Cardiopulmonary Resuscitation

Termination of CPR and ALS measures may be considered in the prehospital setting in the following circumstances[17]:

- Trauma patients with an EMS-witnessed cardiopulmonary arrest and 15 minutes of unsuccessful resuscitation and CPR.
- Patients with traumatic cardiopulmonary arrest who would require transport longer than 15 minutes to reach an ED or trauma center.

Prolonged Transport

Although most urban or suburban EMS transports take 30 minutes or less, many prehospital care providers in rural and frontier settings routinely manage patients for much longer periods of time during transport. Additionally, providers are called on to manage patients during transfer from one medical facility to another, either by ground or air. These transfers may take up to several hours.

Special preparations need to be taken when prehospital care providers are involved in the prolonged transport of a trauma patient. The issues that must be considered before undertaking such a transport can be divided into those dealing with the patient, the prehospital crew, and equipment.

Patient Issues

Of preeminent importance is providing a safe, warm, and secure environment in which the patient is transported. The gurney should be appropriately secured to the ambulance, and the patient secured to the gurney. The patient should be secured in a position that allows maximum access to the patient, especially the injured areas. Before transport, the security of any airway devices placed must be assured, and

adjuncts (e.g., monitors, oxygen tanks) should be secured so that they do not become projectiles in the event that the ambulance has to swerve in an evasive action or is involved in a motor vehicle crash. Equipment should not rest on the patient, because pressure ulcers might be created during a prolonged transport. As emphasized throughout this text, hypothermia is a potentially deadly complication in a trauma patient, and the patient compartment must be sufficiently warm.

The patient should receive serial assessments of the primary survey and vital signs at routine intervals. The prehospital care providers accompanying the patient should be trained at a level appropriate to the anticipated needs of the patient. Critically injured patients should generally be managed by providers with advanced training.

Two management plans should be devised. The first, a medical plan, is developed to manage either anticipated or unexpected problems with the patient during transport. Necessary equipment, medications, and supplies should be readily available. The second plan involves identifying the most expeditious route to the receiving hospital. Weather conditions, road conditions (e.g., construction), and traffic concerns should be identified and anticipated. Additionally, the providers should be knowledgeable about the medical facilities along the transport route in case a problem arises that cannot be managed en route to the primary destination.

Crew

The safety of the EMS crew is as important as that of the patient. The prehospital crew needs to use appropriate safety devices, such as seat belts, and they should be secured during transport unless an issue involving patient care prevents this. The crew members use Standard Precautions and ensure that sufficient gloves and other personal protective equipment are available for the trip.

Equipment

Equipment issues during prolonged transport involve the ambulance, supplies, monitors, and communications. The ambulance must be in good working order, including an adequate amount of fuel and a spare tire. The crew must make sure that sufficient supplies are available and accessible for the transport, including gauze and pads for reinforcing dressings and oxygen. A good rule of thumb is to provision the ambulance with about 50% more supplies and medications than the anticipated need, in case a significant delay is encountered. Patient care equipment must be in good working order, including oxygen regulators and suction devices. Also, success of a prolonged transport may depend on functional communications, including the ability to communicate with other crew members, medical control, and the destination facility.

The management of specific injuries during prolonged transport is discussed in the subsequent corresponding chapters of this text.

SCENARIO 1 SOLUTION

Providing emergency medical care along roadsides ranks as one of the most dangerous situations encountered by prehospital care providers. Assessment of the scene reveals many potential hazards, the most apparent being the environmental conditions. Snow not only obscures vision, but also makes the roadway slippery and increases stopping distances. Lying on the ground in the cold and snow may predispose the patient to hypothermia. If this incident occurred at night, the darkness adds to the risk and makes it imperative that personnel wear reflective clothing. Law enforcement personnel are essential for traffic control along the scene. Fuel spills, chemical cargo, and other vehicle fluids may create a hazardous material situation. Fire department personnel can isolate or neutralize the fluids while monitoring the scene for fires that may erupt. In addition, a bloody patient exposes prehospital care personnel to the risks of bloodborne infections, and the caregivers should wear physical barriers, including gloves, masks, and eye protection.

SCENARIO 2 SOLUTION

You have been on the scene for 1 minute, yet you have obtained much important information to guide further assessment and treatment of the patient. In the first 15 seconds of patient contact, you have developed a general impression of the patient, determining that resuscitation is not necessary. With a few simple actions you have evaluated the A, B, C, and D of the initial assessment. The patient spoke to you without difficulty, indicating that his airway is open and he is breathing with no signs of distress. At the same time, with an awareness of the mechanism of injury, you have stabilized the cervical spine. You have noted no obvious bleeding, your partner has assessed the radial pulse, and you have observed the patient's skin color, temperature, and moisture. These findings indicate no immediate threats to the patient's circulatory status. Additionally, you have simultaneously found no initial evidence of disability because the patient is awake, is alert, and answers questions appropriately. This information, along with information about the fall, will help you determine the need for additional resources, the type of transportation indicated, and to what type of facility you should deliver the patient.

Now that you have completed these steps and no immediate lifesaving intervention is necessary, you will proceed with step E of the primary survey early in the evaluation process and then obtain vital signs. You will expose the patient to look for additional injuries and bleeding that may have been concealed by clothing, then cover the patient to protect him from the environment. During this process, you will perform a more detailed examination, noting less serious injuries. The next steps you will take are packaging the patient, including splinting the entire spine and extremity injuries and bandaging wounds if time allows; initiating transportation; and communicating with medical direction and the receiving facility. During the trip to the hospital, you will continue to reevaluate and monitor the patient. Your knowledge of kinematics and the patient's witnessed loss of consciousness will generate a high index of suspicion for traumatic brain injury, lower extremity injuries, and injuries to the spine. In an advanced life support (ALS) system, IV access will be established en route to the receiving facility.

SUMMARY

- It is important to assess for hazards of all types as a part of assessing the scene for provider safety in each and every patient contact. Hazards include traffic issues, environmental concerns, violence, bloodborne pathogens, and hazardous materials.

- Assessing the scene will ensure that provider personnel and equipment are not compromised and unavailable for others and ensure that other health care professionals are protected from hazards that are not isolated or removed.

- Sometimes hazards will be ruled out quickly, but if they are not looked for, they won't be seen, and this is what can cause harm.
- Certain situations, such as crime scenes or intentional acts including the use of weapons of mass destruction, will affect how the provider deals with the scene and the patients at that scene.
- Incidents will be managed using an Incident Command System structure, and EMS is one of the components in that structure. Providers must know and understand the ICS system and their role within that system.
- Chances of survival for a patient with traumatic injuries depend on the immediate identification and mitigation of conditions that interfere with tissue perfusion.
- The identification of these conditions requires a systematic, prioritized, logical process of collecting information and acting on it. This process is referred to as *patient assessment*.
- Patient assessment begins with scene assessment and includes the formation of a general impression of the patient, a primary survey, and, when the patient's condition and availability of additional EMS personnel permit, a secondary survey.
- The information obtained through this process is analyzed and used as the basis for patient care and transport decisions.

- In the care of the trauma patient, a missed problem is a missed opportunity to aid potentially in an individual's survival.
- After the simultaneous determination of scene safety and general impression of the situation, the focus is on the priorities of patient assessment: the patency of the patient's airway, the ventilatory status, and the circulatory status. This primary survey follows the ABCDE format for evaluation of the patient's airway, breathing, circulation, disability (initial neurologic examination), and exposure (removing the patient's clothing to discover additional significant injuries). Although the sequential nature of language limits the ability to describe the simultaneity of these actions, the primary survey of the patient is a process of actions that occur essentially at the same time.
- Immediate threats to the patient's life are quickly corrected in a "find and fix" manner. Once the provider manages the patient's airway and breathing and controls exsanguinating hemorrhage, he or she packages the patient and begins transportation without additional treatment at the scene. The limitations of field management of trauma require the safe, expedient delivery of the patient to definitive care.

References

1. Maguire BJ, Hunting KL, Smith GS, Levick NR: Occupational fatalities in emergency medical services, *Ann Emerg Med* 40(6):625, 2002.
2. National Highway Traffic and Safety Administration: Traffic safety facts, 2003, www.nrd.nhtsa.dot.gov/pdf/nrd-30/NCSA/TSFAAnn/2003/cov2.htm.
3. Schaeffer J: Prevent run downs: best practices for roadside incident management, 2002, www.jems.com/jems/news02/0903a.html (accessed September 2002).
4. Poland GA, Jacobson RM: Prevention of hepatitis B with the hepatitis B vaccine, *N Engl J Med* 351:2832, 2004.
5. Georgia Emergency Management Agency: Surviving weapons of mass destruction, www.ojp.usdoj.gov/odp/docs/video.htm.
6. Georgia Emergency Management Agency, Department of Justice Bureau of Justice Assistance: Surviving the secondary device: the rules have changed, www.ojp.usdoj.gov/odp/docs/video.htm.
7. Lerner EB, Schwartz RB, Coule PL, et al: Mass casualty triage: an evaluation of the data and development of a proposed national guideline, *Disaster Med Public Health Preparedness*, 2:S25–S34, 2008.
8. Advanced Trauma Life Support (ATLS) Subcommittee, Committee on Trauma: Initial assessment and management. In *Advanced trauma life support course for doctors, student course manual*, ed 7, Chicago, 2004, ACS.
9. Kragh JF, Littrel ML, Jones JA, et al: Battle casualty survival with emergency tourniquet use to stop limb bleeding, *J Emerg Med*, 2009, epub ahead of publication.
10. Beekley AC, Sebesta JA, Blackbourne LH, et al: Prehospital tourniquet use in Operation Iraqi Freedom: effect on hemorrhage control and outcomes, *J Trauma* 64:S28–S37, 2008.
11. Doyle GS, Taillac PP: Tourniquets: a review of current use with proposals for expanded prehospital use, *Prehosp Emerg Care* 12:241–256, 2008.
12. First Aid Science Advisory Board: First aid, *Circulation* 112(III):115, 2005.
13. Swan KG Jr, Wright DS, Barbagiovanni SS, et al: Tourniquets revisited, *J Trauma* 66:672–675, 2009.
14. Teasdale G, Jennett B: Assessment of coma and impaired consciousness: a practical scale, *Lancet* 2:81, 1974.
15. Healey C, Osler TM, Rogers FB, et al: Improving the Glasgow Coma Scale score: motor score alone is a better predictor, *J Trauma* 54:671, 2003.
16. Committee on Trauma: *Resources for optimal care of the injured patient: 1999*, Chicago, 1998, American College of Surgeons.
17. Hopson LR, Hirsh E, Delgado J, et al: Guidelines for withholding or termination of resuscitation in prehospital traumatic cardiopulmonary arrest, *Prehosp Emerg Care* 7:141, 2003.
18. American Heart Association: 2010 guidelines for cardiopulmonary resuscitation and emergency cardiovascular care, Part 12: Cardiac Arrest in Special Situations, *Circulation* 22: S829–S861, 2010.

Suggested Reading

Centers for Disease Control and Prevention: See website for information on Standard Precautions and postexposure prophylaxis, www.cdc.gov.

Rinnert KJ: A review of infection control practices, risk reduction, and legislative regulations for blood-borne disease: applications for emergency medical services, *Prehosp Emerg Care* 2(1):70, 1998.

Rinnert KJ, O'Connor RE, Delbridge T: Risk reduction for exposure to blood-borne pathogens in EMS: National Association of EMS Physicians, *Prehosp Emerg Care* 2(1):62, 1998.

CHAPTER 4

Airway and Breathing

CHAPTER OBJECTIVES

At the completion of this chapter, the reader will be able to do the following:

✓ Integrate the principles of breathing and gas exchange with the pathophysiology of trauma.

✓ Relate the role of oxygen to the pathophysiology of trauma.

✓ Explain the mechanisms by which supplemental oxygen and ventilatory support are beneficial to the trauma patient.

✓ Given a scenario that involves a trauma patient, select the most effective means of providing a patent airway to suit the needs of the patient.

✓ Given a scenario that involves a patient who requires ventilatory support, select the most effective means available to suit the needs of the trauma patient.

✓ Given situations that involve various trauma patients, formulate a plan for airway management and ventilation.

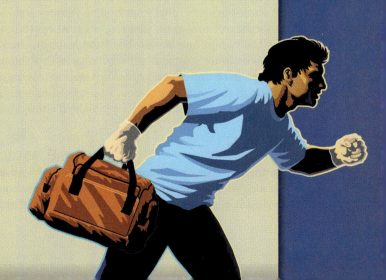

SCENARIO

You and your partner are dispatched to a pedestrian who has been hit by a motor vehicle. You find that your patient has been thrown about 30 feet from the point of impact. The car has damage to the grill and a spider web mark on the windshield. The driver of the car is out of the vehicle, standing by his car. The pedestrian is being attended to by a police officer who is maintaining an open airway for the patient. The patient looks to be in his thirties, weighing around 280 pounds (125 kg). The officer reports that since her arrival the patient has been unconscious. You note bleeding from the scalp, the nose, and ear canals, bruising around both orbits, and an angulated right femur. You also note that the patient is making snoring sounds with each breath that he takes and that his breathing pattern is irregular. You are within 8 minutes of the local trauma center by ground.

What indicators of airway compromise are evident in this patient?

What other information, if any, would you seek from witnesses or the first responders?

Describe the sequence of actions you would take to manage this patient before and during transport.

Airway management and the support of breathing play a prominent role in the management of trauma patients. Its importance is recognized now even more than in years past. The failure to maintain adequate oxygen levels (oxygenation) and breathing (ventilation) causes secondary injury to the brain and other organs, compounding the primary injury produced by the initial trauma. Ensuring an open, clear airway and maintaining the patient's oxygenation and supporting ventilation, when necessary, are critical steps in minimizing the overall injury sustained by the patient and improving the likelihood of good outcome.

Oxygenation of the brain and oxygen delivery to other parts of the body provided by adequate airway management and ventilation remain the most important components of prehospital patient care. Because techniques and adjunct devices for managing the airway are changing and will continue to change, keeping abreast of these changes is important.

The respiratory system serves two primary functions, as follows:

1. The system provides oxygen to the red blood cells, which carry the oxygen to all the cells in the body.
2. The system removes carbon dioxide (CO_2), a waste product of metabolism, from the body.

Inability of the respiratory system to provide oxygen to the cells or inability of the cells to use the oxygen supplied results in *anaerobic (without oxygen) metabolism* and can quickly lead to death. Failure to eliminate CO_2 can lead to coma.

Anatomy

The respiratory system is composed of the upper airway and the lower airway, including the lungs (Figure 4-1). Each part of the system plays an important role in ensuring gas exchange, the process by which oxygen enters the bloodstream and CO_2 is removed.

Upper Airway

The upper airway consists of the nasal cavity and the oral cavity (Figure 4-2). Air entering the nasal cavity is warmed, humidified, and filtered to remove larger particles and other impurities. Beyond these cavities is the area known as the pharynx, which runs from the back of the soft palate to the upper end of the esophagus. The pharynx is composed of muscle lined with mucous membranes. The pharynx is divided into three discrete sections: the nasopharynx (upper portion), the oropharynx (middle portion), and the hypopharynx (lower or distal end of the pharynx). Below the pharynx are the esophagus, which leads to the stomach, and the trachea, at which point the lower airway begins. The entrance to the trachea is the larynx (Figure 4-3), which contains the vocal cords, and the muscles that make them work, housed in a strong "box" made of stiff cartilage. The vocal cords are folds of tissue that move in response to breathing and speaking. Directly above the larynx is a leaf-shaped structure called the *epiglottis*. Acting as a gate or flapper valve, the epiglottis directs air into the trachea and solids and liquids into the esophagus.

Lower Airway

The lower airway consists of the trachea, its branches, and the lungs. On inspiration, air travels through the upper airway and into the lower airway before reaching the alveoli, where the actual gas exchange occurs. The trachea divides into the right and left *mainstem bronchi*. Each of the mainstem bronchi subdivides into several primary bronchi and then into bronchioles. *Bronchioles* (very small bronchial tubes) terminate at the *alveoli*, which are tiny air sacs surrounded by capillaries. The alveoli are the site of gas exchange where the respiratory and circulatory systems meet.

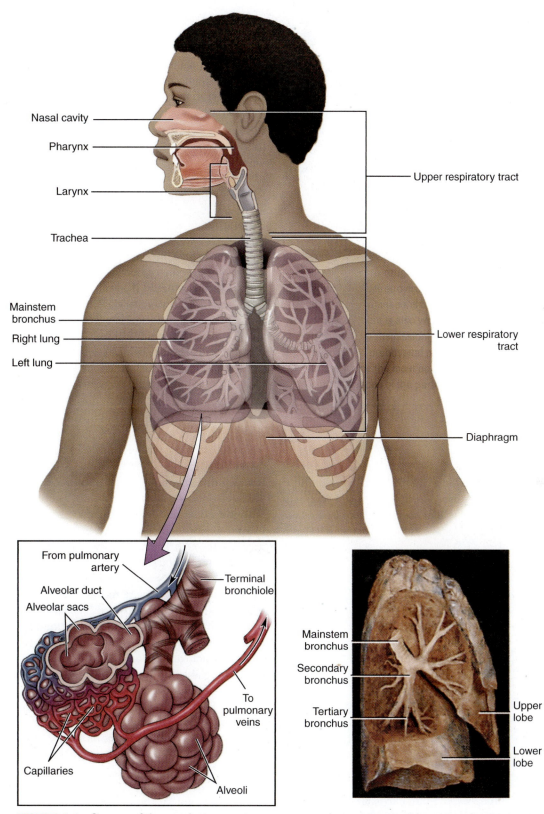

FIGURE 4-1 Organs of the respiratory system: upper respiratory tract and lower respiratory tract. (Modified from Herlihy B, Maebius WK: *The human body in health and disease,* Philadelphia, 2000, Saunders.)

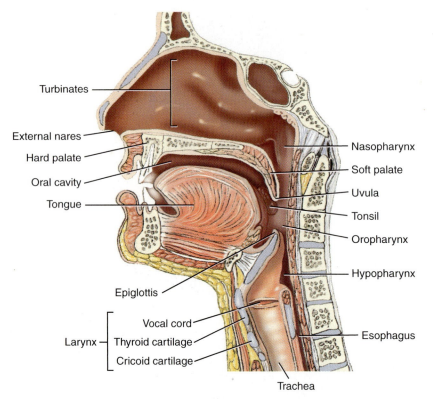

FIGURE 4-2 Sagittal section through the nasal cavity and pharynx viewed from the medial side.

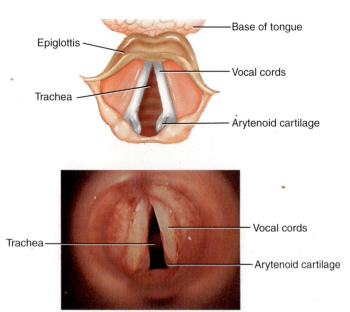

FIGURE 4-3 Vocal cords viewed from above, showing their relationship to the paired cartilages of the larynx and the epiglottis.
(*Bottom,* Custom Medical Stock photo, modified from Thibodeau GA: *Structure and function,* ed 9, St Louis, 1992, Mosby.)

Physiology

The airway is a pathway that leads air through the nose, mouth, pharynx, trachea, and bronchi to the alveoli in the lung. With each breath the average adult takes in approximately 500 mL of air. The airway system holds up to 150 mL of air that never actually reaches the alveoli to participate in the critical gas exchange process. The space in which this air is held is known as *dead space.* The air inside this dead space is not available to the body to be used for oxygenation because it never reaches the alveoli.

With each breath, air is drawn into the lungs. When air reaches the alveoli, oxygen moves from the alveoli, across the alveolar–capillary membrane, and into the red blood cells (RBCs). The circulatory system then delivers the oxygen-carrying RBCs to the body tissues, where oxygen is used in the process of cellular metabolism.

As oxygen is transferred from inside the alveoli to the RBCs, CO_2 is exchanged in the opposite direction, from the plasma to the alveoli. Carbon dioxide, which is carried in the plasma, not in the RBCs, moves from the bloodstream, across the alveolar-capillary membrane, and into the alveoli, where it is eliminated during exhalation (Figure 4-4). On completion of this exchange, the oxygenated RBCs and plasma

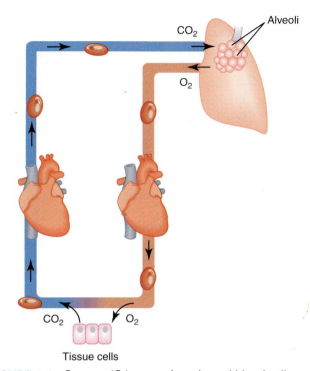

FIGURE 4-4 Oxygen (O_2) moves into the red blood cells from the alveoli. The O_2 is transferred to the tissue cell on the hemoglobin molecule. After leaving the hemoglobin molecule, the O_2 travels into the tissue cell. Carbon dioxide (CO_2) travels in the reverse direction, but not on the hemoglobin molecule. It travels in the plasma as CO_2.

with a low CO_2 level return to the left side of the heart to be pumped to all the cells in the body.

Once at the cell, the oxygenated RBCs deliver their oxygen, which the cells then use for aerobic metabolism. Carbon dioxide, a by-product of aerobic metabolism, is released into the blood plasma. Deoxygenated blood returns to the right side of the heart. The blood is pumped to the lungs, where it is again supplied with oxygen, and the CO_2 is eliminated by diffusion.

The alveoli must be constantly replenished with a fresh supply of air that contains an adequate amount of oxygen. This replenishment of air, known as *ventilation,* is essential for the elimination of CO_2. Ventilation is measurable. The size of each breath, called the *tidal volume,* multiplied by the ventilatory rate for 1 minute equals the *minute volume:*

Minute volume =

Tidal volume × Ventilatory rate per minute

During normal resting ventilation, about 500 mL of air is taken into the lungs. As mentioned previously, part of this volume, 150 mL, remains in the airway system as dead space and does not participate in gas exchange. If the tidal volume

is 500 mL and the ventilatory rate is 14 breaths/minute, the minute volume can be calculated as follows:

Minute volume = 500 mL × 14 breaths/minute

Minute volume = 7000 mL/minute, or 7 L/minute

Therefore, at rest, about 7 L of air must move in and out of the lungs each minute to maintain adequate CO_2 elimination and oxygenation. If the minute volume falls below normal, the patient has inadequate ventilation, a condition called *hypoventilation.* Hypoventilation leads to a buildup of CO_2 in the body. Hypoventilation is common when head or chest trauma causes an altered breathing pattern or an inability to move the chest wall adequately. For example, a patient with rib fractures who is breathing quickly and shallowly because of the pain of the injury may have a tidal volume of 100 mL and a ventilatory rate of 40 breaths/minute. This patient's minute volume can be calculated as follows:

Minute volume = 100 mL × 40 breaths/minute

Minute volume = 4000 mL/minute, or 4 L/minute

If 7 L/minute is necessary for adequate gas exchange in a nontraumatized person at rest, 4 L/minute is much less than what the body requires to eliminate CO_2 effectively, indicating hypoventilation. Furthermore, 150 mL of air is necessary to overcome dead space. If tidal volume is 100 mL, oxygenated air will never reach the alveoli. If left untreated, this hypoventilation will quickly lead to severe distress and ultimately death.

In the previous example, the patient is hypoventilating even though the ventilatory rate is 40 breaths/minute. Evaluating a patient's ability to exchange air involves assessing both ventilatory rate and depth. A common mistake is assuming that any patient with a fast ventilatory rate is hyperventilating. Assessment of ventilatory function always includes an evaluation of how well a patient is taking in, diffusing, and delivering oxygen. Without proper intake and processing of oxygen, anaerobic metabolism will begin. In addition, effective ventilation must also be assured. A patient may accomplish ventilation completely, partially, or not at all. Aggressive assessment and management of these inadequacies in both oxygenation and ventilation are paramount to a successful outcome.

Oxygenation and Ventilation of the Trauma Patient

The oxygenation process within the human body involves the following three phases:

1. *External respiration* is the transfer of oxygen (O_2) molecules from the atmosphere to the blood. Air contains

21% oxygen with most of the remainder made up of nitrogen. When supplemental oxygen is provided, the percent of oxygen in each inspiration increases, causing an increase in the amount of oxygen in each alveolus.

2. *Oxygen delivery* is the result of O_2 transfer from the atmosphere to the RBC during ventilation and the transportation of these RBCs to the tissues via the cardiovascular system. This process primarily involves the heart pumping an adequate number of red blood cells which contain hemoglobin to carry the oxygen.

   One could describe the RBCs as the body's "oxygen tankers." These tankers move along the vascular system "highways" to "off-load" their O_2 supply at the body's distribution points, the capillary beds.

3. *Internal (cellular) respiration* is the movement, or diffusion, of oxygen from the RBCs into the tissue cells. Cellular metabolism normally produces energy. Because the actual exchange of oxygen between the RBCs and the tissues occurs in the thin-walled capillaries, any factor that interrupts a supply of oxygen will disrupt this cycle. Supplemental oxygen can help overcome some of these factors. The tissues cannot consume adequate oxygen if adequate amounts are not available.

Adequate oxygenation depends on all three of these phases. Although the ability to assess tissue oxygenation in prehospital situations is improving rapidly, appropriate ventilatory support for all trauma patients begins by providing supplemental oxygen to help ensure that hypoxia is corrected or averted entirely.

Pathophysiology

Trauma can affect the respiratory system's ability to adequately provide oxygen and eliminate carbon dioxide in the following ways:

1. Hypoventilation can result from loss of ventilatory drive, usually because of decreased neurologic function, most often after a traumatic brain injury.
2. Hypoventilation can result from obstruction of airflow through the upper and lower airways.
3. Hypoventilation can be caused by decreased expansion of the lungs.
4. *Hypoxemia* (decreased oxygen level in the blood) can result from decreased diffusion of oxygen across the alveolar–capillary membrane.
5. *Hypoxia* (deficient tissue oxygenation) can be caused by decreased blood flow to the alveoli.
6. Hypoxia can result from the inability of the air to reach the capillaries, usually because the alveoli are filled with fluid or debris.
7. Hypoxia can be caused by decreased blood flow to the tissue cells.

The first three ways involve hypoventilation as a result of the reduction of minute volume. If left untreated, hypoventilation results in CO_2 buildup, acid buildup, and eventually death.

Management involves improving the patient's ventilatory rate and depth by correcting existing airway problems and assisting ventilation as appropriate.

The following sections discuss the first two causes of inadequate ventilation: decreased neurologic function and mechanical obstruction. These two problems must be recognized by the trauma first responder and corrected in order to minimize complications arising from inadequate oxygenation.

Decreased Neurologic Function

Decreased minute volume can be caused by two clinical conditions related to decreased neurologic function: flaccidity of the tongue and a decreased level of consciousness (LOC).

Flaccidity of the tongue associated with a reduced LOC allows the tongue to fall into a dependent position (toward the lowest area of the body). If a patient is supine, the base of the tongue will fall backward and occlude the hypopharynx (Figure 4-5). This complication commonly presents as snoring with respirations. To prevent the tongue from occluding the hypopharynx or correct the problem when it occurs, maintaining an open airway must be assured in any supine patient with a diminished LOC, regardless of whether signs of ventilatory compromise exist. Such patients may also require periodic suctioning because secretions, saliva, blood, or vomitus may accumulate in the oropharynx. A decreased LOC will also affect ventilatory drive and may reduce the rate of ventilation, the volume of ventilation, or both. This reduction in minute volume may be temporary or permanent.

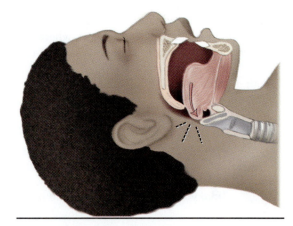

FIGURE 4-5 In an unconscious patient the tongue has lost its muscle tone and falls back into the hypopharnyx, occluding the airway and preventing passage of oxygen into the trachea and lungs.

Mechanical Obstruction

Another cause of decreased minute volume is mechanical airway obstruction. The source of these obstructions may be neurologically influenced or purely mechanical in nature. Neurologic insults that alter the LOC may disrupt the "controls" that normally hold the tongue in an anatomically neutral (nonobstructing) position. If these "controls" are compromised, the tongue falls rearward, occluding the hypopharynx (see Figure 4-5).

Foreign bodies in the airway may be objects that were in the patient's mouth at the time of the injury, such as dentures, chewing gum, tobacco, real teeth, and bone. Outside materials, such as glass from a broken windshield or any object that is near the patient's mouth on injury, may also threaten airway patency. Upper and lower airway obstructions may also be caused by bone or cartilage collapse as a result of a fractured larynx or trachea, by mucous membrane avulsed from the hypopharynx or tongue, or by facial damage in which blood and fragments of bone and tissue create an obstruction.

Management of mechanical airway obstructions can be extremely challenging. Foreign bodies in the oral cavity may become lodged and create occlusions in the hypopharynx or the larynx. Crush injuries to the larynx and edema of the vocal cords may be present. Patients with facial injuries present with two of the most common foreign body obstructions, blood and vomit. Treatment of these problems is aimed at immediate recognition of the obstruction and the steps taken to ensure airway patency.

Assessment of the Airway and Ventilation

The ability to assess the airway is required in order to effectively manage it. Many aspects of assessing the airway are done without even thinking about them. A patient who is alert and talking to us as we walk through the door has an open and clear airway. But when the patients' level of consciousness is decreased it is essential to thoroughly assess the airway prior to moving to other injuries. When examining the airway during the primary survey the following need to be assessed.

Positioning of the Airway and Patient

As you make visual contact with the patient you observe the position of the patient. Patients in a supine position are at risk for airway obstruction from the tongue falling back into the airway. Most trauma patients will be placed in the supine position on a backboard for spinal immobilization. Any patient exhibiting signs of decreased level of consciousness will need constant re-examination for airway obstruction and the placement of an adjunctive device such as a nasopharyngeal (NPA) or oropharyngeal (OPA) airway to ensure an open airway. Patients who present with an open airway while lying on their side may obstruct their airways when placed supine on a backboard. Patients with facial trauma and active bleeding may need to be maintained in the position that they are found if they are maintaining their own airway. Placing these patients supine on a backboard may cause obstruction to the airway and possible aspiration of blood. In these cases, if patients are maintaining their own airway, the best course of action may be to let them continue.

Any Sounds Emanating from the Upper Airway

Noise coming from the upper airway is never a good sign. These noises, such as snoring or gurgling, can often be heard as you approach the patient. These noises are usually a result of a partial airway obstruction caused by either the tongue, vomit or blood, or foreign bodies in the upper airway. Steps must be taken immediately to alleviate the obstructions and maintain an open airway.

Examine the Airway for Obstructions

Look in the mouth for any obvious foreign matter or any gross anatomical malformations. Remove foreign bodies found.

Look for Chest Rise

Limited chest rise as the patient breaths may be a sign of an obstructed airway. The use of accessory muscles (the patient is straining to breath) and the appearance of increased work of breathing may lead to a high index of suspicion of airway compromise.

Listen for Abnormal Breathing Sounds

A wheezing sound while the patient breaths in is called stridor and points to a partially obstructed upper airway. This obstruction may be an anatomical obstruction, such as the tongue, that has fallen back into the airway, or it may be a swollen (edematous) epiglottis or airway. Stridor may also be caused by foreign bodies. An edematous or swollen airway is an emergent situation that demands quick action to prevent total airway obstruction.

Selection of Adjunctive Device

If any problems are found with the airway during the primary survey, the provider needs to take immediate action to establish and maintain an open airway. Once a basic airway has been established using manual maneuvers such as a trauma jaw thrust, it is necessary to use an adjunctive device to maintain the airway in an open position. The particular device should be selected based on the provider's level of training and proficiency with that particular device. This should then be calculated into a risk–benefit analysis for the use of various types of devices and techniques that may be needed for this particular patient. The choice of the airway adjunct should be patient-driven. That is, the provider should ask, "What is the best airway for this particular patient in this particular situation?" The more times a skill is performed, the better the chance for a successful outcome. Careful evaluation of the airway prior to selecting the airway adjunct for any particular patient is essential to the best possible patient outcome.

Management

Airway Control

Ensuring a clear and open airway is the first priority of trauma management and resuscitation, and no action is more crucial in airway management than appropriate assessment of the airway (Figure 4-6). Whenever the airway is managed, the possibility of a cervical spine injury must always be considered. The use of any of method of airway control requires simultaneous manual stabilization of the cervical spine in a neutral position until the patient has been completely immobilized (see Chapter 6).

Essential Skills

Management of the airway in trauma patients takes precedence over all other procedures because without an adequate airway, a positive outcome cannot be achieved. Management of the airway can be challenging, but in most patients, basic procedures may be sufficient initially and are often all that is needed to maintain adequate oxygenation.[1]

Manual Clearing of the Airway. The first step in airway management is a quick visual inspection of the oropharyngeal cavity. Foreign material (e.g., pieces of food) or broken teeth and blood may be found in the mouth of a trauma patient. These are swept out of the mouth using a gloved finger or, in the case of blood or vomitus, may be suctioned away. In addition, positioning of the patient on the side, when not contraindicated by possible spinal trauma, will allow for gravity-assisted clearing of secretions, blood, and vomitus.

Manual Maneuvers. In unresponsive patients the tongue becomes flaccid, falling back and blocking the hypopharynx (see Figure 4-5). The tongue is the most common cause of

airway obstruction. Manual methods to clear this type of obstruction can easily be accomplished because the tongue is attached to the mandible (jaw) and moves forward with it. Any maneuver that moves the mandible forward will pull the tongue out of the hypopharynx:

- *Trauma jaw thrust.* In patients with suspected head, neck, or facial trauma, spine injury is also always suspected, and the cervical spine is maintained in a neutral inline position. The trauma jaw-thrust maneuver allows the prehospital care provider to open the airway with little or no movement of the head and cervical spine (Figure 4-7). The mandible is thrust forward by placing the thumbs on each zygoma (cheekbone), placing the index and long fingers on the mandible (jaw), and, at the same angle, pushing the mandible forward.
- *Trauma chin lift.* The trauma chin-lift maneuver is used to relieve a variety of anatomic airway obstructions in patients who are breathing spontaneously (Figure 4-8). The chin and lower incisors are grasped and then lifted to pull the mandible forward. The prehospital care provider wears gloves to avoid body fluid contamination.

Both these techniques result in movement of the lower mandible anteriorly (upward) and slightly caudal (toward the feet), pulling the tongue forward, away from the posterior airway, and opening the mouth. The trauma jaw thrust pushes the mandible forward, whereas the trauma chin lift pulls the mandible. The trauma jaw thrust and the trauma chin lift are modifications of the conventional jaw thrust and chin lift. The modifications provide protection to the patient's cervical spine while opening the airway by displacing the tongue from the posterior pharynx.

Suctioning. A trauma patient may not be capable of effectively clearing the buildup of secretions, vomitus, blood, or foreign

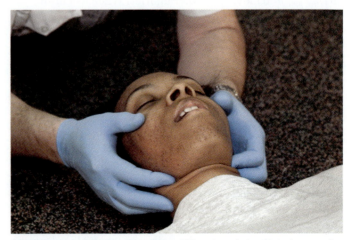

FIGURE 4-7 Trauma jaw thrust. The thumb is placed on each zygoma (cheekbone) with the index and long fingers at the angle of the mandible (jaw). The mandible is lifted superiorly.

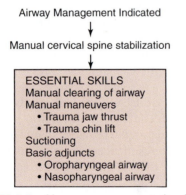

Airway Management Indicated

↓

Manual cervical spine stabilization

↓

ESSENTIAL SKILLS
Manual clearing of airway
Manual maneuvers
  • Trauma jaw thrust
  • Trauma chin lift
Suctioning
Basic adjuncts
  • Oropharyngeal airway
  • Nasopharyngeal airway

FIGURE 4-6 Airway management algorithm.

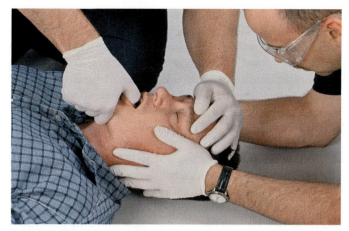

FIGURE 4-8 Trauma chin lift. The chin lift performs a function similar to that of the trauma jaw thrust. It moves the mandible forward by moving the tongue.

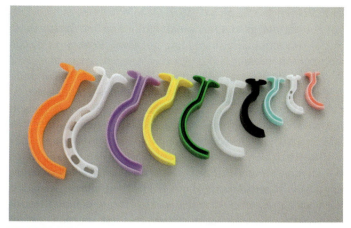

FIGURE 4-9 Oropharyngeal airways.
(From McSwain NE Jr, Paturas JL: *The basic EMT: comprehensive prehospital patient care,* ed 2, St Louis, 2001, Mosby.)

objects from the trachea. Providing suction is an important part of maintaining a clear airway.

The most significant complication of suctioning is that suctioning for prolonged periods will produce low oxygen levels in the blood (hypoxemia), which may manifest as a cardiac abnormality (e.g., tachycardia). Preoxygenation of the trauma patient by providing supplemental oxygen will help prevent hypoxemia. In addition, during an extended period of suctioning, irregular heart rhythms may occur from hypoxemia and lead to hypoxia of the heart or stimulation of the vagus nerve secondary to tracheal irritation. Vagal nerve stimulation may lead to profound bradycardia (slow heart rate) and hypotension.

The trauma patient may require aggressive suctioning of the upper airway. Much larger amounts of blood and vomit may be in the airway on the arrival of emergency medical services (EMS) than a suction unit can quickly clear. If so, the patient may be rolled onto his or her side while maintaining cervical spine stabilization; gravity will then assist in clearing the airway. A rigid suction device is preferred to clear the oropharynx. Although hypoxia can result from prolonged suctioning, a totally obstructed airway will provide no air exchange. Aggressive suctioning and patient positioning are done until the airway is at least partially clear. At that point, hyperoxygenation followed by repeated suctioning can be performed. Hyperoxygenation, like pre-oxygenation, may be accomplished with either a non-rebreather mask on a high flow of supplemental oxygen or with a bag-mask device that has oxygen attached and flowing at 15 LPM.

Basic Adjuncts. When manual airway maneuvers are unsuccessful or when continued maintenance of an open airway is necessary, the use of an artificial airway is the next step.

Oropharyngeal Airway. The most frequently used artificial airway is the oropharyngeal airway (OPA) (Figure 4-9). The OPA

is inserted in either a direct or an inverted manner. (See skills section at the end of this chapter for detailed step-by-step instructions.)

Indications
■ Patient who is unable to maintain his or her airway

Contraindications
■ Patient who is conscious or semiconscious

Complications
■ Because it stimulates the gag reflex, use of the OPA may lead to gagging, vomiting, and laryngospasm in patients who are conscious.

Nasopharyngeal Airway. The nasopharyngeal airway (NPA) is a soft, rubberlike device that is inserted through one of the nares and then along the curvature of the posterior wall of the nasopharynx and oropharynx (Figure 4-10). (See skills section at the end of this chapter for detailed step-by-step instructions.)

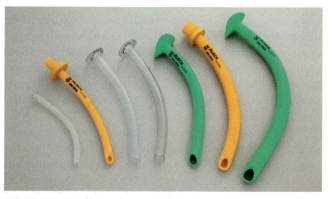

FIGURE 4-10 Nasopharyngeal airways.
(From McSwain NE Jr, Paturas JL: *The basic EMT: comprehensive prehospital patient care,* ed 2, St Louis, 2001, Mosby.)

Indications
- Patient who is unable to maintain his or her airway

Contraindications
- No need for an airway adjunct

Complications
- Bleeding caused by insertion may be a complication.

Ventilatory Devices

All trauma patients should receive appropriate ventilatory support with supplemental oxygen to ensure that hypoxia is corrected or averted entirely. In deciding which method or equipment to use, prehospital care providers should consider the following devices and their respective oxygen concentrations (Figure 4-11).

Pocket Masks

Regardless of which mask is chosen to support ventilation of the trauma patient, the ideal mask has the following characteristics:

1. A good fit
2. Equipped with a one-way valve
3. Made of a transparent material

FIGURE 4-11   Ventilatory Devices and Oxygen Concentration Delivered

Device	Liter Flow (L/Minute)	Oxygen Concentration*
WITHOUT SUPPLEMENTAL OXYGEN		
Mouth-to-mouth	N/A	16%
Mouth-to-mask	N/A	16%
Bag-mask	N/A	21%
WITH SUPPLEMENTAL OXYGEN		
Nasal cannula	1–6	24%–45%
Mouth-to-mask	10	50%
Simple face mask	8–10	40%–60%
Bag-mask without reservoir	8–10	40%–60%
Bag-mask with reservoir	10–15	90%–100%
Nonrebreather mask with reservoir	10–15	90%–100%
Demand valve	N/A	90%–100%
Ventilator	N/A	21%–100%

*Percentages indicated are approximate.
N/A, Not applicable.

4. Has a supplemental oxygen port
5. Available in infant, pediatric, and adult sizes

Mouth-to-mask ventilation satisfactorily delivers adequate tidal volumes by ensuring a tight face seal even when performed by those who do not use this skill often.

Bag-mask Device

The bag-mask device consists of a self-inflating bag and a non-rebreathing device; it can be used with basic (OPA, NPA) or advanced (endotracheal, nasotracheal) airway devices. Most bag-mask devices currently on the market have a volume of 1600 mL and can deliver an O_2 concentration of 90% to 100%. However, a *single* provider attempting to ventilate with a bag-mask may create poor tidal volumes secondary to the inability to create a tight face seal and to squeeze the bag adequately. Ongoing practice of this skill is necessary to ensure that the technique is effective and that the trauma patient receives adequate ventilatory support. (See the skills section at the end of this chapter for detailed step-by-step instructions.)

Regardless of which device is used, it is important to carefully control the rate at which breathes are delivered to the patient. For adults, the rate should be approximately 10 to 12 breaths per minute, and for children 20 per minute. One of the most common errors made in managing patients is to ventilate them too quickly. Hyperventilation has some very serious complications. When a patient is hyperventilated, the CO_2 level in the blood is decreased. This causes the blood vessels, particularly those in the brain, to constrict and thus decrease blood and oxygen delivery. This can cause a secondary injury. In addition, ventilations that are delivered too quickly do not allow enough time for air to exit the lungs, thus causing a buildup of pressure inside the lungs. This leads to decreased blood flow through the heart, again compromising the delivery of oxygen to the rest of the body.

Prolonged Transport

Airway management of a patient before and during a prolonged transport requires complex decision making on the part of the prehospital care provider. Intervention to control and secure the airway, especially with advanced techniques, depends on numerous factors, including the patient's injuries, the clinical skills of the prehospital care provider, the equipment available, and the distance and transport time to definitive care. Involvement of advanced level providers can help assess the risks and benefits of all the airway options available before making a final airway decision. For transports of 15 to 20 minutes, essential skills, including an oral airway and bag-mask ventilation, may be sufficient.

Any patient requiring airway management or ventilatory support requires ongoing patient monitoring. Serial vital signs should also be recorded on patients requiring airway or ventilation interventions.

SCENARIO SOLUTION

Physical evidence at the scene suggests that the pedestrian has likely been subjected to kinetic forces capable of creating life-threatening injuries. The position of the patient suggests that multiple impacts have occurred.

The patient exhibits several signs of airway compromise and ventilatory insufficiency. His ventilations are sonorous and irregular, he has an altered level of consciousness, and he requires frequent suctioning. Bleeding from the nares and ears and the early presence of "raccoon eyes" strongly suggest the presence of a basilar skull fracture. The primary survey indicates a rapidly deteriorating patient who requires aggressive airway care and rapid transport.

You immediately suction his airway and place an OPA. You then administer oxygen with ventilatory assistance using a bag-mask without difficulty. Continue ventilatory support and cervical spine stabilization while further assessing the airway. Be careful to ensure that the airway remains clear and that manual ventilations are effective.

You decide that because of the 4-minute transport time, along with the ease in which bag-mask ventilations are being administered, that you will manage the patient's airway and breathing with the bag-mask device and the OPA.

Take care to maintain the effectiveness of immobilization efforts and frequently reassess the patient's condition. To ensure proper activation of the receiving facility's trauma response, notify the trauma center during transport. On arrival at the trauma center, concisely convey all pertinent information regarding the incident, the patient, and medical interventions to the receiving physician or other appropriate trauma team member. ■

SUMMARY

The trauma patient is susceptible to various injuries that may impair ventilation and gas exchange. Trauma to the chest, airway obstruction, central nervous system injury, and hemorrhage can all result in inadequate tissue perfusion. Proper care for the trauma patient requires that the provider understands or has the following abilities:

- Integrate the principles of ventilation and gas exchange with the pathophysiology of trauma
- Relate the concepts of minute volume and oxygenation to the pathophysiology of trauma
- Explain the mechanisms by which supplemental oxygen and ventilatory support are beneficial to the trauma patient

- Given situations that involve various trauma patients, formulate a plan for airway management and ventilation
- Given current research, understand the risks versus benefits when discussing new invasive procedures
- Given a scenario, can develop a plan for airway management on a given patient in a given location

Managing the airway is not without risks. When applying certain skills and modalities the risk has to be weighed against the potential benefit in that particular patient. What may be the best choice for one patient in a certain situation may not be for another with a similar presentation. Sound critical thinking skills need to be in place to make the best judgments for the trauma patient.

Reference

1. Stockinger ZT, McSwain NE Jr: Prehospital endotracheal intubation for trauma does not improve survival over bag-mask ventilation, *J Trauma* 56(3):531, 2004.

Suggested Reading

American College of Surgeons Committee on Trauma: *Advanced trauma life support for doctors, student course manual*, ed 8, Chicago, 2008, ACS.

Brainard C: Whose tube is it? *JEMS* 31:62, 2006.

Dunford JV, David DP, Ochs M, et al: The incidence of transient hypoxia and heart rate reactivity during paramedic rapid sequence intubation, *Ann Emerg Med* 42:721, 2003.

Soubani AO: Noninvasive monitoring of oxygen and carbon dioxide, *Am J Emerg Med* 19:141, 2001.

Walls RM, Murphy MF (eds): *Manual of Emergency Airway Management*, ed 3, Philadelphia, 2008, Lippincott Williams & Wilkins/Wolters Kluwer Health.

Weitzel N, Kendal J, Pons P: Blind nasotracheal intubation for patients with penetrating neck trauma, *J Trauma* 56(5):1097, 2004.

SPECIFIC SKILLS

Airway Management and Ventilation Skills

Trauma Jaw Thrust

Principle: To open the airway without moving the cervical spine.

In both the trauma jaw thrust and the trauma chin lift, manual neutral inline stabilization of the head and neck is maintained while the mandible is moved anteriorly (forward). This maneuver moves the tongue forward, away from the hypopharynx, and holds the mouth slightly open.

From a position above the patient's head, the prehospital care provider positions his or her hands on either side of the patient's head, fingers pointing caudad (toward the patient's feet).

Depending on the size of the provider's hands, the fingers are spread across the face and around the angle of the patient's mandible.

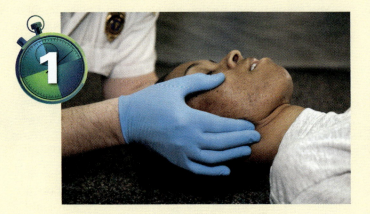

Gentle, equal pressure is applied with these digits to move the patient's mandible anteriorly (forward) and slightly downward (toward the patient's feet).

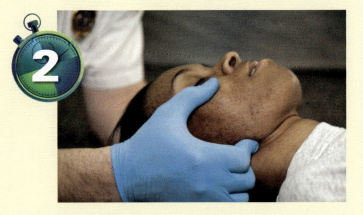

Oropharyngeal Airway

Principle: An adjunct used to maintain an open airway mechanically in a patient without a gag reflex.

The oropharyngeal airway (OPA) is designed to hold the patient's tongue anteriorly out of the pharynx. The OPA is available in various sizes. Proper sizing to the patient is required to ensure a patent airway. *Placement of an OPA in the hypopharynx is contraindicated in patients who have an intact gag reflex.*

Two methods for insertion of the OPA are effective: the tongue jaw-lift insertion method and the tongue blade insertion method. Regardless of which method is used, the first provider stabilizes the patient's head and neck in a neutral inline position while the second provider measures and inserts the OPA.

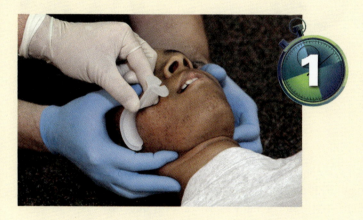

Tongue Jaw-Lift Insertion Method

The first provider brings the patient's head and neck into a neutral inline position and maintains stabilization while opening the patient's airway with a trauma jaw-thrust maneuver. The second provider selects and measures for a properly sized OPA. The distance from the corner of the patient's mouth to the earlobe is a good estimate for proper size.

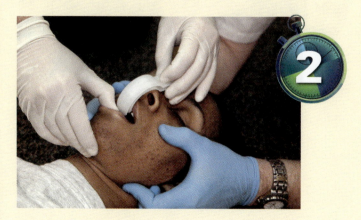

The patient's airway is opened with the chin-lift maneuver. The OPA is turned so that the distal tip is pointing toward the top of the patient's head (flanged end pointing toward patient's head) and tilted toward the mouth opening.

SPECIFIC SKILLS

The OPA is inserted into the patient's mouth and rotated to fit the contours of the patient's anatomy.

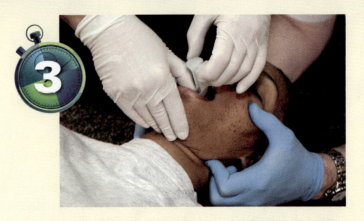

The OPA is rotated until its inside curve is resting against the tongue and holding it out of the posterior pharynx. The flanges of the OPA should be resting against the outside surface of the patient's teeth.

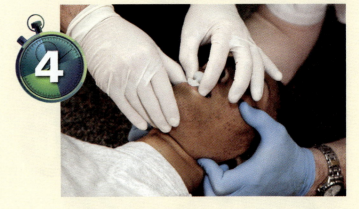

Tongue Blade Insertion Method

The tongue blade insertion method is probably a safer method than the tongue jaw lift because it eliminates the accidental tearing or puncturing of gloves or the skin by sharp, pointed, or broken teeth. This method also eliminates the possibility of being bitten if the patient's level of consciousness (LOC) is not as deep as previously assessed or if any seizure activity occurs.

The first provider brings the patient's head and neck into a neutral inline position and maintains stabilization while opening the patient's airway with the trauma jaw thrust maneuver. The second provider selects and measures for a properly sized OPA.

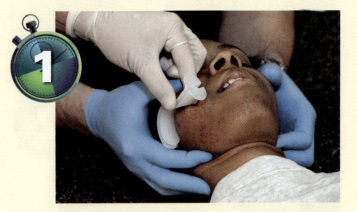

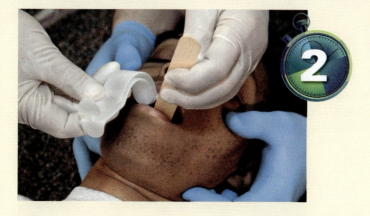

The second provider pulls the patient's mouth open by the chin and places a tongue blade into the patient's mouth to move the tongue forward in place and keep the airway open.

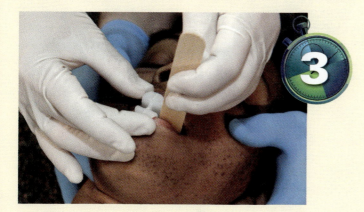

The device is inserted with the flanged end pointing toward the patient's feet and the distal tip pointing into the patient's mouth following the curvature of the airway.

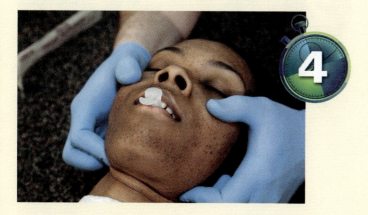

The OPA is advanced until the flanged end of the OPA rests against the outside surface of the patient's teeth.

SPECIFIC SKILLS

Nasopharyngeal Airway

Principle: An adjunct used to maintain an open airway mechanically in a patient with or without a gag reflex.

The nasopharyngeal airway (NPA) is a simple airway adjunct that provides an effective way to maintain a patent airway in patients who may still have an intact gag reflex. Most patients will tolerate the NPA if properly sized. NPAs are available in a range of diameters (internal diameters of 5–9 mm), and the length varies appropriately with the size of the diameter. NPAs are usually made of a flexible, rubberlike material. Rigid NPAs are not recommended for field use.

The first provider brings the patient's head and neck into a neutral inline position and maintains stabilization while opening the patient's airway with the trauma jaw-thrust maneuver. A second provider examines the patient's nostrils with a light and selects the one that is the largest and least deviated or obstructed (usually the right nostril). The second provider selects the appropriately sized NPA for the patient's nostril, a size slightly smaller in diameter than the size of the nostril opening (frequently the diameter of the patient's little finger).

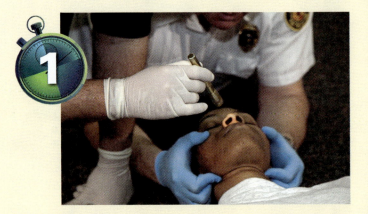

The length of the NPA is also important. The NPA needs to be long enough to supply an air passage between the patient's tongue and the posterior pharynx. The distance from the patient's nose to the earlobe is a good estimate for proper size.

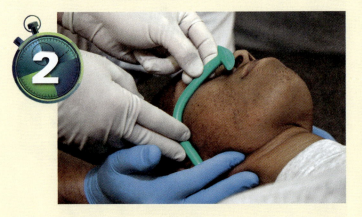

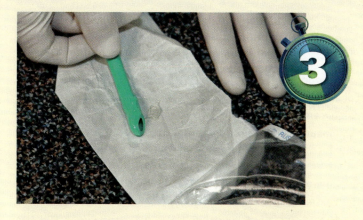

The distal tip (nonflanged end) of the NPA is lubricated liberally with a water-soluble jelly.

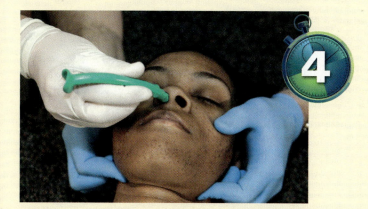

The NPA is slowly inserted into the nostril of choice. Insertion should be in an anterior-to-posterior direction along the floor of the nasal cavity, not in a superior-to-inferior direction. If resistance is met at the posterior end of the nostril, a gentle back-and-forth rotation of the NPA between the fingers will usually aid in passing beyond the turbinate bones of the nasal cavity without damage. Should the NPA continue to meet with resistance, the NPA should not be forced past the obstruction but rather should be withdrawn, and the distal tip should be relubricated and inserted into the other nostril.

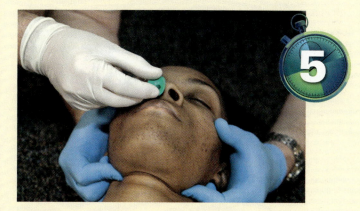

The second provider continues insertion until the flange end of the NPA is next to the anterior nares or until the patient gags. If the patient gags, the NPA is withdrawn slightly.

SPECIFIC SKILLS

Bag-Mask Ventilation

Principle: The preferred method of providing assisted ventilation.

Ventilation using a bag mask system has an advantage over other ventilatory support systems because it gives a prehospital care provider feedback by the feel of the bag (compliance). Positive feedback ensures the operator of successful ventilations; changes in the feedback indicate a loss of mask seal, the presence of a pathologic airway, or a thoracic problem interfering with the delivery of successful ventilations. This "feel" and the control it provides also make the bag-mask device suitable for assisting ventilations. The bag-mask's portability and ability for immediate use make it useful for immediate delivery of ventilations on identification of the need.

Without supplemental oxygen, however, a bag-mask device provides an oxygen concentration of only 21%, a fraction of inspired oxygen (FiO_2) of 0.21; as soon as time allows, an oxygen reservoir and high-concentration supplemental oxygen should be connected to the bag-mask. When oxygen is connected without a reservoir, the FiO_2 is limited to 0.50 or less; with a reservoir, the FiO_2 is 0.85 or greater.

If the patient being ventilated is unconscious without a gag reflex, a properly sized oropharyngeal airway should be inserted before attempting to ventilate with the bag-mask. If the patient has an intact gag reflex, a properly sized nasopharyngeal airway should be inserted before attempting to assist ventilations.

Various bag-mask devices are available, including disposable single-patient-use models that are relatively inexpensive. Different brands have varying bag, valve, and reservoir designs. All the parts used should be of the same model and brand because these parts are usually not safely interchangeable.

Bag-mask units are available in adult, pediatric, and neonatal sizes. Although an adult bag can be used with the properly sized pediatric mask in an emergency, use of the correct bag size is recommended as a safe practice. Adequate ventilations of an adult patient are achieved when a minimum of 800 mL/breath is delivered (1000–1200 mL/breath preferred).

When ventilating with any positive-pressure device, inflation should stop once the chest has risen maximally. When using the bag-mask, the chest should be visualized for maximum inflation and the bag felt to recognize any marked increased resistance in the bag when lung expansion is at its maximum. Adequate time for exhalation is needed (1 : 3 ratio between time for inhalation and time for exhalation). If enough time is not allowed, "stepped or stacked breaths" occur, providing a greater volume of inspiration than expiration. Stepped breaths produce poor air exchange and result in hyperinflation of the lungs, increased pressure within the chest, decreased blood return to the heart causing compromised circulation, opening of the esophagus, and gastric distension.

Two-Provider Method

Two or more prehospital care providers performing ventilations with a bag-mask device is easier than with only one provider. The first provider can focus attention on maintaining an adequate mask seal while the second provides good delivery volume by using both hands to squeeze (deflate) the bag.

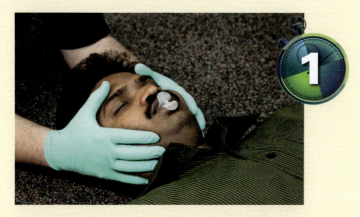

The first provider kneels above the patient's head and maintains manual stabilization of the patient's head and neck in a neutral inline position.

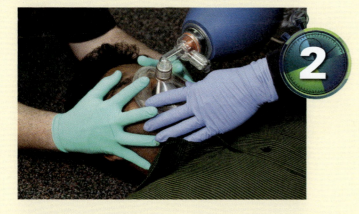

The facemask is placed over the patient's nose and mouth, and the mask is held in place with the thumbs on the lateral portion of the mask while pulling the mandible up into the mask. The other fingers provide the manual stabilization and maintain a patent airway.

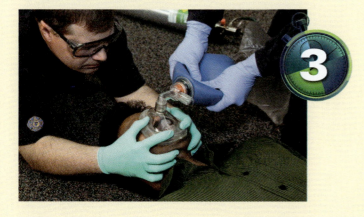

The second provider kneels at the side of the patient and squeezes the bag with both hands to inflate the lungs.

CHAPTER 5

Circulation and Shock

CHAPTER OBJECTIVES

At the completion of this chapter, the reader will be able to do the following:

✓ Define shock.

✓ Classify shock on an etiologic basis.

✓ Explain the pathophysiology of shock and its progression through phases.

✓ Relate shock to energy production, etiology, prevention, and treatment.

✓ Describe common symptoms and assessment findings in shock.

✓ Clinically differentiate the different types of shock.

✓ Discuss the limitations of the field management of shock.

✓ Recognize the need for rapid transport and early definitive management in various forms of shock.

✓ Apply principles of management of shock in the trauma patient.

SCENARIO

You and you partner are dispatched to the scene of a multiple victim shooting. The scene is in the middle of a dark street. Police are already present and state that the scene is secured. You find one person with multiple bullet holes in his upper and lower back. He is breathing rapidly and you see air bubbling out of the holes in his chest. He is lying on top of a woman of similar age (late 20s). He has protected her from the bullets with his body except for some bullet holes in her legs alone. You roll him off her and note that he also has several wounds on his abdomen. A loop of bowel protrudes from one of the wounds in the anterior abdomen. His pulse is weak and very fast. In looking at the woman, you note that a large amount of blood is running onto the pavement from one of her leg wounds, at the knee.

What injuries do you expect in these patients?

How would you manage them in the field?

You are 15 minutes away from the nearest trauma center. How does this alter your management plans?

Although shock following trauma has been recognized for more than three centuries, its description by Samuel Gross in 1872 as a "rude unhinging of the machinery of life"[1] and John Collins Warren as "a momentary pause in the act of death"[2] emphasizes its continuing central role in the causes of major injury and death in the trauma patient. Prompt diagnosis, resuscitation, and definitive management of shock resulting from trauma are all essential in determining patient outcome. The trauma care provider faces significant challenges in accomplishing all these essential actions for shock. To improve survival from shock, a clear understanding of the definition, pathophysiology, and clinical features is essential.

In the prehospital setting the challenge posed by the patient in shock is compounded by the need to assess and manage such patients in a relatively primitive, and sometimes dangerous, environment where sophisticated diagnostic and management tools are either unavailable or impractical to apply. This chapter defines and classifies shock and describes the pathophysiologic changes present in shock to help direct management strategies. It emphasizes the importance of energy production and the preservation of aerobic metabolism in the manufacture of energy, which is the key to life.

the entire pathologic process called shock. The correct definition of shock is a lack of tissue perfusion (blood supply and therefore oxygen) at the cellular level that leads to anaerobic (without oxygen) metabolism and the loss of energy production needed to support life.

If the trauma first responder or any provider, is to understand this abnormal condition and be able to develop a treatment plan to prevent or reverse shock, it is important that he or she knows and understands what is happening to the body at a cellular level. The normal physiologic responses the body uses to protect itself from the development of shock must be understood, recognized, and interpreted. Only then can a rational approach for managing the problems of the patient in shock be developed.

Shock can kill a patient in the field, the emergency department, the operating room, or the intensive care unit. Although actual death may be delayed for several hours to several days or even weeks, the most common cause of that death is the failure of early resuscitation. The lack of perfusion of cells by oxygenated blood results in anaerobic metabolism and decreased function for organ survival. Even when some cells are initially spared, death can occur later, because the remaining cells are unable to carry out the function of that organ indefinitely. This chapter explains this phenomenon and presents methods to prevent such an outcome.

Definition of Shock

Although it has many definitions, shock is most often regarded as a state of generalized decrease in the blood supply to the cells and organs of the body. As a result, the delivery of oxygen to the cells is inadequate to meet their metabolic needs. In addition, the removal of waste products is also impaired.

It is a basic principle of prehospital care that shock is not defined as low blood pressure, rapid pulse rates, or cool, clammy skin; these are merely the systemic manifestations of

Physiology

Metabolism: The Human Motor

The human body consists of more than 100 million cells, and each one of these cells requires oxygen to function and produce energy. The cells take in oxygen and metabolize it through a complicated physiologic process that produces energy. The metabolism of the cell requires energy, and cells must have fuel, glucose, to carry out this process. As in any combustion event, a by-product is also produced. In the body, oxygen and glucose are metabolized to produce energy, water (H_2O), and carbon dioxide (CO_2).

This is similar to the process that occurs in a motor vehicle engine when gasoline and air are mixed and burned to produce energy, and carbon monoxide (CO) is created as a by-product. The motor moves the car, the heater warms the driver, and the electricity generated is used for the lights to show the road, all because of the burning of gasoline to produce energy.

Aerobic metabolism describes the use of oxygen by cells. This form of metabolism is the body's principal combustion process. It produces a lot of energy using oxygen in a complicated process known as the Krebs cycle. Cells in the body do contain an alternate power source. **Anaerobic metabolism** occurs without the use of oxygen. It is the backup power system in the body and uses stored body fat as its energy source; however, it only produces a small amount of energy.

The major by-product of anaerobic metabolism is excessive amounts of acid. In addition, energy production is reduced 15-fold. If anaerobic metabolism is not reversed quickly, cells cannot continue to function and will die because of that lack of energy. If a sufficient number of cells in any one organ die, the entire organ ceases to function. If a large number of cells in an organ die, but not enough cells to kill it, the organ's function will be significantly reduced and the remaining cells in that organ will have to work even harder than usual to keep the organ functioning. These overworked cells may or may not be able to support the function of the entire organ. Even with some cells remaining, the organ may still die. An example is a patient who has suffered a heart attack. Blood flow and oxygen are shut off to one portion of the heart muscle, and some cells of the heart die, thus decreasing cardiac output and the oxygen supply to the rest of the heart. This, in turn, causes a further reduction in oxygenation of the remaining heart cells. If not enough other cells remain, or if they are not strong enough to take over the entire function of the heart to meet the blood flow needs of the body, heart failure can result. Unless major improvement in cardiac output and oxygenation occur, the patient eventually will not survive.

As this systemic deterioration continues, more and more organs die and eventually the entire organism (the human) dies. Depending on the organ initially involved, the progression from cell death to organism death can be rapid or delayed. If the organ involved is the brain, death can occur within minutes. On the other hand, if other organs are involved, it can take as long as 2 or 3 weeks before the damage caused by hypoxia or **hypoperfusion** in the first minutes post-trauma results in the patient's death. The effectiveness of the trauma first responder's actions to reverse or prevent **hypoxia** (insufficient oxygen available to meet cell requirements) and hypoperfusion (inadequate blood passing to tissue cells) in the critical prehospital time period may not be immediately

apparent. However, these resuscitation measures are unquestionably necessary if the patient is to ultimately survive. The sensitivity of cells to the lack of oxygen and the usefulness of anaerobic metabolism varies from organ system to organ system. This sensitivity is called **ischemic** (lack of oxygen) sensitivity and it is greatest in the brain, heart, and lungs. It may take only 4 to 6 minutes of anaerobic metabolism before one or more of these vital organs are injured beyond repair. In contrast, skin and muscle tissue have a significantly longer ischemic sensitivity—as long as 4 to 6 hours. The abdominal organs generally fall between these two groups and are able to survive 45 to 90 minutes of anaerobic metabolism (Figure 5-1).

Long-term survival of the individual organs and the body as a whole requires delivery of important nutrients (oxygen and glucose) to the tissue cells. Other nutrients are also important, but because the resupply of these other materials is not a component of the prehospital EMS system, they are not discussed here. Although these factors are important, they are beyond the scope of the trauma first responder's practice and resources. The most important supply item is oxygen.

A second component that is important to the long-term well-being of the individual organs and the body is the removal of the waste products of metabolism. Hypoperfusion impairs the removal of these waste products, allowing them to build up, which can ultimately lead to damage of the organs.

A crucial part of this entire process is that the patient must have enough red blood cells (RBCs) available to deliver adequate amounts of oxygen to tissue cells throughout the body, so that these cells can produce energy. Additionally, the patient's airway must be patent and adequate volume and depth of respirations present (see Chapter 4, Airway and Breathing).

The prehospital treatment of shock is directed at ensuring that critical components are maintained, with the goal of preventing or reversing anaerobic metabolism, thus avoiding cellular death and, ultimately, patient death. These components should be the major emphasis of the trauma care provider and are implemented in the management of the trauma patient by the following actions:

- Maintaining an adequate airway and ventilation, thus providing adequate oxygen to the red blood cells
- Judicious use of supplemental oxygen as part of ventilating the patient
- Maintaining adequate circulation, thus perfusing tissue cells with oxygenated blood

FIGURE 5-1 Organ Tolerance to Ischemia

Organ	Warm Ischemia Time
Heart, brain, lungs	4–6 minutes
Kidneys, liver, gastrointestinal tract	45–90 minutes
Muscle, bone, skin	4–6 hours

The first component (oxygenation of the lungs and red blood cells) is covered in Chapter 4, Airway and Breathing. The second component involves perfusion, which is the delivery of blood to the tissue cells. A helpful analogy to use in describing perfusion is to think of the RBCs as transport vans, the lungs as oxygen warehouses, the blood vessels as roads and highways, and the body tissue cells as the oxygen's destination. An insufficient number of transport vans, obstructions along the roads and highways, and slow transport vans can all contribute to decreased oxygen delivery and the eventual starvation of the tissue cells.

The fluid component of the circulatory system—blood—contains not only RBCs but infection-fighting factors (white blood cells and antibodies), platelets and factors to support blood clotting in hemorrhage, protein for cellular rebuilding, nutrition in the form of glucose, and other substances necessary for metabolism and survival.

Classification of Shock

The prime determinants of cellular perfusion are the heart (acting as the pump or the motor of the system); fluid volume (acting as the hydraulic fluid); the blood vessels (serving as the conduits or plumbing); and, finally, the cells of the body. Based on these components of the perfusion system, shock may be classified into the following categories:

- *Hypovolemic*, primarily from hemorrhage in the trauma patient, related to loss of circulating blood volume. This is the most common cause of shock in the trauma patient.
- *Distributive* (or vasogenic), related to abnormality in vascular tone arising from several different causes.
- *Cardiogenic*, related to interference with the pump action of the heart.

By far the most common cause of shock in the trauma patient is hemorrhage, and the safest approach in managing the trauma patient in shock is to consider the cause of the shock as being hemorrhagic until proven otherwise.

More detailed descriptions of these different types of shock follow after a discussion of the relevant anatomy and pathophysiology of shock.

Anatomy and Pathophysiology

Cardiovascular, Hemodynamic, and Endocrine Responses

Heart

The heart consists of two receiving chambers *(atria)* and two major pumping chambers *(ventricles)*. The function of the atria is to accumulate and store blood so that the ven-

tricles can fill rapidly, minimizing delay in the pumping cycle. The right atrium receives blood from the veins of the body and pumps it to the right ventricle. With each contraction of the right ventricle (Figure 5-2), blood is pumped through the lungs for loading of oxygen to the red blood cells (Figure 5-3). The oxygenated blood from the lungs is

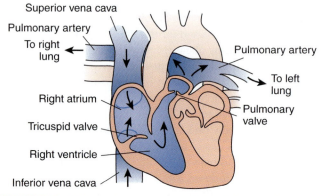

FIGURE 5-2 With each contraction of the right ventricle, blood is pumped through the lungs. Blood from the lungs enters the left side of the heart, and the left ventricle pumps it into the systemic vascular system.

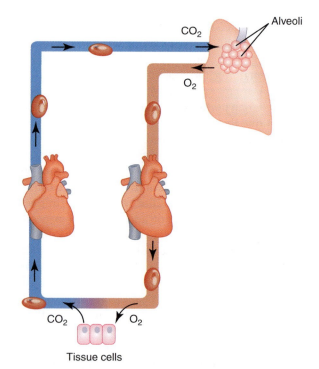

FIGURE 5-3 Although the heart seems to be one organ, it functions as if it were two organs. Unoxygenated blood is received into the "right heart" from the superior and inferior venae cavae and pumped through the pulmonary artery into the lungs. The blood is oxygenated in the lungs, flows back into the heart through the pulmonary vein, and is pumped out of the left ventricle.

returned to the left atrium and is pumped into the left ventricle. Then the RBCs are pumped by the contractions of the ventricle throughout the arteries of the body to the tissue cells (Figure 5-4).

Blood is forced through the circulatory system by the contraction of the left ventricle. This sudden pressure increase produces a pulse wave to push blood through the system. The peak of the pressure increase is the systolic blood pressure and represents the force of the pulse wave produced by ventricular contraction *(systole).* The resting pressure in the vessels between ventricular contractions is the diastolic blood pressure and represents the force that remains in the blood vessels that continues to move blood through the vessels while the ventricle is refilling for the next pulse of blood *(diastole).*

The difference between the systolic and diastolic pressures is called *pulse pressure.* This is the pressure of the blood as it is being pushed out into the circulation. It is the pressure felt against the finger tip when the pulse is checked.

Blood Vessels

The blood vessels contain the blood and route it to the various areas and cells of the body. They are the "highways" of the physiologic process of circulation. The single, large exit tube from the heart, the *aorta,* splits into multiple arteries of decreasing size, the smallest of which are the capillaries (Figure 5-5). A capillary allows only one cell to pass through at a time; therefore, oxygen and nutrients carried by red blood cells (RBCs) and plasma are able to pass (diffuse) easily through the walls of the capillary into the tissue cell (Figure 5-6). Each tissue cell has a membranous covering called the *cell membrane.*

The size of the vascular "container" is controlled by smooth muscles in the walls of the arteries and arterioles and, to a lesser extent, by muscles in the walls of the venules and veins. These muscles respond to signals from the brain primarily to the circulating hormones epinephrine and norepinephrine. These muscle fibers in the walls of the vessels,

depending on whether they are being stimulated or allowed to relax, result in either the constriction or dilation of the blood vessels, thus changing the size of the container component of the cardiovascular system and therefore raising or lowering the patient's blood pressure.

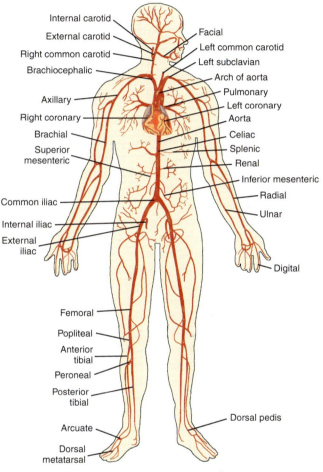

FIGURE 5-5 Principle arteries of the body.

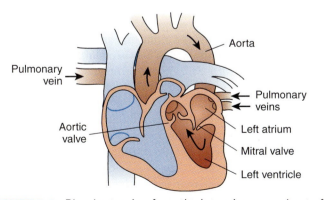

FIGURE 5-4 Blood returning from the lungs is pumped out of the heart and through the aorta to the rest of the body by left ventricular contraction.

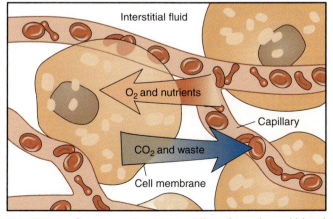

FIGURE 5-6 Oxygen and nutrients diffuse from the red blood cells through the capillary wall, the interstitial fluid, and the cell membrane into the cell.

Blood

The fluid component of the circulatory system, the blood, contains not only RBCs but also infection-fighting factors (white blood cells [WBCs] and antibodies), platelets and clotting factors essential for blood clotting in the event of vascular injury, protein for cellular rebuilding, nutrients such as glucose, and other substances necessary for metabolism and survival. The volume of fluid within the vascular system must equal the capacity of the blood vessels if it is to adequately fill the container and maintain perfusion and blood pressure. Any differences in the volume of the vascular system container compared with the volume of blood in that container will affect the flow of blood either positively or negatively, as well as affecting blood pressure.

Nervous System

The *autonomic nervous system* directs and controls the involuntary functions of the body, such as respiration, digestion, and cardiovascular function. It is divided into two subsystems, the sympathetic and parasympathetic nervous systems. These systems oppose each other to keep vital body systems in balance.

The *sympathetic nervous system* produces the fight-or-flight response. This response simultaneously causes the heart to beat faster and stronger, increases the ventilatory rate, and constricts the blood vessels to nonessential organs (skin and gastrointestinal tract) while dilating vessels and improving blood flow to muscles. The goal of this response is to maintain sufficient amounts of oxygenated blood to critical tissues so that an individual can respond to an emergency situation, while shunting blood away from nonessential areas. In contrast, the parasympathetic system slows the heart rate, decreases the ventilatory rate, and increases gastrointestinal activity.

In patients who are hemorrhaging after sustaining trauma, the body attempts to compensate for the blood loss. The cardiovascular system is regulated by the brain. In response to a fall in blood pressure, stimuli travel to the brain from stretch receptors in the carotid sinus and the aortic arch. This leads to increased sympathetic nervous system activity, with increased peripheral vascular resistance resulting from arteriolar constriction and increased cardiac output from an increased rate and force of cardiac contraction. Increased venous tone enhances circulatory blood volume. Blood is thus diverted from the extremities, bowel, and kidney to more vital areas—that is, the heart and brain.

Types of Shock

There are three types of shock:

1. Hypovolemic shock
   - Vascular volume smaller than normal vascular size
     - Loss of fluid and electrolytes
     - Dehydration
     - Loss of blood
     - Hemorrhagic shock
2. Distributive Shock
   - Vascular space is larger than normal
     - Neurogenic "shock" (hypotension)
     - Psychogenic shock
     - Septic shock
     - Anaphylactic shock
3. Cardiogenic shock
   - Pump failure
     - Intrinsic to the heart
       - Heart muscle damage
       - Dysrhythmias (abnormal beating)
     - Extrinsic to the heart
       - Cardiac tamponade

Hypovolemic Shock

Acute loss of blood volume, either from dehydration (loss of fluid and electrolytes) or hemorrhage (loss of plasma and RBCs), causes an imbalance in the relationship of fluid volume to the size of the container. The container retains its normal size, but the fluid volume is decreased. *Hypovolemic shock* is the most common cause of shock encountered in the prehospital environment, and blood loss is by far the most common cause of shock in trauma patients and the most dangerous for the patient.

When blood is lost from the circulation, the heart is stimulated to increase cardiac output by increasing the strength and rate of contractions. This is caused by the release of *epinephrine* from the adrenal glands located just above the kidneys. The sympathetic nervous system also releases *norepinephrine* to trigger constriction of the blood vessels to reduce the size of the container and bring it more into proportion with the volume of remaining fluid. Vasoconstriction results in closing of the peripheral capillaries, reducing oxygen delivery, and forces the switch from aerobic to anaerobic metabolism at the cellular level.

These defense mechanisms work well up to a point. When the defense mechanisms can no longer compensate for the lost volume, a patient's blood pressure will drop. A decrease in blood pressure marks the switch from compensated to decompensated shock—a sign of impending death. A patient who has signs of compensation such as tachycardia is already in shock, not "going into shock." Unless aggressive resuscitation occurs, the patient who enters decompensated shock has only one more stage of decline left—irreversible shock leading to death.

Hemorrhagic Shock

Hemorrhagic shock (hypovolemic shock resulting from blood loss) can be categorized into four classes, depending on the severity of hemorrhage, as follows (Figure 5-7):

1. *Class I hemorrhage* represents a loss of up to 15% of blood volume in the adult (up to 750 mL). This stage has few clinical manifestations. Increase in heart rate (tachycardia) is often minimal, and no measurable changes in

FIGURE 5-7 Classifications of Hemorrhagic Shock

	Class I	Class II	Class III	Class IV
Amount of blood loss (% total blood volume)	<750 mL (<15%)	750–1500 mL (15%–30%)	1500–2000 mL (30%–40%)	>2000 mL (>40%)
Heart rate (beats/minute)	Normal or minimally increased	>100	>120	>140
Ventilatory rate (breaths/minute)	Normal	20–30	30–40	>35
Systolic blood pressure (mm Hg)	Normal	Normal	Decreased	Greatly decreased

Modified from American College of Surgeons Committee on Trauma: *Advanced trauma life support for doctors, student course manual,* ed 8, Chicago, 2008, ACS.

blood pressure, pulse pressure, or ventilatory rate occur. Most healthy patients sustaining this amount of hemorrhage will recover without any problem as long as no further blood loss occurs. The body's compensatory mechanisms restore the intravascular container/fluid volume ratio and assist in the maintenance of blood pressure.

2. *Class II hemorrhage* represents a loss of 15% to 30% of blood volume (750–1500 mL). Most adults are capable of compensating for this amount of blood loss by activation of the sympathetic nervous system and maintaining their blood pressure. Clinical findings include increased ventilatory rate and tachycardia. The clinical clues to this phase are tachycardia, tachypnea (increased ventilatory rate), and normal systolic blood pressure. Because the blood pressure is normal, this is "compensated shock"; the patient is in shock and able to compensate for the time being. The patient often demonstrates anxiety or fear. On occasion, these patients may require blood transfusion after arrival to the hospital; however, most will respond well to intravenous fluids given by advanced level providers if hemorrhage is controlled at this point.

3. *Class III hemorrhage* represents a loss of 30% to 40% of blood volume (1500–2000 mL). When blood loss reaches this point, most patients are no longer able to compensate for the volume loss, and hypotension (low blood pressure) occurs. The classic findings of shock are obvious and include tachycardia (heart rate > 120 beats/minute), tachypnea (ventilatory rate 30–40 breaths/minute), and severe anxiety or confusion. Many of these patients will require blood transfusion and surgical intervention for adequate resuscitation and control of hemorrhage.

4. *Class IV hemorrhage* represents a loss of more than 40% of blood volume (>2000 mL). This stage of severe shock is characterized by marked tachycardia (heart rate > 140 beats/minute), tachypnea (ventilatory rate > 35 breaths/minute), profound confusion or lethargy, and greatly decreased systolic blood pressure, typically

in the range of 60 mm Hg. These patients truly have only minutes to live. Survival depends on immediate control of hemorrhage (surgery for internal hemorrhage) and aggressive resuscitation, including blood and plasma transfusions.

The rapidity with which a patient develops shock depends on how fast blood is lost from the circulation.

The *definitive management for volume deficit* is to stop the fluid loss and replace the lost fluid. A *dehydrated patient* needs fluid replacement with water and salt, whereas a *trauma patient* who has lost blood needs to have the source of blood loss stopped and, if significant blood loss has occurred, blood replacement needs to be accomplished. Blood replacement is usually not available in the prehospital environment; therefore, trauma patients with hemorrhagic shock must have measures to control external blood loss instituted and rapid transportation to the hospital where blood, plasma, and clotting factors are available and emergent operative steps as necessary to control internal blood loss can be performed.

Distributive (Vasogenic) Shock

Distributive shock, or vasogenic shock, occurs when the vascular container enlarges without a proportional increase in fluid volume to keep the now larger container filled. Although the amount of intravascular fluid has not changed, relatively less fluid is available for the now larger size of the container. As a result, the volume of fluid available for the heart to pump decreases, thus reducing cardiac output. In most situations, fluid has not been lost from the vascular system. This form of shock is not a cause of hypovolemia, where fluid has been lost through hemorrhage, vomiting, or diarrhea. Instead, the problem is the size of the container which is now larger than the fluid available to fill it. For this reason, this condition is sometimes referred to as *relative hypovolemia*. The net result is a decrease in both systolic and diastolic blood pressures. Although some of the presenting signs and symptoms may closely mimic those of hypovolemic shock, the cause of the two conditions is different.

FIGURE 5-8   Signs Associated with Types of Shock

Vital Sign	Hypovolemic	Neurogenic	Septic	Cardiogenic
Skin temperature	Cool, clammy	Warm, dry	Cool, clammy	Cool, clammy
Skin color	Pale, cyanotic	Pink	Pale, mottled	Pale, cyanotic
Blood pressure	Drops	Drops	Drops	Drops
Level of consciousness	Altered	Lucid	Altered	Altered

Distributive shock can result from loss of autonomic nervous system control of the smooth muscles that control the size of the blood vessels or release of chemicals that result in peripheral vasodilation. This loss of control can stem from spinal cord trauma, simple fainting, severe infections, or allergic reactions. Management of distributive shock is directed toward improving oxygenation of the blood and improving or maintaining blood flow to the brain and vital organs.

Neurogenic "Shock"

Neurogenic shock, or more appropriately neurogenic hypotension, occurs when a spinal cord injury interrupts the sympathetic nervous system pathway. Because of the loss of sympathetic control of the vascular system, which controls the smooth muscles in the walls of the blood vessels, the peripheral vessels dilate below the level of injury. This vasodilation that occurs causes the container for the blood volume to increase in size and results in relative hypovolemia. The patient is not really hypovolemic, but the normal blood volume insufficiently fills the expanded container. This decrease in blood pressure does not alter perfusion or compromise energy production and therefore is *not* shock since energy production remains unaffected. However, because there is less resistance to blood flow, the systolic and diastolic pressures are lower.

Decompensated hypovolemic shock and neurogenic shock both produce a decreased systolic blood pressure. However, the other vital and clinical signs, as well as the treatment for each, are different (Figure 5-8). Hypovolemia produces cold, clammy, pale, or cyanotic (blue-colored) skin and delayed capillary refilling time. In neurogenic shock the patient has warm, dry skin, especially below the area of injury. The pulse in hypovolemic shock patients is weak, thready, and rapid. In neurogenic shock, because of unopposed parasympathetic activity on the heart, bradycardia is typically seen rather than tachycardia, but the pulse quality may be weak. Hypovolemia produces a decreased level of consciousness (LOC), or at least anxiety and often combativeness. In the absence of a traumatic brain injury, the patient with neurogenic shock is usually alert, oriented, and lucid when in the supine position (Figure 5-9).

Patients with neurogenic shock often have associated injuries that produce significant hemorrhage. Therefore, a patient who has neurogenic shock and signs of hypovolemia, such as tachycardia, should be treated as if blood loss is present.

FIGURE 5-9   Neurogenic Shock Versus Spinal Shock

As discussed in this chapter, the term *neurogenic shock* refers to a disruption of the sympathetic nervous system, typically from injury to the spinal cord, that results in significant dilation of the peripheral arteries. If untreated, this may result in impaired perfusion to the body's tissues. This condition should not be confused with *spinal shock,* a term that refers to an injury to the spinal cord resulting in *temporary* loss of sensory and motor function. Thus, spinal shock indicates that the spinal cord has been damaged ("shocked") and is not working properly. Strictly speaking, spinal shock does not represent a defect in organ or tissue perfusion. The prehospital care provider should be aware that both neurogenic shock and spinal shock can simultaneously occur in the same patient.

Psychogenic (Vasovagal) "Shock"

Psychogenic shock typically results from overstimulation of the parasympathetic nervous system, which produces bradycardia (slow heart rate). The increased parasympathetic activity may also result in transient peripheral vasodilation and hypotension. If the bradycardia and vasodilation are severe enough, cardiac output falls dramatically, resulting in insufficient blood flow to the brain. Vasovagal syncope (fainting) occurs when the patient loses consciousness. Compared with neurogenic shock, the periods of bradycardia and vasodilation are generally very brief and limited to no more than a few minutes, whereas neurogenic shock may last up to several days. In psychogenic shock patients, normal blood pressure is quickly restored when the patient is placed in a horizontal position. Because it is self-limited, a vasovagal episode is unlikely to result in true "shock" and the body quickly recovers before significant systemic impairment of perfusion occurs.

Septic Shock

Septic shock, seen in patients with life-threatening infections, is another condition that exhibits vascular dilation. Thus, septic shock has characteristics of both distributive shock and hypovolemic shock. Septic shock is virtually never encountered within minutes of an injury; however, the trauma care provider may be called on to care for a trauma patient in septic shock during an interfacility transfer, or if a patient sustains an injury to the gastrointestinal tract and did not promptly seek medical attention.

Anaphylactic Shock

Anaphylactic shock is a severe, life-threatening allergic reaction that involves numerous body organ systems. When individuals are exposed to an allergen for the first time, they become sensitized to it. If they are later re-exposed to that same allergen, a systemic response occurs involving the entire body. In addition to the more common symptoms of allergic reaction such as redness (erythema) of the skin, development of hives (urticaria), and itching, more serious findings are noted, including respiratory distress, airway obstruction, and vasodilation leading to shock. Airway management may be needed in some cases. Treatment involves administration of epinephrine, antihistamines, and steroids by ALS providers or in the hospital.

Cardiogenic Shock

Cardiogenic shock, or failure of the heart's pumping activity, results from causes that can be categorized as either intrinsic (a result of direct damage to the heart itself) or extrinsic (related to a problem outside the heart).

Intrinsic Causes

Heart Muscle Damage. Any process that weakens the cardiac muscle will affect its output. The damage may result from an acute interruption of the heart's own blood supply (as in a myocardial infarction from coronary artery disease) or from a direct bruise to the heart muscle (as in a blunt cardiac injury). A recurring cycle will ensue: Decreased oxygenation causes decreased contractility, which results in decreased ability to pump and therefore decreased systemic perfusion. Decreased perfusion results in a continuing decrease in oxygenation and thus a continuation of the cycle. As with any muscle, the cardiac muscle does not work as efficiently when it becomes bruised or damaged.

Dysrhythmia. The development of an abnormal heart rhythm (dysrhythmia) can affect the efficiency of contractions, resulting in impaired circulation to the body. Hypoxia may lead to lack of oxygen to the heart (myocardial ischemia) and cause dysrhythmias, such as premature contractions and tachycardia. Because cardiac output is a result of the volume ejected with each contraction (stroke volume), any dysrhythmia that results in a slow rate of contractions (bradycardia) or shortens the left ventricle's filling time (tachycardia) can decrease stroke volume and cardiac output. Blunt cardiac injury may also result in dysrhythmias, the most common of which is a mild, persistent tachycardia.

Extrinsic Causes

Cardiac Tamponade. Fluid in the pericardial sac surrounding the heart will prevent the heart from refilling completely during the diastolic (relaxation) phase. In the case of trauma, blood leaks into the pericardial sac and the walls of the ventricle cannot fully expand. In the case of penetrating cardiac trauma (stab or gunshot wounds), more blood may be squeezed out of the cardiac wound and enter the pericardial sac with each contraction, further compromising cardiac output. Severe shock and death may rapidly follow.

Complications of Shock

Several complications may result in patients with persistent or inadequately resuscitated shock, which is why early recognition and aggressive management of shock are essential. The quality of care delivered in the prehospital setting can alter a patient's hospital course and outcome. *Failure to recognize shock and initiate proper treatment in the prehospital setting may extend the patient's hospital length of stay.* The following complications of shock are not often seen in the prehospital setting, but they are a result of shock in the field and in the ED. In addition they may be encountered while transferring patients between facilities. Knowing the outcome of the process of shock helps in the understanding of the severity of the condition, the importance of rapid hemorrhage control, and appropriate fluid replacement.

Acute Renal Failure

Impaired circulation to the kidneys, resulting from prolonged shock, can result in temporary or permanent renal failure. These patients often require dialysis for several weeks to months.

Acute Respiratory Distress Syndrome

Acute respiratory distress syndrome (ARDS) is the result of damage to the lining of the capillaries in the lung. This leads to leakage of fluid into the lungs, making it much more difficult for oxygen to diffuse across the alveolar walls and into the capillaries and bind with the RBCs. ARDS is associated with a mortality rate of about 40%, and the patients who survive may require mechanical ventilation for up to several months.

Hematologic Failure

The term *coagulopathy* refers to impairment in the normal blood-clotting capabilities of the circulatory system and the body. This may result from hypothermia (decreased body temperature), dilution of clotting factors from transfusion of fluids, or depletion of the clotting substances as they are used in an effort to control bleeding (*consumptive* coagulopathy).

Hepatic Failure

Severe damage to the liver is a less common result of prolonged shock. Liver failure is manifested by persistent hypoglycemia (low blood sugar), persistent lactic acidosis, and jaundice. Because the liver produces many of the clotting factors necessary for hemostasis, a coagulopathy may accompany liver failure.

Overwhelming Infection

An increased risk of infection is associated with severe shock. This is thought to be from several causes:

1. A marked decrease in the number of WBCs, predisposing the shock patient to infection, is another manifestation of hematologic failure.
2. The ischemia and reduction in energy production in the cells of the wall of the bowel in the patient with shock may allow bacteria to leak out into the peritoneal cavity.
3. There is decreased function of the immune system in the face of ischemia and loss of energy production.

Multiple Organ Failure

Shock, if not successfully treated, can lead to dysfunction first in one organ, then followed by several organs simultaneously, with sepsis being a common accompaniment, leading to the multiple organ dysfunction syndrome.

Failure of one major body system (e.g., lungs, kidneys, blood-clotting cascade, liver) is associated with a mortality rate of about 40%. As an organ system fails, the shock state worsens. By the time four organ systems fail, the mortality rate is essentially 100%.[3] Cardiovascular failure, in the form of cardiogenic and septic shock, can only occasionally be reversed.

Assessment

As was discussed earlier, shock is a condition resulting from decreased perfusion that leads to diminished energy production and heralds the potential onset of death. If not quickly treated, this lack of energy production can become irreversible. The body responds to this decrease in energy production by selectively decreasing perfusion in nonessential parts of the body and increasing cardiovascular function to compensate and better perfuse other, more critical organs. When shock develops, the physiologic response results in clinical signs that indicate the body has responded and is attempting to compensate.

The body's response is identified by the reduction of perfusion to nonvital organs such as the skin, which will feel cold and may look mottled; decreased pulse character in the extremities; cold, cyanotic (bluish coloration) extremities; and decreased mentation as a result of the decline in oxygenated blood perfusion to the brain. The accumulation of acid from anaerobic metabolism produces rapid ventilations as the body attempts to blow off the carbon dioxide by-product. Decreased energy production is identified by sluggish body responses, cold skin, and decreased body temperature. The patient may be shivering in an effort to maintain body heat.

The assessment for the presence of shock must include looking for the subtle early evidence of this state of hypoperfusion. In the prehospital setting, this requires the assessment of organs and systems that are easily examined. Signs of hypoperfusion manifest as malfunction of these accessible organs or systems. Such systems are the brain and central nervous system (CNS), heart and cardiovascular system, respiratory system, skin, and extremities. The signs of decreased perfusion and energy production and the body's response include the following:

- Decreased LOC, anxiety, disorientation, belligerence, bizarre behavior (brain and CNS)
- Tachycardia and decreased systolic pressure (heart and cardiovascular system)
- Rapid, shallow breathing (respiratory system)
- Cold, pale, clammy, diaphoretic, or even cyanotic skin (skin and extremities)

Because hemorrhage is the most common cause of shock in the trauma patient, all shock should be considered to be hemorrhagic until proven otherwise. The first priority is to examine for external sources of hemorrhage and control them as quickly and completely as possible. This may involve such techniques as application of pressure dressing, tourniquets, or splinting of extremity fractures. If there is no evidence of external hemorrhage, internal hemorrhage should be suspected. Although definitive management of internal hemorrhage is not practical in the prehospital setting, identification of an internal source mandates rapid transport to the definitive care institution. Internal hemorrhage can occur in the chest, abdomen, pelvis, or retroperitoneum. Evidence of blunt or penetrating chest injury would suggest a thoracic source. The abdomen, pelvis, and retroperitoneum can be a source of bleeding with evidence of blunt trauma (e.g., bruising, ecchymosis) or penetrating trauma, abdominal distension or tenderness, pelvic instability, leg length inequality, pain in the pelvic area aggravated by movement, perineal ecchymosis, and blood at the urethral meatus. As a general rule, patients who meet National Trauma Triage Protocol (NTTP) criteria 1 or 2 (or both) need rapid transport to the nearest trauma center (Figure 5-10).

If the assessment does not suggest hemorrhage as the cause of the shock, nonhemorrhagic causes should be suspected. These include cardiac tamponade and neurogenic shock.

Areas of patient evaluation include status of the airway, ventilation, perfusion, skin color and temperature, and blood pressure. Each is presented separately here in the context of both the primary survey (initial assessment) and the secondary survey (focused history and physical examination). Simultaneous evaluation is an important part of patient assessment to gather and process information from different sources simultaneously.

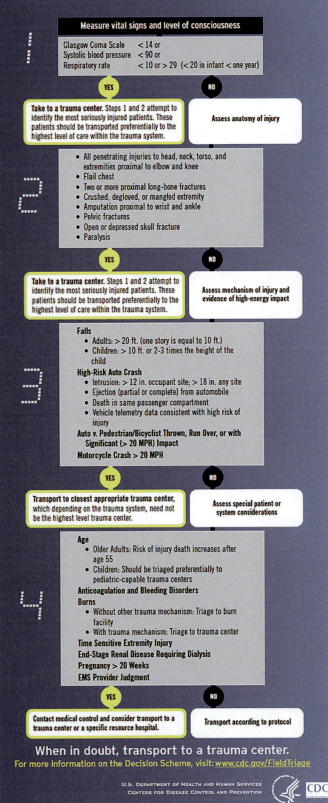

FIGURE 5-10 National Trauma Triage Protocol.
(Courtesy U.S. Department of Health and Human Services, Centers for Disease Control and Prevention.)

Primary Survey

The first step in patient assessment is to get a general impression of the patient's condition as quickly as possible. The following signs identify the need for suspicion of life-threatening conditions:

- Mild anxiety, progressing to confusion or altered LOC
- Mild tachypnea, leading to rapid, labored ventilations
- Mild tachycardia, progressing to marked tachycardia
- Weakened radial pulse, progressing to an absent radial pulse
- Pale or cyanotic skin color
- Loss of pulses in the extremities
- Hypothermia

Any compromise or failure of the airway, breathing, or circulatory system must be managed before proceeding. The following steps are described in an ordered series; however, all these assessments are carried out more or less simultaneously.

Airway

Assessment should include evaluation of the airway to ensure its patency (see Chapter 4).

Breathing. As noted earlier, the anaerobic metabolism associated with decreased cellular oxygenation will produce an increase in lactic acid. The hydrogen ions (H^+) from the acidosis and hypoxia lead to stimulation of the respiratory center to increase the rate and depth of ventilation. Thus, tachypnea is often one of the earliest signs of shock. In the primary survey, time is not taken to measure a ventilatory rate. Instead, ventilations should be estimated to be slow, normal, fast, or very fast. A slow ventilatory rate, in conjunction with shock, generally indicates that a patient is in profound shock and may be moments away from cardiac arrest. Any fast ventilatory rate is a concern and should serve as an impetus to search for the cause of shock. A patient who tries to remove an oxygen mask, particularly when such action is associated with anxiety and belligerence, is displaying another sign of cerebral ischemia. This patient has "air hunger" and feels the need for more ventilation. The presence of a mask over the nose and mouth creates a psychological feeling of ventilatory restriction. This action should be a clue that the patient is not receiving enough oxygen and is hypoxic.

Circulation. There are two components in the assessment of circulation:

- Hemorrhage
- Perfusion with oxygenated blood
  - Total body
  - Regional

The information obtained during the cardiac assessment helps to make a quick initial determination of the patient's total blood volume and perfusion status and, secondarily, provide a similar assessment of specific regions of the body. For example, the pulse, skin color, and temperature of a lower extremity may show compromised perfusion while the same signs may be normal in the upper extremity. This does not mean the signs are inaccurate, only that one part is different from another. The immediate question that must be answered is "Why?" It is important to check for these circulatory and perfusion findings in more than one part of the body and to remember that the assessment of the total body condition should not be based on a single part.

Hemorrhage. Assessment of circulation begins with a rapid scan for significant external hemorrhage. The patient may be lying on the major source of the hemorrhage if the injury is located on the back, or it may be hidden by the patient's clothes. Efforts at restoring perfusion will be much less effective in the face of ongoing hemorrhage. The patient can lose a significant volume of blood from scalp lacerations because of the high concentration of blood vessels or from wounds that damage major blood vessels (subclavian, axillary, brachial, radial, ulnar, carotid, femoral, or popliteal). Examine the entire body to identify external hemorrhage sources.

Pulse. The next important assessment point for perfusion is the pulse. Initial evaluation of the pulse determines whether it can be felt at the artery being examined. In general, loss of a radial pulse indicates severe hypovolemia (or vascular damage to the arm), especially when a central pulse, such as the carotid or femoral artery, is weak, thready, and extremely fast, indicating the status of the total body circulatory system. If the pulse is palpable, its character and strength should be noted, as follows:

- Is the rate strong or weak and thready?
- Is the rate normal, too fast, or too slow?
- Is the rate regular or irregular?

Although many individuals involved in the management of trauma patients focus on blood pressure, precious time should not be spent during the primary survey to obtain a blood pressure. The exact level of the blood pressure is much less important in the primary survey than other signs. Significant information can be determined from the pulse rate and character. In one study of trauma patients, a radial pulse characterized by prehospital care providers as "weak" was associated with blood pressure that averaged 26 mm Hg lower than a pulse thought to be "normal." More importantly, trauma patients with a weak radial pulse were 15 times more likely to die than those with a normal pulse.[4] Although generally obtained at the beginning of the secondary survey, blood pressure can be palpated or auscultated earlier in the assessment if sufficient assistance is present, or once the primary survey has been completed and life-threatening issues are being addressed during transport.

Level of Consciousness. Mental status is part of the disability evaluation, but altered mental status can represent impaired cerebral perfusion. An anxious, belligerent patient should be assumed to have cerebral ischemia and anaerobic metabolism until another cause is identified. Drug and alcohol overdose and cerebral contusion are conditions that cannot be treated rapidly, but cerebral ischemia can be treated. Therefore, all patients in whom cerebral ischemia might be present should be managed as if it is present.

Skin Color. Pink skin color generally indicates a well-oxygenated patient without anaerobic metabolism. Blue (cyanotic) or mottled skin indicates unoxygenated blood and a lack of adequate oxygenation to the periphery. Pale, mottled, or cyanotic skin has inadequate blood flow resulting from one of the following three causes:

1. Peripheral vasoconstriction (most often associated with hypovolemia)
2. Decreased supply of RBCs (acute anemia)
3. Interruption of blood supply to that portion of the body, such as might be found with a fracture or injury of a blood vessel supplying that part of the body.

Pale skin may be a localized or generalized finding with different implications. Other findings, such as tachycardia, should be used to resolve these differences and to determine if the pale skin is a localized, regional, or systemic condition. Also, cyanosis may not develop in hypoxic patients who have lost a significant number of their RBCs from hemorrhage. In patients who have dark-pigmented skin, cyanosis may be difficult to detect in the skin; instead, examine the lips, gums, and palms.

Skin Temperature. As the body shunts blood away from the skin to more important parts of the body, skin temperature decreases. Skin that is cool to the touch indicates decreased cutaneous perfusion and decreased energy production, and therefore shock. Because a significant amount of heat can be lost during the assessment phase, steps should be taken to preserve the patient's body temperature.

A good sign of adequate resuscitation is a warm, dry, pink toe. The environmental conditions in which the determination is made can affect the results, as can an isolated injury that affects perfusion.

Disability

One regional system that can be readily evaluated in the field is brain function. At least five conditions can produce an altered LOC or change in behavior (combativeness or belligerence) in trauma patients, as follows:

1. Hypoxia
2. Shock with impaired cerebral perfusion
3. Traumatic brain injury

4. Intoxication with alcohol or drugs
5. Metabolic processes such as diabetes, seizures, and eclampsia

Of these five conditions, the easiest to treat—and the one that will kill the patient most quickly if not treated—is hypoxia. Any patient with an altered LOC should be treated as if decreased cerebral oxygenation is the cause. An altered LOC is usually one of the first visible signs of shock. Brain injury may be considered primary (caused by direct trauma to brain tissue) or secondary (caused by the effects of hypoxia, hypoperfusion, edema, loss of energy production, etc.). There is no effective treatment in the prehospital setting for the primary brain injury, but secondary brain injury can essentially be prevented or significantly reduced by maintaining oxygenation and perfusion.

Brain function decreases as perfusion and oxygenation drop and ischemia develops. This decreased function evolves through various stages as different areas of the brain become affected. Anxiety and belligerent behavior are usually the first signs, followed by a slowing of the thought processes and a decrease of the body's motor and sensory functions.

The level of cerebral function is an important and measurable prehospital sign of shock. A belligerent, combative, anxious patient or one with a decreased LOC should be assumed to have a hypoxic, hypoperfused brain until another cause can be identified. Hypoperfusion and cerebral hypoxia frequently accompany brain injury and make the long-term result even worse. Even brief episodes of hypoxia and shock may worsen the original brain injury and result in poorer outcomes.

Body Exposure/Environment

The patient's body is exposed to assess for less obvious sites of external blood loss and clues that may indicate internal hemorrhage. The possibility of hypothermia is also considered. This exposure is best done in the patient compartment of a warm ambulance in order to protect the patient from the environment and prying eyes of the public.

Secondary Survey

In some cases, the patient's injuries may be too severe and the condition too critical for an adequate secondary survey to be completed in the field. If time permits, the secondary survey can be done while en route to the hospital if no other issues need to be addressed.

Vital Signs

Measurement of an accurate set of vital signs is one of the first steps in the secondary survey or, after reassessing the primary survey, when a few minutes are available during transport.

Ventilatory Rate. A rate of 20 to 30 breaths/minutes indicates a borderline abnormal rate and the need for supplemental oxygen. A rate greater than 30 breaths/minute indicates a late stage of shock and the need for assisted ventilation. Both these ventilatory rates indicate the need to look for the potential sources of impaired perfusion.

Pulse. In the secondary survey the pulse rate is determined more precisely. The normal pulse range for an adult is 60 to 100 beats/minute. With lower rates, except in extremely athletic individuals, an ischemic heart or a pathologic condition such as complete heart block should be considered. A pulse in the range of 100 to 120 beats/minute identifies a patient who has early shock, with an initial cardiac response of tachycardia. A pulse above 120/minute is a definite sign of shock unless it is caused by pain or fear, and a pulse over 140/minute is considered extremely critical and near death.

Blood Pressure. Blood pressure is one of the least sensitive signs of shock. Blood pressure does not begin to drop until a patient is profoundly hypovolemic (from either true fluid loss or container-enlarged relative hypovolemia). Decreased blood pressure indicates that the patient can no longer compensate for the hypovolemia and hypoperfusion. In otherwise healthy patients, blood loss must exceed 30% of blood volume before the patient's compensatory mechanisms fail and systolic blood pressure drops below 90 mm Hg. For this reason, ventilatory rate, pulse rate and character, capillary refilling time, and LOC are more sensitive indicators of hypovolemia than is blood pressure.

When the patient's pressure has begun to drop, an extremely critical situation exists, and rapid intervention is required. In the prehospital environment, a patient who is found to be hypotensive already has lost a significant volume of blood and ongoing blood loss is likely. The development of hypotension as a first sign of shock means that earlier signs may have been overlooked.

The severity of the situation and the appropriate type of intervention vary based on the cause of the condition. For example, low blood pressure associated with neurogenic shock is not nearly as critical as low blood pressure from hypovolemic shock. Figure 5-11 presents the signs used to assess compensated and decompensated hypovolemic shock.

FIGURE 5-11 Shock Assessment in Compensated and Decompensated Hypovolemic Shock

Vital Sign	Compensated	Decompensated
Pulse	Increased; tachycardia	Greatly increased; marked tachycardia that can progress to bradycardia
Skin	White, cool, moist	White, cold, waxy
Blood pressure range	Normal	Decreased
Level of consciousness	Unaltered	Altered, ranging from disoriented to coma

Ideally, shock will be recognized and treated in the earlier stages before decompensation occurs.

Musculoskeletal Injuries

Significant internal hemorrhage can occur with fractures (Figure 5-12). Of greatest concern are fractures of the femur and pelvis. A single femoral fracture may be associated with up to 1000 to 2000 mL of blood loss into a thigh. This injury alone could potentially result in the loss of 30% to 40% of an adult's blood volume, resulting in decompensated hypovolemic shock. Pelvic fractures, especially those resulting from significant falls or crushing mechanisms, can be associated with massive internal hemorrhage into the retroperitoneal space. A victim of blunt trauma can have multiple fractures and class III or IV shock but no evidence of external blood loss. For example, an adult pedestrian struck by a vehicle and sustaining four rib fractures, a humerus fracture, a femur fracture, and bilateral tibia/fibula fractures may experience internal bleeding of 3000 to 5500 mL of blood. This potential blood loss is enough for the patient to die from shock if it is unrecognized and inappropriately treated.

Confounding Factors

Numerous factors can confound the assessment because they obscure the usual signs of shock in the trauma patient.

Age

Patients at the extremes of life—the very young (neonates) and the elderly—have diminished capability to compensate for acute blood loss and other shock states. Thus, a relatively minor injury may produce decompensated shock in these individuals. On the other hand, children and young adults have a tremendous ability to compensate for blood loss and may appear relatively normal on a quick scan. A closer look may reveal subtle signs of shock, such as mild tachycardia and tachypnea, pale skin with delayed capillary refilling time, and anxiety. Because of their powerful compensatory mechanisms, children found in decompensated shock repre-

FIGURE 5-12 Approximate Internal Blood Loss Associated with Fractures

Type of Fracture	Internal Blood Loss (mL)
Rib	125
Radius or ulna	250–500
Humerus	500–750
Tibia or fibula	500–1000
Femur	1000–2000
Pelvis	1000–Massive

sent dire emergencies. Elderly individuals may be more prone to certain complications of prolonged shock, such as acute renal failure.

Athletic Status

Well-conditioned athletes often have enhanced compensatory capabilities. Many have resting heart rates in the range of 40 to 50 beats/minutes. Thus, a heart rate of 100 to 110 beats/minute or hypotension in a well-conditioned athlete may be warning signs that indicate significant hemorrhage.

Pregnancy

During pregnancy, a woman's blood volume may increase 45% to 50%. Heart rate and cardiac output during pregnancy are also increased. Because of this, a pregnant female may not demonstrate signs of shock until her blood loss exceeds 30% to 35% of her total blood volume. Also, well before the mother demonstrates signs of hypoperfusion, the fetus may be adversely affected because the placental circulation is more sensitive to vasoconstriction in response to the shock state. During the third trimester (months 6 to 9 of pregnancy), the gravid uterus may compress the inferior vena cava, greatly diminishing venous return to the heart and resulting in hypotension. Elevation of the patient's right side once she has been immobilized to a long backboard may alleviate this. Hypotension in a pregnant female that persists after performing this maneuver typically represents life-threatening blood loss.

Preexisting Medical Conditions

Patients with serious preexisting medical conditions, such as coronary artery disease and chronic obstructive pulmonary disease (COPD), are typically less able to compensate for hemorrhage and shock. These patients may experience angina as their heart rate increases in an effort to maintain their blood pressure. Patients with implanted fixed-rate pacemakers are typically unable to develop the compensatory tachycardia necessary to maintain blood pressure.

Medications

Numerous medications may interfere with the body's compensatory mechanisms.

Time Between Injury and Treatment

In situations where the emergency medical services (EMS) response time has been brief, patients may be encountered who have life-threatening internal hemorrhage but have not yet lost enough blood to manifest severe shock (class III or IV hemorrhage). Even patients with penetrating wounds to their aorta, venae cavae, or iliac vessels may arrive at the receiving facility with a normal systolic blood pressure if the EMS response, scene, and transport times are brief. The assumption that patients are not bleeding internally just because they "look good" is frequently very wrong. If a patient "looks good," it may well be because the patient's condition is compensated shock or because not enough time has elapsed for the signs of shock to manifest themselves. Patients should be thoroughly assessed for even the subtlest signs of shock, and internal hemorrhage should be assumed to be present until it is definitively ruled out. This is one reason why continued reassessment of trauma patients is essential.

Management

Steps in the management of shock are as follows:

1. Ensure oxygenation (adequate airway and ventilation)
2. Identify hemorrhage (control external bleeding)
3. Transport to definitive care

In addition to securing the airway and providing ventilation to maintain oxygenation, the primary goals of treatment of shock include identifying the source or cause, treating the cause as specifically as possible, and supporting the circulation. In the prehospital setting, external sources of bleeding should be identified and directly controlled immediately. Internal causes of shock usually cannot be definitively treated in the prehospital setting; therefore, the approach is to transport the patient rapidly (and safely) to the definitive care setting while supporting the circulation in the best way possible. Resuscitation in the prehospital setting includes the following:

- Improve oxygenation of the RBCs in the lungs:
    - Use appropriate airway management.
    - Provide ventilatory support with a bag-mask device, and deliver a high concentration of supplemental oxygen.
- Control both external hemorrhage and internal hemorrhage, to the extent possible in the prehospital setting. *Every red blood cell counts.*
- Improve circulation to deliver the oxygenated RBCs more efficiently to the systemic tissues, and improve oxygenation and energy production at the cellular level.
- Maintain body heat.
- Reach definitive care as soon as possible for operative hemorrhage control and replacement of lost RBCs, plasma, coagulation factors, and platelets.

Without appropriate measures, a patient will continue to deteriorate rapidly until he or she reaches the ultimate "stable" condition—death.

The following four questions need to be addressed when deciding what treatment to provide for a patient in shock:

1. What is the cause of the patient's shock?
2. What is the definitive care for the patient's shock?
3. Where can the patient best receive this definitive care?
4. What interim steps can be taken to support the patient and manage the condition while the patient is being transported to definitive care?

Although the first question may be difficult to answer accurately in the field, identification of the possible source of the shock assists in defining which facility is best suited to meet the patient's need and what measures may be necessary during transport to improve the patient's chances of survival.

Airway

The airway should be evaluated initially in all patients. Patients in need of immediate management of their airway include those with the following conditions, in order of importance:

1. Patients who are not breathing
2. Patients who have obvious airway compromise
3. Patients who have ventilatory rates greater than 20 breaths/minute
4. Patients who have noisy sounds of ventilation

Techniques for securing the airway and maintaining ventilation may be required in the prehospital setting, as outlined in Chapter 4. The importance of essential airway skills, especially when transport times are brief, should not be underestimated.

Breathing

Once a patent airway is ensured, patients in shock or those at risk for developing shock (almost all trauma patients) should initially receive supplemental oxygen.

A nonbreathing patient, or one who is breathing without an adequate depth and rate, needs ventilatory assistance using a bag-mask unit immediately. The rate at which a patient is assisted is important and generally should be no faster than 10 to 12 breaths/minute (one breath every 5–6 seconds). Hyperventilation during assisted ventilation produces a negative physiologic response, especially in the patient with hypovolemic shock.

Circulation: Hemorrhage Control

Control of obvious external hemorrhage immediately follows securing the airway and initiating oxygen therapy and ventilatory support, or it is performed simultaneously with these steps if sufficient assistance is present. If the hemorrhage is clearly life threatening and a rapid initial survey reveals that the patient is breathing, then efforts to control the hemorrhage can take priority. Early recognition and control of external bleeding in the trauma patient help preserve the patient's blood volume and RBCs and ensure continued perfusion of tissues. Even a small trickle of blood can add up to substantial blood loss if it is ignored for a long period. Thus, in the multisystem trauma patient, *no bleeding is minor, and every red blood cell counts* toward ensuring continued perfusion of the body's tissues.

External Hemorrhage

Steps in the field management of external hemorrhage are as follows:

- Handheld direct pressure
- Compression dressings
  - Elastic wrap
  - Air splint
- Tourniquet—extremities

Control of external hemorrhage should proceed in a stepwise fashion, escalating if initial measures fail to control bleeding.

Pressure. Direct hand pressure, applied over a bleeding site, is the initial technique employed to control external hemorrhage. The ability of the body to respond to and control bleeding from a lacerated vessel is a function of (1) the size of the vessel, (2) the pressure within the vessel, (3) the presence of clotting factors, and (4) the ability of the injured vessel to go into spasm. Vessels, especially arteries, that are completely divided (transected) often retract and go into spasm. There is often less hemorrhage from the stump of an extremity with a complete amputation than from an extremity with severe trauma but with blood vessels that are damaged but not completely transected.

For damaged blood vessels, the rate of blood loss is directly related to the size of the hole in the blood vessel and the *transmural pressure* (difference between the pressure inside the vessel and the pressure outside the vessel). Direct pressure over the site of hemorrhage increases the pressure outside the vessel and therefore reduces the transmural (internal vs. external) pressure, helping to slow or stop bleeding. Direct pressure also serves a second and equally important function. Compressing the sides of the torn vessel reduces the size (area) of the opening and further reduces blood flow out of the vessel. Even if blood loss is not completely stemmed, it may be diminished to the point that the blood-clotting system can stop the hemorrhage. This is why direct pressure is almost always successful at controlling bleeding.

Direct pressure on the open wound is followed by a pressure dressing. This is accomplished by (1) putting direct hand pressure over the bleeding site and (2) applying a pressure dressing onto the bleeding area to maintain the increased external pressure.

Two additional points about direct pressure should be emphasized. First, when managing a wound with an impaled object, pressure should be applied on either side of the object rather than over the object. Impaled objects should not be removed in the field because the object may have damaged a vessel, and the object itself could be occluding the hole in the blood vessel and preventing bleeding. Removal of the object

could result in uncontrolled internal hemorrhage. Second, if hands are required to perform other lifesaving tasks, a pressure (compression) dressing can be created using gauze pads and an elastic roller bandage or a blood pressure cuff inflated until hemorrhage stops. This dressing is placed directly over the bleeding site.

Tourniquets. In the past, emphasis has been placed on elevation of an extremity and compression on a pressure point (proximal to the bleeding site) as intermediate steps in hemorrhage control. No research has been published on whether or not elevation of a bleeding extremity slows hemorrhage. Similarly, the use of pressure points for hemorrhage control has not been studied. Thus, in the absence of compelling data, these interventions can no longer be recommended for situations where direct pressure or a pressure dressing has failed to control hemorrhage.

If external bleeding from an extremity cannot be controlled by pressure, application of a tourniquet is the reasonable next step in hemorrhage control (Figure 5-13). Tourniquets had fallen out of favor because of concern about potential complications, including damage to nerves and blood vessels and potential loss of the limb if the tourniquet is left on too long. None of these have been proven and, in fact, data from the Iraq and Afghanistan wars have demonstrated just the opposite.[5,6] Although there is a small risk that all or part of a limb may be sacrificed, given the choice between losing a limb or saving the patient's life, the obvious decision is to preserve life. Data from the military experience suggest that appropriately applied tourniquets could potentially have prevented 7 of 100 combat deaths.[7,8] *Used properly, tourniquets are not only safe but also lifesaving.*[9]

Device Options. Traditionally, a tourniquet has been devised from a cravat folded into a width of about 4 inches (10 cm)

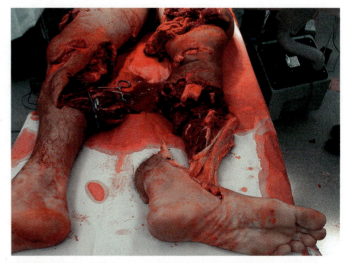

FIGURE 5-13 A fisherman who was run over by a motorboat suffered severe damage to his lower extremities. His life was saved by first responders who applied tourniquets to both thighs.

and wrapped twice around the extremity—the "Spanish windlass." A knot is tied in the bandage, and a metal or wooden rod is placed on top of the knot, and a second knot is tied. The rod is twisted until hemorrhage ceases, and the rod is then secured in place. Tourniquets that are narrow and bandlike should be avoided. Wider tourniquets are more effective at controlling bleeding, and they control hemorrhage at a lower pressure. An inverse relationship exists between tourniquet width and the pressure required to occlude arterial inflow. In addition, a very narrow band is also more likely to result in damage to arteries and superficial nerves. A blood pressure cuff represents another alternative that can be used as a tourniquet although air may leak out of the cuff, diminishing its effectiveness.

Because of the military's interest in an effective, easy-to-use tourniquet (especially one that a soldier could apply with one hand if the other arm was injured), many commercial tourniquets have been developed and marketed. Three products were 100% effective in occluding distal arterial blood flow in a laboratory study: the Combat Application Tourniquet (C-A-T, Phil Durango, Golden, Colo.), the Emergency Military Tourniquet (EMT, Delfi Medical Innovations, Vancouver, Can.), and the Special Operations Force Tactical Tourniquet (SOFTT, Tactical Medical Solutions, Anderson, S. C.).[10]

Application Site. A tourniquet should be applied just above the hemorrhaging wound. If one tourniquet does not completely stop the hemorrhage, then another one should be applied just above the first. Once applied, the tourniquet site should not be covered so that it can be easily seen and monitored for recurrent hemorrhage.

Application Tightness. A tourniquet should be applied tight enough to block arterial flow and occlude the distal pulse. A device that only occludes venous outflow from a limb will actually increase hemorrhage from a wound. A direct relationship exists between the amount of pressure required to control hemorrhage and the size of the limb. Thus, on average, a tourniquet will need to be placed more tightly on a leg to achieve hemorrhage control than on an arm.

Time Limit. Arterial tourniquets have been used safely for up to 120 to 150 minutes in the hospital operating room without significant nerve or muscle damage. Even in suburban or rural settings, many EMS transport times are significantly less than this period. In general, a tourniquet placed in the prehospital setting should remain in place until the patient reaches definitive care at the closest appropriate hospital. Military use has not shown significant deterioration with prolonged application times.[5] If application of a tourniquet is required, the patient will most likely need emergent surgery to control hemorrhage. Thus, the ideal receiving facility for such a patient is one with surgical capabilities. Figure 5-14 provides a sample protocol for tourniquet application. Another study[11] from the military in Iraq and Afghanistan showed a marked difference in survival when the tourniquet was applied before

FIGURE 5-14   Protocol for Tourniquet Application

1. Attempt to control hemorrhage with direct pressure or pressure dressing must fail.
2. A commercially manufactured tourniquet, blood pressure cuff, or "Spanish windlass" is applied to the extremity just proximal to the bleeding wound.
3. The tourniquet is tightened until hemorrhage ceases, and then it is secured in place.
4. The time of tourniquet application is written on a piece of tape and secured to the tourniquet ("TK 21:45" indicates that the tourniquet was applied at 9:45 PM).
5. The tourniquet should be left uncovered so that the site can be seen and monitored for recurrent hemorrhage.
6. Pain management should be considered unless the patient is in class III or IV shock.
7. The patient should ideally be transported to a facility that has surgical capability.

the patient decompensated into shock compared with applying it after blood pressure had dropped.

Internal Hemorrhage

Internal hemorrhage from damaged organs such as the liver or spleen cannot be managed in the field. Instead, the care revolves around recognition of the likelihood of such an injury and immediate transport to an appropriate destination. Internal hemorrhage from fractured bones should also be considered. Rough handling of an injured extremity not only may convert a closed fracture to an open one but also may significantly increase internal bleeding from bone ends, adjacent muscle tissue, or damaged vessels. All suspected extremity fractures should be immobilized in an effort to minimize this hemorrhage. Time may be taken to splint several fractures individually if the patient has no evidence of life-threatening conditions. If the primary survey identifies threats to the patient's life, however, the patient should be immobilized rapidly on a long backboard, thereby immobilizing all the extremities in an anatomic manner, and transported to a medical facility.

Disability

There are no unique, specific interventions for altered mental status in the shock patient. If the patient's abnormal neurologic status is the result of cerebral hypoxia and poor perfusion, efforts to restore perfusion throughout the body should result in improved mental status. In assessing a patient's prognosis after traumatic brain injury, an "initial" Glasgow Coma Scale (GCS) score is typically considered the score following adequate resuscitation and restoration of cerebral perfusion. Assessing a patient's GCS score while still in shock may result in an overly grim prognosis (see Chapter 6, Disability: Brain and Spine Trauma).

Body Exposure and Environment

Maintaining the patient's body temperature within a normal range is important. Hypothermia results from exposure to colder environments and from loss of energy production with anaerobic metabolism. Hypothermia is detrimental and negatively affects a patient's chance of survival.[12]

In the prehospital setting, increasing the core temperature once hypothermia has developed can be difficult; therefore, all steps that can be taken in the field to preserve normal body temperature should be initiated. After being exposed and examined, the patient must be protected from the environment and body temperature maintained. Any wet clothing, including that saturated with blood, is removed from the patient because wet clothing increases heat loss. The patient is covered with warm blankets. An alternative involves covering the patient with plastic sheets, such as heavy, thick garbage bags. They are inexpensive, easily stored, disposable, and effective devices for heat retention. Heated, humidified oxygen, if available, may help preserve body heat.

Once assessed and packaged, the shock patient is moved into the warmed patient compartment of the ambulance. Ideally, the patient compartment of an ambulance is kept at 85° F (29° C) or more when transporting a severely injured trauma patient. The patient's rate of heat loss into a cold compartment is very high. The conditions must be ideal for the patient, not for the providers, because the patient is the most important person in any emergency. A good rule of thumb to follow is that if the provider is comfortable in the patient compartment, it is too cold for the patient.

Patient Transport

Effective treatment of a patient in severe hemorrhagic shock requires a surgeon with access to an OR and blood. Because neither is routinely available in the prehospital trauma setting, rapid transportation to a facility that is capable of managing the patient's injuries is extremely important. Rapid transport does not mean disregarding or neglecting the treatment modalities that are important in patient care (doing the old-fashioned "scoop and run"). It also does not mean driving to the receiving hospital at breakneck speed. However, it does mean that the trauma care provider quickly institutes key, potentially lifesaving measures, such as airway management, ventilatory support, and hemorrhage control, while at the same time expediting the transport process in a safe fashion. Time must not be wasted on an inappropriate assessment or with unnecessary immobilization maneuvers. When caring for a critically injured patient, many steps, such as warming the patient and performing the secondary survey, are accomplished in the ambulance while en route.

Patient Positioning

In general, trauma patients who are in shock should be transported in the supine position, immobilized on a long backboard. Special positioning, such as the Trendelenburg position (placed on an incline with the feet elevated above the head) or the "shock" position (head and torso supine with legs elevated), although used for 150 years, has not been proven to be effective. The Trendelenburg position may aggravate already impaired ventilatory function by placing the weight of the abdominal organs on the diaphragm and may increase intracranial pressure in patients with traumatic brain injury.

Prolonged Transport

During prolonged transport, it is important that perfusion is maintained to the vital organs. Airway management should be optimized before a long transport. Ventilatory support is provided, with care taken to ensure that ventilations are of a reasonable tidal volume and rate so as not to compromise a patient with already tenuous perfusion.

Direct pressure by hand is impractical during a long transport, so significant external hemorrhage should be controlled with pressure dressings. If these efforts fail, a tourniquet should be applied. In situations where a tourniquet has been applied and transport time is expected to exceed 4 hours, attempts should be made to remove the tourniquet after more aggressive attempts at local hemorrhage control. The tourniquet should be slowly loosened while observing the dressing for signs of hemorrhage. If no rebleeding occurs, the tourniquet is completely loosened but left in place in case hemorrhage recurs. Conversion of a tourniquet back to a dressing should not be attempted in the following situations:

1. Presence of class III or IV shock
2. Complete amputation
3. Inability to observe the patient for rebleeding
4. Tourniquet in place longer than 6 hours[9]

Internal hemorrhage control should be optimized by splinting all fractures and applying the pneumatic antishock garment (PASG) or pelvic binder as indicated for intra-abdominal or retroperitoneal hemorrhage.

Techniques for maintaining normal body temperature, as previously described, are even more important in the setting of prolonged transport time. In addition to a warmed patient compartment, the patient should be covered with blankets or materials that preserve body heat; even large, plastic garbage bags help prevent loss of heat. Vital signs should be reassessed frequently to monitor response to resuscitation. The following should be documented at serial intervals: ventilation rate, pulse rate, blood pressure, skin color, and temperature. During prolonged transport, assessing the patient's clinical status and the response to resuscitation is key in determining outcome.

SCENARIO SOLUTION

Based on the mechanism, you should have a high suspicion for thoracic and abdominal injuries leading to hemorrhagic shock in the male patient and significant blood loss from the female patient's leg. No cervical spine immobilization is required in either of these patients. You apply hand pressure dressings to the hemorrhaging leg of the female and anticipate using a tourniquet if the bleeding is not controlled. Both patients should be loaded into the ambulance and transported as quickly as possible to the trauma center. High oxygen concentration should be delivered to the most appropriate airway device based on the level of consciousness and ability to maintain a secure airway after suctioning the airway.

The major focus of management is rapid extrication and transport to the trauma center, where definitive control of hemorrhage would prevent progression through the various stages of shock, leading to death or complications of hypoperfusion, such as renal failure, respiratory failure, and multiorgan dysfunction syndrome. ■

SUMMARY

- Shock causes a state of generalized hypoperfusion, resulting in cellular hypoxia, anaerobic metabolism, loss of energy production, lactic acidosis, hypothermia, and death if not appropriately treated.
- In the trauma patient, hemorrhage is the most common cause of this shock state.
- Care of the patient in shock or one who may go into shock begins with appropriate and complete assessment of the patient, starting with a history of the event and quick visual examination of the patient looking for obvious signs of shock and blood loss.
- The primary goal of therapy is to identify the likely source of hemorrhage and treat it specifically if possible. In the prehospital setting, this approach is most effective when the bleeding source is external. Internal hemorrhage can be treated definitively only by rapidly transporting the patient to the appropriate hospital.
- External hemorrhage should be controlled with direct pressure, followed by application of a pressure dressing. If this is ineffective, a tourniquet may be applied to the extremity proximal to the bleeding site.
- All trauma patients in shock, in addition to maintenance of adequate oxygenation, require rapid extrication and expeditious transport to a definitive care institution where the cause of the shock can be specifically identified and treated.

References

1. Gross SD: *A system of surgery: pathological, diagnostic, therapeutic, and operative,* Philadelphia, 1859, Blanchard and Lea.
2. Thal AP: *Shock: a physiologic basis for treatment,* Chicago, 1971, Yearbook Medical Publishers.
3. Marshall JC, Cook DJ, Christou NV, et al: The multiple organ dysfunction score: a reliable descriptor of a complex clinical syndrome, *Crit Care Med* 23:1638, 1995.
4. McManus J, Yershov AL, Ludwig D, et al: Radial pulse character relationship to systolic blood pressure and trauma outcomes, *Prehosp Emerg Care* 9:423, 2005.
5. Beekley AC, Sebesta JA, Blackbourne LH et al: Prehospital tourniquet use in Operation Iraqi Freedom: effect on hemorrhage control and outcomes members of the 31st Combat Support Hospital Research Group, *The Journal of Trauma* 64(2):S28-S37, February 2008
6. Kragh JF Jr, Walters TJ: Practical use of emergency tourniquets to stop bleeding in major limb trauma Baer, et al. *The Journal of Trauma* 64(2):S38-S50, February 2008.
7. Bellamy RF: The causes of death in conventional land warfare: implications for combat casualty care research, *Mil Med* 149:55, 1984.
8. Mabry RL, Holcomb JB, Baker AM, et al: United States Army Rangers in Somalia: an analysis of combat casualties on an urban battlefield, *J Trauma* 49:515, 2000.
9. Walters TJ, Mabry RL: Use of tourniquets on the battlefield: a consensus panel report, *Mil Med* 170:770, 2005.
10. Walters TL, Wenke JC, Kauvar DS, et al: Laboratory evaluation of battlefield tourniquets in human volunteers, US Army Institute of Surgical Research (unpublished).
11. Kragh JF Jr, Littrel ML, Jones JA, et al. [Epub ahead of print] Battle casualty survival with emergency tourniquet use to stop limb bleeding, *J Emerg Med* 2009 Aug 28.
12. Gentilello LM: Advances in the management of hypothermia, *Surg Clin North Am* 75:2, 1995.

Suggested Reading

American College of Surgeons Committee on Trauma: Shock. In *Advanced trauma life support for doctors, student course manual,* ed 8, Chicago, 2008, ACS.

CHAPTER 6

Disability: Brain and Spine Trauma

CHAPTER OBJECTIVES

At the completion of this chapter, the reader will be able to do the following:

✓ Relate the kinematics of trauma to the potential for traumatic brain injury (TBI).

✓ Incorporate the physical examination and historical data significant for TBI into assessment of the trauma patient.

✓ Formulate a plan of field intervention for both short and prolonged transport times for patients with TBI.

✓ Compare and contrast the specific types of primary TBI and secondary brain injury.

✓ Identify criteria for patient care decisions with regard to mode of transport, level of prehospital care, and hospital resources needed for the appropriate management of the TBI patient.

✓ Understand the role of hyperventilation in the TBI patient.

✓ Describe the epidemiology of spinal injuries.

✓ Compare and contrast the most common mechanisms that produce spinal injury in adults with those in children.

✓ Recognize patients with the potential for spinal trauma.

✓ Relate the signs and symptoms of spinal injury and neurogenic shock with their underlying pathophysiology.

✓ Integrate principles of anatomy and pathophysiology with assessment data and principles of trauma management to formulate a treatment plan for the patient with obvious or potential spinal injury.

✓ Describe the indications for spinal immobilization.

✓ Discuss factors associated with prehospital findings and interventions that may affect spinal injury morbidity and mortality.

Brain Trauma

SCENARIO

You and your partner are dispatched to an alleyway where a 30-year-old man was found lying unconscious and bleeding from the head. Bystanders state that he was assaulted by another man who ran away after striking the patient with a 2 × 4 piece of wood. They report he was unconscious for about 5 minutes but has now awakened. The scene appears safe. The primary survey reveals that the patient is maintaining his airway and breathing normally. A 3¼-inch (8-cm) laceration on the right side of his scalp is bleeding copiously but is readily controlled with direct pressure and a pressure dressing. His pulse rate is 116 beats/minute, and his skin is warm, pink, and well perfused. He opens his eyes spontaneously and follows commands; however, he does not recall the events leading up to the assault. He exhibits some confusion as he attempts to answer questions (Glasgow Coma Scale score [GCS] 14). You apply oxygen using a nonrebreather mask. During spinal immobilization, he speaks incomprehensible words and now only opens his eyes and withdraws his extremities to painful stimuli (GCS 9).

How should you alter your care based on the change in the patient's level of consciousness?

What injury is most likely present given the patient's presenting signs?

What are your management priorities at this point?

What actions may you need to take to combat increased intracranial pressure and maintain cerebral perfusion during a prolonged transport?

Approximately 1.4 million emergency department (ED) visits for traumatic brain injury (TBI) occur each year in the United States.[1] Although 80% of these patients are categorized as having only mild injuries, approximately 235,000 patients are hospitalized annually and about 50,000 patients with TBI die as a result of their TBI.[1] TBI contributes significantly to the death of about half of all trauma victims. Moderate to severe brain injuries are identified in about 100,000 trauma patients annually. Mortality rates for moderate and severe brain injuries are about 10% and 30%, respectively. Of those who survive moderate and severe brain injuries, between 50% and 99% have some degree of permanent neurologic disability.

Motor vehicle crashes (MVCs) remain the leading cause of TBI in those between the ages of 5 and 65 years of age, and falls are the leading cause of TBI in pediatric patients up to the age of 4 years and the elderly population. The head is the most frequently injured part of the body in patients with multisystem injuries. The incidence of gunshot wounds to the brain has increased in recent years in urban areas, and up to 60% of these victims die from their injury.

Patients with TBI represent some of the most challenging trauma patients to treat. They may be combative, and attempts to treat them can be extremely difficult. Intoxication with drugs or alcohol or the presence of shock from other injuries can hinder assessment. Occasionally, serious intracranial injuries can be present with only minimal evidence of external trauma. Skilled care in the prehospital setting focuses on ensuring the adequate delivery of oxygen and nutrients to the brain and rapidly identifying patients at risk for brain herniation and elevated intracranial pressure. This approach can decrease mortality from TBI and also the incidence of permanent neurologic disability.

Anatomy

Knowledge of head and brain anatomy is essential to understand the pathophysiology of TBI. The scalp is the outermost covering of the head and offers some protection to the skull and brain. The scalp is comprised of several layers, including skin, connective tissue, galea aponeurotica, and the periosteum of the skull. The galea is important because it provides the structural support to the scalp and is the key to its integrity. The scalp and soft tissues overlying the face contain many blood vessels and bleed profusely if lacerated.

The skull, or cranium, comprises a number of bones that fuse into a single structure during childhood (see Figure 6-1). Several small openings (*foramina*) through the base of the skull provide pathways for blood vessels and cranial nerves. One large opening, the foramen magnum, is located on the skull base and serves as a passageway for the brainstem to the spinal cord (Figure 6-1). In infancy, "soft spots" (*fontanelles*)

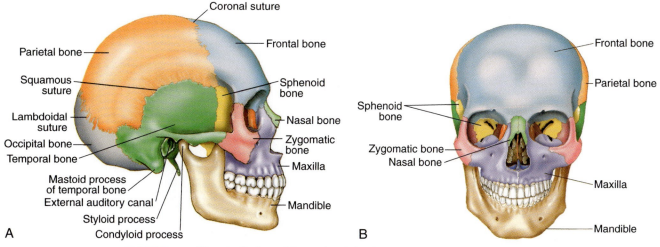

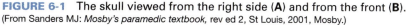

FIGURE 6-1   The skull viewed from the right side (**A**) and from the front (**B**).
(From Sanders MJ: *Mosby's paramedic textbook,* rev ed 2, St Louis, 2001, Mosby.)

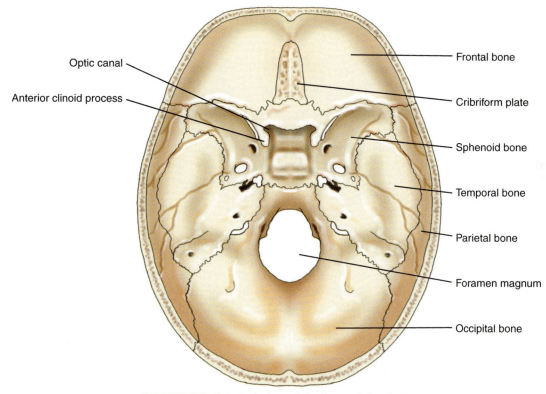

FIGURE 6-2   Internal view of the base of the skull.

can often be identified between the bones. The infant has no bony protection over these portions of the brain until the bones fuse, typically by 2 years of age.

Although most of the bones forming the cranium are thick and strong, the skull is especially thin in the temporal and ethmoid regions, which are more prone to fracture. The cranium provides significant protection to the brain, but the interior surface of the skull base is rough and irregular (see

Figure 6-2). When exposed to a blunt force, the brain may slide across these irregularities, producing cerebral contusions or lacerations.

Three separate membranes, the *meninges,* cover the brain (Figure 6-3). The outermost layer, the *dura mater,* is composed of tough fibrous tissue and is applied to the inside of the skull similar to a laminate. Under normal circumstances, the space between the dura and the inside of the skull, the

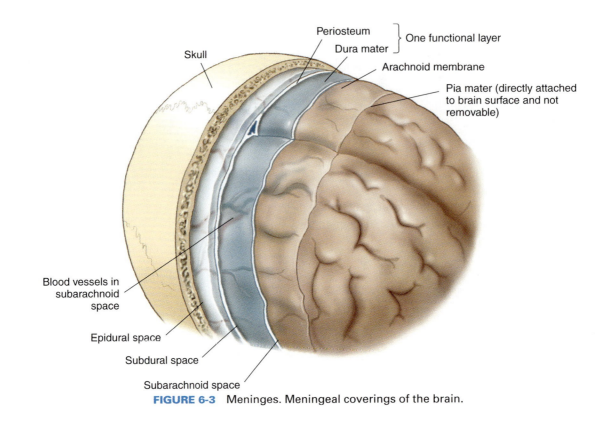

FIGURE 6-3   Meninges. Meningeal coverings of the brain.

epidural space, does not exist; it is a potential space. The middle meningeal arteries are located in grooves in the temporal bones on either side of the head, outside the dura. A blow to the thin temporal bone can create a fracture and tear the middle meningeal artery, resulting in bleeding inside the skull, the common etiology for epidural hematomas.

Unlike the epidural space, which is a potential space, the subdural space is an actual space, between the dura and the brain. This space is spanned in places by veins, which create a vascular communication between the skull and brain. The traumatic rupture of these veins often creates subdural hematomas, which, unlike epidural hematomas, are venous, of lower pressure, and often associated with brain injury. On the other side of the subdural space lies the brain, which is closely covered with two additional meningeal layers, the arachnoid and the pia. The *pia mater* is closely adhered to the brain, again similar to a laminate, and is the final brain covering. On top of the pia run cerebral blood vessels, which emerge from the base of the brain and then cover its surface. Layered on top of these blood vessels is the *arachnoid membrane,* which more loosely covers the brain and its blood vessels, giving the appearance of a "cellophane wrap" around the brain when it is viewed from the subdural space. Before cellophane existed, this covering was thought to resemble a spider web; thus, the name *arachnoid.* Because the cerebral blood vessels run on the surface of the brain but beneath the arachnoid membrane, their rupture (usually from trauma or a ruptured cerebral aneurysm) will result in bleeding into the subarachnoid space. This blood normally does not enter the subdural space

but is contained beneath the arachnoid; it can be seen at surgery as a thin layer of blood on the surface of the brain, contained beneath this translucent membrane. Unlike epidural and subdural hematomas, subarachnoid blood does not normally create mass effect but can be symptomatic of other serious injury to the brain.

The brain also is surrounded by *cerebrospinal fluid* (CSF), which is produced in the ventricular system of the brain and also surrounds the spinal cord. CSF helps cushion the brain and is contained in the subarachnoid space as well.

The brain occupies about 80% of the cranial vault in the skull and is divided into three main regions: the cerebrum, cerebellum, and brainstem (Figure 6-4). The *cerebrum* consists of right and left hemispheres that can be subdivided into several lobes. The cerebrum houses sensory functions, motor functions, and higher intellectual functions such as intelligence and memory. The *cerebellum* is located in the posterior fossa of the cranium, behind the brainstem and beneath the cerebrum, and coordinates movement. The *brainstem* contains the medulla, an area that controls many vital functions, including breathing and heart rate. Much of the reticular activating system (RAS), the portion of the brain responsible for arousal and alertness, is also found in the brainstem. Blunt trauma can impair the RAS, leading to a transient loss of consciousness. The 12 cranial nerves originate from the brain and brainstem (Figure 6-5). The oculomotor nerve, cranial nerve III, controls pupillary constriction and provides an important tool in the assessment of a patient with a suspected brain injury.

FIGURE 6-4   The Brain

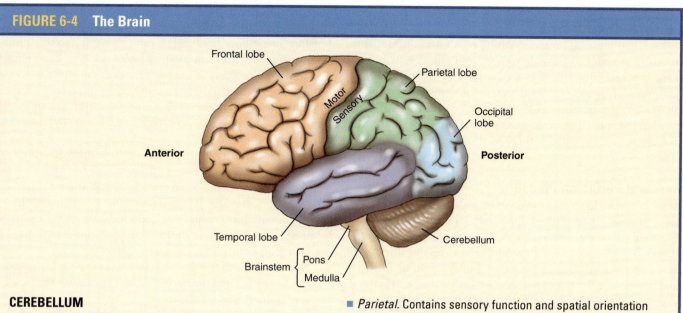

CEREBELLUM
- Controls coordination and balance

CEREBRUM
The cerebrum is composed of the right and left cerebral hemispheres. The dominant hemisphere is the one that contains the language center. This is the left hemisphere in virtually all right-handed individuals and about 85% of left-handed individuals. The cerebrum is composed of the following lobes:

- *Frontal.* Contains emotions, motor function, and expression of speech on the dominant side

- *Parietal.* Contains sensory function and spatial orientation
- *Temporal.* Regulates certain memory functions; contains the area for speech reception and integration in all right-handed and the majority of left-handed individuals
- *Occipital.* Contains vision

BRAINSTEM
- *Midbrain and upper pons.* Contain the reticular activating system (RAS), which is responsible for arousal and alertness
- *Medulla.* Contains the cardiorespiratory centers

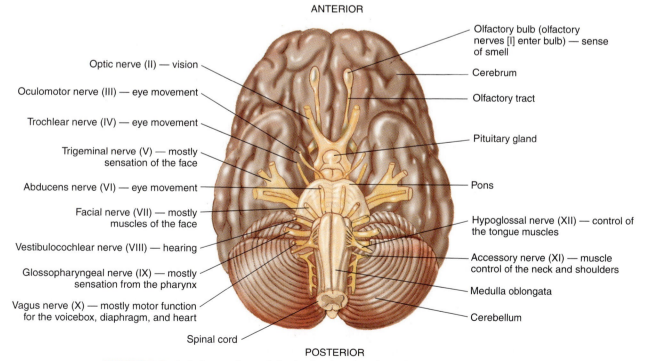

FIGURE 6-5   Inferior surface of the brain showing the origins of the cranial nerves.

Physiology

Cerebral Blood Flow

It is critical that the brain's neurons receive a constant flow of blood in order to provide oxygen and glucose. This constant cerebral blood flow is maintained by ensuring (1) an adequate pressure (cerebral perfusion pressure) to force blood into the head and (2) a regulatory mechanism (autoregulation), which ensures a constant blood flow by varying the resistance to blood flow as the perfusion pressure changes.

Cerebral Perfusion Pressure

Cerebral perfusion pressure (CPP) is the amount of pressure it takes to push blood through the cerebral circulation and thus maintain blood flow and oxygen and glucose delivery to the energy demanding cells of the brain. This relates directly to the amount of pressure inside the cranial vault, or intracranial pressure (ICP). Because the space inside the skull is fixed, anything that occupies additional space within the cranial vault will cause the intracranial pressure to start to increase. As the ICP increases, the amount of pressure needed to push blood through the brain also increases. If the patient's blood pressure cannot keep up with the increase in ICP, or if treatment to decrease the ICP is not rapidly instituted, the amount of blood flowing through the brain will start to decrease, leading to ischemic brain damage.

Autoregulation of CBF

The most important factor for the brain, however, is not CPP itself, but rather cerebral blood flow (CBF). The brain works very hard at keeping its cerebral blood flow constant over a wide range of changing conditions. This is known as autoregulation. Autoregulation is crucial to the brain's normal function.

Pathophysiology

TBI can be divided into two categories: primary and secondary.

Primary Brain Injury. Primary brain injury is the direct trauma to the brain and associated vascular injuries that occur at the moment of the original insult. It includes contusions, hemorrhages, and lacerations and other direct mechanical injury to the brain and its vasculature and coverings. Because neural tissue does not regenerate well, there is minimal expectation of recovery of the structure and function lost due to primary injury. Also, little possibility exists for repair.

Secondary Brain Injury. *Secondary brain injury* refers to the ongoing injury processes that are set in motion by the primary injury. At the time of injury, pathophysiologic processes are initiated that continue to injure the brain for hours, days, and weeks after the initial insult. The primary focus in the prehospital management of TBI is to identify and limit or stop these secondary injury mechanisms.

Large studies in the late 1980s demonstrated that unrecognized and untreated hypoxia (low blood oxygen) and hypotension (low blood pressure) were as damaging to the injured brain as elevated ICP. Subsequent observations have shown that impaired delivery of oxygen or energy substrate (e.g., glucose) to the injured brain has a much more devastating impact than in the normal brain. Therefore, in addition to hematoma, two other sources of secondary injury are hypoxia and hypotension.[2-6]

Secondary injury mechanisms include the following:

1. Compression of the brain from bleeding and swelling leading to elevated ICP and mechanical shifting of the brain, which can cause the brain to be squeezed through the foramen magnum (herniation) and significant morbidity and mortality if not addressed.
2. Hypoxia, which results from inadequate delivery of oxygen to the injured brain caused by ventilatory or circulatory failure or mass effect.
3. Hypotension and inadequate cerebral blood flow (CBF), which can cause inadequate oxygen delivery to the brain. Low CBF also reduces delivery of glucose to the injured.
4. Cellular mechanisms, including energy failure, inflammation, and "suicide" cascades, which can be triggered at the cellular level and can lead to cell death.

Intracranial Causes

Mass Effect and Herniation. The secondary injury mechanisms most often recognized are those related to *mass effect.* The brain is encased in a space that is fixed in size. All the space within the cranium is taken up by brain, blood, or CSF. If any other mass, such as a hematoma, cerebral swelling, or a tumor, occupies any space within the cranial vault, some other structure needs to be forced out (Figure 6-6).

At first, in response to the expanding mass, the volume of CSF surrounding the brain is reduced. The CSF naturally circulates within and around the brain, brainstem, and spinal cord; however, as the mass expands, more CSF is forced out of the head, and the total CSF volume within the skull is reduced. Blood volume in the cranial vault is also reduced in a similar manner, with venous blood the principal volume reduced in the head.

As a result of the CSF and blood volumes being reduced, the pressure in the head does not rise during the early phases of the expansion of intracranial masses. During this phase, if the growing mass is the only intracranial pathology, patients can appear to be asymptomatic. Once the ability to force out CSF and blood has been exhausted, however, the pressure inside the cranium, the ICP, starts to rise rapidly, and causes brain shift and various herniation syndromes, which can compress vital centers and jeopardize arterial blood supply to the brain. The consequences of this movement toward the foramen magnum are described as the various herniation syndromes.

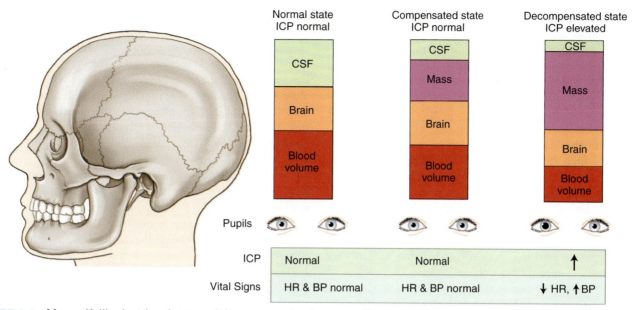

	Normal state ICP normal	Compensated state ICP normal	Decompensated state ICP elevated
ICP	Normal	Normal	↑
Vital Signs	HR & BP normal	HR & BP normal	↓ HR, ↑ BP

FIGURE 6-6 Monro-Kellie doctrine: intracranial compensation for expanding mass. The volume of the intracranial contents remains constant. If the addition of a mass such as a hematoma results in the squeezing out of an equal volume of cerebrospinal fluid *(CSF)* and venous blood, the intracranial pressure *(ICP)* remains normal. However, when this compensatory mechanism is exhausted, an exponential increase occurs in ICP for even a small additional increase in the volume of the hematoma.
(From McSwain NE Jr, Paturas JL: *The basic EMT: comprehensive prehospital patient care,* ed 2, St Louis, 2001, Mosby.)

If the expanding mass is along the convexity of the brain, as in the typical position for a temporal lobe epidural hematoma, the temporal lobe will be forced toward the center of the brain at the tentorial opening. This movement forces the medial portion of the temporal lobe, the *uncus,* into the third nerve, the motor tract, and the brainstem and RAS on that side. This is called *uncal herniation* and results in malfunction of the third cranial nerve, causing a dilated or blown pupil on the side of the herniation (Figure 6-7). It also results in loss of function of the motor tract on the same side, which causes muscle weakness on the opposite of the body from the lesion. In the last stages of uncal herniation, the RAS is affected and the patient lapses into coma, an event associated with a much poorer prognosis.

Another type of herniation, called *tonsillar herniation,* occurs as the brain is pushed down toward the foramen magnum and pushes the cerebellum and medulla ahead of it. This can ultimately result in the most caudal part of the cerebellum, the cerebellar tonsils, and the medulla becoming wedged in the foramen magnum, with the medulla subsequently being crushed. Injury to the lower medulla results in

cardiac and respiratory arrest, a common final event for patients with herniation. The process of forcing the posterior fossa contents into the foramen magnum is referred to as "coning"[7] (Figure 6-8).

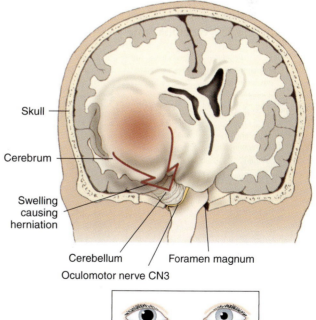

FIGURE 6-8 The skull is a large, bony structure that contains the brain. The brain cannot escape the skull if it expands because of edema or if there is hemorrhage in the skull that presses on the brain.

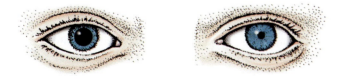

FIGURE 6-7 Suspect injury to the brain whenever a patient's pupils are unequal in size.

Clinical Herniation Syndromes. Clinical features of the herniation syndromes can help identify a patient who is herniating. Traditionally, as just mentioned, uncal herniation will often result in dilation or sluggishness of the pupil, referred to as a "blown pupil." Abnormal motor findings can also accompany herniation. Muscle weakness on the side opposite the abnormal pupil may be associated with uncal herniation. More extensive herniation can result in destruction of structures in the brainstem. This can result in *decorticate posturing*, which involves flexion of the upper extremities and rigidity and extension of the lower extremities. A more ominous finding is *decerebrate posturing*, in which all extremities are extended, and arching of the spine may occur. Decerebrate posturing occurs with injury and damage to the brainstem (Figure 6-9). After herniation, a terminal event may ensue and the extremities become flaccid, and motor activity is absent.[8,9]

In the final stages, herniation often produces abnormal ventilatory patterns or apnea (respiratory arrest), with worsening hypoxia and significantly altered blood CO_2 levels. *Cheyne-Stokes ventilations* are a repeating cycle of slow, shallow breaths that become deeper and more rapid and then return to slow, shallow breaths. Brief periods of apnea may occur between cycles. *Central neurogenic hyperventilation* refers to consistently rapid, deep breaths, and *ataxic breathing* refers to erratic ventilatory efforts that lack any discernible pattern. Spontaneous respiratory function ceases with compression of the brainstem, a common final pathway for herniation.[7]

As tissue hypoxia develops in the brain, reflexes are activated in an effort to maintain cerebral oxygen delivery. To overcome rising ICP, the autonomic nervous system is activated to increase systemic blood pressure. Systolic pressures can reach up to 250 mm Hg. However, as the receptors in the carotid arteries and aortic arch sense a greatly increased blood pressure, messages are sent to the brainstem to activate the parasympathetic nervous system. A signal is then sent to slow the heart rate. *Cushing's phenomenon* refers to this ominous combination of greatly increased arterial blood pressure and the resultant bradycardia that can occur with severely increased ICP.

Ischemia and Herniation. The herniation syndromes describe how the swelling brain, because it is contained in a fully enclosed space, can sustain mechanical damage. However, elevated ICP from cerebral swelling can also cause injury to the brain by creating cerebral ischemia as well as the resulting decreased oxygen delivery. As cerebral swelling increases, ICP also increases. Increases in ICP threaten cerebral blood flow. In addition to mechanical injury to the brain, cerebral swelling also can cause ischemic injury to the brain, compounding the ischemic insults the brain might sustain from other causes, such as systemic hypotension.

To complicate matters further, as these mechanical and ischemic insults create injury to the brain, they create more cerebral swelling. In this way, cerebral edema can cause injury that creates more cerebral edema, which in turn leads to further injury and edema in a downward spiral that can lead to herniation and death if not interrupted. Limiting this secondary injury and breaking this cycle of injury is the principal goal of TBI management.

Cerebral Edema. Cerebral edema (brain swelling) often occurs at the site of a primary brain injury. Injury to the nerve cell membranes allows fluid to collect within damaged neurons, leading to cerebral edema. In addition, injury can lead to inflammatory responses that injure the neurons and the cerebral capillaries, leading to additional fluid collection. As the edema develops, the mechanical and ischemic injury previously described occurs, which aggravates these processes and leads to further edema and injury.

Cerebral edema can occur in association with or as a result of intracranial hematomas, as a result of injury to the brain parenchyma in the form of cerebral contusion, or as a result of diffuse brain injury from hypoxia or hypotension.

Intracerebral Hematomas. In trauma, mass effect results from actual accumulation of blood in the intracranial space. Intracranial hematomas, such as epidural, subdural, or intracerebral hematomas, are major sources of mass effect. Because the mass effect from these hematomas is caused by their size, rapid removal of these hematomas can break the cycle of edema and injury described earlier. Unfortunately, these hematomas often have associated cerebral edema, and other means, in addition to removing the hematoma, are required to stop the cycle of injury and edema. (Specific cerebral hematomas are described later.)

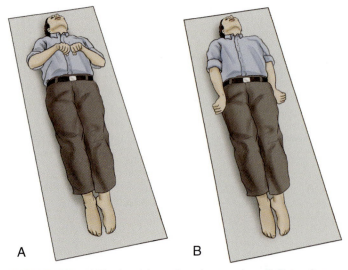

FIGURE 6-9 **A**, Flexion (decorticate) posturing. **B**, Extention (decerebrate) posturing.
(From Aehlert B: *Paramedic practice today: above and beyond*, St Louis, 2010, Mosby.)

Extracranial Causes

Hypotension. In the national TBI database, one of the most significant predictors of poor outcome from TBI was the amount of time spent with a systolic blood pressure (SBP) less than 90 mm Hg. In fact, a single episode of SBP less than 90 mm Hg can lead to a poorer outcome.[10] Several studies have confirmed the profound impact of low SBP on the outcome after TBI. Many patients with TBI sustain other injuries, often involving hemorrhage and subsequent low blood pressure.

Hypoxia. One of the most critical substrates delivered to the injured brain by the circulation is oxygen. Irreversible brain damage can occur after only 4 to 6 minutes of cerebral anoxia. Several studies have demonstrated that significant numbers of TBI victims present with low or inadequate oxygen levels.[5] The emphasis on prehospital airway management and oxygen delivery for brain-injured patients has partly been the result of these studies. Limiting hypotension is a key component in ensuring that the brain receives an adequate supply of oxygen during the post-injury phase.[11]

Hemorrhage is common in patients with TBI, resulting not only in shock but also in loss of blood and therefore hemoglobin.

For oxygenated blood to be delivered to the brain, the lungs must be properly functioning, which they often are not after trauma. Patients with an inadequate airway, aspiration of blood or gastric contents, pulmonary contusions, or pneumothoraces have pathologic conditions that will interfere with good respiratory function and the ability to transfer oxygen from the inspired air to the blood. In addition to ensuring oxygen transport to the brain through adequate hemoglobin and circulation, providers must ensure adequate oxygenation through an adequate airway and with adequate ventilation.

As with hypotension, aggressive limitation of cerebral hypoxia with appropriate management of airway, breathing, and circulation is essential for limiting secondary brain injury.

Seizures. A patient with acute TBI is at risk for seizures for several reasons. Hypoxia from either airway or breathing problems can induce generalized seizure activity, as can hypoglycemia and electrolyte abnormalities. Ischemic or damaged brain tissue can serve as an irritable focus to produce grand mal seizures or status epilepticus. Seizures, in turn, can aggravate preexisting hypoxia caused by impairment of respiratory function. Additionally, the massive neuronal activity associated with generalized seizures rapidly depletes oxygen and glucose levels, further worsening cerebral ischemia.

Assessment

A quick survey of the kinematics of the injury, combined with a rapid primary survey, will help identify potential life-threatening problems in a patient with a suspected TBI.

Kinematics

As with all trauma patients, assessment must include consideration of the mechanism of injury. Because many patients with severe TBI have an altered level of consciousness (LOC), key data about the kinematics will often come from observation of the scene or from bystanders. The windshield of the patient's vehicle may have a spider web pattern, suggesting an impact with the patient's head, or a bloody object may be present that was used as a weapon during an assault. A lateral impact on the side of the head can cause fracture of the skull with injury to the underlying middle meningeal artery, leading to epidural hematoma, or it can cause a coup/contrecoup injury with venous damage and subdural hemorrhage. This important information should be reported to personnel at the receiving facility because it may be essential for proper diagnosis and management of the patient.

Primary Survey

Airway. The patency of the patient's airway should be examined and assured. In unconscious individuals the tongue may completely occlude the airway. Noisy ventilations indicate partial obstruction by either the tongue or foreign material. Emesis, hemorrhage, and swelling from facial trauma are common causes of airway compromise in patients with TBI.

Breathing. Evaluation of respiratory function must include an assessment of the rate, depth, and adequacy of breathing. As noted previously, several different breathing patterns can result from severe brain injury. In multisystem trauma patients, chest (thoracic) injuries can further impair both oxygenation and ventilation. Cervical spine fractures occur in about 2% to 5% of patients with TBI and may result in spinal cord injuries that significantly interfere with ventilation.

Adequate oxygen delivery to the injured brain is an essential part of the effort to limit secondary brain injury. Failure to maintain adequate amounts of oxygen appears to result in poorer outcomes for brain-injured patients. Assessing for adequate airway and ventilatory effort is crucial in the early stages of managing TBI.

Circulation. As noted previously, maintaining an SBP greater than 90 mm Hg is critical for limiting secondary brain injury in the victims of TBI. Therefore, the control of hemorrhage and the prevention and treatment of shock are critical. The prehospital care provider will note and quantify evidence of external bleeding, if possible. In the absence of significant external blood loss, a weak, rapid pulse in a victim of blunt trauma suggests life-threatening internal hemorrhage in the chest, abdomen, pelvis, or soft tissues surrounding long-bone fractures. In an infant with open fontanelles, sufficient blood loss can occur inside the skull to produce hypovolemic shock. A slow, forceful pulse may result from intracranial hypertension and indicate impending herniation (Cushing's phenomenon). In a patient with potentially life-threatening injuries, transport should not be delayed to measure blood pressure but should be performed en route as time permits.

Disability. During the primary survey and after the initiation of appropriate measures to treat problems identified in the airway, breathing, and circulation assessments, a baseline Glasgow Coma Scale (GCS) score should be calculated to assess the patient's LOC accurately (Figure 6-10). As described in Chapter 3, the GCS score is calculated by using the best response noted while evaluating the patient's eyes, verbal response, and motor response. Each component of the score should be recorded individually, rather than just providing a total so that specific changes can be noted over time. If a patient lacks spontaneous eye opening, a verbal command (e.g., "Open your eyes") should be used. If the patient does not respond to a verbal stimulus, a painful stimulus, such as nail bed pressure with a pen or squeezing of anterior axillary tissue, should be applied.

FIGURE 6-10   Glasgow Coma Scale

Evaluation	Points
EYE OPENING	
Spontaneous eye opening	4
Eye opening on command	3
Eye opening to painful stimulus	2
No eye opening	1
BEST VERBAL RESPONSE	
Answers appropriately (oriented)	5
Gives confused answers	4
Inappropriate response	3
Makes unintelligible noises	2
Makes no verbal response	1
BEST MOTOR RESPONSE	
Follows command	6
Localizes painful stimuli	5
Withdrawal to pain (nonlocalizing movement to pain)	4
Responds with abnormal flexion to painful stimuli (decorticate)	3
Responds with abnormal extension to pain (decerebrate)	2
Gives no motor response	1

Note that the lowest possible score is 3 and the highest possible score is 15.

The patient's verbal response can be examined using a question such as, "What happened to you?" If fully oriented, the patient will supply a coherent answer. Otherwise, the patient's verbal response is scored as confused, inappropriate, unintelligible, or absent. If the patient's airway is managed, the score is calculated from only the eye and motor scales.

The last component of the GCS is the motor score. A simple, unambiguous command should be given to the patient, such as, "Hold up two fingers" or "Show me a hitchhiker's sign." A patient who squeezes the finger of a prehospital care provider may simply be demonstrating a grasping reflex as opposed to following a command purposefully. A painful stimulus is used if the patient fails to follow a command and the patient's *best* motor response is scored. A patient who attempts to push away a painful stimulus is considered to be "localizing." Other possible responses to pain include withdrawal from the stimulus, abnormal flexion (decorticate) or extension (decerebrate) of the upper extremities, and absence of a motor function.

The pupils are examined quickly for symmetry and response to light. A difference of greater than 1 mm in pupil size is considered abnormal. A significant portion of the population has *anisocoria,* inequality of pupil size, either from birth or acquired as the result of eye trauma. It is not always possible in the field to distinguish between pupillary inequality caused by trauma and congenital or pre-existing post-traumatic anisocoria. Pupillary inequality should always be treated as secondary to the acute trauma until the appropriate workup has ruled out cerebral edema or motor or ophthalmic nerve injury.[12]

Expose/Environment. Patients who have sustained a TBI often have other injuries that threaten life and limb as well as the brain. All such injuries must be identified. The entire body should be examined for other potentially life-threatening problems.

Secondary Survey

Once life-threatening injuries have been identified and managed, a thorough secondary survey should be completed if time permits. The patient's head and face should be palpated carefully for wounds, depressions, and crepitus. Any drainage of clear fluid from the nose or ear canals may be CSF, indicating an open skull fracture.

The pupillary size and response should be rechecked at this time. Because of the incidence of cervical spine fractures in patients with TBI, as noted previously, the neck should be examined for tenderness and bony deformities.

In a cooperative patient, a more thorough neurologic examination should also be performed. This will include assessing the cranial nerves, sensation, and motor function in all extremities. Neurologic deficits, such as hemiparesis (weakness) or hemiplegia (paralysis), present on only one side of the body are considered to be indicative of TBI.

History. An AMPLE (*a*llergies, *m*edications, *p*ast history, *l*ast meal, *e*vents) history can be obtained from the patient, family members, or bystanders. Diabetes mellitus, seizure disorders, and drug or alcohol intoxication can mimic TBI. Any evidence of drug use or overdose should be noted. The patient may have a history of prior head injury and may complain of persistent or recurring headache, visual disturbances, nausea and vomiting, or difficulty speaking.[13]

Serial Examinations. About 3% of patients with apparently mild brain injury (GCS 14 or 15) may experience an unexpected deterioration in their mentation. During transport, both the primary survey and assessment of the GCS should be repeated at frequent intervals. Patients whose GCS deteriorates by more than 2 points during transport are at particularly high risk for an ongoing pathologic process.[12,14,15] These patients need rapid transport to an appropriate facility. The receiving facility will use GCS trends during transport in the patient's early management. Trends in the GCS or vital signs should be reported to the receiving facility and documented on the patient care report. Responses to management should also be recorded.[16]

Specific Head and Neck Injuries

Scalp

As noted in the anatomy section, the scalp is composed of multiple layers of tissue and contains numerous blood vessels; even a small laceration may result in copious hemorrhage. More complex injuries, such as a degloving injury, in which a large area of the scalp is torn back from the skull, can result in hypovolemic shock and even exsanguination (Figure 6-11). These types of injury often occur in an unrestrained front-seat occupant of a vehicle whose head impacts the windshield, as well as in workers whose long hair becomes caught in machinery. A serious blow to the head may result in the formation of a scalp hematoma, which may be confused with a depressed skull fracture while palpating the scalp.

Skull Fractures

Fractures of the skull can result from either blunt or penetrating trauma. *Linear fractures* account for about 80% of skull fractures; however, a powerful impact may produce a *depressed* skull fracture, where fragments of bone are driven toward or into the underlying brain tissue (Figure 6-12). Although simple linear fractures can be diagnosed only with a radiographic study, depressed skull fractures can often be felt during a careful physical examination. A closed, nondepressed skull fracture by itself is of little clinical significance, but its presence increases the risk of an intracranial hematoma. Closed, depressed skull fractures may require neurosurgical intervention. Open skull fractures can result from a particularly severe impact or from a gunshot wound and serve as an entry site for bacteria, predisposing the patient to meningitis. If the dura mater is torn, brain tissue or CSF may leak from an open skull fracture. Because of the risk of meningitis, these wounds require immediate neurosurgical evaluation.

Basilar skull fractures (fractures of the floor of the cranium) should be suspected if CSF is draining from the nostrils or ear canals. Periorbital bruising (ecchymosis) ("raccoon eyes") and Battle's sign, in which ecchymosis is noted behind the ears, often occur with basilar skull fractures, although they may take several hours after injury to become apparent.

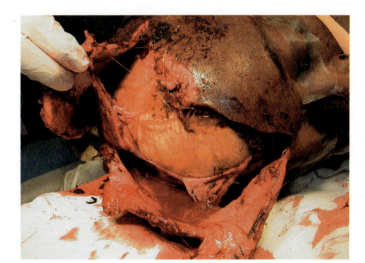

FIGURE 6-11 Extensive scalp injuries may result in massive external hemorrhage.

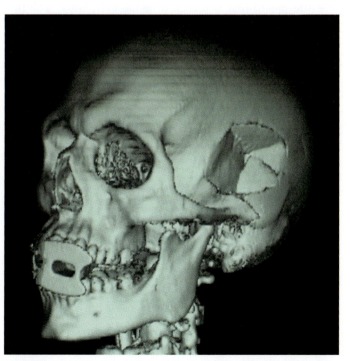

FIGURE 6-12 Depressed skull fracture may force particles of bone into the brain tissue.

Facial Injuries

Injuries to the face range from minor soft tissue trauma to severe injuries associated with airway compromise or hypovolemic shock. The airway may be compromised by either structural changes resulting from the trauma or from fluid or other objects in the airway itself. Structural changes may result from deformities of the fractured facial bones or from hematomas that develop in the tissues. Because the head has a high concentration of blood vessels, many injuries to this region result in significant hemorrhage. Blood and blood clots may interfere with the patency of the airway. Facial trauma is often associated with alterations in consciousness and even severe trauma to the brain. Trauma to the face may result in fractures or displacement of teeth into the airway lumen. TBIs and swallowed blood from facial injuries may lead to vomiting, which also leads to airway obstruction.

Trauma to the Eye and Orbit

Injury to the structures of the orbit and eye are not uncommon and often result from direct trauma to the face either from intentional (assault) or unintentional causes. Although injury of the globe (eyeball) itself is not often encountered, it must be a consideration whenever trauma to the face and orbit is noted because proper management of a globe injury may result in salvage of the patient's vision.

Eyelid Laceration. In the prehospital setting, laceration of an eyelid must cause consideration of the possibility that the globe has been penetrated. Field treatment consists of immediately covering the eye with a protective rigid shield (*not* a pressure patch) that is placed over the bony orbit. The primary consideration is to avoid any pressure on the eye that might do further harm by forcing intraocular contents out through a corneal or scleral laceration.

Corneal Abrasion. A corneal abrasion is a disruption of the protective covering of the cornea. This results in intense pain, tearing, light sensitivity (photophobia), and increased susceptibility to infection until the defect has healed (usually in 2 to 3 days). There is typically a history of trauma or contact lens wear. Prehospital management for this disorder in the urban setting is to cover the eye with a patch, shield, or sunglasses to reduce the discomfort caused by light sensitivity.

Subconjunctival Hemorrhage. Subconjunctival hemorrhage is a bright red area over the sclera of the eye that results from bleeding between the conjunctiva and the sclera. It is easily visible (Figure 6-13). This injury is innocuous and resolves over a period of several days to several weeks without treatment. In the presence of antecedent trauma, one should be alert for another, more serious injury. In particular, if hemorrhage results in massive swelling of the conjunctiva (chemosis), an occult globe rupture should be suspected. Prehospital

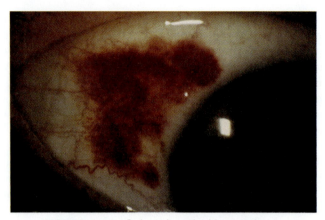

FIGURE 6-13 Subconjunctival hemorrhage.

management of this disorder consists solely of transporting the patient to the hospital so that the diagnosis can be confirmed and other associated disorders ruled out.

Hyphema. *Hyphema* is defined as blood in the anterior chamber of the globe between the iris and the cornea. This is usually seen in the setting of acute trauma. The eye should be examined with the victim sitting upright. If enough blood is present, it collects at the bottom of the anterior chamber and is visible as a layered hyphema (Figure 6-14). This may not be appreciated if the victim is examined while in a supine position or if the amount of blood is very small. Hyphema patients should have a protective shield placed over the eye and be transported to the hospital in a sitting position (if there is no other contraindication) so that a complete eye examination can be performed.

Open Globe. If there is a history of trauma and penlight inspection of the eye reveals an obvious damaged eyeball (globe), the examination should be discontinued and a protective shield placed onto the bony orbit over the eye. Do *not* apply a pressure patch or instill any eye drops. There are two primary concerns in the management of this condition. The first is to mini-

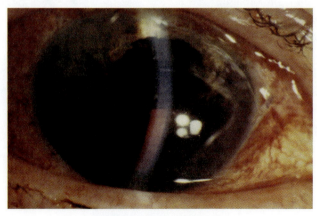

FIGURE 6-14 Hyphema.

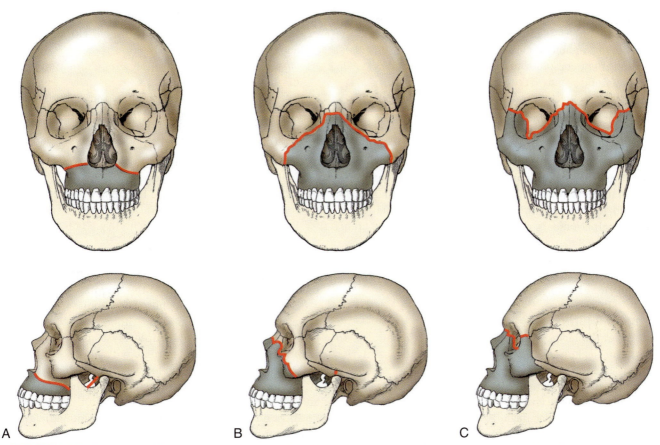

FIGURE 6-15 Types of Le Fort fractures of the midface. **A,** Le Fort I fracture. **B,** Le Fort II fracture. **C,** Le Fort III fracture. (From Sheehy S: *Emergency nursing,* ed 3, St Louis, 1992, Mosby.)

mize manipulation of or additional trauma to the eye that might raise intraocular pressure and result in expulsion of intraocular contents through the corneal or scleral defect. The second is to prevent development of post-traumatic endophthalmitis, an infection of the aqueous and vitreous humors of the eye. This typically has devastating visual results, with only 30% of victims in one study retaining visual acuity greater than or equal to 20/400.[17] Expeditious transport to the hospital is warranted for ophthalmologic evaluation and surgical repair.

A penetrating injury to the eye or a ruptured globe may not always be obvious. Clues to occult rupture include large subconjunctival hemorrhage with chemosis, dark uveal tissue (the colored iris) present at or protruding through the limbus (junction of the cornea and the sclera), distorted pupil, leak from a linear or punctate corneal epithelial defect, mechanism of injury (hammering metal on metal, impaling injury, etc.), or decrease in vision. If an occult globe rupture is suspected, the victim should be treated as described previously for an obvious open globe. The relatively less severe appearance of the injury does not eliminate the threat of endophthalmitis, so again rapid transport to the hospital is warranted.

Nasal Fractures

Fracture of the nasal bones is the most common fracture in the face. Indications that a nasal fracture is present include ecchymosis, edema, nasal deformity, swelling, and bloody nose (epistaxis). On palpation, bony crepitus may be noted.

Midface Fractures

Midfacial fractures can be categorized as follows (Figure 6-15):

Le Fort I fracture involves a horizontal detachment of the maxilla from the nasal floor. Although air passage through the nares may not be affected, the oropharynx may be compromised by a blood clot or edema in the soft palate.

Le Fort II fracture, also known as a *pyramidal fracture,* includes the right and left maxillae, the medial portion of the orbital floor, and the nasal bones. The sinuses are well vascularized, and this fracture may be associated with airway compromise from significant hemorrhage.

Le Fort III fracture involves the facial bones being fractured off the skull (craniofacial disjunction). Because of the forces involved, this injury may be associated with airway compromise, presence of TBI, injuries to the tear ducts, malocclusion of teeth, and CSF leakage from the nares.

Patients with a midface fracture generally have loss of normal facial symmetry. The face may appear flattened, and the patient may be unable to close the jaws or teeth. If conscious, the patient may complain of facial pain and numbness. On palpation, crepitus may be noted over fracture sites.

Mandibular Fractures

Following fractures of the nasal bones, mandibular (jaw) fractures are the second most common type of facial fracture. In more than 50% of cases the mandible is broken in more than one location. The most common complaint of a patient with a mandibular fracture is malocclusion of the teeth; that is, the upper and lower teeth no longer meet in their usual alignment. On palpation, a "step-off" type of deformity and crepitance may be noted.

In a supine patient with a mandible fracture, the tongue may occlude the airway because the bony support structure of the tongue is no longer intact.

Laryngeal Injuries

Fractures of the larynx typically result from a blunt blow to the anterior neck, or a motorcycle or bicycle rider's anterior neck may be struck by an object. The patient may complain of a change in voice (usually lower in tone). On inspection, the provider may note a neck contusion or loss of the prominence of the thyroid cartilage (Adam's apple). A fracture of the larynx may result in the development of subcutaneous emphysema (air) in the neck, which may be detected on palpation.

Injuries to Cervical Vessels

A carotid artery and internal jugular vein traverse the anterior neck on either side of the trachea. The carotid arteries supply blood to the majority of the brain, and the internal jugular veins drain this region. Injury to one of these vessels can produce profound hemorrhage. An added danger from internal jugular vein injuries is air embolism. If a patient is sitting up or the head is elevated, venous pressure may fall below atmospheric pressure during inspiration, permitting air to enter the venous system. A large air embolus can be fatal because it can interfere with both cardiac function and cerebral perfusion.

Brain Injuries
Cerebral Concussion. The diagnosis of a "concussion" is made when an injured patient shows any transient alteration in neurologic function. Although most people associate a loss of consciousness with the diagnosis of concussion, loss of consciousness is not required to make a diagnosis of concussion; rather, post-traumatic amnesia is the hallmark of concussion. Other neurologic changes include the following[18]:

- Vacant stare (befuddled facial expression)
- Delayed verbal and motor responses (slow to answer questions or follow instructions)

- Confusion and inability to focus attention (easily distracted and unable to follow through with normal activities)
- Disorientation (walking in the wrong direction; unaware of time, date, and place)
- Slurred or incoherent speech (making disjointed or incomprehensible statements)
- Lack of coordination (stumbling, inability to walk tandem/straight line)
- Inappropriate emotions to the circumstances (distraught, crying for no apparent reason)
- Memory deficits (exhibited by patient repeatedly asking the same question that has already been answered)
- Inability to memorize and recall (e.g., 3 of 3 words or 3 of 3 objects in 5 minutes)

In all patients with only a simple concussion, head computed tomography (CT) scan at the hospital will be normal.

Severe headache, dizziness, and nausea and vomiting often accompany a concussion. Although most of these findings last several hours to a couple days, some patients experience a post-concussive syndrome with headaches, dizziness, and difficulty concentrating for weeks and even months after a severe concussion. Patients exhibiting signs of concussion and especially patients with nausea, vomiting, or neurologic findings on secondary survey should be immediately transported for further evaluation.

Intracranial Hematoma. Intracranial hematomas are divided into three general types: epidural, subdural, and intracerebral. Because the signs and symptoms of each of these have significant overlap, specific diagnosis clinically in the prehospital setting (as well as the ED) is almost impossible, although the prehospital care provider may suspect one type over another based on the characteristic clinical presentation. Even so, a definitive diagnosis can only be made after a CT scan is performed at the receiving facility. Because these hematomas occupy space inside the rigid skull, they may produce rapid increases in ICP, especially if they are sizable.

Epidural Hematoma. Epidural hematomas account for about 2% of TBIs that require hospitalization. These hematomas often result from a low-velocity blow to the temporal bone, such as the impact from a punch or baseball. A fracture of this thin bone damages the middle meningeal artery, which results in arterial bleeding that collects between the skull and dura mater (Figure 6-16). This high-pressure arterial blood can start to peal the dura off of the inner table of the skull, creating an epidural space full of blood. Such an epidural hematoma has a characteristic lens shape, as seen on the CT scan, created by the dura holding the hematoma against the inner table of the skull. The principal threat to the brain is from the expanding mass of blood displacing the brain and threatening herniation. For this reason, patients whose epidural hematoma is rapidly evacuated often have excellent recoveries.

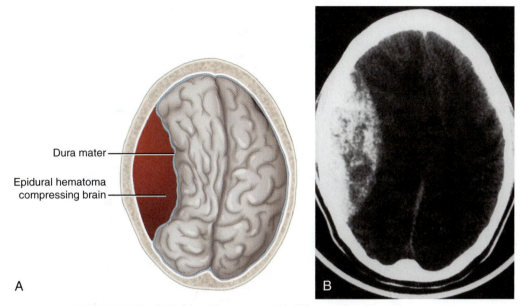

FIGURE 6-16 **A,** Epidural hematoma. **B,** CT scan of epidural hematoma. (**B** from Cruz J: *Neurologic and neurosurgical emergencies,* Philadelphia, 1998, Saunders.)

The classic history for an epidural hematoma is a patient experiencing a brief loss of consciousness, then regaining consciousness, and then experiencing a rapid decline in consciousness. During the period of consciousness, the *lucid interval,* the patient may be oriented, lethargic, or confused or may complain of a headache. Only about one third of patients with epidural hematomas actually experience this "lucid interval," however, and it may also occur with other types of intracranial hemorrhages, making it nonspecific for epidural hematoma. Nonetheless, a patient who experiences a "lucid interval," followed by a decline in GCS, is at risk for a progressive intracranial process and needs emergency evaluation.

As a patient's LOC worsens, examination may reveal a dilated and sluggish or nonreactive pupil on the side of the herniation (ipsilateral side). Because motor nerves cross over to the other side above the spinal cord, hemiparesis or hemiplegia typically occurs on the side opposite the impact (contralateral side). The mortality rate for an epidural hematoma is about 20%; however, with rapid recognition and evacuation, the mortality rate can be as low as 2%. This is because an epidural hematoma is usually a "pure" space-occupying lesion, with little injury to the brain beneath. Once the hematoma is removed, the pathologic effect is also removed, and the patient can make an excellent recovery. Such rapid removal reduces not only mortality but also subsequent, significant neurologic morbidity. Epidural hematomas often occur in young people, who are just beginning their careers, emphasizing the societal value as well as the human value of their rapid identification and removal.

Subdural Hematoma. Subdural hematomas account for about 30% of severe brain injuries. In addition to being more common than epidural hematomas, they also differ in etiology, location, and prognosis. Unlike the epidural hematoma caused by arterial hemorrhage, a subdural hematoma generally results from a venous bleed from bridging veins that are torn during a violent blow to the head. In this injury the blood collects in the subdural space, between the dura mater and the arachnoid membrane (Figure 6-17).

The disruption of the bridging veins usually results in relatively rapid accumulation of blood in the subdural space, with rapid onset of mass effect. Adding to this morbidity is injury to the brain tissue itself beneath the subdural hematoma, which occurs as part of the injury leading to the venous disruption. As a result, unlike epidural hematomas, the mass effect of subdural hematomas is often caused by both the accumulated blood and the swelling of the injured brain beneath. Patients presenting with such acute mass effect will have an acutely depressed mental status and will need emergency ICP monitoring and management and possibly surgery.

Cerebral Contusions. Damage to the brain itself may produce cerebral contusions and, if this damage includes injury to the blood vessels within the brain, actual bleeding into the substance of the brain, or *intracerebral hematomas.* Cerebral contusions are relatively common, occurring in about 20% to 30% of severe brain injuries, but in a significant percentage of moderate head injuries as well. Although typically the result of blunt trauma, these injuries may also occur from penetrating trauma, such as a gunshot wound to the brain. In blunt trauma, cerebral contusions may be numerous. Cerebral contusions result from a complex pattern of transmission and reflection of forces within the skull. As a result, contusions often occur in locations remote from the site of impact, often on the opposite side of the brain, commonly referred to as "contrecoup" injury.

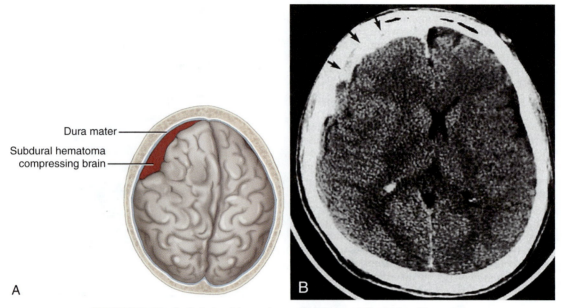

FIGURE 6-17 **A,** Subdural hematoma. **B,** CT scan of subdural hematoma. (**B** from Cruz J: *Neurologic and neurosurgical emergencies,* Philadelphia, 1998, Saunders.)

Cerebral contusions often take 12 to 24 hours to appear on CT scans, and thus a patient with a cerebral contusion may have an initially normal head CT scan. The only clue to its presence may be a depressed GCS, with many patients showing moderate head injuries (GCS 9–13). As the contusion evolves after injury, it not only becomes more apparent on head CT but also can cause increased mass effect and create increasing headache, or cause moderate head injuries to deteriorate to severe head injuries in about 10% of patients.[19]

Subarachnoid Hemorrhage. Subarachnoid hemorrhage is bleeding beneath the arachnoid membrane, which lies under the subdural space covering the brain. Many of the brain's blood vessels are located in the subarachnoid space, so injury to these vessels will cause subarachnoid bleeding, a layering of blood beneath the arachnoid membrane on the surface of the brain. This layering of blood is usually very thin and rarely causes mass effect.

Subarachnoid hemorrhage is usually thought to be associated with ruptured cerebral aneurysms. In fact, post-traumatic subarachnoid hemorrhage is the most common cause of subarachnoid bleeding. Because subarachnoid bleeding rarely causes mass effect, it does not require surgery for decompression. It is a marker for potentially severe brain injury, however, and its presence increases the risk for other space-occupying lesions. Patients with traumatic subarachnoid hemorrhage (tSAH) have a 63% to 73% increased risk of a cerebral contusion, and 44% will develop subdural hematomas. Patients with tSAH have an increased risk of elevated ICP and intraventricular hemorrhage. Patients with large amounts of tSAH have a 72% to 78% chance for a poor outcome, and in the Trauma Coma Data Bank the presence of tSAH doubled the incidence of death in brain-injured patients.[17,20]

Management

Effective management of a patient with TBI begins with orderly interventions focused on treating any life-threatening problems identified in the primary survey. Once these problems are addressed, the patient should be rapidly packaged and transported to the nearest facility capable of caring for patients with TBI.

Airway

Patients with a depressed LOC may be unable to protect their airway, and adequate oxygenation of the injured brain is critical to preventing secondary injury. As noted earlier, facial injuries can be associated with hemorrhage and edema that may compromise the airway. Hematomas in the floor of the mouth or in the soft palate may occlude the airway. The essential skills are appropriate initial airway interventions (see Chapter 4). Both oral and nasal airways may become occluded by edema or blood clots, and intermittent suctioning may be necessary. Patients with facial fractures and laryngeal or other neck injuries will typically assume a position that maintains their airway. Attempts to force a patient to lie supine or wear a cervical collar may be met with extreme combativeness if they become hypoxic as a result of positional airway impairment. In these situations, airway patency takes precedence over spinal immobilization, and patients may be transported in a sitting or semisitting position, as tolerated.

Cervical collars may be deferred if thought to compromise the airway while manual stabilization is performed. Conscious patients can often assist in managing their airway by suctioning when they feel it is needed; the provider can allow them to hold and use the suction device. Facial trauma, including those injuries caused by gunshot wounds, is not a contraindication to endotracheal intubation.

Breathing

All patients with suspected TBI should receive supplemental oxygen. Oxygen should be provided via a non-rebreather facemask for a spontaneously breathing patient.

The degree of ventilation is judged by counting breaths per minute. Normal ventilatory rates should be used when assisting ventilation in patients with TBI: 10 breaths/minute for adults, 20 breaths/minute for children, and 25 breaths/minute for infants. Overaggressive hyperventilation produces cerebral vasoconstriction, which in turn leads to a decrease in cerebral oxygen delivery. For adult patients, ventilating with a tidal volume of 350 to 500 mL at a rate of 10 breaths/minute should be sufficient to maintain adequate oxygenation without inducing hypocarbia.[21]

Hyperventilation of a patient in a controlled fashion may be considered in the specific circumstance of signs of herniation. These signs include asymmetric pupils, dilated and nonreactive pupils, extensor posturing or no response on motor examination, or progressive neurologic deterioration, defined as a decrease in the GCS of more than 2 points in a patient whose initial GCS was 8 or less. In such cases, mild, controlled hyperventilation in the field may be performed during the prehospital phase of care. Mild hyperventilation is defined as careful control of the breathing rate (20 breaths/minute for adults, 25 breaths/minute for children, and 30 breaths/minute for infants less than 1 year of age).[22]

Circulation

Both blood loss and hypotension are important causes of secondary brain injury, so efforts should be taken to prevent or treat these conditions. Hemorrhage control is essential. Direct pressure or pressure dressings should be applied to any external hemorrhage. Complex scalp wounds can produce significant external blood loss. Several gauze pads held in place by an elastic roller bandage creates an effective pressure dressing to control bleeding. If this fails to control bleeding, it can often be controlled by applying direct pressure along the wound edges, thereby compressing the scalp vasculature between the skin and the skull. Dramatic bleeding can often be controlled with this maneuver. A pressure dressing should not be applied to a depressed or open skull fracture unless significant hemorrhage is present, because it may aggravate brain injury and lead to an increase in ICP. Direct gentle pressure may also limit the size of extracranial (scalp) hematomas. Gentle handling and immobilization to a long backboard in anatomic alignment can minimize blood loss around fractures.

Hemorrhage from the carotid arteries and internal jugular veins may be massive. In most circumstances, direct pressure will control such external hemorrhage. Injuries to these vessels from penetrating trauma may be associated with internal bleeding presenting as an expanding hematoma. These hematomas may compromise the airway, and airway management may be necessary. Because hypotension further worsens brain ischemia, standard measures should be employed to combat shock. In patients with TBI, the combination of hypoxia and

hypotension is associated with a mortality rate of about 75%. If shock is present and major internal hemorrhage is suspected, prompt transport to a trauma center takes priority over brain injuries.

Disability

Assessment using the Glasgow Coma Scale (GCS) should be integrated into the routine evaluation of all trauma patients after circulation is addressed. Use of the GCS helps evaluate the patient's status and may impact transport and triage decisions, depending on the system in which the provider is working.

Prehospital management of TBI patients primarily consists of measures aimed at reversing and preventing factors that cause secondary brain injury. Because of the significant incidence of cervical spine fractures, patients with suspected TBI should be placed in spinal immobilization. Some degree of caution must be exercised when applying a cervical collar to a patient with TBI. Some evidence suggests that a tightly fitted cervical collar can impede venous drainage of the head, thereby increasing ICP. *Application of a cervical collar is not mandatory as long as the head and neck are sufficiently immobilized.*

Transportation

To achieve the best possible outcome, patients with moderate and severe TBI should be transported directly to a trauma center that can perform a CT scan and ICP monitoring and provide prompt neurosurgical intervention. If such a facility is not available, aeromedical transport from the scene to an appropriate trauma center should be considered.[16]

The patient's pulse rate, blood pressure, and GCS should be reassessed and documented every 5 to 10 minutes during transport. The patient's body heat should be preserved during transport.

The receiving facility should be notified as early as possible so that appropriate preparations can be made before the patient's arrival. The radio report should include information regarding the mechanism of injury, initial GCS score and any changes en route, focal signs (e.g., motor exam asymmetry, unilaterally or bilaterally dilated pupils) and vital signs, other serious injuries, and response to management.[16]

Prolonged Transport. As with all patients with suspected TBI, efforts should focus on preventing secondary brain injury. A prolonged transport time may lower the threshold for performing airway management. Efforts to control the airway should be performed while cervical spine stabilization is being applied. Oxygen should be administered. Because of the risk of developing pressure ulcers from lying on a hard backboard, the patient may be placed on a padded long backboard, especially if the anticipated transport time is lengthy. Serial vital signs, including ventilations, pulse, blood pressure, and GCS score, should be measured. Pupils should be periodically checked for response to light and symmetry.

The rapid decrease in this patient's GCS score is extremely worrisome, so you need to transport the patient to a facility with neurosurgical coverage immediately on completion of spinal immobilization. Given the lucid interval demonstrated by this patient, suspect the presence of an epidural hematoma. Examination of the eyes may reveal an enlarged, sluggishly reactive pupil on the right side, and weakness or paralysis may develop on the left side of the body. A CT scan at the receiving trauma center can confirm the diagnosis.

Once en route, reevaluate the patient's airway and breathing. You supply supplemental oxygen and assist ventilations as necessary with a bag-mask device. Reassess the scalp wound to ensure that hemorrhage is adequately controlled. Measure the patient's vital signs and take a blood pressure reading. Perform a complete secondary survey to rule out additional injuries, and determine blood glucose level. During transport, you frequently assess the patency of the patient's airway, measure his vital signs, and check his GCS score and pupillary response. Notify the receiving facility of the patient's condition and update it if any significant changes occur.

Consider controlled hyperventilation if signs of herniation are present. When combined with appropriate neurosurgical intervention, aggressive prehospital care should improve the outcome of patients with moderate to severe TBI. ■

External hemorrhage should be controlled. Associated injuries should be managed while en route to the receiving facility. Fractures should be appropriately splinted to control both internal hemorrhage and pain.

Warning signs of possible increased ICP and herniation include the following:

- Decline in GCS score of two points or more
- Development of a sluggish or nonreactive pupil
- Development of hemiplegia or hemiparesis
- Cushing's phenomenon

Controlled, mild therapeutic hyperventilation may be considered for obvious signs of herniation. The following ventilatory rates should be used: 20 breaths/minute for adults, 25 breaths/minute for children, and 30 breaths/minute for infants. *Prophylactic hyperventilation has no role in TBI, and therapeutic hyperventilation, if instituted, should be stopped if signs of intracranial hypertension resolve.* The primary focus for the TBI patient during prolonged transport or in austere environments is the best possible maintenance of cerebral oxygenation and perfusion and the best efforts possible to control cerebral edema.

Spinal Trauma

You have been dispatched to the scene of a gymnastics event. On arrival, you find a 19-year-old woman lying supine on a gym mat underneath exercise bars. The scene is safe. Her gymnastics coach is sitting next to her trying to talk to her, but she is not responding.

As you begin your primary survey, you find an unresponsive female patient who fell while performing her gymnastics routine. She has abrasions on her forehead and an obvious deformity of the right wrist. Her airway is open, and she is breathing regularly. She shows no obvious signs of external blood loss. Her skin appears dry and warm with normal color. As you are performing your primary assessment, she begins to awaken, but remains confused as what happened.

What pathologic processes explain the patient's presentation?

What intermediate interventions and further assessments are needed?

What are the management goals for this patient?

Spinal trauma, if not recognized and properly managed, can result in irreparable damage to the spinal cord and leave a patient paralyzed for life. Some patients sustain immediate spinal cord damage as a result of trauma. Others sustain an injury to the spinal column that does not initially damage the cord; cord damage may result later with movement of the spine. Because the central nervous system (CNS) is incapable of regeneration, a severed spinal cord cannot be repaired. The consequences of inappropriately moving a patient with a spinal column injury, or allowing the patient to move, can be devastating. Failure to detect and immobilize a fractured spine properly may produce a much worse outcome than, for example, failure to immobilize a fractured femur properly. Conversely, spinal immobilization of the patient who has no indications of injury also has consequences and should not be done without careful consideration of the risks versus the benefits.

Spinal cord injury can have profound effects on human physiology, lifestyle, and financial circumstances. Human physiology is affected because the use of extremities or other areas is severely limited or completely impaired as a result of cord damage. Lifestyle is affected because spinal cord injury usually results in profound changes to daily activity levels and independence. Spinal cord injury also impacts the financial circumstances of the patient as well as the population in general.[23] A patient with this injury requires both acute and long-term care. The lifetime cost of this care is estimated at approximately $1.35 million per patient for a permanent spinal cord injury.[24]

About 32 people per 1 million population will sustain some type of spinal cord injury annually. An estimated 250,000 to 400,000 people live with spinal cord injuries in the United States. Spinal cord injury can occur at any age; however, it usually occurs in those 16 to 35 years of age because this age group is involved in the most violent and high-risk activities. Most trauma patients are 16 to 20 years of age. The second largest group of patients is 21 to 25 years, and the third largest group is 26 to 35 years of age. Common causes are motor vehicle crashes (48%), falls (21%), penetrating injuries (15%), sports injuries (14%), and other injuries (2%). Overall, approximately 11,000 people sustain spinal cord injuries annually in the United States.[25]

Sudden violent forces acting on the body can force the spine beyond its normal limits of motion by either impacting on the head or neck or driving the torso out from under the head. The following four concepts help clarify the possible effect of energy on the spine when evaluating the potential for injury:

1. The head is similar to a bowling ball perched on top of the neck, and its mass often moves in a different direction from the torso, resulting in strong forces being applied to the neck (cervical spine, spinal cord).
2. Objects in motion tend to stay in motion, and objects at rest tend to stay at rest.

3. Sudden or violent movement of the upper legs displaces the pelvis, resulting in forceful movement of the lower spine. Because of the weight and inertia of the head and torso, force in an opposite (contra) direction is applied to the upper spine.
4. Normal neurologic function does not rule out bone or ligament injury to the spine or conditions that have stressed the spinal cord to the limit of its tolerance.

Some trauma patients with neurologic deficit will have a temporary or permanent spinal cord injury. Other patients have neurologic deficit caused by either a peripheral nerve injury or an extremity injury not associated with spinal cord injury. It should be assumed that any patient who has sustained any of the following injuries has a potential spinal injury[26,27]:

- Any blunt mechanism that produced a violent impact on the head, neck, torso, or pelvis
- Incidents that produce sudden acceleration, deceleration, or lateral bending forces to the neck or torso
- Any fall from a height, especially in elderly persons
- Ejection or a fall from any motorized or otherwise powered transportation device
- Any victim of a shallow-water diving incident

Any such patient should be manually stabilized in a neutral inline position (unless contraindicated) until the need for spinal immobilization has been assessed.

Anatomy and Physiology
Vertebral Anatomy
The spinal column is composed of 33 bones called *vertebrae*, which are stacked on top of one another. Except for the first (C1) and second (C2) vertebrae (cervical) at the top of the spine and the fused sacral and coccygeal vertebrae at the lower spine, all the vertebrae are almost alike in form, structure, and motion (Figure 6-18). The largest part of each vertebra is the anterior part, called the *body*. Each vertebral body bears most of the weight of the vertebral column and torso superior to it. Two curved sides called the *neural arches* are formed by the pedicle and posteriorly by the lamina. The posterior part of the vertebra is a tail-like structure called the *spinous process*. In the lower five cervical vertebrae, this posterior process points directly posterior, whereas in the thoracic and lumbar vertebrae, it points slightly downward toward the feet.

Most vertebrae also have similarly styled protuberances called *transverse processes* at each side. The transverse and spinous processes serve as attachment points for muscles and are therefore fulcrums for movement. The neural arches and the posterior part of each vertebral body form a near-circular shape with an opening in the center called the *vertebral foramen* (spinal canal). The spinal cord passes

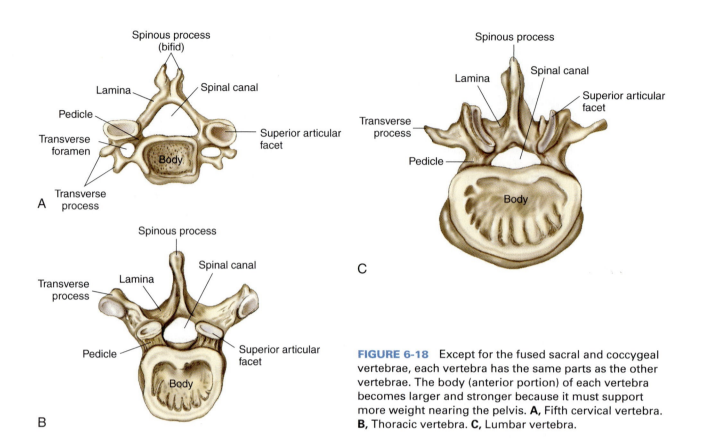

FIGURE 6-18 Except for the fused sacral and coccygeal vertebrae, each vertebra has the same parts as the other vertebrae. The body (anterior portion) of each vertebra becomes larger and stronger because it must support more weight nearing the pelvis. **A,** Fifth cervical vertebra. **B,** Thoracic vertebra. **C,** Lumbar vertebra.

through this opening. The cord is protected somewhat from injury by the bone surrounding it. Each vertebral foramen lines up with that of the vertebrae above and the vertebrae below to form the hollow spinal canal through which the spinal cord passes.

As mentioned previously, the first and second cervical vertebrae are uniquely shaped. The first cervical vertebra, C1, is a simple ring of bone. The second cervical vertebra has a projection of bone that sticks up to form a special joint with C1 that allows the head to move about (see Figure 6-19).

Vertebral Column. The individual vertebrae are stacked in an S-like shape (Figure 6-20). This organization allows extensive multidirectional movement while imparting maximum strength. The spinal column is divided into five individual regions for reference. Beginning at the top of the spinal col-

umn and descending downward, these regions are the cervical, thoracic, lumbar, sacral, and coccygeal regions. Vertebrae are identified by the first letter of the region in which they are found and their sequence from the top of that region. The first cervical vertebra is called *C1*, the third thoracic vertebra *T3*, the fifth lumbar vertebra *L5*, and so on throughout the entire spinal column. Each vertebra supports increasing body weight as the vertebrae progress down the spinal column. Appropriately, the vertebrae from C3 to L5 become progressively larger to accommodate the increased weight and workload (see Figure 6-18).

Located at the top end of the spinal column are the seven cervical vertebrae that support the head. The cervical region is flexible to allow for total movement of the head. Next are 12 thoracic vertebrae. Each pair of ribs connects posteriorly to one of the thoracic vertebrae. Unlike the cer-

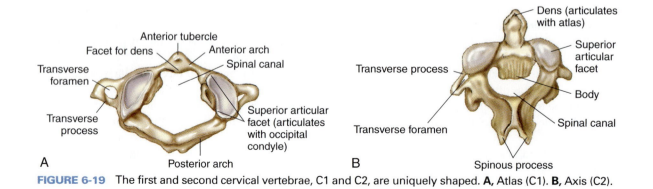

FIGURE 6-19 The first and second cervical vertebrae, C1 and C2, are uniquely shaped. **A,** Atlas (C1). **B,** Axis (C2).

vical spine, the thoracic spine is relatively rigid. Below the thoracic vertebrae are the five *lumbar* vertebrae. These are the most massive of all the vertebrae. The lumbar area is also flexible, allowing for movement in several directions. The five *sacral* vertebrae are fused, forming a single structure known as the *sacrum.* The four *coccygeal* vertebrae are also fused, forming the *coccyx* (tailbone). Approximately 55% of spinal injuries occur in the cervical region, 15% in the thoracic region, 15% at the thoracolumbar junction, and 15% in the lumbosacral area.

Ligaments and muscles tether the spine from the base of the skull to the pelvis. These ligaments and muscles form a web that sheathes the entire bony part of the spinal column, holding it in normal alignment and allowing for movement (Figure 6-21). If these ligaments and muscles are torn, excessive movement of one vertebra in relation to another occurs. In the presence of torn spinal ligaments, this excessive movement may result in dislocation of the vertebrae, which can compromise the space inside the spinal canal and thus damage the spinal cord.

The head balances on top of the spine, and the spine is supported by the pelvis. The human head weighs between 16 and 22 pounds (7–10 kg), somewhat more that the average weight of a bowling ball. The weight and position of the head atop the thin and flexible neck, the forces that act on the head, the small size of the supporting muscle, and the lack of ribs or other bones help make the cervical spine particularly susceptible to injury.

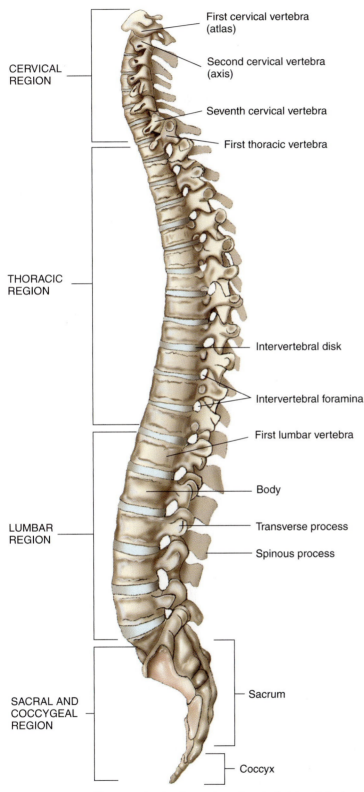

CERVICAL REGION

First cervical vertebra (atlas)

Second cervical vertebra (axis)

Seventh cervical vertebra

First thoracic vertebra

THORACIC REGION

Intervertebral disk

Intervertebral foramina

First lumbar vertebra

Body

Transverse process

Spinous process

LUMBAR REGION

SACRAL AND COCCYGEAL REGION

Sacrum

Coccyx

FIGURE 6-20   The vertebral column is not a straight rod, but a series of blocks that are stacked to allow for several bends or curves. At each of the curves, the spine is more vulnerable to fractures, thus the origin of the phrase "breaking the S in a fall."

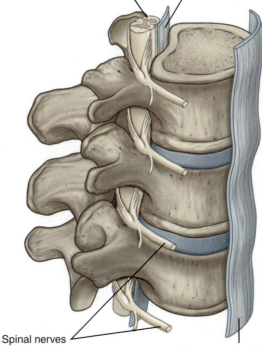

Spinal cord   Posterior longitudinal ligament

Spinal nerves

Anterior longitudinal ligament

FIGURE 6-21   Anterior and posterior longitudinal ligaments of vertebral column.

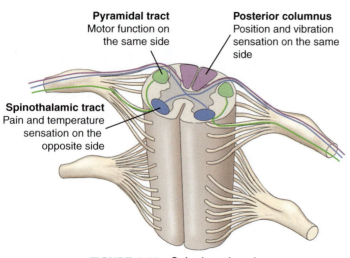

Pyramidal tract
Motor function on the same side

Posterior columnus
Position and vibration sensation on the same side

Spinothalamic tract
Pain and temperature sensation on the opposite side

FIGURE 6-22 Spinal cord tracks.

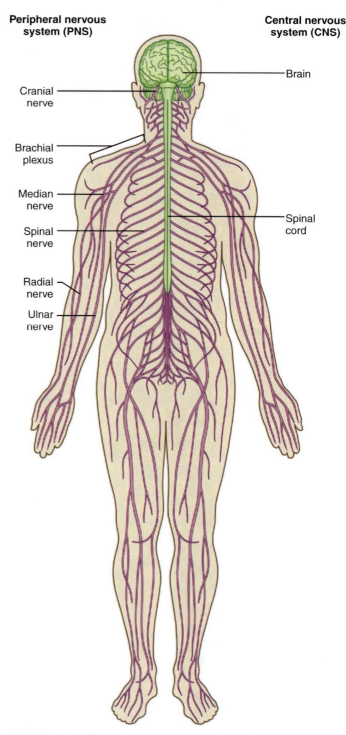

Peripheral nervous system (PNS)

Central nervous system (CNS)

Brain

Cranial nerve

Brachial plexus

Median nerve

Spinal nerve

Radial nerve

Ulnar nerve

Spinal cord

FIGURE 6-23 Central nervous system (green) and peripheral nervous system (purple).

At the level of C3, the spinal cord occupies approximately 95% of the spinal canal (the spinal cord occupies approximately 65% of the spinal canal area at its end in the lumbar region), and only 3 mm of clearance exists between the cord and the canal wall. Even a minor dislocation at this point can produce compression of the spinal cord. The posterior neck muscles are strong, permitting up to 60% of the range of flexion and 70% of the range of extension of the head without any stretching of the cord. However, when sudden violent acceleration, deceleration, or lateral force is applied to the body, the significant weight of the head on the narrow cervical spine can amplify the effects of sudden movement. An example of this would be a rear-end collision without the headrest properly adjusted.

The *sacrum* is the base of the spinal column, the platform on which the spinal column rests. Between 70% and 80% of the body's total weight rests on the sacrum. The sacrum is a part of both the spinal column and the pelvic girdle, and it is joined to the rest of the pelvis by immovable joints.

Spinal Cord Anatomy

The spinal cord is continuous with the brain and starts from the base of the brainstem, passing through the foramen magnum (the hole at the base of the skull) and through each vertebra to the level of the second lumbar (L2) vertebra. The spinal cord is surrounded by cerebrospinal fluid (CSF) and is encased in a dural sheath. This dural sheath covers the brain and continues down to the second sacral vertebra. CSF performs the same function for the cord as for the brain, acting as a cushion against injury during rapid and severe movement.

The spinal cord itself consists of gray matter and white matter. The white matter contains the anatomic spinal tracts. Spinal tracts are divided into two types: ascending and descending (Figure 6-22).

Ascending nerve tracts carry sensory impulses from body parts through the cord up to the brain. Ascending nerve tracts can be further divided into tracts that carry the different sensations of pain and temperature; touch and pressure; and sensory impulses of motion, vibration, position, and light touch. The nerve tracts that carry pain and temperature sensation "cross over" in the body, meaning that the nerve root with that information from the right side of the body crosses over to the left side of the spinal cord and then goes up to the brain. In contrast, the nerve tract that carries the sensory information for position, vibration, and light touch does *not* cross over in the spinal cord. Thus, this sensory information is carried up to the brain on the same side of the spinal cord as the nerve roots.

Descending nerve tracts are responsible for carrying motor impulses from the brain through the cord down to the body, and they control all muscle movement and muscle tone. These descending tracts also do not cross over in the spinal cord. Therefore, the motor tract on the right side of the cord controls motor function on the right side of the body. These motor tracts *do* cross over in the brainstem, however, so the left side of the brain controls motor function on the right side of the body, and vice versa.

As the spinal cord continues to descend, pairs of nerves branch off from the cord at each vertebra and extend to the various parts of the body (Figure 6-23). The spinal cord has 31 pairs of spinal nerves, named according to the level from which they arise. These nerve branches have multiple control functions, and their level in the spinal cord is represented by dermatomes. A *dermatome* is the sensory area on the body for which a nerve root is responsible. Collectively, dermatomes allow the body areas to be mapped out for each spinal level (Figure 6-24).

Dermatomes help determine the level of a spinal cord injury. Two landmarks to keep in mind are the *nipple level,*

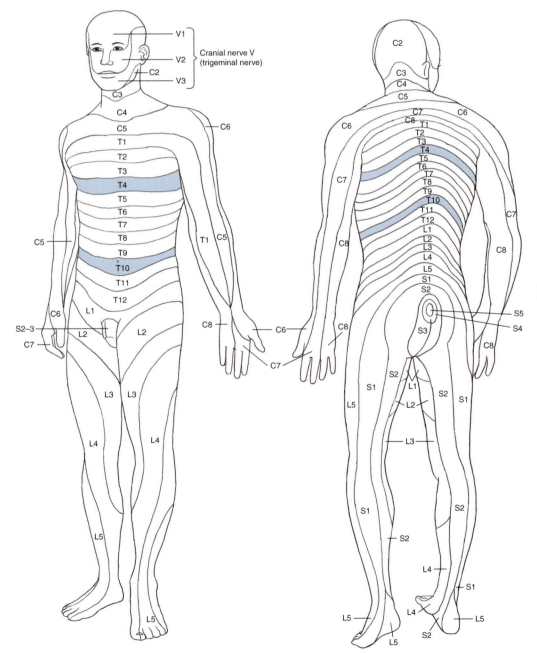

FIGURE 6-24 Dermatome map shows the relationship between areas of touch sensation on the skin and the spinal nerves that correspond to these areas. Loss of sensation in a specific area may indicate injury to the corresponding spinal nerve.

which is the T4 dermatome, and the *umbilicus level,* which is the T10 dermatome.

The process of inhalation and exhalation requires both chest excursion and proper changes in the shape of the diaphragm. The diaphragm is innervated by the phrenic nerves, which originate from the nerves arising from the cord between levels C2 and C5. If the cord above the level of C2 or the phrenic nerves are cut or the nerve impulses are otherwise disrupted, a patient will lose the ability to breathe spontaneously. A patient with this injury may asphyxiate before the arrival of providers unless bystanders initiate rescue breathing. Positive-pressure ventilation will need to be continued during transport.

Skeletal Injuries

Various types of injuries can occur to the spine, including the following[28]:

- Compression fractures that produce wedge compression or total flattening of the body of the vertebra.
- Fractures that produce small fragments of bone that may lie in the spinal canal near the cord.
- *Subluxation,* which is a partial dislocation of a vertebra from its normal alignment in the spinal column.
- Overstretching or tearing of the ligaments and muscles, producing instability between the vertebrae.

Any of these skeletal injuries may immediately result in the irreversible transection of the cord, or the injury may compress or stretch the cord. In some patients, however, damage to the vertebrae or ligaments results in an *unstable* spinal column injury but does not produce an immediate spinal cord injury. In addition, patients who have cervical spine injuries also have a 10% chance of having another spinal fracture. Therefore, the entire spine must be immobilized in patients who have indications for cervical spinal immobilization.

Normal neurologic function does not rule out a bony fracture or an unstable spine. Although the presence of good motor and sensory responses in the extremities indicates that the cord is currently intact, it does not exclude a damaged vertebra or associated bony or soft tissue injury. A significant percentage of patients with spine fractures have no neurologic deficit. A full assessment is required to determine the need for immobilization.

Specific Mechanisms of Injury That Cause Spinal Trauma

Axial loading can occur in several ways. Most often, this compression of the spine occurs when the head strikes an object and the weight of the still-moving body bears against the stopped head, such as when the head of an unrestrained occupant strikes the windshield or when the head strikes an object in a shallow-water diving incident. Compression and axial loading also occur when a patient sustains a fall from a substantial height and lands in a standing position. This drives the weight of the head and thorax down against the lumbar spine while the sacral spine remains stationary. About 20% of falls from a height greater than 15 feet involve an associated lumbar spine fracture. During such an extreme energy exchange, the spinal column tends to exaggerate its normal curves, and fractures and compressions occur at such areas.

Excessive flexion (hyperflexion), excessive extension (hyperextension), and *excessive rotation (hyperrotation)* can cause bone damage and tearing of muscles and ligaments, resulting in impingement on or stretching of the spinal cord.

Sudden or excessive lateral bending requires much less movement than flexion or extension before injury occurs. During lateral impact, the torso and the thoracic spine are moved laterally. The head tends to remain in place until it is pulled along by the cervical attachments. The center of gravity of the head is above and anterior to its seat and attachment to the cervical spine; therefore, the head will tend to roll sideways. This movement often results in dislocations and bony fractures.

Distraction (overelongation of the spine) occurs when one part of the spine is stable and the rest is in longitudinal motion. This pulling apart of the spine can easily cause stretching and tearing of the cord. Distraction injury is a common mechanism in children's playground injuries and in hangings.

Although any one of these types of violent movements may be the dominant cause of spinal injury in a given patient, one or more of the others will usually also be involved.

Spinal Cord Injuries

Primary injury occurs at the time of impact or force application and may cause cord compression, direct cord injury (usually from sharp unstable bony fragments or projectiles), and interruption of the cord's blood supply. Secondary injury occurs after the initial insult and can include swelling, ischemia, or movement of bony fragments.[29]

Assessment

Spinal injury, as with other conditions, should be assessed in the context of other injuries and conditions present. The primary survey is the first priority. However, often the patient first needs to be moved in order to ensure the safety of all individuals at the scene. Therefore, a rapid scene assessment and history of the event should determine if the possibility of a spinal injury exists, in which case the patient's spine must be manually protected. The patient's head is brought into a neutral inline position, unless contraindicated (see page 158). The head is maintained in that position until the assessment reveals no indication for immobilization or the manual stabilization is replaced with a spine immobilization device, such as a half-spine board, long backboard, or vest-type device.

Neurologic Examination

In the field, a rapid neurologic examination is performed to identify obvious deficits related to a spinal cord injury. The patient is asked to move the arms, hands, and legs, and any inability to do so is noted. Then the patient is checked for the presence or absence of sensation, beginning at the shoulders and moving down the body to the feet. A complete neurologic examination does not need to be performed in the prehospital setting because it will not provide additional information that will affect the decisions about needed prehospital care and only serves to expend precious time on scene and delay transport.

The rapid neurologic examination should be repeated after the patient has been immobilized, anytime the patient is moved, and upon arrival to the receiving facility. This will help identify any changes in patient condition that may have occurred after the initial assessment.

Using Mechanism of Injury to Assess Spinal Cord Injury

In addition to the mechanism of injury and the kinematics involved, assessment of the neck for spinal immobilization should also include assessment of the motor and sensory function, presence of pain or tenderness, and patient reliability as predictors of spinal cord injury. In addition, the patient may not complain of pain in the spinal column because of pain associated with a more distracting painful injury, such as a fractured femur.[30] Alcohol or drugs that the patient may have ingested may also blunt the patient's perception of pain and mask serious injury.

Providers should focus on appropriate indications for performing spinal immobilization.[31-38] If no indications are present after a careful and thorough examination, there may be no need for spinal immobilization. The cornerstone to proper spinal care is the same as with all trauma care: superior assessment, with appropriate and timely treatment.

Blunt Trauma

Major causes of spinal injury in adult patients include the following:

1. Motor vehicle crashes (MVCs)
2. Shallow-water incidents
3. Motorcycle crashes
4. Falls
5. Sports injuries

Major causes of spinal injury in pediatric patients include the following:

1. Falls from heights (generally two to three times the patient's height)
2. Falls from a tricycle or bicycle
3. Being struck by a motor vehicle

As a guideline, the provider should assume the presence of spinal injury and an unstable spine with the following situations, and an assessment of the spine should be conducted to determine the need for immobilization:

- Any blunt mechanism that produced a violent impact on the head, neck, torso, or pelvis (e.g., assault, entrapment in a structural collapse)
- Incidents that produce sudden acceleration, deceleration, or lateral bending forces to the neck or torso (e.g., moderate- to high-speed MVCs, pedestrians struck by vehicle, involvement in explosion)
- Any fall, especially in elderly persons
- Ejection or a fall from any motorized or otherwise powered transportation device (e.g., scooters, skateboards, bicycles, motor vehicles, motorcycles, recreational vehicles)
- Any victim of a shallow-water incident (e.g., diving, body surfing)

Other situations often associated with spinal damage include the following:

- Head injuries with any alteration in level of consciousness
- Significant helmet damage
- Significant blunt injury to the torso
- Impacted or other deceleration fractures of the legs or hips
- Significant localized injuries to the area of the spinal column

These mechanisms of injury should mandate a thorough and complete examination to determine if indications are present to necessitate spinal immobilization.

The wearing of proper seat belt restraints has proved to save lives and reduce head, face, and thoracic injuries. However, the use of proper restraints does not rule out the possibility of spinal injury. In significant frontal-impact collisions when sudden severe deceleration occurs, the restrained torso stops suddenly but the unrestrained head attempts to continue its forward movement. Held by the strong posterior neck muscles, the head can move forward only slightly. If the force of deceleration is strong enough, the head then rotates down until the chin strikes the chest wall, often rotating across the diagonal strap of the shoulder restraint. Such rapid, forceful hyperflexion and rotation of the neck can result in compression fractures of the cervical vertebrae, dislocation, and stretching of the spinal cord. Different mechanisms can also cause spinal trauma in restrained victims of rear or lateral collisions. The amount of damage to the vehicle and the patient's other injuries are the key factors in determining if a patient needs to be immobilized.

The patient's ability to walk should not be a factor in determining whether a patient needs to be treated for spinal injury. A significant number of patients who require surgical repair of unstable spinal injuries were found "walking around" at the scene or walked into the emergency department at the hospital.

Penetrating Trauma

Penetrating injury represents a special consideration regarding the potential for spinal trauma.[39] In general, if a patient did not sustain definite neurologic injury at the moment that the trauma occurred, there is little concern for subsequent development of a spinal cord injury. This is because of the mechanism of injury and the kinematics associated with the force involved. Penetrating objects generally do not produce unstable spinal fractures because penetrating trauma produces minimal risk of unstable ligamentous or bony injury, unlike blunt injury. A penetrating object causes injury along the path of penetration. If the object did not directly injure the spinal cord as it penetrated, the patient is unlikely to develop a spinal cord injury. Numerous studies have shown that unstable spinal injuries rarely occur from penetrating trauma to the head, neck, or torso[40–45] and that penetrating injuries are *not* indications for spinal immobilization. Because of the very low risk of an unstable spinal injury and because the other injuries created by the penetrating trauma often require a higher priority in management, patients with penetrating trauma need not undergo spinal immobilization.

Indications for Spinal Immobilization

The mechanism of injury can be used as an aid to determine indications for spinal immobilization (Figure 6-25). The key point always is that a complete physical assessment coupled with good clinical judgment will guide decision making, and *if in doubt, immobilize.*

Patients with a penetrating injury (e.g., gunshot or stab wounds) to the head, neck, or torso should be considered to have a concerning mechanism of injury when they complain of neurologic symptoms or display such findings as numbness, tingling, and loss of motor or sensory function or actual loss of consciousness. However, if patients with penetrating injury have no neurologic complaints, secondary mechanism of injury, or findings, the spine does not need to be immobilized (although the backboard may still be used for lifting and transport purposes).

In the patient with blunt trauma, the following conditions should mandate spinal immobilization:

1. *Altered level of consciousness* (LOC), with Glasgow Coma Scale (GCS) score less than 15. Any factor that alters the patient's perception of pain will hinder the responder's assessment for injury; this includes the following:
   - Traumatic brain injury (TBI)
   - Altered mental status (AMS) other than TBI. For example, patients with psychiatric illness, with Alzheimer's disease, or under the influence of intoxicants may have impaired pain perception.
   - Acute stress reactions (ASRs) may cause "pain masking."

2. *Spinal pain or tenderness.* This includes pain or pain on movement, point tenderness, and deformity and guarding of the spinal area.
3. *Neurologic deficit or complaint.* This includes bilateral paralysis, partial paralysis, paresis (weakness), numbness, prickling or tingling, and neurogenic spinal shock below the level of the injury. In males, a continuing erection of the penis (priapism) may be an additional indication of spinal cord injury.
4. *Anatomic deformity of the spine.* This includes any deformity noted on physical examination of the patient.

However, the absence of these signs does not rule out bony spinal injury (Figure 6-26).

When a patient has a concerning mechanism of injury in the absence of the conditions just listed, the reliability of the patient must be assessed. A reliable patient is calm, cooperative, and sober. An unreliable patient may exhibit any of the following:

- *Intoxication.* Patients who are under the influence of drugs or alcohol are immobilized and managed as if they had spinal injury until they are calm, cooperative, and sober.
- *Distracting painful injuries.* Injuries that are severely painful may prevent the patient from giving reliable responses during the assessment.[30] Examples would include a fractured femur or a large burn (see Figure 6-25).
- *Communication barriers.* Communication problems include language barriers, deafness, very young patients, or patients who for any reason cannot communicate effectively.

The patient should be continually rechecked for reliability at all phases of an assessment. If at any time the patient exhibits these signs or symptoms or the reliability of the examination is in question, it should be assumed that the patient has a spinal injury, and full immobilization management techniques should be implemented.

In many situations the mechanism of injury is not suggestive of neck injury (e.g., falling on outstretched hand and producing Colles fracture). In these patients, in the presence of a normal examination and proper assessment, spinal immobilization is not indicated.

Management

In the United States, the first step in the management of a potentially unstable spine is to immobilize the patient in a supine position, usually on a rigid long backboard in a neutral inline position. In many other countries, a full-body vacuum mattress splint is often used instead of the backboard. The head, neck, torso, and pelvis should each be immobilized

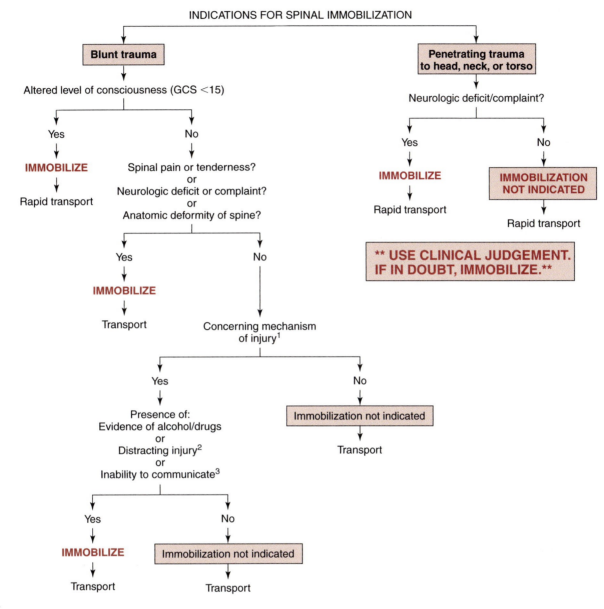

INDICATIONS FOR SPINAL IMMOBILIZATION

Notes:

[1]Concerning mechanisms of injury
• Any mechanism that produced a violent impact to the head, neck, torso, or pelvis (e.g., assault, entrapment in structural collapse, etc.)
• Incidents producing sudden acceleration, deceleration, or lateral bending forces to the neck or torso (e.g., moderate- to high-speed MVC, pedestrian struck, involvement in an explosion, etc.)
• Any fall, especially in elderly persons
• Ejection or fall from any motorized or otherwise-powered transportation device (e.g., scooters, skateboards, bicycles, motor vehicles, motorcycles, or recreational vehicles)
• Victim of shallow-water diving incident

[2]Distracting injury
  Any injury that may have the potential to impair the patient's ability to appreciate other injuries. Examples of distracting injuries include a) long bone fracture; b) a visceral injury requiring surgical consultation; c) a large laceration, degloving injury, or crush injury; d) large burns or e) any other injury producing acute functional impairment.
  (Adapted from Hoffman JR, Wolfson AB, Todd K, Mower WR: Selective cervical spine radiography in blunt trauma: methodology of the National Emergency X-Radiography Utilization Study [NEXUS], *Ann Emerg Med* 461, 1998.)

[3]Inability to communicate. Any patient who, for reasons not specified above, cannot clearly communicate so as to actively participate in their assessment. Examples: speech or hearing impaired, those who only speak a foreign language, and small children.

FIGURE 6-25   Indications for spinal immobilization.

FIGURE 6-26 Signs and Symptoms of Spinal Trauma

- Pain in the neck or back
- Pain on movement of the neck or back
- Pain on palpation of the posterior neck or midline of the back
- Deformity of the spinal column
- Guarding or splinting of the muscles of the neck or back
- Paralysis, paresis, numbness, or tingling in the legs or arms at any time after the incident
- Signs and symptoms of neurogenic shock
- Priapism (sustained penile erection in male patients)

in a neutral inline position to prevent any further movement of the unstable spine that could result in damage to the spinal cord. Spinal immobilization follows the common principle of fracture management: immobilizing the joint above and the joint below an injury. Because of the anatomy of the spine, this principle of immobilization must be extended beyond just the joint above and below a suspected vertebral injury. The joint above the spine means the head and the joint below means the pelvis.

Fractures of one area of the spine are often associated with fractures of other areas of the spine.[45] Therefore, the entire weight-bearing spine (cervical, thoracic, lumbar, and sacral) should be considered as one entity and the entire spine immobilized and supported to achieve proper immobilization. The supine position is the most stable position to ensure continued support during handling, carrying, and transporting a patient. It also provides the best access for further examination and additional resuscitation and management of a patient. When the patient is supine, the airway, mouth and nose, eyes, chest, and abdomen can be accessed simultaneously.

Patients usually present in one of four general postures: sitting, semiprone, supine, or standing. The patient's spine needs to be protected and stabilized immediately and continuously from the time the patient is discovered until the patient is mechanically secured to a long backboard. Techniques and equipment such as manual stabilization, half-spine boards, immobilization vests, standing take-down, scoop stretchers, proper logroll methods, and rapid extrication with full manual stabilization are interim management strategies used to protect a patient's spine. These techniques allow for a patient's safe movement from the position in which the patient was found until full supine immobilization on a rigid long backboard can be implemented.

Often, too much focus is placed on particular immobilization devices without an understanding of the principles of immobilization and how to modify these principles to meet individual patient needs. Specific devices and immobilization methods can be safely used only with an understanding of the anatomic principles that are generic to all methods and equipment. Any inflexible, detailed method for using a device will not meet the varying conditions found in the field. Regardless of the specific equipment or method used, the management of any patient with an unstable spine should follow the general steps described in the next section.

General Method

When the decision is made to immobilize a trauma patient, follow these principles:

1. Move the patient's head into a proper neutral inline position (unless contraindicated; see next section). Continue manual support and inline stabilization without interruption.
2. Evaluate the patient by performing the primary survey, and provide any immediately required intervention.
3. Check the patient's motor ability, sensory response, and circulation in all four extremities if the patient's condition allows.
4. Examine the patient's neck, and measure and apply a properly fitting, effective cervical collar.
5. Depending on the situation, position a shortboard or vest-type device on the patient, or place the patient on a long backboard.
6. Immobilize the patient's torso to the device so that it cannot move up, down, left, or right.
7. Evaluate and pad behind the adult patient's head or pediatric patient chest as needed.
8. Immobilize the patient's head to the device, maintaining a neutral inline position.
9. Once the patient is on the long backboard, immobilize the legs so that they cannot move anteriorly or laterally.
10. Fasten the patient's arms to the backboard.
11. Reevaluate the primary survey, and reassess the patient's motor ability, sensory response, and circulation in all four extremities if the patient's condition allows.

Manual Inline Stabilization of the Head

Once it has been determined from the mechanism of injury that an injured spine potentially exists, the first step is to provide manual inline stabilization. The patient's head is grasped and carefully moved into a neutral inline position unless contraindicated (see below). A proper neutral inline position is maintained without any significant traction on the head and neck. Only enough pull should be exerted on a sitting or standing patient to cause *axial unloading* (taking the weight of the head off the axis and the rest of the cervical spine). The head should be constantly maintained in the manually stabilized, neutral inline position until mechanical immobilization of the torso and head is completed or the examination reveals no need for spinal immobilization. In this way the patient's head and neck are immediately immobilized and remain so until after examination at the hospital. Moving the head into a neutral inline position presents less risk than if the patient were carried and transported with the head left in an angulated position. In addition, both immobilization and transport of the patient are much simpler with the patient in a neutral position.

Movement of the patient's head into a neutral inline position is contraindicated in a few cases. If careful movement of the head and neck into a neutral inline position results in any of the following, *the movement must be stopped:*

- Resistance to movement is noted
- Neck muscle spasm
- Increased pain
- Commencement or increase of a neurologic deficit, such as numbness, tingling, or loss of motor ability
- Compromise of the airway or ventilation

Neutral inline movement should not be attempted if a patient's injuries are so severe that the head presents with such misalignment that it no longer appears to extend from the midline of the shoulders. In these situations the patient's head must be immobilized in the position in which it was initially found. Fortunately, such cases are rare.

Rigid Cervical Collars

Rigid cervical collars alone do not provide adequate immobilization; they simply aid in supporting the neck and promote a lack of movement. Rigid cervical collars limit flexion by about 90% and limit extension, lateral bending, and rotation by about 50%. A rigid cervical collar is an important adjunct to immobilization but must always be used with manual stabilization or mechanical immobilization provided by a suitable spine immobilization device. A soft cervical collar is of no use as an adjunct to spinal immobilization in the field.

The unique primary purpose of a cervical collar is to protect the cervical spine from compression. Prehospital methods of immobilization (using a vest, shortboard, or a long backboard device) still allow some slight movement of the patient and the spine because these devices only fasten externally to the patient, and the skin and muscle tissue move slightly on the skeletal frame even when the patient is extremely well immobilized. Most rescue situations involve some movement of the patient and spine when extricating, carrying, and loading the patient. This type of movement also occurs when an ambulance accelerates and decelerates in normal driving conditions.

An effective cervical collar sits on the chest, posterior thoracic spine and clavicle, and trapezius muscles, where the tissue movement is at a minimum. This still allows movement at C6, C7, and T1 but prevents compression of these vertebrae. The head is immobilized under the angle of the

FIGURE 6-27   Guidelines for Rigid Cervical Collars

- Do not adequately immobilize by their use alone
- Must be properly sized for each patient
- Must not inhibit a patient's ability to open the mouth or the prehospital care provider's ability to open the patient's mouth if vomiting occurs
- Should not obstruct or hinder ventilation in any way

mandible and at the occiput of the skull. The rigid collar allows the unavoidable loading between the head and the torso to be transferred from the cervical spine to the collar, eliminating or minimizing the cervical compression that could otherwise result.

The collar must be the correct size for the patient. A collar that is too short will not be effective and will allow significant flexion. A collar that is too large will cause hyperextension or full motion if the chin is inside of it. A collar must be applied properly. A collar that is too loose will be ineffective in limiting head movement and can accidentally cover the anterior chin, mouth, and nose, obstructing the patient's airway. A collar that is too tight can compress the veins of the neck, causing increased intracranial pressure.

A collar should be applied after bringing the patient's head into a neutral inline position. If the head cannot be returned to a neutral inline position, use of any collar is difficult and should not be considered. In this case the use of an improvised blanket or towel roll may assist in stabilization. A collar that does not allow the mandible to move down and the mouth to open without motion of the spine will produce aspiration of gastric contents into the lungs if the patient vomits and therefore should not be used. Alternative methods to immobilize a patient when a collar cannot be used may include use of such items as blankets, towels, and tape. In the prehospital setting the care provider may need to be creative when presented with these types of patients. Whatever method is used, the basic concepts of immobilization should be followed (Figure 6-27).

Immobilization of Torso to the Board Device

Regardless of the specific board device used, the patient must be immobilized so that the torso cannot move up, down, left, or right. The rigid device is strapped to the torso and the torso to the device. The device is secured to the patient's torso so that the head and neck will be supported and immobilized when affixed to it. The patient's torso and pelvis are immobilized to the device so that the thoracic, lumbar, and sacral sections of the spine are supported and cannot move. **The torso should be immobilized to the device before the head is secured.** In this way, any movement of the device that may occur when fastening the torso straps is prevented from angulating the cervical spine.

Many different methods exist for attaching the device to the torso. Protection against movement in any direction—up, down, left, or right-should be achieved at both the upper torso (shoulders or chest) and the lower torso (pelvis) to avoid compression and lateral movement of the vertebrae of the torso. Immobilization of the upper torso can be achieved with several specific methods; an understanding of the basic anatomic principles common to each method must be applied. Cephalad movement of the upper torso is prohibited by use of a strap on each side, fastened to the board below the upper margin of each shoulder, which then passes over the shoulder and is fastened at a lower point. Caudad movement of the torso can be prohibited by use of straps that pass snugly around the pelvis and legs.

In one method, two straps (one going from each side of the board over the shoulder, then across the upper chest and through the opposite armpit, to fasten to the board on the armpit side) produce an X, which stops any upward, downward, left, or right movement of the upper torso. The same immobilization can be achieved by fastening one strap to the board and passing it through one armpit, then across the upper chest and through the opposite armpit, to fasten to the second side of the board. A strap or cravat is then added to each side and passed over the shoulder to fasten it to the armpit strap, similar to a pair of suspenders.

Immobilization of the upper torso of a patient with a fractured clavicle is accomplished by placing backpack-type loops around each shoulder through the armpit and fastening the ends of each loop in the same handhold. The straps remain near the lateral edges of the upper torso and do not cross the clavicles. With any of these methods, the straps are over the upper third of the chest and can be fastened tightly without producing the ventilatory compromise typically produced by tight straps placed lower on the thorax.

Immobilization of the lower torso can be achieved by use of a single strap fastened tightly over the pelvis at the iliac crests. If the long backboard will have to be upended or carried on stairs or over a distance, a pair of groin loops will provide stronger immobilization than the single strap across the iliac crests.

Lateral movement or anterior movement away from the rigid device at the midtorso can be prevented by use of an additional strap around the midtorso. Any strap that surrounds the torso between the upper thorax and the iliac crests should be snug but not so tight that it inhibits chest excursion impairing ventilatory function or causes a significant increase in intra-abdominal pressure.

Maintenance of Neutral Inline Position of the Head

In many patients, when the head is placed in a neutral inline position, the posterior-most portion of the occipital region at the back of the head is between ½ and 3½ inches anterior to the posterior thoracic wall (Figure 6-28, A). Therefore, in most adults, a space exists between the back of the head and the device when the head is in a neutral inline position, so suitable padding should be added before securing the head to the board device (Figure 6-28, B). To be effective, this padding must be made of a material that does not readily compress. Firm, semirigid pads designed for this purpose or folded towels can be used. The amount of padding needed must be individualized for each patient; a few individuals require none. If too little padding is inserted or if the padding is of an unsuitable spongy material, the head will be hyperextended when head straps are applied. If too much padding is inserted, the head will be moved into a flexed position. Both hyperextension and flexion of the head can increase spinal cord damage and are contraindicated.

The same anatomic relationship between the head and back applies when most people are supine, whether on the ground or on a backboard. When most adults are supine, the head falls back into a hyperextended position. On arrival, the head should

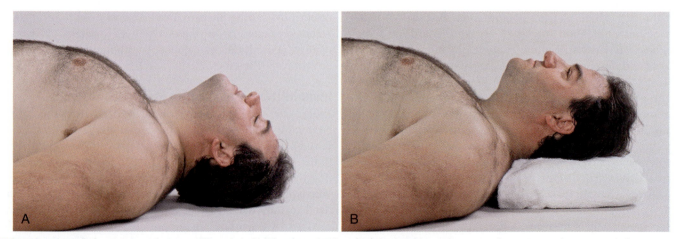

FIGURE 6-28 A, In some patients, pulling the skull back to the level of the backboard can produce severe hyperextension. **B,** Padding is needed between the back of the head and the backboard to prevent such hyperextension.

FIGURE 6-29   Athletic Equipment Removal

A number of recent publications, including a position paper, have advocated the immobilization of helmeted athletes to a long backboard with the helmet in place.[32–39] A search of the medical literature for supporting evidence reveals that these recommendations are based on, at best, class III research. Studies criticizing the practice of helmet removal have primarily been done in cadavers. These studies report that extreme hyperextension of the cervical spine occurs when the helmet alone is removed and the shoulder pads are left in place; however, all the studies were done without the placement of appropriate padding under the head to prevent it from falling back onto the backboard. Adherence to proper spinal precautions and application of treatment principles will best accomplish the task of spinal immobilization whether or not the helmet or shoulder pads are removed.

Athletic equipment should be removed by personnel trained and experienced in the removal of sports equipment. Historically, these trained and experienced personnel generally have been those individuals, usually athletic trainers, present at the athletic event site. Emergency medical services (EMS) responders, however, need to receive training in such removal, because access to the airway, if needed, can be accomplished only by appropriate access to the patient's face and head, which requires removal of the facemask at a minimum and the helmet in many cases. If the decision is made *not* to remove the equipment at the scene, someone knowledgeable in sports equipment removal should accompany the patient to the hospital.

Although special care for helmeted athletes is needed, the general principles of spinal immobilization taught in Prehospital Trauma Life Support (PHTLS) courses are appropriate and need to be followed. Ideally, the helmet and shoulder pads should be removed as one unit. However, it is still possible to immobilize a player to a long backboard without causing hyperextension of the cervical spine when the helmet alone is removed. This is accomplished by the appropriate use of padding behind the head to maintain the head in neutral alignment with the rest of the spine if the shoulder pads are not removed. EMS responders must determine the specific medical needs for an injured athlete and take appropriate steps to meet those needs, which may often include immediate removal of the athletic equipment.

---

be moved into a neutral inline position and manually maintained in that position, which in many adults will require holding the head up off the ground. Once the patient is placed on the long backboard and the head is about to be fastened to the board, proper padding (as described) should be inserted between the back of the head and the board to maintain the neutral position. These principles should be used with all patients, including athletes with shoulder pads and patients with abnormal curvature of the spine (Figure 6-29).

In small children, generally those with the body size of a 7 year old or younger, the size of the head is much larger relative to the rest of the body than in adults, and the muscles of the back are less developed.[46] When a small child's head is in a neutral inline position, the back of the head usually extends 1 to 2 inches (2.5–5 cm) beyond the posterior plane of the back. Therefore, if a small child is placed directly on a rigid surface, the head will be moved into a position of flexion (Figure 6-30, A).

Placing small children on a standard long backboard results in unwanted flexion of the head and neck. The long backboard needs to be modified by either creating a recess in the board or inserting padding under the torso to maintain the head in a neutral position (Figure 6-30, B). The padding placed under the torso should be of the appropriate thickness so that the head lies on the board in a neutral position; too much will result in extension, too little in flexion. The padding under the torso must also be firm and evenly shaped. Use of irregularly shaped or insufficient padding, or placing it under only the shoulders, can result in movement and misalignment of the spine.

Completing Immobilization

Head

Once the patient's torso has been immobilized to the rigid device and appropriate padding inserted behind the head as needed, the head should be secured to the device. Because of its rounded shape, the head cannot be stabilized on a flat surface with only straps or tape. Use of these alone will still allow the head to rotate and move laterally. Also, because of the angle of the forehead and the slippery nature of moist skin and hair, a simple strap over the forehead is unreliable and can easily slide off. Although the human head weighs about the same as a bowling ball, it has a significantly different shape. The head is ovoid, being longer than it is wide and having almost completely flat lateral sides, resembling a bowling ball with about 2 inches (5 cm) cut off to form left and right sides. Adequate external immobilization of the head, regardless of method or device, can be achieved only by placing pads or rolled blankets on these flat sides and securing them with straps or tape. In the case of vest-type devices, this is accomplished with hinged side flaps that are part of the vest.

The side supports, whether they are preshaped foam blocks or rolled blankets, are placed next to both sides of the head. The sidepieces should be at least as wide as the patient's ears, or

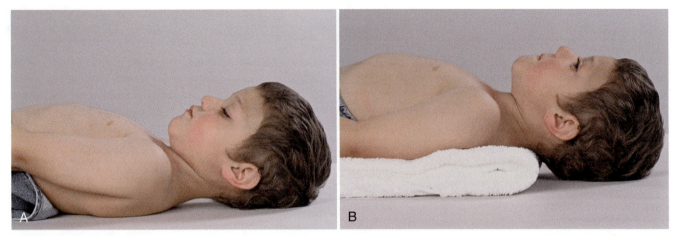

FIGURE 6-30 **A,** The larger size of a child's head relative to body size, combined with the reduced development of the posterior thoracic muscles, produces hyperflexion of the head when a child is placed on a backboard. **B,** Padding beneath the shoulders and torso will prevent this hyperflexion.

larger, and be at least as high as the level of the patient's eyes. Two straps or pieces of tape surrounding these headpieces draw the sides together. When it is packaged between the blocks or blankets, the head now has a flat posterior surface that can be realistically fixed to a flat board. The upper forehead strap is placed tightly across the front of the lower forehead (across the supraorbital ridge) to help prevent anterior movement of the head. This strap should be pulled tightly enough to just indent the blocks or blankets and rest firmly on the forehead. Sandbags are not recommended for use as side supports because of the weight that may be placed on the head and neck when the immobilized patient is turned on his side or the fact that they may shift during sudden acceleration or deceleration of the ambulance, causing the head and neck to move.[47]

The use of chin cups or straps encircling the chin prevents opening of the mouth to vomit, so these devices should not be used. The device that holds the head, regardless of type, also requires a lower strap to help keep the sidepieces firmly pressed against the lower sides of the head and to anchor the device further and prevent anterior movement of the lower head and neck. The lower strap passes around the sidepieces and across the anterior rigid portion of the cervical collar. This strap should not place too much pressure on the front of the collar, which could produce an airway or venous return problem at the neck.

Legs

Significant outward rotation of the legs may result in anterior movement of the pelvis and movement of the lower spine; tying the feet together eliminates this possibility. Placing a rolled blanket or piece of padding between the legs will increase comfort for the patient.

The patient's legs are immobilized to the board with two or more straps: one strap proximal to the knees at about midthigh and one strap distal to the knees.

The average adult measures 14 to 20 inches (35–50 cm) from one side to the other at the hips and only 6 to 9 inches (15–23 cm) from one side to the other at the ankles. When the feet are placed together, a **V** shape is formed from the hips to the ankles. Because the ankles are considerably narrower than the board, a strap placed across the lower legs can prevent anterior movement but will not prevent the legs from moving laterally from one edge of the board to the other. If the board is angled or rotated, the legs will fall to the lower edge of the board, which can angulate the pelvis and produce movement of the spinal column.

The legs can be kept in the middle of the board by placing blanket rolls between each leg and the edges of the board before strapping. It is important to ensure that the straps are not so tight as to impair distal circulation.

Arms

For safety, the patient's arms should be secured to the board or across the torso before moving the patient. One way to achieve this is with the arms placed at the sides on the board with the palms in, secured by a strap across the forearms and torso. This strap should be snug but not so tight as to compromise the circulation in the hands.

The patient's arms should not be included in the strap at the iliac crests or in the groin loops. If the straps are tight enough to provide adequate immobilization of the lower torso, they can compromise the circulation in the hands. If the straps are loose, they will not provide adequate immobilization of the torso or arms. Use of an additional strap exclusively to hold the arms allows the strap to be opened for taking a blood pressure measurement or starting an intravenous line once the patient is in the ambulance without compromising the immobilization. If the arm strap is also a torso strap, loosening it to free just an arm has the side effect of loosening the torso immobilization as well.

FIGURE 6-31   Criteria for Evaluating Immobilization Skills

Practice is needed using immobilization skills in hands-on sessions using mock patients before use with real patients. At least one study has shown that appropriate immobilization was not performed in a significant number of patients with potential spinal injury.[44] When practicing or when evaluating new methods or equipment, the following criteria will serve as good tools for measuring how effectively the "patient" has been immobilized:

1. Initiate manual inline stabilization immediately and maintain until it is replaced mechanically.
2. Check neurologic function distally.
3. Apply an effective, properly sized cervical collar.
4. Secure the torso before the head.
5. Prevent movement of the torso up or down the board device.
6. Prevent movement of the upper and lower torso left or right on the board device.
7. Prevent anterior movement of the torso off the rigid device.
8. Ensure that ties crossing the chest do not inhibit chest excursion or result in ventilatory compromise.
9. Effectively immobilize the head so that it cannot move in any direction, including rotation.
10. Provide padding behind the head, if necessary.
11. Maintain the head in a neutral inline position.
12. Ensure that nothing inhibits or prevents the mouth from being opened.
13. Immobilize the legs so that they cannot move anteriorly, rotate, or move from side to side, even if the board and patient are rotated to the side.
14. Maintain the pelvis and legs in a neutral inline position.
15. Ensure that the arms are appropriately secured to the board or torso.
16. Ensure that any ties or straps do not compromise distal circulation in any limb.
17. Reevaluate the patient if bumped, jostled, or in any way moved in a manner that could compromise an unstable spine while the device was being applied.
18. Complete the procedure within an appropriate time frame.
19. Recheck distal neurologic function.

Many methods and variations can meet these objectives. The selection of a specific method and specific equipment will be based on the situation, the patient's condition, and available resources.

Most Common Mistakes

The following are the four most common immobilization errors:

1. *Inadequate immobilization.* The torso can move significantly up or down on the board device, or the head can still move excessively.
2. *Immobilization with the head hyperextended.* The most common cause is a lack of appropriate padding behind the head.
3. *Immobiling the head before the torso or readjusting the torso straps after the head has been secured.* This causes movement of the device relative to the torso, which results in movement of the head and cervical spine.
4. *Inadequate padding.* Failure to fill the voids under a patient can allow for inadvertent movement of the spine with additional injury as well as increased discomfort for the patient.

Complete spine immobilization is generally not a comfortable experience for the patient. As the degree and quality of the immobilization increase, the patient's comfort decreases. Spine immobilization is a balance between the need to protect and immobilize the spine completely and the need to make it tolerable for the patient. This is why proper evaluation of the need for spinal immobilization is indicated (Figure 6-31).

Obese Patients

With the increasing size of many patients, care of the *bariatric* (overweight, obese) patient is becoming more common. Transport of a 400-pound (182-kg) patient is becoming an everyday occurrence, and special bariatric transport cots have been developed for this purpose. However, a review of commercially available backboards shows that most long backboards measure 16 × 72 inches, with a few measuring 18 inches wide. The weight limit for these long backboards varies from 250 pounds (113 kg) to 600 pounds (272 kg). When using backboards on bariatric trauma patients, special care is needed to ensure that the safe operating limits are not exceeded. Also, additional personnel must be used to lift and extricate bariatric patients, without further injury to the patient or provider. This subgroup of trauma patients presents challenges of safe packaging and moving procedures balanced against short scene times normally recommended in the critically injured trauma patients.

Prolonged Transport

As with other injuries, the prolonged transport of patients with suspected or confirmed spinal and spinal cord injuries presents special considerations. Keeping in mind the goal to move patients with a suspected spinal cord injury only once, care should be taken to pad a long backboard prior to securing the patient. Cervical spine stabilization and spinal movement precautions should be utilized as the patient is moved to the padded backboard. Such efforts should help reduce the risk for the development of pressure ulcers in a patient with spinal cord injury. Any areas where there could be pressure on the patient's body, especially over bony prominences, should be sufficiently padded.

Patients who are immobilized to long backboards are at risk for aspiration should they regurgitate. In the event the patient begins to vomit, the backboard and patient should immediately be tipped onto the side. Suction should be kept near the head of the patient so it is readily accessible should vomiting occur.

Patients with high spinal cord injuries may have involvement of their diaphragm and accessory respiratory muscles (i.e., intercostal muscles), predisposing them to respiratory failure. Impending respiratory failure may be aggravated and hastened by straps placed for spinal immobilization that further restrict respiration. Before initiating a prolonged transport, double check to make sure that the patient's torso is secured at the shoulder girdle and at the pelvis and that any straps do not limit chest wall excursion.

The presence of tachycardia combined with hypotension should raise suspicion for the presence of hypovolemic, rather than neurogenic, shock. Careful assessment may pinpoint the source of hemorrhage, although intra-abdominal sources and pelvic fractures are most likely. The loss of sensation that accompanies a spinal cord injury may prevent a conscious patient from perceiving peritonitis or other injuries below the level of the sensory deficit.

Patients with spinal cord injuries lose some ability to regulate body temperature, and this effect is more pronounced with higher injuries. Thus, these patients are sensitive to the development of hypothermia, especially when they are in a cold environment. Patients should be kept warm (normothermic), but remember that covering them with too many blankets may lead to hyperthermia.

Spine and spinal cord injuries are best managed at facilities that have excellent orthopedic or neurosurgical service and are experienced in the management of these injuries. All level I and II trauma centers should be capable of managing the spinal cord injury and any associated injuries. Some facilities that specialize in the management of spine and spinal cord injuries may directly accept a patient who has suffered only a spinal cord injury (i.e., a shallow-water diving injury no with evidence of aspiration).

SUMMARY

- Preventing the development of or recognizing and treating hypoxia and reduced cerebral blood flow in the field can make the difference between a good or an unacceptable outcome.
- The severity of TBI may not be immediately apparent; therefore, serial neurologic evaluations of the patient, including Glasgow Coma Scale scores and pupillary response, are necessary to recognize changes in the patient's condition.
- TBI is often found in association with multisystem trauma, so all problems are addressed in the appropriate order of priority. Not only are airway, breathing, and circulation always the priorities of patient care, but they are specifically important in the management of TBI in preventing secondary brain injury.
- Prehospital management of the TBI patient involves controlling hemorrhage from other injuries, maintaining a systolic blood pressure of at least 90 mm Hg, and providing oxygen.
- Hyperventilation of patients is performed only when objective signs of brain herniation are noted.
- The vertebral column is composed of 24 separate vertebrae plus the sacrum and coccyx stacked on top of one another.
- The major functions of the spinal column are to support the weight of the body and allow movement.

- The spinal cord is enclosed within the vertebral column and is vulnerable to injury from abnormal movement and positioning. When support for the vertebral column has been lost as a result of injury to the vertebrae or to the muscles and ligaments that help hold the spinal column in place, injury to the spinal cord can occur.
- Because the cord does not regenerate, permanent neurologic injury, often involving paralysis, can result. The presence of spinal trauma and the need to immobilize the patient may be indicated by other injuries that could occur only with sudden, violent forces acting on the body or by specific signs and symptoms of vertebral or spinal cord injury.
- Damage to the bones of the spinal column is not always evident. If an initial injury to the cord has not occurred, neurologic deficit will not be present, even though spinal column is unstable.
- Immobilization of spinal fractures, as with other fractures, requires immobilization of the joint above and the joint below the injury. For the spine, the joints above are the head and neck, and the joint below is the pelvis. The device selected should immobilize the head, chest, and pelvis areas in a neutral inline position without causing or allowing movement.

SCENARIO SOLUTION

The patient's vital signs are pulse 66, respirations 14, and blood pressure 96/70. As you continue your examination, you note that the patient is not moving her arms or legs. This patient is exhibiting signs of neurogenic shock. Interruption of the sympathetic nervous system and unopposed parasympathetic influence on the vascular system below the point of spinal injury result in an increased size of the vascular container and a relative hypovolemia. The patient's response to the spinal cord injury is a low blood pressure and bradycardia.

The first priorities of care are to continue to maintain a patent airway and oxygenation and assist ventilation as necessary to ensure an adequate minute volume while concurrently providing manual stabilization of the cervical spine. Immobilize the patient effectively and efficiently on a long backboard and transport the patient to an appropriate facility. Splint the fractured arm while en route.

The goals of prehospital management for this patient are to prevent additional spinal cord trauma, maintain tissue perfusion, and care for extremity trauma en route and transport without delay to a trauma center for definitive care. ■

References

1. Centers for Disease Control and Prevention: Traumatic Brain Injury. Available at www.cdc.gov/ncipc/tbi/TBI.htm. Accessed August 18, 2010.
2. Marmarou A, Anderson RL, Ward JL, et al: Impact of ICP instability and hypotension on outcome in patients with severe head trauma, *J Neurosurg* 75:S59, 1991.
3. Miller JD, Becker DP: Secondary insults to the injured brain, *J R Coll Surg Edinb* 27:292, 1982.
4. Miller JD, Sweet RC, Narayan RK, et al: Early insults to the injured brain, *JAMA* 240:439, 1978.
5. Silverston P: Pulse oximetry at the roadside: a study of pulse oximetry in immediate care, *BMJ* 298:711, 1989.
6. Stochetti N, Furlan A, Volta F: Hypoxemia and arterial hypotension at the accident scene in head injury, *J Trauma* 40:764, 1996.
7. Plum F: *The diagnosis of stupor and coma,* ed 3, New York, 1982, Oxford University Press.
8. Langfitt TW, Weinstein JD, Kassell NF, Simeone FA: Transmission of increased intracranial pressure. I. Within the craniospinal axis, *J Neurosurg* 21:989, 1964.
9. Langfitt TW: Increased intracranial pressure, *Clin Neurosurg* 16:436, 1969.
10. Marmarou A, Anderson RL, Ward JL, et al: Impact of ICP instability and hypotension on outcome in patients with severe head trauma, *J Neurosurg* 75:S59, 1991.
11. Manley GT, Pitts LH, Morabito D, et al: Brain tissue oxygenation during hemorrhagic shock, resuscitation, and alterations in ventilation, *J Trauma Injury Infect Crit Care* 46:261, 1999.
12. Brain Trauma Foundation: Glasgow Coma Score. In *Guidelines for prehospital management of traumatic brain injury,* New York, 2000, The Foundation.
13. American College of Surgeons: *Advanced trauma life support,* Chicago, 2004, The College.
14. Servadei F, Nasi MT, Cremonini AM: Importance of a reliable admission Glasgow Coma Scale score for determining the need for evacuation of post-traumatic subdural hematomas: a prospective study of 65 patients, *J Trauma* 44:868, 1998.
15. Winkler JV, Rosen P, Alfrey EJ: Prehospital use of the Glasgow Coma Scale in severe head injury, *J Emerg Med* 2:1, 1984.
16. Brain Trauma Foundation: Hospital transport decisions. In *Guidelines for prehospital management of traumatic brain injury,* New York, 2000, The Foundation.
17. Kihtir T, Ivatury RR, Simon RJ, et al: Early management of civilian gunshot wounds to the face, *J Trauma* 35:569, 1993.
18. American Academy of Neurology: The management of concussion in sports (summary statement), *Neurology* 48:581, 1997.
19. Rimel RW, Giordani B, Barth JT: Moderate head injury: completing the clinical spectrum of brain trauma, *Neurosurgery* 11:344, 1982.
20. Brain Trauma Foundation: CT scan features. In *Management and prognosis of severe traumatic brain injury,* ed 2, New York, 2000, The Foundation.
21. Davis DP, Dunford JV, Poste JC, et al: The impact of hypoxia and hyperventilation on outcome after paramedic rapid sequence intubation of severely head injured patients, *J Trauma* 57:1, 2004.
22. Badjatia N, Carney N, Crocco TJ, et al: Treatment: Cerebral Herniation. In *Guidelines for prehospital management of traumatic brain injury, 2nd Edition.* Prehosp Emergency Care 12:Suppl 1:1-52, 2008.
23. DeVivo MJ: Causes and costs of spinal cord injury in the United States, *Spinal Cord* 35:809, 1997.
24. Spinal Cord Injury Information Pages: www.sci-info-pages.com/facts.html. Accessed November 15, 2009.
25. Jackson AB, Dijkers M, Devivo MJ, Poczatek RB: A demographic profile of new traumatic spinal cord injuries: change and stability over 30 years, *Arch Phys Med Rehabil* 85:1740, 2004.
26. Meldon SW, Moettus LN: Thoracolumbar spine fractures: clinical presentation and the effect of altered sensorium and major injury, *J Trauma* 38:1110, 1995.
27. Ross SE, O'Malley KF, DeLong WG, et al: Clinical predictors of unstable cervical spine injury in multiply injured patients, *Injury* 23:317, 1992.

28. Marion DW, Pryzybylski G: Injury to the vertebrae and spinal cord. In Mattox KL, Feliciano DV, Moore EE, editors: *Trauma,* New York, 2000, McGraw-Hill.

29. Tator CH, Fehlings MG: Review of the secondary injury theory of acute spinal cord trauma with special emphasis on vascular mechanisms, *J Neurosurg* 75:15, 1991.

30. Bilello JP, Davis JW, Cunningham MA, et al: Cervical spinal cord injury and the need for cardiovascular intervention, *Arch Surg* 138:1127, 2003.

31. Ullrich A, Hendey GW, Geiderman J, et al: Distracting painful injuries associated with cervical spinal injuries in blunt trauma, *Acad Emerg Med* 8:25, 2001.

32. Domeier RM, Evans RW, Swor RA, et al: Prospective validation of out-of-hospital spinal clearance criteria: a preliminary report, *Acad Emerg Med* 4:643, 1997.

33. Domeier RM, Swor RA, Evans RW, et al: Multicenter prospective validation of prehospital clinical spinal clearance criteria, *J Trauma* 53:744, 2002.

34. Hankins DG, Rivera-Rivera EJ, Ornato JP, et al: Spinal immobilization in the field: clinical clearance criteria and implementation, *Prehosp Emerg Care* 5:88, 2001.

35. Stroh G, Braude D: Can an out-of-hospital cervical spine clearance protocol identify all patients with injuries? An argument for selective immobilization, *Ann Emerg Med* 37:609, 2001.

36. Dunn TM, Dalton A, Dorfman T, Dunn WW: Are emergency medical technician-basics able to use a selective immobilization of the cervical spine protocol? A preliminary report, *Prehosp Emerg Care* 8:207, 2004.

37. Domeier RM, Frederiksen SM, Welch K: Prospective performance assessment of an out-of-hospital protocol for selective spine immobilization using clinical spine clearance criteria, *Ann Emerg Med* 46:123, 2005.

38. Domeier RM, National Association of EMS Physicians Standards and Practice Committee: Indications for prehospital spinal immobilization, *Prehosp Emerg Care* 3:251, 1997.

39. Connell RA, Graham CA, Munro PT: Is spinal immobilization necessary for all patients sustaining isolated penetrating trauma? *Injury* 34:912, 2003.

40. Chong CL, Ware DN, Harris JH: Is cervical spine imaging indicated in gunshot wounds to the cranium? *J Trauma* 44:501, 1998.

41. Kaups KL, Davis JW: Patients with gunshot wounds to the head do not require cervical spine immobilization and evaluation, *J Trauma* 44:865, 1998.

42. Lanoix R, Gupta R, Leak L, Pierre J: C-spine injury associated with gunshot wounds to the head: retrospective study and literature review, *J Trauma* 49:860, 2000.

43. Barkana Y, Stein M, Scope A, et al: Prehospital stabilization of the cervical spine for penetrating injuries of the neck: is it necessary? *Injury* 34:912, 2003.

44. Cornwell EE, Chang, DC, Boner JP, et al: Thoracolumbar immobilization for trauma patients with torso gunshot wounds-is it necessary? *Arch Surg* 136:324, 2001.

45. American College of Surgeons Committee on Trauma: *Advanced trauma life support for doctors, student course manual,* ed 7, Chicago, 2004, American College of Surgeons.

46. DeBoer SL, Seaver M: Big head, little body syndrome: what EMS providers need to know, *Emerg Med Serv* 33:47, 2004.

47. Nesathurai S: Steroids and spinal cord injury: revisiting the NASCIS 2 and NASCIS 3 trials, *J Trauma* 45:1088, 1998.

Suggested Reading

American College of Surgeons Committee on Trauma: Head trauma. In *Advanced trauma life support for doctors, student course manual,* ed 7, Chicago, 2004, ACS.

Atkinson JLD: The neglected prehospital phase of head injury: apnea and catecholamine surge, *Mayo Clin Proceed* 75:37, 2000.

Bertz JE: Maxillofacial injuries, *Clin Symp* 33:2, 1981.

Chi JH, Nemani V, Manley GT: Prehospital treatment of traumatic brain injury, *Sem Neurosurg* 14:71, 2003.

Guidelines for the determination of brain death, *JAMA* 246:2184, 1981.

Kolb JC, Summer RL, Galli L: Cervical collar-induced changes in intracranial pressure, *Am J Emerg Med* 17:135, 1999.

Muizelaar JP, Marmarou A, Ward JD, et al: Adverse effects of prolonged hyperventilation in patients with severe brain injury: a randomized clinical trial, *J Neurosurg* 75:731, 1991.

Pennardt AM, Zehner WJ: Paramedic documentation of indicators for cervical spine injury, *Prehosp Disaster Med* 9:40, 1994.

Rosner MJ, Coley IB: Cerebral perfusion pressure, intracranial pressure and head elevation, *J Neurosurg* 65:636, 1986.

Teasdale G, Jennett B: Assessment of coma and impaired consciousness: a practical scale, *Lancet* 2:81, 1974.

Valadka AB: Injury to the cranium. In Mattox KL, Feliciano DV, Moore EE: *Trauma,* ed 4, Norwalk, Conn, 2000, Appleton & Lange.

SPECIFIC SKILLS

Spine Management

Logroll

Principle: To turn a patient while maintaining manual stabilization with minimal movement of the spine. The logroll is indicated for (1) positioning a patient onto a long backboard or other device to facilitate movement of the patient and (2) turning a patient with suspected spinal trauma to examine the back.

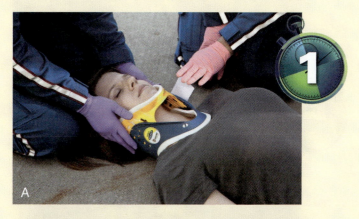

A

A. Supine Patient

While one prehospital care provider maintains neutral inline stabilization at the patient's head, a second provider applies a properly sized cervical collar.

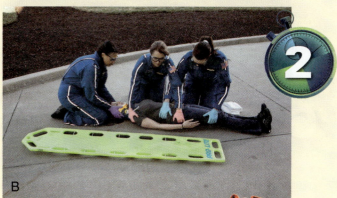

B

While one provider maintains neutral inline stabilization, a second provider kneels at the patient's midthorax, and a third provider kneels at the level of the patient's knees. The patient's arms are straightened and placed palms-in next to the torso while the patient's legs are brought into neutral alignment. The patient is grasped at the shoulder and hips in such a fashion as to maintain a neutral inline position of the lower extremities. The patient is "logrolled" slightly onto his or her side. The long backboard is placed with the foot end of the board positioned between the patient's knees and ankles (the head of the long backboard will extend beyond the patient's head).

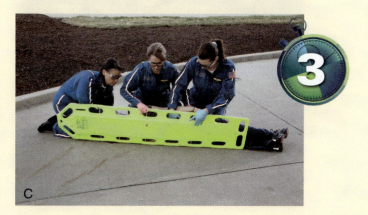

C

The long backboard is held against the patient's back and the patient is logrolled back onto the long backboard, and the board is lowered to the ground with the patient.

SPECIFIC SKILLS

Once on the ground, the patient is grasped firmly by the shoulders, the pelvis, and the lower extremities.

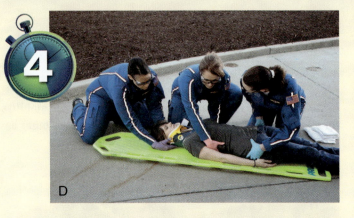

D

The patient is moved upward and laterally onto the long backboard. Neutral inline stabilization is maintained without pulling on the patient's head and neck.

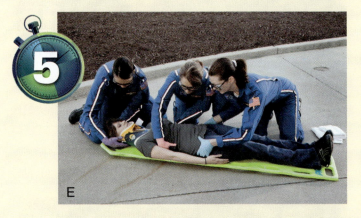

E

The patient is positioned onto the long backboard with the head at the top of the board and the body centered.

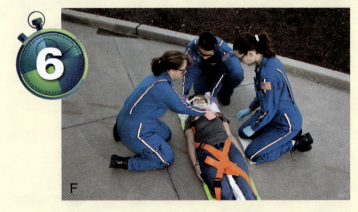

F

B. Prone or Semiprone Patient

When a patient presents in a prone or semiprone position, a stabilization method similar to that used for the supine patient can be used. The method incorporates the same initial alignment of the patient's limbs, the same positioning and hand placement of the prehospital care providers, and the same responsibilities for maintaining alignment.

The patient's arms are positioned in anticipation of the full rotation that will occur. With the semiprone logroll method, a cervical collar can be safely applied only after the patient is in an inline position and supine on the long backboard, not before.

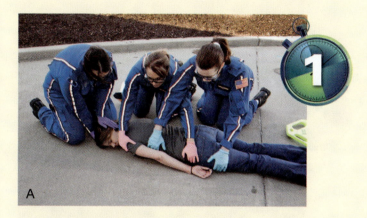

Whenever possible, the patient should always be rolled away from the direction in which the patient's face initially points. One provider establishes inline manual stabilization of the patient's head and neck. Another provider kneels at the patient's thorax and grasps the patient's opposite shoulder and wrist and pelvis area. A third provider kneels at the patient's knees and grasps the patient's wrist and pelvis area and lower extremities.

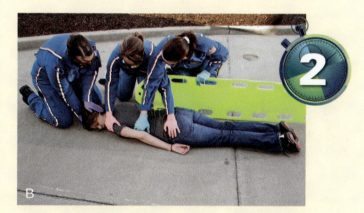

The long backboard is placed on the lateral edge with the foot of the board between the patient's knees and ankles.

SPECIFIC SKILLS

The patient is logrolled onto his or her side. The patient's head rotates less than the torso, so by the time the patient is on his or her side (perpendicular to the ground), the head and torso have come into proper alignment.

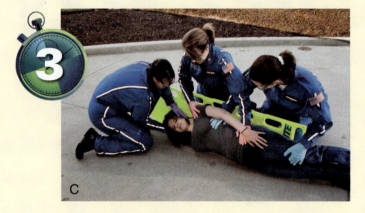

C

Once the patient is supine on the long backboard, the patient is moved upward and toward the center of the board. The prehospital care providers should take care not to pull the patient but to maintain neutral inline stabilization. Once the patient is positioned properly on the long backboard, a properly sized cervical collar can be applied, and the patient can be secured to the backboard.

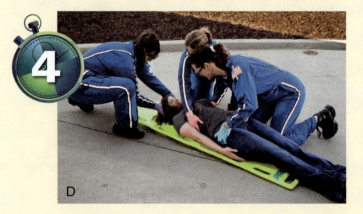

D

Standing Longboard Application

Principle: To fully immobilize a standing patient to a long backboard while maintaining the head and neck in a neutral position and minimizing the risk of additional injury.

This application is indicated for spinal immobilization of a trauma patient who is ambulatory but is found to have an indication for spinal immobilization (see Figure 6-25).

Two general methods exist for immobilizing a standing patient to a long backboard. The first method involves securing the standing patient's torso and head to the board before lowering the board to the ground. This method causes some discomfort to the patient and may not allow the patient to be lowered to the ground without movement. The second method involves manual stabilization of the patient to the board while lowering the board and patient to the ground and then securing the patient to the board. This second method is the preferred method and can be accomplished with two or three rescuers.

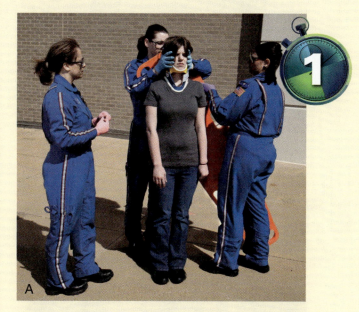

A. Three or More Providers

Prehospital care providers can apply manual inline stabilization from either behind the patient or in front of the patient. Once manual inline stabilization of the patient's head and neck is applied, a properly sized rigid cervical collar can be applied. A long backboard is placed behind the patient from the side and pressed against the patient. Manual inline stabilization is maintained throughout the procedure until the patient is secured to the long backboard.

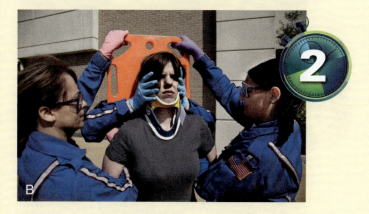

Two prehospital care providers stand on either side of the patient, turned slightly toward the patient. Each provider inserts the hand closest to the patient under the patient's armpit and grasps the nearest handhold of the backboard without moving the patient's shoulders. The other hand grasps a higher handhold on the board. While manual inline stabilization is maintained, the patient and backboard are lowered to the ground.

SPECIFIC SKILLS

As the patient is lowered to the ground the provider behind the patient providing the manual stabilization must rotate their hands to maintain the stabilization.

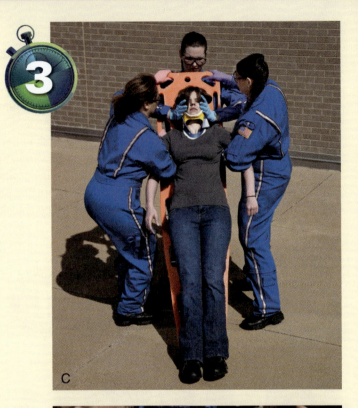

As the patient is lowered to the ground each provider on the side of the patient one at a time will need to release their hold on the upper portion of the board and reposition their hand under the provider's arm maintaining manual stabilization of the patient's head and neck.

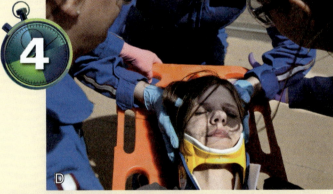

Once the patient and board are on the ground, the patient is secured to the long backboard.

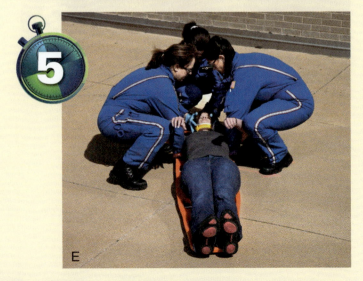

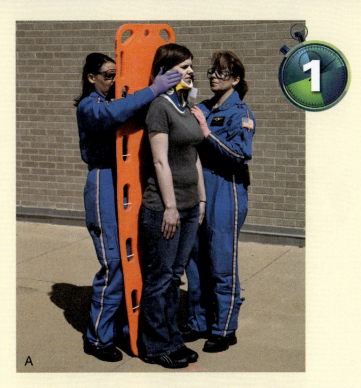

B. Two Providers

When three or more prehospital care providers are not available, two providers can still achieve immobilization. The first provider establishes and maintains manual stabilization of the patient's head and neck while the second provider measures and applies an appropriate sized cervical collar. Once the collar has been applied, the second provider places a backboard behind the patient and in front of the first provider.

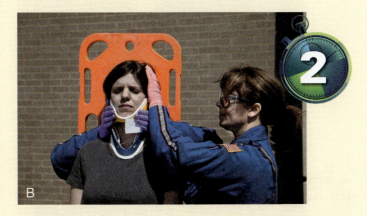

The second provider holds the backboard with their hand closest to the board. The second provider now places their other hand, palm surface with fingers extended, on the patient's head and applies light pressure to assist in maintaining manual stabilization.

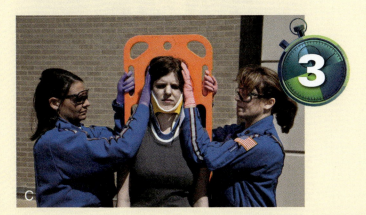

The first provider now can release the patient's head with the hand closest to the second provider. With the other hand, the first provider repositions it to the side of the patient's head to apply lateral pressure while moving to the patient's side and grasping the backboard at the level of the patient's head or higher.

SPECIFIC SKILLS

The patient is lowered, along with the backboard, to the ground while both providers maintain manual stabilization with equal lateral pressure against the side of the patient's head. The prehospital care providers need to work together during this move to ensure maximum manual stabilization.

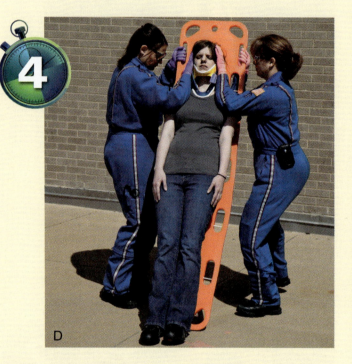

D

Once the patient and backboard are on the ground, manual in-line stabilization can be maintained by one provider from above the patient's head until the patient is secured to the long backboard.

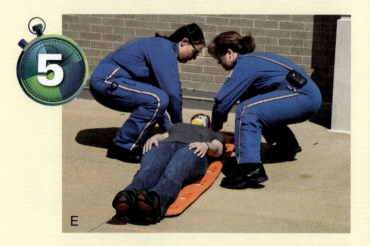

E

Sitting Immobilization (Vest-Type Extrication Device)

Principle: To immobilize a trauma patient without critical injuries before moving the patient from a sitting position.

This type of immobilization is used when spinal stabilization is indicated for a sitting trauma patient without life-threatening conditions.

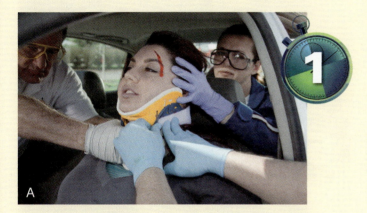

Several brands of vest-type extrication devices are available. Each model is slightly different in design, but any model can serve as a general example. The Kendrick Extrication Device **(KED)** is used in this demonstration. The details (but not the general sequence) are modified when using a different model or brand of extrication device. Also, during this demonstration, the windshield of the vehicle has been removed for clarification purposes. Manual inline stabilization is initiated and a properly sized cervical collar applied.

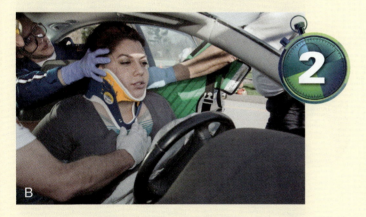

The patient is maintained in an upright position slightly forward to provide an adequate amount of space between the patient's back and the vehicle seat for placement of the vest-type device. *Note:* Before placing the vest-type device behind the patient, the two long straps (groin straps) are unfastened and placed behind the vest device.

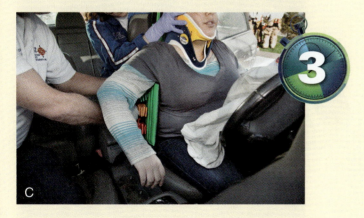

After placing the vest device behind the patient, the side flaps are placed around the patient and moved until the side flaps are touching the patient's armpits.

SPECIFIC SKILLS

The torso straps are positioned and fastened, starting with the middle chest strap and followed by the lower chest strap. Each strap is tightened after attachment. Use of the upper chest strap at this time is optional. If the upper chest strap is used, the provider should ensure that it is not so tight that it impedes the patient's ventilations. The upper chest strap should be tightened just before moving the patient.

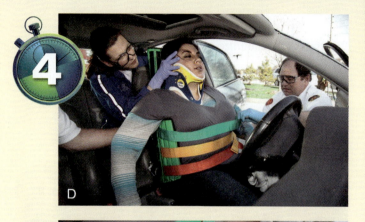

Each groin strap is positioned and fastened. Using a back-and-forth motion, each strap is worked under the patient's thigh and buttock until it is in a straight line in the intergluteal fold from front to back. Each groin strap is placed under the patient's leg and attached to the vest on the same side as the strap's origin. Once in place, each groin strap is tightened. The patient's genitalia should not be placed under the straps but to the side of each strap.

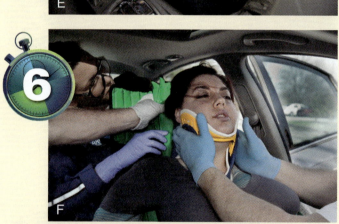

Padding is placed between the patient's head and the vest to maintain neutral alignment.

The patient's head is secured to the head flaps of the vest device. The provider should be careful not to seat the patient's mandible or obstruct the airway. *Note:* The torso straps should be evaluated and readjusted as needed.

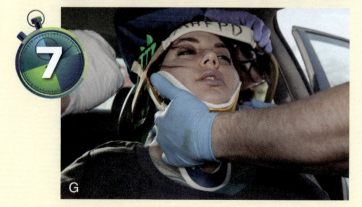

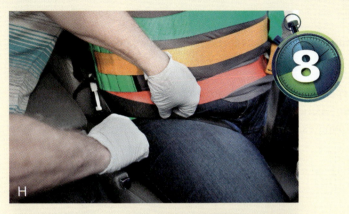

All straps should be rechecked before moving the patient. If the upper chest strap has not been secured, it should be attached and tightened.

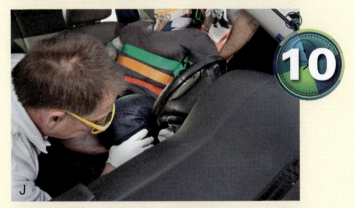

If possible, the ambulance cot with a long backboard should be brought to the opening of the vehicle door. The long backboard is placed under the patient's buttocks so that one end is securely supported on the vehicle seat and the other end on the ambulance cot. If the ambulance cot is not available or the terrain will not allow the placement of the cot, other prehospital care providers can hold the long backboard while the patient is rotated and lifted out of the vehicle.

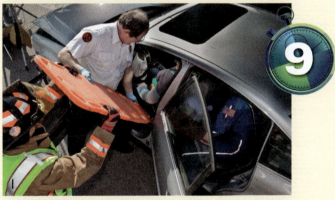

While rotating the patient, the patient's lower extremities must be elevated onto the seat. If the vehicle has a center console, the patient's legs should be moved over the console one at a time.

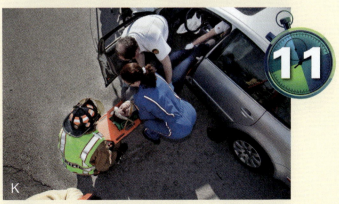

Once the patient is rotated with his or her back to the center of the long backboard, the patient is lowered to the board while keeping the legs elevated. After placing the patient onto the long backboard, the two groin straps are released and the patient's legs are lowered. The patient is positioned by moving him or her up on the board with the vest device in place. The provider should consider releasing the upper chest strap at this time.

Once the patient is positioned on the long backboard, the vest device is left secured in place to continue to immobilize the patient's head, neck, and torso. The patient and vest device are secured to the long backboard. The patient's lower extremities are immobilized to the board, and the long backboard is secured to the ambulance cot.

SPECIFIC SKILLS

Rapid Extrication

Principle: To manually stabilize a patient with critical injuries before and during movement from a sitting position.

A. Three or More Providers

Sitting patients with life-threatening conditions and indications for spinal immobilization (see Figure 6-14) can be rapidly extricated. Immobilization to an interim device before moving the patient provides more stable immobilization than when using only the manual (rapid extrication) method. However, it requires an additional 4 to 8 minutes to complete. The prehospital care provider will use the vest or half-board methods in the following situations:

- When the scene and patient's condition are stable and time is not a primary concern

or

- When a special rescue situation involving substantial lifting or technical rescue hoisting exists, and significant movement or carrying of the patient is involved before it is practical to complete the supine immobilization to a long backboard

Rapid extrication is indicated in the following situations:

- When the patient has life-threatening conditions identified during the primary survey that cannot be corrected where the patient is found
- When the scene is unsafe and clear danger to the prehospital care provider and patient exists, necessitating rapid removal to a safe location
- When the patient needs to be moved quickly to access other, more seriously injured patients

Note: Rapid extrication is only selected when life-threatening conditions are present and not on the basis of personal preference.

Once the decision is made to extricate a patient rapidly, manual inline stabilization of the patient's head and neck in a neutral position is initiated. This is best accomplished from behind the patient. If a provider is unable to get behind the patient, manual stabilization can be accomplished from the side. Whether from behind the patient or the side, the patient's head and neck are brought into a neutral alignment, a rapid assessment of the patient is performed, and a properly sized cervical collar is applied.

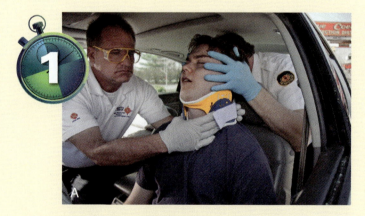

While manual stabilization is maintained, the patient's upper torso and lower torso and legs are controlled. The patient is rotated in a series of short, controlled movements.

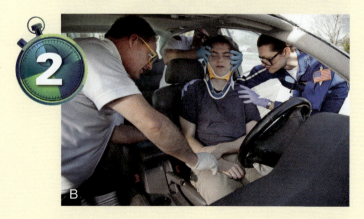

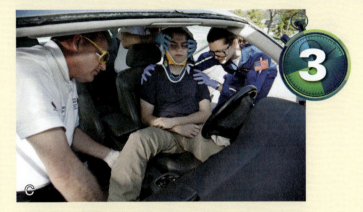

If the vehicle has a center console the patient's legs should be moved one at a time over the console.

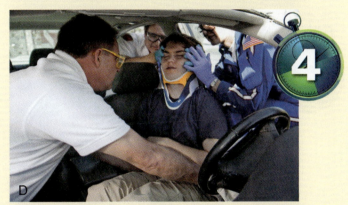

The patient is continued to be rotated in short controlled movements until control of manual stabilization can no longer be maintained by the first provider. A second provider assumes manual stabilization from the first provider while standing outside of the vehicle.

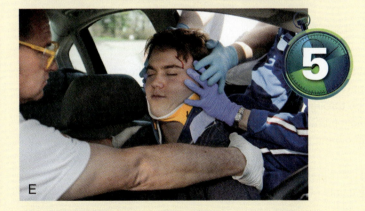

The first provider can now move outside the vehicle and reassume manual stabilization from the second provider.

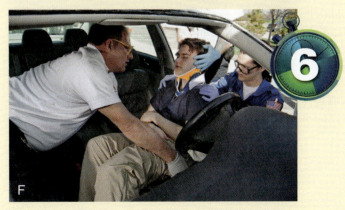

The rotation of the patient is continued until the patient can be lowered out of the vehicle door opening and onto the long backboard.

SPECIFIC SKILLS

The long backboard is placed with the foot end of the board on the vehicle seat and the head end on the ambulance cot. If the cot cannot be placed next to the vehicle, other prehospital care providers can hold the long backboard while the patient is lowered onto the backboard.

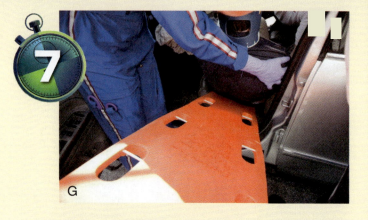

Once the patient's torso is down on the board, the weight of the patient's chest is controlled while the patient's pelvis and lower legs are controlled. The patient is moved upward onto the long backboard. The prehospital care provider who is maintaining manual stabilization is careful not to pull the patient but to support the patient's head and neck.

After the patient is positioned onto the long backboard, the prehospital care providers can secure the patient to the board and the board to the ambulance cot. The patient's upper torso is secured first, then the lower torso and pelvis area, then the head. The patient's legs are secured last. If the scene is unsafe, the patient should be moved to a safe area before being secured to the board or cot.

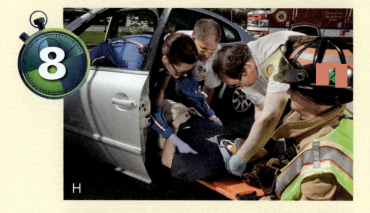

Note: This represents only one example of rapid extrication. Because very few field situations are ideal, prehospital care providers may need to modify the steps for extrication for the particular patient and situation. The principle of rapid extrication should remain the same regardless of the situation: maintain manual stabilization throughout the extrication process without interruption, and maintain the entire spine in an inline position without unwanted movement. Any positioning of the prehospital care providers that works can be successful. However, numerous position changes and hand position takeovers should be avoided because they invite a lapse in manual stabilization.

The rapid extrication technique can effectively provide manual inline stabilization of the patient's head, neck, and torso throughout a patient's removal from a vehicle. The following are three key points of rapid extrication:

1. One prehospital care provider maintains stabilization of the patient's head and neck at all times, another rotates and stabilizes the patient's upper torso, and a third moves and controls the patient's lower torso, pelvis, and lower extremities.
2. Maintaining manual inline stabilization of the patient's head and neck is impossible if attempting to move the patient in one continuous motion. The prehospital care providers need to limit each movement, stopping to reposition and prepare for the next move. Undue haste will cause delay and may result in movement of the spine.
3. Each situation and patient may require adaptation of the principles of rapid extrication. This can only work effectively if the maneuvers are practiced. Each provider needs to know the actions and movements of the other providers.

B. Two Providers

In some situations an adequate number of providers may not be available to extricate a critical patient rapidly. In these situations a two-provider technique is useful.

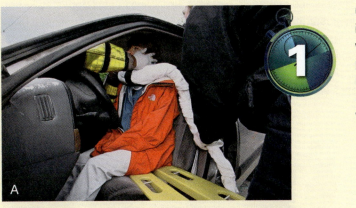

One prehospital care provider initiates and maintains manual inline stabilization of the patient's head and neck. A second provider places a properly sized cervical collar on the patient and places a prerolled blanket around the patient. The center of the blanket roll is placed at the patient's midline on the rigid cervical collar. The ends of the blanket roll are wrapped around the cervical collar and placed under the patient's arms.

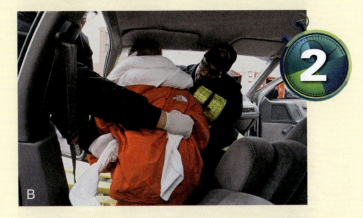

The patient is turned using the ends of the blanket roll and until the patient's back is centered on the door opening.

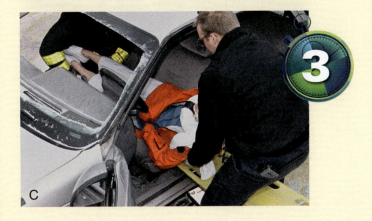

The first provider takes control of the blanket ends, moving them under the patient's shoulders, and moves the patient by the blanket while the second provider moves and controls the patient's lower torso, pelvis, and legs.

SPECIFIC SKILLS

Helmet Removal

Principle: To remove a safety helmet while minimizing the risk of additional injury.

Patients who are wearing full-face helmets must have the helmet removed early in the assessment process (see Figure 6-29). This provides immediate access for the prehospital care provider to assess and manage a patient's airway and ventilatory status. Helmet removal ensures that hidden bleeding is not occurring into the posterior helmet and allows the provider to move the head (from the flexed position caused by large helmets) into neutral alignment. It also permits complete assessment of the head and neck in the secondary survey and facilitates spinal immobilization when indicated (see Figure 6-25). The prehospital care provider explains to the patient what will occur. If the patient verbalizes that the provider should not remove the helmet, the provider explains that properly trained personnel can remove it by protecting the patient's spine. Two providers are required for this maneuver.

One provider takes position above the patient's head. With palms pressed on the sides of the helmet and fingertips curled over the lower margin, the first provider stabilizes the helmet, head, and neck in as close to a neutral inline position as the helmet allows. A second provider kneels at the side of the patient, opens or removes the face shield if needed, remove eyeglasses if present, and unfastens or cuts the chin strap.

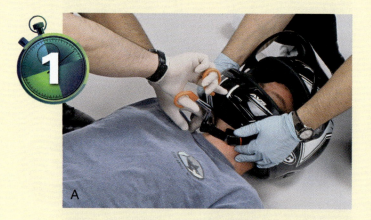

A

The patient's mandible is grasped between the thumb and the first two fingers at the angle of the mandible. The other hand is placed under the patient's neck on the occiput of the skull to take control of manual stabilization. The provider's forearms should be resting on the floor or ground or on the provider's thighs for additional support.

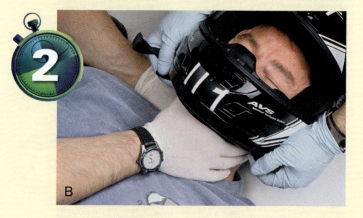

B

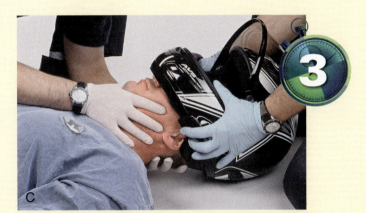

The first provider pulls the sides of the helmet slightly apart, away from the patient's head, and rotates the helmet with up-and-down rocking motions while pulling it off of the patient's head. Movement of the helmet is slow and deliberate. The provider takes care as the helmet clears the patient's nose.

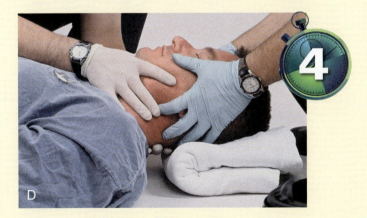

Once the helmet is removed, padding should be placed behind the patient's head to maintain a neutral inline position. Manual stabilization is maintained, and a properly sized cervical collar is placed on the patient.

Note: Two key elements are involved in helmet removal, as follows:

1. While one provider maintains manual stabilization of the patient's head and neck, the other provider moves. At no time should both providers be moving their hands.
2. The provider rotates the helmet in different directions, first to clear the patient's nose and then to clear the back of the patient's head.

CHAPTER 7

Musculoskeletal Trauma

CHAPTER OBJECTIVES

At the completion of this chapter, the reader will be able to do the following:

✓ Define fracture, sprain, and strain.

✓ List the three categories used to classify patients with extremity injuries, and relate this classification to priority of care.

✓ Describe the primary and secondary surveys as related to extremity trauma.

✓ Discuss the significance of hemorrhage in both open and closed fractures of the long bones, pelvis, and ribs.

✓ List the five major pathophysiologic problems associated with extremity injuries that may require management in the prehospital setting.

✓ Explain the management of extremity trauma as an isolated injury and in the presence of multisystem trauma.

✓ Given a scenario involving an extremity injury, select an appropriate splint and splinting method.

✓ Describe the special considerations involved in femur fracture management.

✓ Describe the management of amputations.

SCENARIO

You are called to a construction site where a worker is complaining of pain to his right mid-thigh after a fork lift pinned him against a container. Once you determine the scene is safe to enter, you discover the patient lying on the ground. He is able to describe the sequence of events leading up to his injury but appears tired and is in a great deal of pain; he is diaphoretic and pale. You've determined that his airway is open and he is breathing without difficulty or obstruction at a rate of 24 breaths/minute. The patient complains only of pain to the right mid-thigh and loss of sensation and the ability to move beyond the injury. He has a pulse of 120 and blood pressure is 104/76. On exposing the right leg you note swelling mid-thigh and shortening of the limb, which is rotated outward.

What do the kinematics of this event tell you about the potential injuries for this patient?

What type of injury does this patient have and what would your management priorities be?

Musculoskeletal injury, although common in trauma patients, rarely poses an immediate life-threatening condition. Skeletal trauma can be life threatening, however, when it produces severe blood loss (hemorrhage), either externally or from internal bleeding into the extremity, or the retroperitoneum in the case of the pelvis.

When caring for a critical trauma patient, the prehospital care provider has three primary considerations with regard to extremity injuries, as follows:

1. Maintain assessment priorities. Do not be distracted by dramatic, non–life-threatening musculoskeletal injuries (Figure 7-1).
2. Recognize potentially life-threatening musculoskeletal injuries.
3. Recognize the kinematics that created the musculoskeletal injuries and the potential for other life-threatening injuries caused by that energy transfer.

If a life-threatening or potentially life-threatening condition is discovered anywhere in the body during the primary survey (initial assessment), the secondary survey (detailed history and physical examination) should not be started. Any problems found during the primary survey should be corrected in ABC order before moving to the secondary survey (see later discussion). This may mean delaying the secondary survey until the patient is en route or even until arrival at the emergency department (ED).

Critical trauma patients should be transported on longboards to allow for resuscitation and treatment of both critical and noncritical injuries. Using a longboard allows for immobilization of the patient's entire body on a single platform that makes it possible to move the victim without disturbing the splinting. Although some injuries are more obvious than others, the prehospital care provider should treat every painful musculoskeletal injury as a possible fracture and immobilize it to limit the potential for further injury and to provide some comfort and reduction of pain.

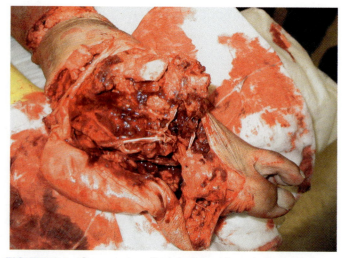

FIGURE 7-1 Some extremity injuries, although dramatic in appearance, are not life threatening.

Anatomy and Physiology

Understanding the gross anatomy and physiology of the human body is an important piece of the prehospital care provider's fund of knowledge. Anatomy and physiology are the foundations on which assessment and management are based. Without a good grasp of the structures of the bones and muscles, one will not be able to relate kinematics and superficial injuries to injuries that are internal. Although this textbook does not discuss all the anatomy and physiology of the musculoskeletal system, it reviews some of the basics.

The mature human body has approximately 206 bones separated into categories by shape: long, short, flat, sutural, and sesamoid. *Long* bones include the femur, humerus, ulna, radius, tibia, and fibula. *Short* bones include metacarpals, metatarsals, and phalanges. *Flat* bones are usually thin and compact, such as the sternum, ribs, and scapulae. *Sutural* bones are part of the skull and are located between the joints of certain cranial bones. *Sesamoid* bones are bones located within tendons; the patella is the largest sesamoid bone (Figure 7-2).

The human body has more than 700 individual muscles, which are categorized by function. The muscles that are specific to this chapter are the voluntary, or skeletal, muscles. They are termed *skeletal* because they move the skeletal system. Muscles in this category voluntarily move the structures of the body (Figure 7-3). When a muscle contracts, it shortens and thus is able to move the bones that make up a joint.

Other important structures discussed in this chapter are tendons and ligaments. A *tendon* is a band of tough, inelastic, fibrous tissue. It is the white part at the end of a muscle that directly attaches a muscle to the bone that it will move. A *ligament* is a band of tough, fibrous tissue connecting bone to bone; its function is to hold joints together.

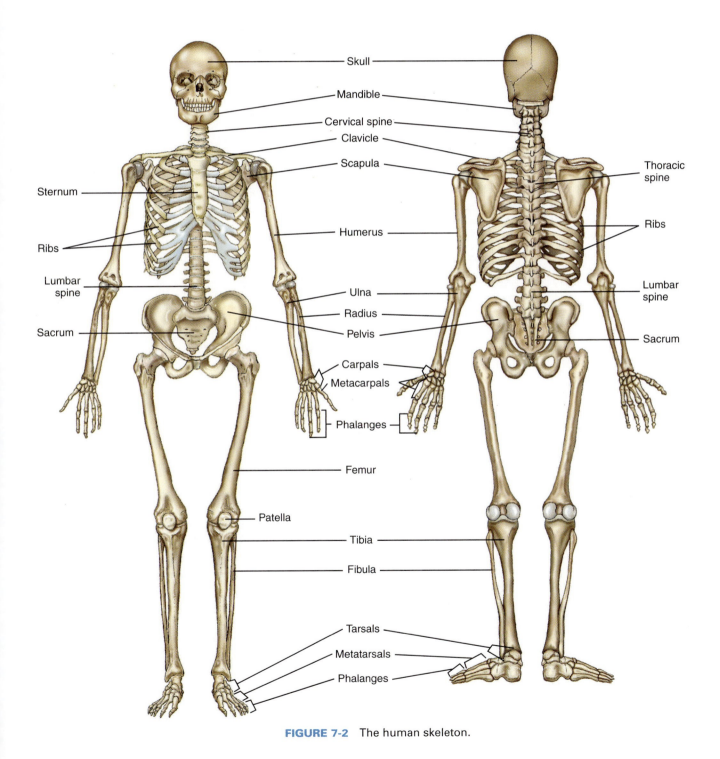

FIGURE 7-2   The human skeleton.

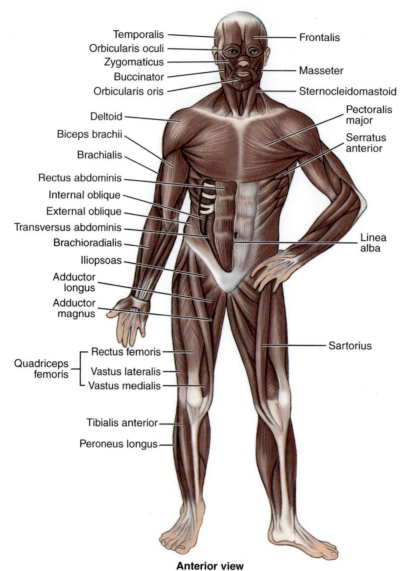

Anterior view

FIGURE 7-3   Major muscles of the human body.
(From Herlihy B, Maebius NK: *The human body in health and illness,* ed 2, St Louis, 2003, WB Saunders.)

Assessment

Musculoskeletal trauma can be categorized into the following three main types:

1. Life-threatening injuries resulting from musculoskeletal trauma, such as external hemorrhage, or internal hemorrhage associated with pelvic or femur fractures with life-threatening blood loss
2. Non–life-threatening musculoskeletal trauma associated with multisystem life-threatening trauma (life-threatening injuries plus limb fractures)
3. Isolated non–life-threatening musculoskeletal trauma (isolated limb fractures)

The purpose of the primary survey is to identify and treat life-threatening injuries. The presence of a non–life-threatening musculoskeletal injury can be an indicator of possible multisystem trauma and should not distract the prehospital care provider from performing a complete primary assessment. Although the presence of musculoskeletal trauma should not divert from the care of more life-threatening conditions, the injuries should be looked at as possible indicators for potential life-threatening conditions. Evaluating the kinematics that created the obvious injuries may point to occult serious injuries.

Kinematics

Understanding the kinematics involved in an injury is one of the most important functions of the assessment and manage-

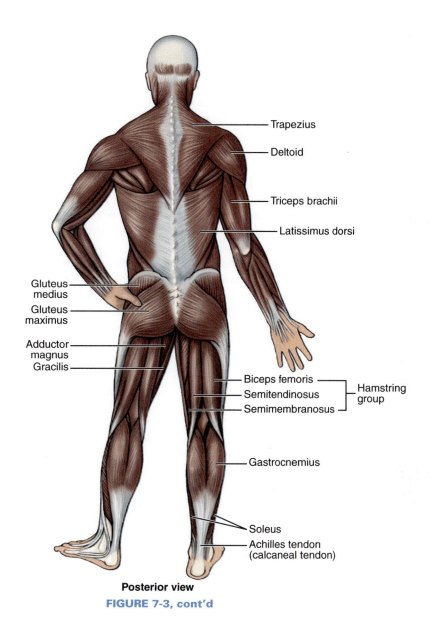

Trapezius

Deltoid

Triceps brachii

Latissimus dorsi

Gluteus medius

Gluteus maximus

Adductor magnus

Gracilis

Biceps femoris

Semitendinosus

Semimembranosus

Hamstring group

Gastrocnemius

Soleus

Achilles tendon (calcaneal tendon)

Posterior view

FIGURE 7-3, cont'd

ment of a trauma patient. Rapidly determining the kinematics and whether it involved low-energy versus high-energy transference (e.g., falling from a bike vs. being thrown from a motorcycle) will lead the prehospital care provider to the recognition of most critical injuries. The best source for determining the kinematics is directly from the patient. If the patient is unresponsive, details of the injury mechanism can be obtained from witnesses. Often a "best guess" approach to the events based on injuries can be used if no one was present at the incident. This information should be reported to the receiving facility and documented on the patient care record.

Based on the kinematics, the prehospital care provider may develop a high index of suspicion for the injuries that a patient might have sustained. Consideration of the kinematics may bring to mind additional injuries for which the pro-

vider should assess, given knowledge of various injury patterns. For example:

- If a patient jumps out of a window and lands feet first, the primary injury suspicion would be fractures of the calcaneus (heel), tibia, fibula, femur, pelvis, and spine and aortic shear injuries. However, secondary injuries might include abdominal injury or head injury from tumbling forward after hitting the ground.
- If a patient is involved in a motorcycle collision with a telephone pole and hits his or her head on the pole, primary injuries will include head, cervical spine, and thoracic injury. A secondary injury might include a femur fracture from striking the femur on the handlebars.

Another example involves a patient riding in the passenger side of a vehicle that sustains a side-impact collision. The door of the target vehicle is pushed against the upper arm, which can then be pushed into the chest wall, while at the same time the door can hit the pelvis or femur on the same side. Given the kinematics of this crash, suspicion for musculoskeletal injury would include humerus, pelvis, and femur fractures. Further injury suspicion would include rib fractures, chest wall muscle injury, lung and heart injuries, and abdominal organ injury. Another secondary injury to consider is abrasion from a deployed air bag.

Another possible injury from a side-impact collision results from an unrestrained passenger becoming a missile (object) inside the vehicle. The other vehicle striking the passenger side sets the passenger in motion until he or she is stopped by another object, such as the driver. However, near-side injuries are more severe than far-side injuries. In this case the kinematics to consider for the driver is the energy delivered by the unrestrained passenger's body.

A basic understanding of kinematics guides the provider's assessment for the less obvious injuries.

Primary and Secondary Surveys

Primary Survey

The first step of any assessment is to ensure scene safety and evaluate the situation. Once the scene is safe, the patient can be assessed. The primary survey addresses the immediately life-threatening conditions that are identified. Although angulated fractures or partial amputations may draw the provider's attention, life-threatening conditions should take priority. Airway, breathing, and circulation, disability, and exposure (ABCDE) remain the most important parts of assessment. For a patient with life-threatening conditions identified in the primary survey, management of musculoskeletal trauma is delayed until those problems are corrected; however, external hemorrhage is included in the primary survey and must be controlled when deemed life threatening. If the patient has no life-threatening injuries, the prehospital care provider proceeds to the secondary survey.

Secondary Survey

Assessment of the extremities occurs during the secondary survey. To facilitate examination, the provider considers removing any clothing that was not removed during the primary survey, as allowed by the environment. If the mechanism of injury is not obvious, the patient or bystanders can be questioned about how the injuries occurred. The patient should also be queried about the presence of pain in the extremities. Most patients with significant musculoskeletal injuries have pain, unless a spinal cord or peripheral nerve injury is present. Assessment of the extremities also includes evaluating for pain, weakness, or abnormal sensations in the extremities.

Bones and Joints. Evaluation of bones and joints is accomplished by inspecting for deformities that may represent fractures or dislocations, and palpating the extremity for tenderness and crepitus (Figure 7-4). *Crepitus* is the grinding feeling that bones make when the fractured ends rub against one another. Crepitus can be elicited by palpating the site of injury and by movement of the extremity. Crepitus sounds like a crackling or popping noise or the popping of plastic bubble wrap used for packing. This feeling of bones grating against one another during the assessment of a patient can produce further injury; therefore, once the crepitus is noted, no additional or repetitive steps should be taken to produce it. Crepitus is a distinct feeling that is not easily forgotten.

Soft Tissue Injuries. The provider visually inspects for swelling, lacerations, abrasions, hematomas, skin color, and wounds. Any wound adjacent to a fracture may indicate the presence of an open fracture. Firmness and tenseness of the soft tissues may indicate presence of a compartment syndrome.

Circulation. Circulation is checked by feeling for distal pulses (radial in the upper extremity and dorsalis pedis or posterior tibial in the lower extremity) and noting capillary refill time in the fingers or toes. Absence of distal pulses in the extremities can indicate disruption of an artery, compression of the vessel by a hematoma or bone fragment, or a compartment syndrome. Large or expanding hematomas may indicate the presence of an injury to a large vessel.

Neurologic Function. The provider assesses both motor and sensory function in the extremities. If a long-bone fracture is suspected, do not ask the patient to move the extremity, because such movement can induce significant pain and pos-

FIGURE 7-4   Common Joint Dislocation Deformities

Joint	Direction	Deformity
Shoulder	Anterior	Squared off
	Posterior	Locked in internal rotation
Elbow	Posterior	Olecranon prominent posteriorly
Hip	Anterior	Flexed, abducted, externally rotated
	Posterior	Flexed, adducted, internally rotated
Knee	Anteroposterior	Loss of normal contour, extended
Ankle	Lateral is most common	Externally rotated, prominent medial malleolus
Subtalar joint	Lateral is most common	Laterally displaced os calcis

FIGURE 7-5 Peripheral Nerve Assessment of Upper Extremities

Nerve	Motor	Sensation	Injury
Ulnar	Index finger abduction	Little finger	Elbow injury
Median, distal	Thenar contraction with opposition	Index finger	Wrist dislocation
Median, anterior interosseous	Index tip flexion		Supracondylar fracture of humerus (children)
Musculocutaneous	Elbow tip flexion	Lateral forearm	Anterior shoulder dislocation
Radial	Thumb, finger metocarpophalangeal extension	First dorsal web space	Distal humeral shaft, anterior shoulder dislocation
Axillary	Deltoid	Lateral shoulder	Anterior shoulder dislocation, proximal humerus fracture

(From American College of Surgeons Committee on Trauma: *Advanced trauma life support,* ed 8, Chicago, 2009, ACS.)

FIGURE 7-6 Peripheral Nerve Assessment of Lower Extremities

Nerve	Motor	Sensation	Injury
Femoral	Knee extension	Anterior knee	Pubic rami fractures
Obturator	Hip adduction	Medial thigh	Obturator ring fractures
Posterior tibial	Toe flexion	Sole of foot	Knee dislocation
Superficial peroneal	Ankle eversion	Lateral dorsum of foot	Fibular neck fracture, knee dislocation
Deep peroneal	Ankle/toe dorsiflexion	Dorsal first to second web space	Fibular neck fracture, compartment syndrome
Sciatic nerve	Plantar dorsiflexion	Foot	Posterior hip dislocation
Superior gluteal	Hip abduction	—	Acetabular fracture
Inferior gluteal	Gluteus maximus hip extension	—	Acetabular fracture

(From American College of Surgeons Committee on Trauma: *Advanced trauma life support,* ed 8, Chicago, 2009, ACS.)

sibly convert a closed fracture to an open fracture. For most situations in the prehospital setting, evaluating gross neurologic functioning is sufficient.

Motor function can be assessed by first asking the patient if any weakness is noted. Motor function in the upper extremity is evaluated by having the patient open and close a fist and by testing grip strength (the patient squeezes the providers fingers). Lower extremity motor function is tested by having the patient wiggle the toes.

Sensory function is evaluated by asking about the presence of any abnormal sensations or numbness and testing to see if the patient feels the provider touching various locations on the extremities, including the fingers and toes. Figures 7-5 and 7-6 provide information on performing more detailed evaluations of motor and sensory function of the extremities.

Repeat evaluation of extremity perfusion and neurologic functioning should be performed after any splinting procedure.

Associated Injuries. While performing the secondary survey, clues to the kinematics may be uncovered and an injury pattern may be suspected. Such injury patterns can prompt the provider to assess for occult injuries associated with specific fractures. An example would be a thoracic injury associated with a shoulder injury. Thorough examination of the entire body will ensure injuries are not missed. Figure 7-7 provides some examples of associated injuries.

Specific Musculoskeletal Injuries

Injuries to the extremities result in two primary problems that require management in the prehospital setting: hemorrhage and instability (fractures and dislocations).

FIGURE 7-7 **Injuries Associated with Musculoskeletal Injuries**

Injury	Missed/Associated Injury
Clavical fracture Scapular fracture Fracture and/or dislocation of shoulder	Major thoracic injury, especially pulmonary contusion and rib fractures
Displaced thoracic spine fracture	Thoracic aorta rupture
Spine fracture	Intraabdominal injury
Fracture/dislocation of elbow	Brachial artery injury Median, ulnare, and radial nerve injury
Major pelvic disruption (motor vehicle occupant)	Abdominal, thoracic, or head injury
Major pelvic disruption (motorcyclist or pedestrian)	Pelvic vascular hemorrhage
Femur fracture	Femoral neck fracture Posterior hip dislocation
Posterior knee dislocation	Femoral fracture Posterior hip dislocation
Knee dislocation or displaced tibial plateau fracture	Popliteal artery and nerve injuries
Calcaneal fracture	Spine injury or fracture Fracture-dislocation of hindfoot Tibial plateau fracture
Open fracture	70% incidence of associated nonskeletal injury

FIGURE 7-8 **Approximate Internal Blood Loss Associated with Fractures**

Bone Fractured	Internal Blood Loss (mL)
Rib	125
Radius or ulna	250–500
Humerus	500–750
Tibia or fibula	500–1000
Femur	1000–2000
Pelvis	1000–massive

experienced individuals tend to overestimate the amount of external hemorrhage, underestimation is also possible because overt signs of external blood loss may not always be apparent. A recent study suggested that prehospital estimates of blood loss were inaccurate and not clinically beneficial.[1] The reasons for these inaccurate blood loss estimates are many and include the fact that the patient may have been moved from the site of injury and that lost blood may have been absorbed by clothing or soil or washed away in water or by rain.

Internal hemorrhage is also common with musculoskeletal trauma. It may result from damage to major blood vessels, from disrupted muscle, and from the bone marrow of fractured bones. Continued swelling of an extremity or a cold, pale, pulseless extremity could indicate internal hemorrhage from major arteries or veins. Significant internal blood loss can be associated with fractures (Figure 7-8). The prehospital care provider considers both the potential internal and the external blood loss associated with extremity trauma. This will help the provider anticipate the development of shock, prepare for the possibility of systemic deterioration, and to intervene appropriately to minimize its occurrence.

Hemorrhage

Bleeding can be dramatic or subtle. Whether it is the capillary ooze of a large abrasion, the dark red blood flowing from a superficial laceration, or the bright red spurting of an open artery, the amount of blood lost and the rate of its loss will determine the patient's ability to compensate or descend into shock. A good rule to remember is, "No bleeding is minor; every red blood cell counts." Even a small trickle of blood can add up to substantial blood loss if it is ignored for a long period.

External arterial bleeding should be identified during the primary survey. Generally, this type of bleeding is easily recognized, but assessment can be difficult when blood is hidden under a patient or in heavy or dark clothing. Ideally, obvious hemorrhage is controlled while the patient's airway and breathing are being managed, if sufficient assistance is present; otherwise, it is controlled when identified during assessment of circulation or when the patient's clothing is removed. Estimation of external blood loss is extremely difficult. Although less

Management

The initial management of external hemorrhage involves the application of direct pressure. Elevation of an extremity has not been shown to slow hemorrhage, and in musculoskeletal trauma it may aggravate injuries that are present. If hemorrhage is not controlled with direct pressure or a pressure dressing, a tourniquet should be applied.

After controlling bleeding in patients with life-threatening hemorrhage from an extremity, prehospital care providers can reassess the primary survey and focus on resuscitation and rapid transport to the facility that can best treat the condition.

Instability (Fractures and Dislocations)

Tears of the supporting structures of a joint, fracture of a bone, and major muscle or tendon injury affect the ability of an extremity to support itself. The two injuries that cause instability of bones or joints are fractures and dislocations.

Fractures

If a bone is broken (fractured), immobilizing it will reduce the potential for further injury and pain. Movement of the sharp ends of the fractured bone may damage blood vessels, resulting in internal and external hemorrhage. Additionally, fractures can damage muscle tissue and nerves.

In general, fractures are classified as either closed or open. In a *closed fracture* the skin is not punctured by the bone ends, whereas in an *open fracture* the integrity of the skin has been interrupted (Figure 7-9, *A*). Physicians may classify fractures by their pattern (e.g., greenstick, comminuted), but these types cannot be differentiated without an x-ray, and knowledge of the fracture pattern really does not alter field management.

Closed fractures are fractures in which the bone has been broken but the patient has no loss of skin integrity (i.e., the skin is not broken or lacerated over the fracture site) (Figure 7-9, *B*). Signs of a closed fracture include tenderness, deformity, hematomas, swelling, and crepitus, although in some patients, tenderness may be the only finding. Pulses, skin color, and motor and sensory function should be assessed below the suspected fracture site. Asking a patient to move the fractured extremity could result in an open fracture. It is not always true that an extremity is not fractured because the patient can voluntarily move it; adrenalin from a traumatic event may motivate patients to do things they normally would not tolerate. Additionally, some patients have a remarkably high pain tolerance.

Open fractures usually occur when a sharp bone end penetrates the skin from the inside or an injury lacerates the skin and muscle down to a fracture site (Figure 7-9, *C*). When a bone punctures the skin, the end can be contaminated with

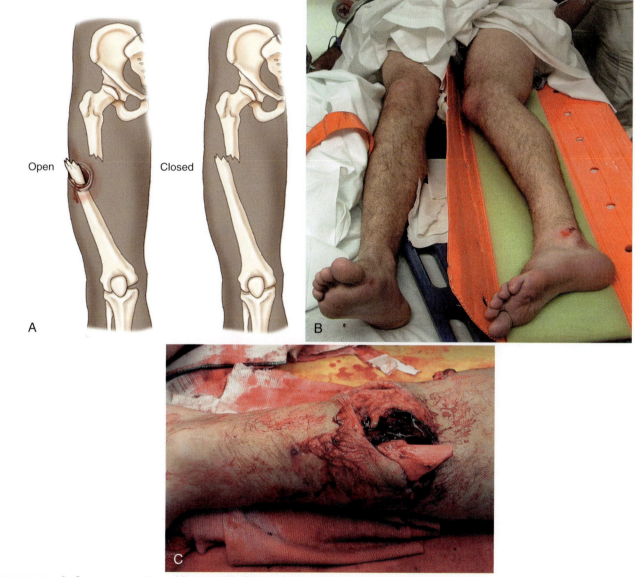

FIGURE 7-9 **A,** Open versus closed fracture. **B,** Closed fracture of the femur. Note the internal rotation and shortening of the left leg. **C,** Open fracture of the tibia.

bacteria from the skin or environment. This can lead to the serious complication of a bone infection *(osteomyelitis)*, which can interfere with healing of the fracture and require months or even years of treatment. Although the skin wound associated with an open fracture often is not associated with significant hemorrhage, persistent bleeding may come from the marrow cavity of the bone or as a hematoma deep inside the tissue decompresses through the skin opening. Any open wound near a possible fracture needs to be considered an open fracture and treated as such. A protruding bone or bone end should generally not be intentionally replaced; however, the bones occasionally return to a near-normal position when they are realigned or by the muscle spasms that usually occur with fractures. Inadequate splinting or rough handling of a fractured extremity may convert a closed fracture into an open one. Open fractures may be easy to locate on a trauma patient. Although bone protruding from a wound is pretty obvious, soft tissue injuries in proximity to a fracture/deformity may have resulted from a bone end that broke through the surface of the skin only to recede back into the tissue.

As noted earlier, fractures may result in significant internal hemorrhage into the tissue planes surrounding the fracture. The two most common fractures associated with the greatest hemorrhage are femur and pelvic fractures. An adult can lose 1000 to 2000 mL of blood per thigh. Thus, internal hemorrhage associated with bilateral femur fractures may be sufficient to result in death from hypovolemic shock.

Pelvic fractures also are a common cause of significant hemorrhage (Figure 7-10). Multiple small arteries and veins are located next to the pelvis and may be torn by bone ends or as the sacroiliac joints fracture or open up. Overaggressive palpation or manipulation of the pelvis (pelvic rock) can sig-nificantly increase blood loss when an unstable pelvic fracture is present. To assess the pelvis, gentle palpation is acceptable but should only be performed once. Gentle manual pressure anterior to posterior and from the sides may identify crepitus or instability. Because of the amount of space in the pelvic cavity, hemorrhage may occur with few external signs of compromise. Open fractures of the pelvis, often resulting when a pedestrian is struck by a car or when an occupant is ejected from a motor vehicle, are particularly deadly. Falls can also result in pelvic fracture, so it is important to consider pelvic fracture with any mechanism that involves energy absorbed by the pelvis or complaints of pain around the pelvis. Often, massive external rather than internal hemorrhage results, and bone ends may lacerate the rectum or vagina, resulting in severe pelvic infection.

Management

Open and Closed Fractures. The first consideration in managing fractures is to control hemorrhage and treat for shock. Direct pressure and pressure dressings will control virtually all external hemorrhage encountered in the field. Open wounds or exposed bone ends should be covered with a sterile dressing moistened with sterile normal saline or water. Internal hemorrhage from a fracture is primarily controlled by immobilization, which has the added benefit of providing pain relief. If the bone ends of an open fracture retract into the wound during splinting, this information must be documented on the patient care record and reported to ED personnel.

An injured extremity should be moved as little as possible, both during the secondary survey and application of a splint. Before splinting, an injured extremity should generally be returned to normal anatomical position, including the use of gentle traction to restore an extremity to its normal length. The two primary contraindications for doing this include either significant pain or resistance to movement experienced during an attempt to normal anatomical position. Traditional teaching was to splint a suspected fracture "in the position found;" however, there is good rationale for restoring normal anatomical position. First, a "reduced fracture," one that is returned to normal anatomical position and alignment, is easier to splint. Second, reducing a fracture may alleviate compression on arteries or nerves and result in improved blood circulation and neurologic functioning. Reduction of fractures also decreases hemorrhage. If the fracture is open and bone is exposed, the bone end should be gently rinsed with sterile water or normal saline to remove obvious contamination before an attempt to restore normal anatomical position. It is not of major concern if the bone ends retract back into the skin during this manipulation, because open fractures require treatment in the operating room regardless. However, the fact that the bone was exposed before reduction is key information that should be passed on during patient report at the receiving facility. No more than two attempts should be made to restore an extremity to normal position, and if unsuccessful, the extremity should be splinted "as is."

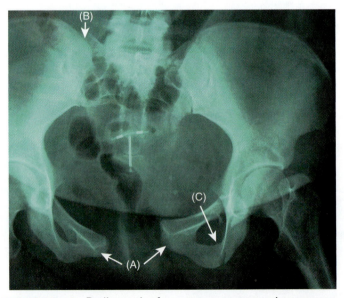

FIGURE 7-10 Radiograph of a severe anteroposterior compression fracture of the pelvis. There is marked widening of the symphysis pubis **(A)**, disruption of the sacroiliac joint **(B)**, and fractures of the pubic rami **(C)**.

The primary objective of splinting is to prevent movement of the body part. This will help decrease the patient's pain and prevent further soft tissue damage and hemorrhage. To immobilize any long bone in an extremity effectively, the entire limb should be immobilized. To do this, the injured site should be supported manually while the joint and bone above (proximal to) and the joint and bone below (distal to) the injury site are immobilized. Numerous types of splints are available, and most can be used with both open and closed fractures (Figure 7-11). With virtually all splinting techniques, further inspection of the extremity is limited, and a thorough assessment should be performed before splinting.

FIGURE 7-11   Types of Splints

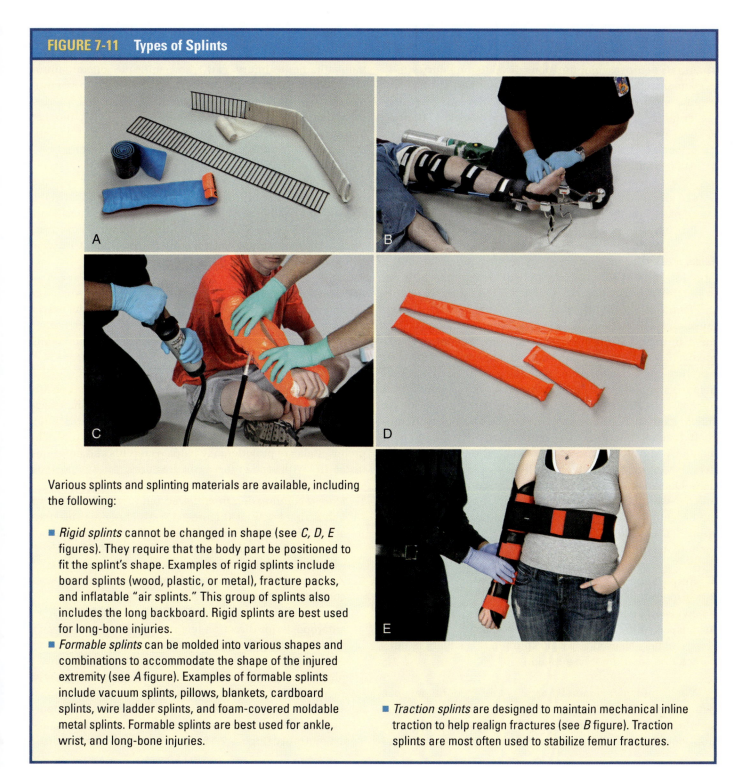

Various splints and splinting materials are available, including the following:

- *Rigid splints* cannot be changed in shape (see *C, D, E* figures). They require that the body part be positioned to fit the splint's shape. Examples of rigid splints include board splints (wood, plastic, or metal), fracture packs, and inflatable "air splints." This group of splints also includes the long backboard. Rigid splints are best used for long-bone injuries.
- *Formable splints* can be molded into various shapes and combinations to accommodate the shape of the injured extremity (see *A* figure). Examples of formable splints include vacuum splints, pillows, blankets, cardboard splints, wire ladder splints, and foam-covered moldable metal splints. Formable splints are best used for ankle, wrist, and long-bone injuries.
- *Traction splints* are designed to maintain mechanical inline traction to help realign fractures (see *B* figure). Traction splints are most often used to stabilize femur fractures.

A, Formable splint. **B,** Traction splint. **C,** Vacuum splint. **D,** Board splint. **E,** Fracpac.
(**B** and **C** from Sanders MJ: *Mosby's paramedic textbook,* ed 3, St Louis, 2006, Mosby.)

Four additional points are important to remember when applying any type of splint:

1. Pad rigid splints to prevent movement of the extremity inside the splint, to help increase the patient's comfort, and to prevent pressure sores.
2. Remove jewelry and watches so that these objects will not inhibit circulation as additional swelling occurs. Lubrication with lotion or a water-soluble jelly may facilitate removal of tight rings.
3. Assess neurovascular functions distal to the injury site before and after applying any splint and periodically thereafter. A pulseless extremity indicates either a vascular injury or a compartment syndrome, and rapid transport to an appropriate facility becomes even more of a priority.
4. After splinting, consider elevating the extremity, if possible, to decrease edema and throbbing. Ice or cold packs can also be used to decrease pain and swelling and may be placed on the splinted extremity near the suspected fracture site.

Femur Fractures. Femur fractures represent a unique splinting situation because of the musculature of the thigh. In addition to providing key structural support for the lower extremity, the femur also provides resistance to the powerful thigh muscles, keeping them out to length. When the femur is fractured in the midshaft area, this resistance to contraction is removed. As these muscles contract, the sharp bone ends tear through muscle tissue, producing additional internal hemorrhage and pain and predisposing the patient to an open fracture. In the absence of life-threatening conditions, a *traction splint* should be applied to stabilize suspected midshaft femoral fractures. The application of traction, both manually and by the use of a mechanical device, will help decrease internal bleeding as well as decrease the patient's pain. One study of prehospital use of traction splints documented that almost 40% of the patients had an injury that either complicated or contraindicated use of a traction splint.[2] Contraindications to the use of a traction splint include the following:

■ Suspected pelvic fracture
■ Suspected femoral neck (hip) fracture
■ Avulsion or amputation of the ankle and foot
■ Suspected fractures adjacent to the knee (A traction splint may be used as a rigid splint in this situation, but traction should not be applied.)

When midshaft femoral fractures are encountered in a patient with additional injuries that are life threatening, time should not be taken to apply a traction splint. Instead, attention should be focused on the critical problems, and the suspect lower extremity fractures will be sufficiently stabilized when the patient is immobilized to a long backboard.

Pelvic Fractures. Pelvic fractures can range from minor, relatively insignificant fractures to complex injuries associated with massive internal and external hemorrhage. Fractures of the pelvic ring are associated with overall mortality of 6%, whereas mortality from open pelvic fractures may exceed 50%. Blood loss accounts for the leading cause of death in patients with pelvic fractures; the remaining deaths are from traumatic brain injury (TBI) and multiple organ failure. Because the pelvis is a strong bone and difficult to fracture, patients with pelvic fractures often have associated injuries, including TBIs (51%), long-bone fractures (48%), thoracic injuries (20%), urethral disruption in men (15%), splenic trauma (10%), and liver and kidney trauma (7% each).

Rami Fractures. Isolated fractures of the inferior or superior rami are generally minor and do not require surgical stabilization. Individuals who fall forcibly on their perineum may fracture all four rami ("straddle" injury). These fractures typically are not associated with significant internal hemorrhage.

Acetabular Fractures. Acetabular fractures occur when the head of the femur is driven into the acetabulum of the pelvis. Surgical intervention is generally needed to optimize normal hip function. These injuries may be associated with significant internal hemorrhage.

Pelvic Ring Fractures. Fractures of the pelvic ring are typically classified into three categories. Life-threatening hemorrhage is probably most common with vertical shear fractures, but it may be associated with each type of pelvic ring fracture. The prehospital care provider may palpate crepitus and note bony instability with each of these ring fractures.

1. *Lateral compression fractures* account for the majority of pelvic ring fractures (Figure 7-12, *A*). These injuries may occur when forces are applied to the lateral aspects of the pelvis (e.g., pedestrian is struck by a car). The volume of the pelvis is decreased in these fractures.
2. *Anteroposterior compression fractures* account for about 15% of pelvic ring fractures (Figure 7-12, *B*). These injuries occur when forces are applied in an anteroposterior direction (e.g., person pinned between a vehicle and wall). These injuries are also known as "open book" pelvic fractures because usually the symphysis is separated and the volume of the pelvis greatly increased.
3. *Vertical shear fractures* account for the smallest proportion of pelvic ring fractures but tend to cause the highest mortality (Figure 7-12, *C*). They occur when a verti-

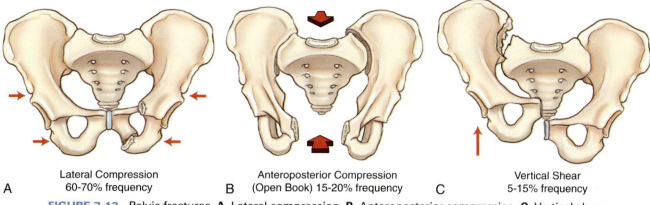

A	B	C
Lateral Compression 60-70% frequency	Anteroposterior Compression (Open Book) 15-20% frequency	Vertical Shear 5-15% frequency

FIGURE 7-12 Pelvic fractures. **A,** Lateral compression. **B,** Anteroposterior compression. **C,** Vertical shear.

cal force is applied to the hemipelvis (e.g., fall from a height, landing on one leg first). Because one half of the pelvis is sheared off the remaining portion, blood vessels are often torn, resulting in severe internal hemorrhage.

Severe pelvic fractures present two challenging problems for prehospital care providers. The greatest concern is internal hemorrhage, which can be very difficult to manage. A second and related concern is that patients with grossly unstable pelvic fractures may be difficult to move, and even turning using a modified logroll procedure can shift bone fragments, causing additional hemorrhage. The best way to move a patient with an unstable fracture identified on palpation may be with a scoop stretcher. If a scoop stretcher is not available, the patient should be turned using a modified logroll procedure only enough to slide a long backboard under the patient. This action should be carried out expeditiously.

Dislocations

Joints are held together by ligaments. The bones are attached to muscles by tendons. Movement of an extremity is accomplished by the contraction (shortening) of muscles. This reduction of muscle length pulls the tendons that are attached to a bone and moves the extremity at a joint. A *dislocation* is a separation of two bones at the joint, resulting from significant disruption to the ligaments that normally provide stability at a joint (Figures 7-13 and 7-14). A dislocation, similar to a fracture, produces an area of instability that the prehospital care provider needs to secure. Dislocations can produce great pain. A dislocation can be difficult to distinguish from a fracture and may be associated with fractures as well (fracture-dislocation). Individuals with prior dislocations have more

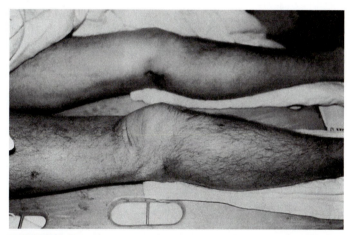

FIGURE 7-13 Right anterior knee dislocation with overriding tibia on the femur.
(From Ferrera PC, Colucciello SA, Marx JA, et al: Trauma management: An emergency medicine approach, St Louis, 2001, Mosby.)

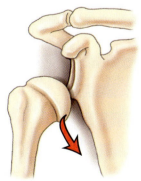

FIGURE 7-14 A dislocation is a separation of a bone from a joint.

lax ligaments and may be prone to more frequent dislocations unless the problem is corrected surgically. Unlike those sustaining a dislocation for the first time, these patients are often familiar with their injury and can help in assessment and stabilization. Deformity of a joint provides a clue to the type of dislocation.

Management. As a general rule, suspected dislocations should be splinted in the position found. Gentle manipulation of the joint can be done to try to restore blood flow when the pulse is absent or weak. When faced with a brief transport time to the hospital, however, the better decision may be to initiate transport rather than attempt manipulation. This manipulation will cause the patient great pain, so the patient should be prepared before moving the extremity. A splint should be used to immobilize the injury. Documentation of how the injury was found and of the presence of pulses, movement, sensation, and color before and after splinting is important. During transport, ice or cold packs can be used to decrease pain and swelling. Analgesia should also be provided to reduce pain.

A position paper from the National Association of EMS Physicians (NAEMSP) recommends reduction of dislocations when transport time is prolonged.[3] The rationale is that joints are more difficult to reduce if they are left in a dislocated position for a prolonged period. Attempted reduction of a dislocation should only be undertaken when permitted by written protocols or online medical control, and when the provider has been properly trained in the appropriate techniques. All attempts at reduction of a dislocation should be properly documented.

Special Considerations

Critical Multisystem Trauma Patient

Adherence to the primary assessment priorities in patients with multisystem trauma that includes injured extremities does not imply that extremity injuries should be ignored or that injured extremities should not be protected from further harm. Rather, it means that when faced with a critically injured trauma patient with extremity injuries that are not bleeding, *life takes precedence over limb.* The focus should be on maintaining vital functions through resuscitation, and only limited measures should be taken to address the extremity injuries, regardless of how dramatic the injuries appear. By properly immobilizing a patient to a long backboard, all extremities are essentially splinted in an anatomic position. A secondary survey need not be completed if the life-threatening problems identified in the primary survey require ongoing interventions and if transport time is short. If a secondary survey is deferred for this reason, the prehospital care provider can simply docu-

ment the findings that precluded performing the secondary survey.

Amputations

When tissue has been totally separated from an extremity, the tissue is completely without nutrition and oxygenation. This type of injury is termed amputation or avulsion. An *amputation* is the loss of part or all of a limb, and an *avulsion* involves the tearing away of soft tissue. Initially, bleeding may be severe with these injuries; later, vessels at the injured site may retract and constrict and clotting may combine to diminish the blood loss. However, subsequent movement may disrupt the blood clot, and bleeding can recur. All amputations may be accompanied by significant bleeding but more so with partial amputations. This is because when vessels are completely transacted, they retract and constrict and blood clots may form decreasing or stopping hemorrhage. On the other hand, when a vessel is only partially transacted, the two ends cannot retract and blood continues to pour out of the hole.

Amputations are often evident on the scene (Figure 7-15). This type of injury receives great attention from bystanders, and the patient may or may not even know that the extremity is missing. Psychologically, the prehospital care provider needs to deal with this injury cautiously. The patient may not be ready to confront the loss of a limb and should be told after being assessed and treated. The missing extremity should be located for possible reattachment. Even if it is not possible to regain complete function of the extremity, the patient may regain partial function. The primary survey should be performed before looking for a missing extremity. The appearance of an amputation may be

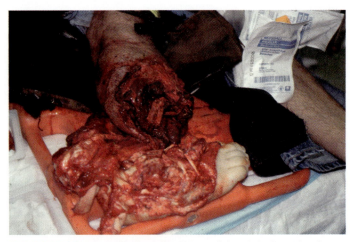

FIGURE 7-15 Complete amputation of the right leg after it became entangled in machinery.

horrifying, but if the patient is not breathing, the loss of the limb is secondary.

Principles of managing an amputated part include the following[4]:

1. Clean the amputated part by gentle rinsing with lactated Ringer's (LR) solution or sterile saline (NS).
2. Wrap the part in sterile gauze moistened with LR or NS solution and place it in a plastic bag or container.
3. After labelling the bag or container, place it in an outer container filled with crushed ice.
4. *Do not* freeze the part by placing it directly on the ice or by adding another coolant such as dry ice.
5. Transport the part along with the patient to the closest appropriate facility.

The longer the amputated portion is without oxygen, the less likely that it can be replaced successfully. Cooling the amputated body part, without freezing it, will reduce the metabolic rate and prolong this critical time. However, replantation is not a guarantee of successful attachment or ultimate function. Because lower extremity prostheses generally allow the patient to resume a near-normal life, lower extremities are rarely considered for replantation. Furthermore, only cleanly separated amputations in otherwise healthy, younger individuals are usually considered for replantation. Smokers are less likely to have successful replantation because the nicotine in tobacco is a potent vasoconstrictor and may compromise blood flow to the replanted segment. Patients who are candidates for replantation of fingers or a hand/forearm should be transported to a level I trauma center because level II and III facilities often lack replantation capability.

Transport of a patient should not be delayed to locate a missing amputated part. If the amputated part is not readily found, law enforcement officials or other responders should remain at the scene to search for it while the patient is being transported. When the amputated part is being transported in a separate vehicle from the patient, the prehospital care provider ensures that the transporters of the amputated part understand clearly where the patient is being transported and how to handle the part once it is located. The receiving facility should be notified as soon as the part is located, and transportation of the part should be initiated as soon as possible.

Crush Syndrome

Crush syndrome, also known as traumatic rhabdomyolysis, is a clinical entity characterized by renal failure and death after severe muscle trauma. Crush syndrome was first described in World War I in German soldiers rescued from collapsed trenches, then again in World War II in patients of the London Blitz. In World War II, crush syndrome had a mortality rate in excess of 90%. During the Korean War, mortality was 84%, but after the advent of hemodialysis, mortality decreased to 53%. In the Vietnam War the mortality rate was approximately the same, at 50%.

The importance of crush syndrome, however, should not be limited to historical or military interest. Approximately 3% to 20% of the survivors of earthquakes have sustained a crush injury, and approximately 40% of survivors from collapsed buildings will have crush injuries.[5,6] In 1978 an earthquake near Beijing, China, injured more than 350,000 persons, with 242,769 deaths. More than 48,000 of these people died from crush syndrome. More commonly, mechanisms of crush syndrome include prolonged entrapment from a trench collapse, construction collapse, or motor vehicle collision.

Crush syndrome arises from a crushing type injury to large muscle masses commonly involving the thigh or calf. Crush syndrome occurs when destruction of muscle releases the molecule known as myoglobin. *Myoglobin* is a protein found in muscle that is responsible for giving meat its characteristic red color. The function of myoglobin in muscle tissue is to serve as an intracellular storage site for oxygen. When myoglobin is released from damaged muscle, however, it is capable of causing damage to the kidneys and acute renal failure (ARF).

Patients with crush syndrome are identified by the following:

- Prolonged entrapment
- Traumatic injury to muscle mass
- Compromised circulation to the injured area

Traumatic injury to the muscle causes release of not only myoglobin but also potassium. Once the patient has been extricated, the affected limb becomes reperfused with new blood, but the old blood, with elevated levels of myoglobin and potassium, is washed out of the injured area and into the rest of the body. Elevated potassium can result in life-threatening cardiac dysrhythmias, and free myoglobin will produce tea- or cola-colored urine and will eventually result in renal failure.

The key to improving outcomes in crush syndrome is early and aggressive fluid resuscitation. It is important for the prehospital care provider to remember that toxins are accumulating within the entrapped limb during the extrication. On freeing the entrapped limb, the accumulated toxins wash into the central circulation, similar to a bolus of poison. Therefore, success will depend on minimizing the toxic effects of accumulated myoglobin and potassium before release of the limb. Resuscitation needs to occur before extrication.[7] Some authors have advocated that final extrication be delayed until the patient has been adequately resuscitated.[8] A delay in fluid resuscitation will result in renal failure in 50% of the patients, and a delay of 12 hours or more produces renal failure in almost 100% of patients.

A poorly resuscitated patient may go into cardiac arrest during extrication because of the sudden release of metabolic acid and potassium into the bloodstream when the compression on the extremity is released.[9] Therefore, providers capable of initiating an intravenous (IV) line and administering IV fluids to the patient should be called to the scene.

Mangled Extremity

A "mangled extremity" refers to a complex injury resulting from high-energy transfer in which significant injury occurs to two or more of the following: (1) skin and muscle, (2) tendons, (3) bone, (4) blood vessels, and (5) nerves (Figure 7-16). Common mechanisms producing mangled extremities include motorcycle crashes, ejection from a motor vehicle crash (MVC), and a pedestrian struck by an automobile. When encountered, patients may be in shock from either external blood loss or hemorrhage from associated injuries, which are common because of the high-energy mechanism. Most mangled extremities involve severe open fractures, and amputation may be necessary in 50% to 75% of patients. Limb salvage is possible in some patients, typically involving six to eight procedures, and success often depends on the experience of the trauma and orthopedic surgeons.

Even with a mangled extremity, the focus is still on the primary survey to rule out or address life-threatening conditions. Hemorrhage control, including the use of a tourniquet, may be required. The mangled extremity should be splinted if the patient's condition allows. These patients are probably best cared for at high-volume, level I trauma centers.

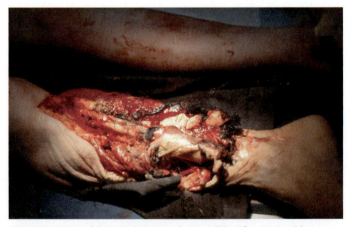

FIGURE 7-16 Mangled extremity resulting from crushing injury between two vehicles. The patient has fractures and extensive soft tissue injury.

Sprains

A *sprain* is an injury in which ligaments are stretched or torn. Sprains are caused by a sudden twisting of the joint beyond its normal range of motion. They are characterized by significant pain, swelling, and possible hematoma. Externally, sprains may resemble a fracture or dislocation. Definitive differentiation between a sprain and a fracture is accomplished only through a radiographic study. In the prehospital setting, it is reasonable to splint a suspected sprain in case it turns out to be a fracture or dislocation. An ice or cold pack may help relieve pain, as well as use of narcotic pain medication.

Strains

A strain is an injury that involves stretching or tearing of muscle tissue. It usually occurs near the point where a muscle in transitioning into a ligament. Like sprains, these injuries cause pain, swelling, and hemorrhage.

Prolonged Transport

Patients with extremity trauma often have coexisting injuries. Ongoing internal blood loss may be from abdominal or thoracic injuries, and during a prolonged transport the primary survey will need to be assessed frequently to ensure that all life-threatening conditions are identified and no new ones have emerged. Vital signs should be obtained at regular intervals.

During long transports, the prehospital care provider needs to focus greater attention on extremity circulation. In limbs with compromised vascular supply, the provider can attempt to restore normal anatomical positioning to optimize the chance for improved blood flow. Similarly, dislocation with impaired distal circulation should be considered for reduction in the field. Distal perfusion, including pulses, color, and temperature, as well as motor and sensory function, should be examined in a serial manner. Measures to ensure patient comfort should be taken. Splinting devices should be comfortable and well padded. The limbs should be assessed for any potential points inside the splint where pressure could contribute to the creation of an ulcer, especially in an extremity with compromised perfusion. Contaminated wounds should be flushed with normal saline (tap water may be used if nothing else is available) so that gross particulate matter (e.g., soil, grass) is removed. If a body part has been amputated, it should also be periodically assessed so that it remains cool but does not freeze or become macerated by soaking in water.

SCENARIO SOLUTION

With your partner's help, you were able to apply a traction splint to the mid-shaft femur fracture of the right leg. After securing your patient to the backboard, you were able to move the patient to the ambulance for transport to the hospital. Once in the ambulance, oxygen via mask was administered. The patient's vital signs remained unchanged throughout the transport. ■

SUMMARY

- In patients with multisystem trauma, attention is directed toward the primary survey and the identification and management of all life-threatening injuries, including internal or external hemorrhage in the extremities.
- Prehospital care providers must be careful not to be distracted from addressing life-threatening conditions by the gross, dramatic appearance of any noncritical injuries or by the patient's request for their management.
- Once the patient has been fully assessed and found to have only isolated injuries without systemic implication, those injuries should be addressed.

- Musculoskeletal injuries, in the order of their threat to life, should be immobilized in order to prevent further injury and provide comfort and some relief from pain.
- When the mechanism of injury indicates sudden, violent changes in motion, multisystem trauma, or spinal trauma, potential systemic decline needs to be anticipated and the patient's age, physical condition, and medical history included in the evaluation.

References

1. Williams B, Boyle M: Estimation of external blood loss by paramedics: Is there any point? *Prehosp Disaster Med* 22(6):502-506, 2007.
2. Wood SP, Vrahas M, Wedel S: Femur fracture immobilization with traction splints in multisystem trauma patients, *Prehosp Emerg Care* 7:241, 2003.
3. Goth P, Garnett G: Clinical guidelines for delayed or prolonged transport: II. Dislocations. Rural Affairs Committee, National Association of Emergency Medical Services Physicians, *Prehosp Disaster Med* 8(1):77, 1993.
4. Seyfer AE: *Guidelines for management of amputated parts*, Chicago, 1996, American College of Surgeons Committee on Trauma.
5. Pepe E, Mosesso VN, Falk JL: Prehospital fluid resuscitation of the patient with major trauma, *Prehosp Emerg Care* 6:81, 2002.
6. Better OS: Management of shock and acute renal failure in casualties suffering from crush syndrome, *Ren Fail* 19:647, 1997.
7. Michaelson M, Taitelman U, Bshouty Z, et al: Crush syndrome: experience from the Lebanon war, 1982, *Isr J Med Sci* 20:305, 1984.
8. Pretto EA, Angus D, Abrams J, et al: An analysis of prehospital mortality in an earthquake, *Prehosp Disaster Med* 9:107, 1994.
9. Collins AJ, Burzstein S: Renal failure in disasters, *Crit Care Clin* 7:421, 1991.

Suggested Reading

Ashkenazi I, Isakovich B, Kluger Y, et al: Prehospital management of earthquake casualties buried under rubble, *Prehosp Disast Med* 20:122, 2005.
American College of Surgeons Committee on Trauma: Musculoskeletal trauma. In *Advanced trauma life support*, ed 8, Chicago, 2009, ACS.
Coppola PT, Coppola M: Emergency department evaluation and treatment of pelvic fractures, *Emerg Med Clin North Am* 18(1):1, 2003.
Gregory RT, Gould RJ, Peclet M, et al: The mangled extremity syndrome: a severity grading system for multisystem injury of the extremity, *J Trauma* 25:1147, 1985.
Howe HR, Poole GV, Hansen KJ, et al: Salvage of lower extremities following combined orthopedic and vascular trauma: a predictive salvage index, *Am Surg* 53:205, 1987.
McSwain NE Jr, Paturas JL, editors: *The basic EMT: comprehensive prehospital patient care*, ed 2, St Louis, 2001, Mosby.
Roessler MS, Wisner DH, Holcroft JW: The mangled extremity: when to amputate? *Arch Surg* 126:1243, 1991.

SPECIFIC SKILLS

Rigid Splinting

Check distal pulses and stabilize the extremity above and below the fracture site before manipulating the extremity

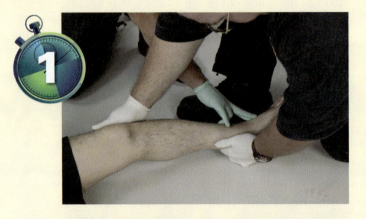

Apply rigid splints on at least 2 sides of the extremity

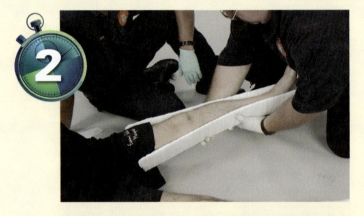

Wrap the splints securely to the extremity wrapping distal to proximal
    Re-check distal pulses after splint is applied.

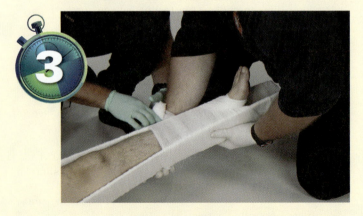

(Chapleau W, Pons P: *Emergency medical technician: making the difference,* ed 2, St Louis, 2007, Mosby.)

Traction Splinting

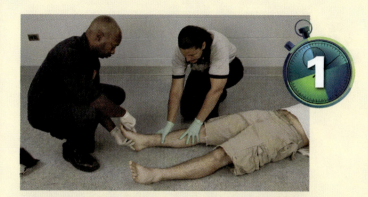

Check distal pulses while supporting the injured extremity

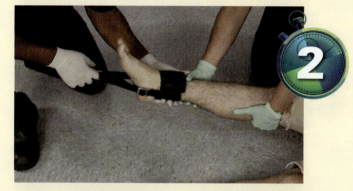

Attach the ankle strap and apply manual traction, check distal pulse after applying traction

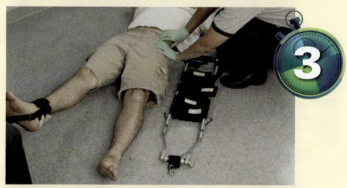

Adjust the traction splint to the proper length using the uninjured extremity as a guide

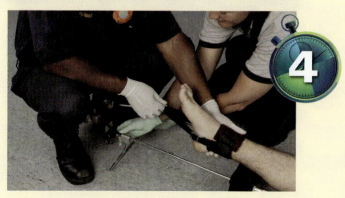

Slide the splint under the injured extremity, fasten the strap at the top of the splint and re-check the distal pulse

SPECIFIC SKILLS

Attach the traction device to the ankle strap and ratchet up the traction until the device takes the traction away from the EMT applying manual traction

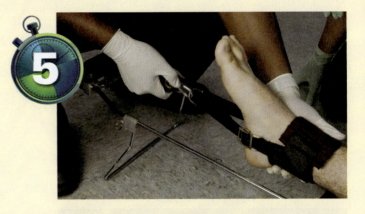

Recheck the pulse after traction is turned over to the device

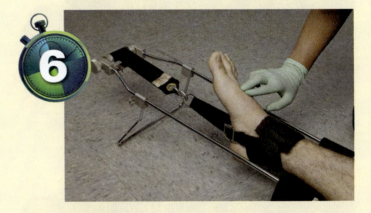

Attach the leg straps to secure the leg in the splint

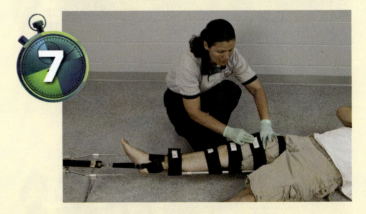

(Chapleau W, Pons P: *Emergency medical technician: making the difference,* ed 2, St Louis, 2007, Mosby.)

Vacuum Splinting

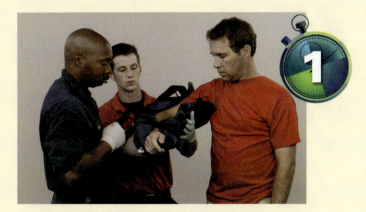

Lay the splint on a flat area. Smooth it out until the plastic beads are evenly distributed. Evacuate some air from the splint so the sides will not collapse when the splint is shaped.

Place the splint underneath the extremity, and bend it in a u-shape around the extremity. Fasten the Velcro fasteners. Then, form each major curve around any bend in the extremity so that the extremity is held completely in place.

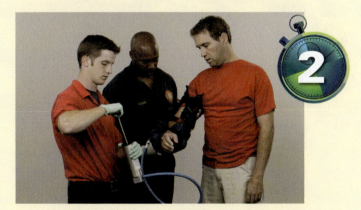

Finally, use the pump to remove the remaining air to leave the splint rigid.

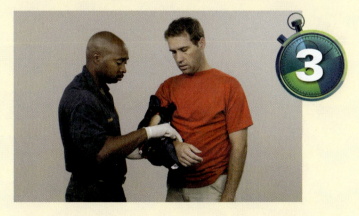

Check distal circulation on the extremity.

(Chapleau W, Pons P: *Emergency medical technician: making the difference,* ed 2, St Louis, 2007, Mosby.)

SPECIFIC SKILLS

Sling and Swathe Application

After checking distal pulse and sensation, apply the sling to the patient

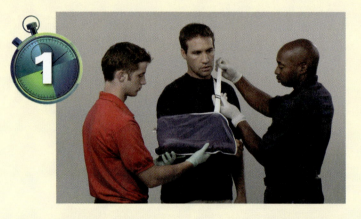

Wrap the upper arm to the chest without restricting breathing

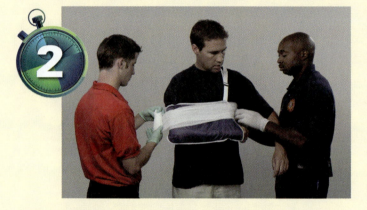

Re-check the distal pulse and sensation after the sling is secured

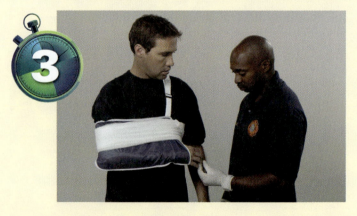

(Chapleau W, Pons P: *Emergency medical technician: making the difference,* ed 2, St Louis, 2007, Mosby.)

CHAPTER 8

Burn Trauma

CHAPTER OBJECTIVES

At the completion of this chapter, the reader will be able to do the following:

- ✓ Define the various depths of burns.
- ✓ Define the zones of burn injuries.
- ✓ Understand how ice can deepen the depth of burns.
- ✓ Estimate burn size using the "rule of nines."
- ✓ Describe initial burn care.
- ✓ Discuss the unique concerns of electrical injuries.
- ✓ Discuss the concerns in patients with circumferential burns.
- ✓ Discuss the three elements of smoke inhalation.
- ✓ Discuss criteria for the transfer of patients to burn centers.

SCENARIO

You are called to a residential structure fire. When your unit arrives, you witness a two-story house that is fully involved with fire and with thick black smoke pouring out of the roof and windows. You are directed to an injured person (Patient 1) who is being cared for by bystanders. They tell you that the patient reentered the burning building in an attempt to rescue his dog, and he was carried out unconscious by firefighters. When you arrive at the side of the patient you find a male who is likely in his thirties. The majority of his clothes have been burned off. He has obvious burns to his face and his hair has been singed. He is unconscious; he is breathing spontaneously but labored. On exam, his airway is patent with assistance, and he ventilates easily. You administer oxygen to the patient with a non–rebreathing mask. The sleeves of his shirt have been burned back. His arms have circumferential burns, but his pulse is easily palpable. His heart rate is 118 beats/minute, blood pressure 148/94 mm Hg, and respirations 22 breaths/minute; the pulse oximeter reading is SaO_2 92%. On examination, you determine that the patient has burns on his entire head, anterior chest, and abdomen and his entire right and left arm and hand. Several feet away is the patient's brother (Patient 2), who is frantic about Patient 1's condition. Patient 2 has burns to his entire right arm and hand from the tips of the finger to his shoulder.

What is the extent of burns for each patient?

What are the initial steps for managing these patients?

How does the trauma first responder recognize an inhalation injury?

Introduction

Many people consider burns to be the most frightening and dreaded of all injuries. In the course of our daily lives, we have all sustained a burn of some degree and have experienced the intense pain and anxiety associated with even a small burn. Burns are common in industrialized and agricultural cultures and in civilian and military settings. Burns can range from small to catastrophic injuries covering large regions of the body. Regardless of size, all burns are serious. Even minor burns can result in serious disability.

A common misconception is that burn injuries are isolated to the skin. On the contrary, large burns are capable of life-threatening effects involving the heart, lungs, kidneys, gastrointestinal (GI) tract, and immune system. The most common cause of death in a fire patient is not from the direct complications of the burn wound but from complications of respiratory failure.

Although considered a form of trauma, burns have some significant differences that merit consideration. After a trauma, such as a motor vehicle crash (MVC) or a fall, the patient's body tries to respond to preserve life. These responses can include the shunting of blood away from less critical body functions, increase in output from the heart (increased pulse), and increase in production of various proteins in the serum that can help protect body tissues. In contrast, after a burn, the patient's body essentially attempts to shut down, go into shock, and die.

Recognition of the cause of burns will prevent the rescuer from entering an unsafe situation and sustaining unnecessary injury, as well as provide optimal care for the patient. Trauma first responders also need to consider the circumstances in which the burn occurred, because a large percentage of burns in both children and adults result from an intentional injury.

Smoke inhalation is a life-threatening injury that is often more dangerous than the burn injury. Inhalation of toxic fumes from smoke is a greater predictor of burn mortality than the age of the patient or the size of the burn.[1] A patient need not inhale a large quantity of smoke to cause severe injury. In addition, life-threatening complications may not become apparent for several days.

Approximately 20% of all burn patients are children, and 20% of these children are the victims of intentional injury or child abuse.[2,3] Most health care providers are surprised to learn that intentional burn injury is second only to beating in the forms of physical violence inflicted on children. Burns as a form of abuse are not limited to children. It is common to see women burned in cases of domestic violence, as well as elderly persons in cases of elder abuse.

Anatomy of Skin

The skin covers about 1.5 to 2.0 square meters (approximately 16 to 22 square feet) in the average adult. It is made up of three layers, the epidermis, the dermis, and the subcutaneous tissues such as fat (Figure 8-1). The outermost layer is the epidermis, which is about 0.05 mm thick in areas such as the eyelids and can be as thick as 1 mm on the sole of the foot.

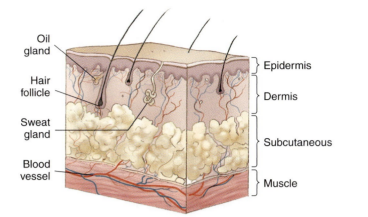

FIGURE 8-1 Normal skin. The skin is composed of three tissue layers—epidermis, dermis, and subcutaneous layer—and associated muscle. Some layers contain structures such as glands, hair follicles, blood vessels, and nerves. All these structures are interrelated to the maintenance, loss, and gain of body temperature.

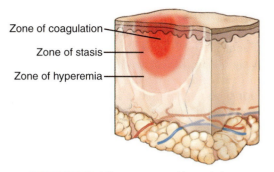

FIGURE 8-2 Three zones of burn injury.

The deeper dermis is on average 10 times thicker than the epidermis.

The skin of males is thicker than the skin of females, and the skin of children and elderly persons is thinner than that of the average adult. These facts explain how an individual can suffer burns of varying depths when exposed to a single burning agent, and how a child might experience a deep burn whereas an adult with the same exposure would have only a superficial injury.

The skin serves several complex functions, including protection from the external environment, prevention of infection, regulation of fluids, temperature control, and sensation.

Burn Characteristics

The creation of a burn is similar to frying an egg. When one breaks an egg into a hot skillet, the egg is initially liquid and transparent. As the egg is exposed to the high temperatures, it rapidly becomes opaque and solidifies. A virtually identical process occurs in human tissue when a patient is burned. In the case of the egg, the proteins of the egg change shape and are destroyed in a process known as denaturation. When a burn occurs to patients, the elevated (or freezing) temperature, radiation, or chemical agent causes the proteins in the skin to be severely damaged, resulting in protein denaturation. Injury to the skin can occur in two phases: immediate and delayed.

Skin is capable of tolerating temperatures of up to 40° C (104° F) for brief periods. However, once temperatures exceed this point, there is a dramatic increase in the magnitude of tissue destruction.[4]

A third-degree (full thickness of the skin) burn has three zones of tissue injury[5] (Figure 8-2). The central zone is known as the zone of coagulation or zone of necrosis, and this is the region of greatest tissue destruction. This tissue in this zone is dead and is not capable of repairing itself.

Next to the zone of necrosis is a region of lesser injury, the zone of stasis. The cells in this zone are injured but not irreversibly. If the tissue in this zone is deprived of its oxygen or blood flow, these cells will die and become necrotic. This area is called the zone of stasis because immediately after injury, the blood flow to this region is stagnant. Timely and appropriate burn care will preserve blood flow and oxygen delivery to these injured cells. Proper care and resuscitation of the patient will eliminate this stasis and reestablish delivery of oxygen to these injured and susceptible cells. A common error that results in damage to this area is the application of ice by a well-meaning bystander or provider. When ice is used to stop the burning process, the ice causes blood vessels to constrict, thus preventing reestablishment of blood flow. The result is a partial-thickness burn that then converts to a full-thickness burn, which is much more difficult to treat. Although the application of ice will improve a patient's pain, the pain relief will be at the expense of additional tissue destruction. For these reasons, ongoing burning should be stopped with the use of room temperature water. The outermost zone is known as the zone of hyperemia. This zone has minimal cellular injury and is characterized by increased blood flow due to the inflammation caused by the burn injury.

Burn Depth

Estimating how deep a burn is can be very difficult to even the most experienced provider. Often, a burn that initially appears to be second degree will prove to be third degree in 24 to 48 hours. The surface of a burn may appear to be a first-degree or second-degree burn at first glance, but later when the superficial epidermis separates off, a white, third-degree burn injury is discovered. Because the burn may change over time, it is often wise to withhold final judgment of burn depth for up to 48 hours after injury. Often it is best simply to tell patients that the injury is either superficial or deep and that time is required to determine ultimate burn depth.

First-Degree Burns

First-degree burns involve only the epidermis and are typically red and painful (Figure 8-3). These injuries are rarely clinically significant, other than the pain they cause, with the exception of large areas of sunburn, where the patient risks dehydration without attention to appropriate oral fluid hydration. These wounds typically heal within a week, and the patient will not scar.

Second-Degree Burns

Second-degree burns, also known as partial-thickness burns, are those that involve the epidermis and varying portions of the underlying dermis (Figure 8-4). Second-degree burns can be further classified as either superficial or deep. Second-degree burns appear as blisters (Figure 8-5) or as burned areas with a glistening or wet appearance because the epidermis has come off. These wounds will be painful. Because remnants of the dermis survive, these burns are often capable of healing in 2 to 3 weeks. In partial-thickness burns the zone of stasis involves the entire epidermis and varying depths of the superficial dermis. If not well cared for, the zone of stasis in these injuries can progress to necrosis, making these burns larger and perhaps converting the wound to a third-degree burn. A superficial second-degree burn will heal with careful wound care. Deep second-degree burns may require surgery.

FIGURE 8-5   Blisters

Much discussion has been generated about blisters, including whether or not to remove them and how to approach the blister associated with partial-thickness burn. A blister occurs when the epidermis separates off the underlying dermis and fluid that is leaking from nearby vessels fills the blister. The presence of osmotically active proteins in the blister fluid draws additional fluid into the blister space, causing the blister to continue to enlarge. As the blister enlarges, it creates pressure on the injured tissue of the wound bed, which increases the patient's pain. Many think that the skin of the blister acts as a dressing and prevents contamination of the wound. However, the skin of the blister is not normal and therefore cannot serve as a protective barrier. Additionally, maintaining the blister intact prevents one from applying topical antibiotics directly on the injury. For these reasons, most burn specialists open and debride blisters after arrival of the patient to the hospital.[6]

Third-Degree Burns

Third-degree burns involve complete damage to the epidermis and dermis and may have several appearances (Figure 8-6). Most often these wounds will appear as thick, dry, white, leathery burns, regardless of race or skin color (Figure 8-7). In severe cases the skin will have a charred appearance (Figure 8-8). This leathery skin is referred to as an eschar. It has often been said that third-degree burns are painless because the nerve endings in the burned tissue have been destroyed. Patients with third-degree burns have pain. Third-degree burns are typically surrounded by areas of partial and superficial thickness burns, which are extremely painful. Burns of this depth can be disabling and life threatening. Prompt surgical excision and intensive rehabilitation at a specialized center is required.

Fourth-Degree Burns

Fourth-degree burns are those that not only burn all layers of the skin but also burn underlying fat, muscles, bone, or internal organs (Figures 8-9 and 8-10).

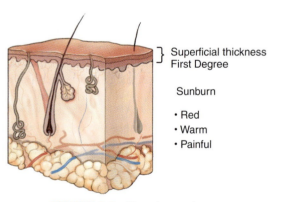

Superficial thickness
First Degree

Sunburn

• Red
• Warm
• Painful

FIGURE 8-3   First-degree burn.

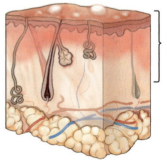

Partial thickness
Second Degree

• Blistering
• Painful
• Glistening wound bed

FIGURE 8-4   Second-degree burn.

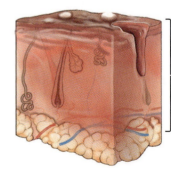

Full thickness
Third Degree

• Leathery
• White to charred
• Dead tissue
• Victims will have pain from burned areas adjacent to the third degree burn.

FIGURE 8-6   Third-degree burn.

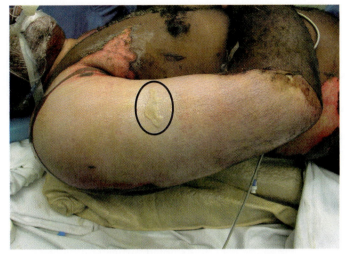

FIGURE 8-7 This patient has suffered a full-thickness burn, characterized as white and leathery in appearance.

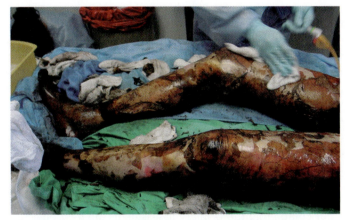

FIGURE 8-8 Example of deep full-thickness burn with charring of the skin and visible thrombosis of blood vessels.

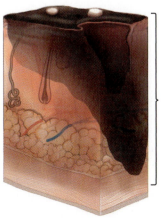

Fourth Degree

FIGURE 8-9 Fourth-degree burn.

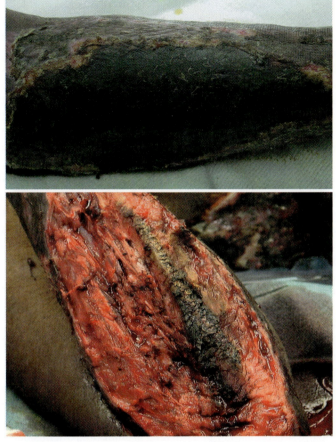

FIGURE 8-10 Fourth-degree burns to the arm, with burns not only to the skin but also to the subcutaneous fat, muscle, and bone.

Assessment and Management

Primary Survey and Resuscitation

The goal of the primary assessment is to systematically evaluate and treat life-threatening disorders in order of importance to preserve life. The ABCDE method of trauma care applies to the management of the burn patient. Although major burns are often an ultimately lethal injury, burns by themselves are not typically an immediately life-threatening problem unless there is burn-related impairment of airway or breathing. The overall appearance of the burns can be dramatic and even grotesque. However, the knowledgeable trauma first responder will be mindful that the patient may also have suffered from a mechanical trauma and have less apparent internal injuries that are more rapidly lethal.

Airway

Preservation of an open airway is the highest priority in caring for a burn patient. The heat from the fire can cause swelling of the airway and block the opening. Therefore, careful initial, as well as continuous, evaluation is required. It is a mistake to believe that once the ABC assessment is completed that all is well with the airway. For example, a burned patient might well have an open airway on the first airway evaluation. In the time that follows, the face as well as the airway will likely swell. As a result, an airway that was satisfactory initially may become critically narrowed 30 or 60 minutes later. The airway can narrow to the degree that the airway becomes completely obstructed and air cannot pass down into the trachea and lungs. To avoid catastrophic airway narrowing or blockage, early involvement of advanced providers who can control the airway if necessary is prudent. Often, patients are the individuals best suited to manage their own airway by assuming a position that maintains an open airway and allows for comfortable respiration. In those instances where intervention is required, the airway should be managed by the most experienced personnel available.

Breathing

As with any trauma patient, breathing can be adversely affected by such problems as fractured ribs, pneumothoraces, and open chest wounds. In the event of circumferential chest wall burns, the burned skin will start to harden and contract while the deeper soft tissues will simultaneously swell. The net result is that the burns constrict the chest wall similarly to having several leather belts tighten around the patient's chest wall. At time progresses, the patient cannot move the chest wall to breath.

Circulation

Evaluation and management of circulation includes looking for other injuries that can produce blood loss, the measurement of blood pressure, and evaluation of circumferential burns. Accurate measurement of blood pressure may be difficult or impossible with burns to the extremities. Even if a blood pressure can be obtained, in some cases it may not correctly reflect systemic arterial blood pressure because of the effect of full-thickness burns and swelling of the extremities. Even if the patient has adequate arterial blood pressure, blood flow into an extremity may be critically reduced because of swelling associated with circumferential injuries. Burned extremities should be elevated to help reduce the degree of swelling in the affected limb.

Disability

Burn patients are trauma patients and may have sustained injuries in addition to the thermal injuries. Burns are obvious and sometimes intimidating injuries, but it is vital to assess for other, less obvious internal injuries that may be more immediately life threatening than the burn injuries. In an effort to escape being burned, patients will leap from the windows of buildings; elements of the burning structure may collapse and fall on the patient; or the patient may be trapped in the burning wreckage of an MVC. Evaluate the patient for neurologic and movement deficits. Identify and splint fractures of long bones. Perform spinal immobilization if a potential spine injury is suspected. A source of life-threatening neurologic disability that is unique to burn patients (and potentially rescuers and trauma first responders) is the effect of inhaled toxins such as carbon monoxide and hydrogen cyanide gas.

Exposure/Environment

The next priority is to expose the patient completely so that every square inch of the patient can be inspected. All clothing and jewelry should be promptly removed. In a patient with mechanical trauma, all of the patient's clothes are removed in order to identify injuries that might be concealed by the clothing. In a burn patient, removal of the clothing can potentially have a therapeutic benefit. As noted earlier, clothing and jewelry can retain residual heat that may continue to burn the patient. In addition, jewelry can be constricting and lead to impaired circulation as burned areas begin to swell. After chemical burns, the patient's clothing may be soaked with the potentially hazardous material that burned the patient, and improper handling of the clothing can result in injury to both the patient and responders.

Controlling the environmental temperature is critical when caring for patients with large burns. Burn patients are not able to retain their own body heat and are extremely susceptible to hypothermia. Make every effort to keep the patient warm and to preserve body temperature. Apply several layers of blankets. As a general rule, if you as a trauma responder are comfortable, then the ambient temperature is not warm enough for the patient.

Secondary Survey

After completing the primary assessment, the next objective is completion of the secondary assessment. The secondary assessment of a burn patient is no different than that in any other trauma patient. The provider should complete a head-to-toe evaluation, attempting to identify additional injuries or medical conditions.

Burn Size Estimation (Assessment)

Estimation of burn size is necessary to determine the severity of the injury, the best place to treat the patient, and, when indicated, the need to resuscitate the patient and prevent complications associated with fluid loss and shock from the burn injury. The most widely applied method is known as the "rule of nines." This method applies the principle that major regions of the body in adults are considered to be 9% of the total body surface area (Figure 8-11). The perineum or genital area represents 1%.

Children have different proportions than adults. Children's heads are proportionally larger than adults, and their legs are shorter in proportion than adults. Because these proportions vary with differing age groups, it is not appropriate to apply the rule of nines to pediatric patients.

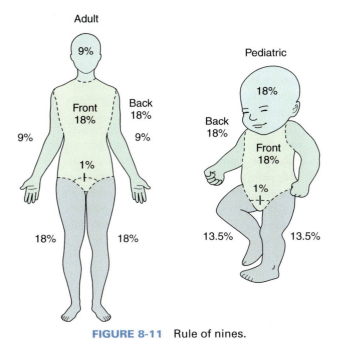

FIGURE 8-11   Rule of nines.

The Lund-Browder chart is a diagram that takes into account age-related changes in children. Using these charts, a provider first maps the burn and then determines burn size based on an accompanying reference table (Figure 8-12).

The complexity of this method makes it difficult to use in a prehospital situation.

Dressings

Before transport of a patient, the burn wounds should be dressed. The goal of the dressings is to prevent ongoing contamination and prevent airflow over the wounds, which will help with pain control.

Dressings in the form of a sterile sheet or towel are sufficient. Several layers of blankets are then placed over the sterile burn sheets to help keep the patient warm. Topical antibiotics and other burn ointments should not be applied until the patient has been evaluated by the burn center.

Transportation

Patients who have multiple injuries in addition to their burns should first be transported to a trauma center, where immediately life-threatening injuries can be identified and surgically treated, if necessary. Once stabilized at a trauma center, the patient with burns should be transported to a burn center for definitive burn care and rehabilitation. The American Burn Association and the American College of Surgeons have identified criteria for transport or transfer of burn patients to a burn center, as outlined in Figure 8-13. In those geographic areas without easy access to a burn center, local medical direction will determine the preferred choice of destination for such cases.

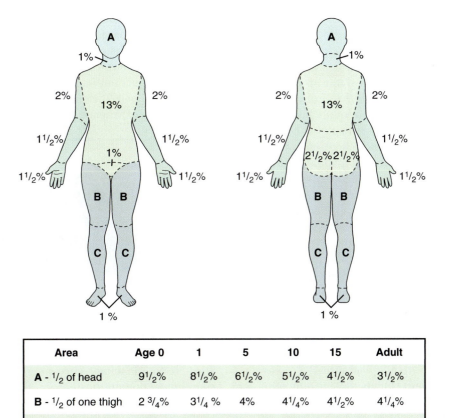

Area	Age 0	1	5	10	15	Adult
A - 1/2 of head	9 1/2 %	8 1/2 %	6 1/2 %	5 1/2 %	4 1/2 %	3 1/2 %
B - 1/2 of one thigh	2 3/4 %	3 1/4 %	4%	4 1/4 %	4 1/2 %	4 1/4 %
C - 1/2 of one leg	2 1/2 %	2 1/2 %	2 3/4 %	3%	3 1/4 %	3 1/2 %

FIGURE 8-12   Lund-Browder chart.

FIGURE 8-13   Injuries Requiring Burn Unit Care

Patients with serious burns should receive care at centers that have special expertise and resources. Initial transport or early transfer to a burn unit should result in a lower mortality rate and fewer complications. A burn unit may treat adults, children, or both. The Committee on Trauma of the American College of Surgeons recommends referral to a burn unit for patients with burn injuries who meet the following criteria:

1. Inhalation injury.
2. Partial- or full-thickness burns over greater than 10% of the total body surface area (TBSA) in patients under the age of 10 years or over the age of 50 years.
3. Partial- or full-thickness burns over greater than 20% BSA in patients age 10 to 50 years.
4. Full-thickness (third-degree) burns greater than 5% BSA in any age group.

5. Burns that involve the face, hands, feet, genitalia, perineum, or major joints.
6. Electrical burns, including lightning injury.
7. Significant chemical burns.
8. Burn injury in patients with preexisting medical disorders that could complicate management, prolong recovery, or affect mortality.
9. Any patients with burns and concomitant trauma (e.g., fractures) in which the burn injury poses the greatest risk of morbidity or mortality; if trauma poses the greater immediate risk, the patient may be initially stabilized in a trauma center before transfer to a burn unit.
10. Burned children in hospitals without qualified personnel or equipment for the care of children.
11. Burn injury in patients who will require special social, emotional, or long-term rehabilitative intervention.

(From the American College of Surgeons Committee on Trauma: *Advanced Trauma Life Support for Doctors,* 8th ed, Chicago, 2008.

Management

Initial Burn Care

The initial step in the care of a burn patient is to stop the burning process. The most effective and appropriate method of stopping the burning is cooling with large amounts of room temperature water. Use of cold water or ice is contra-indicated. As previously mentioned, the application of ice will stop the burning and provide pain relief, but it also will increase the extent of tissue damage in the zone of stasis. Remove all clothing and jewelry; these items maintain resid-ual heat and will continue to burn the patient. In addition, jewelry may constrict digits or extremities as the tissues begin to swell.

Effective dressing of the burn is the application of sterile, nonadherent dressings. Cover the area with a clean sheet. If a sheet is not readily available, substitute a sterile surgical gown, drapes, or towels. The dressing will prevent ongoing environmental contamination while helping to prevent the patient from experiencing pain from air flowing over the exposed nerve endings (Figure 8-14).

Prehospital providers have often been unsatisfied and frustrated with the simple application of sterile sheets to a burn. However, topical ointments and conventional topical antibiotics should not be applied because they prevent a direct inspection of the burn. Such topical ointments and antibiotics will be removed on admission to the burn center to allow direct visualization of the burn and determination of burn severity. Unfortunately, the removal of ointments applied in the field will increase pain and discomfort the patient is

FIGURE 8-14   Prevent Airflow over Patient's Burn

Most of us have experienced the pain associated with a dental cavity. The pain is intensified when we inhale air over the exposed nerve. With a partial-thickness burn, thousands of the nerves are exposed, and the air currents in the environment produce pain in the patient when the currents come into contact with the exposed nerves of the wound bed. Therefore, by keeping burns covered, the patient will experience less pain.

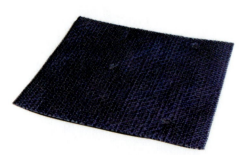

FIGURE 8-15   Acticoat dressing.
(Courtesy Smith & Nephew Wound Management.)

already experiencing. Also, some topical medications may complicate the application of tissue-engineered products used to aid wound healing.

High-concentration antimicrobial-coated dressings (e.g., Silverlon or Acticoat) have become the mainstay of wound care in burn centers (Figure 8-15). These dressings are coated with silver, which is time-released over several days when applied to an open burn wound. The released silver provides rapid antimicrobial coverage of the common bacteria contaminating and infecting wounds. Recently, these dressings have been adapted from burn center use to prehospital applications. These large antimicrobial sheets can be rapidly applied to the burn and can help to eradicate any contaminating organisms. This method of wound care allows prehospital providers to apply a nonpharmaceutical device that greatly reduces burn wound contamination within 30 minutes after application.[7–9]

Fluid Resuscitation

Administration of large amounts of intravenous (IV) fluids is needed over the course of the first day after the burn to prevent a burn patient from going into shock. After a burn, the patient loses a substantial amount of fluid in the form of swelling of the entire body, as well as evaporation of fluid at the site of the burn.

Intravenous access and fluid administration will be performed by advanced level providers and should be considered for those situations involving long transport time to the hospital. In urban settings with short transport times, the need for obtaining IV access is based not on the burn but rather as other conditions warrant.

Special Considerations

Electrical Burns

Electrical injuries are devastating injuries that are easy to underappreciate. In many cases the extent of externally visible tissue damage does not accurately reflect the magnitude of the injury. Tissue destruction is greater than the apparent trauma because most of the destruction occurs internally as the electricity is conducted through the patient. The patient will have external burns at the points of contact with the electrical source as well as grounding points. As the electricity courses through the patient's body, deep layers of tissue are destroyed despite seemingly minor injuries on the surface (Figure 8-16).

Electrical injuries may cause massive destruction of muscles, which results in the release of both potassium and myoglobin. The release of muscle potassium causes a significant increase in the serum level, which can result in abnormal cardiac rhythms. Myoglobin is a molecule found in the muscle that assists the muscle tissue use oxygen. When released into the bloodstream in large amounts, myoglobin is toxic to the kidneys and can cause kidney failure. This condition, myoglobinuria, is evidenced by tea- or cola-colored urine (Figure 8-17).

The electrical burn patient may have associated injuries as well. Approximately 15% of patients with electrical injuries will also have traumatic injuries. This is a rate that is

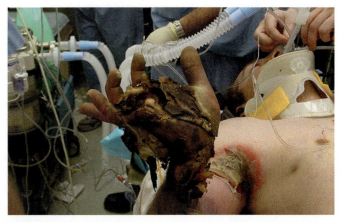

FIGURE 8-16 Patient after electrical injury from high-tension wires.

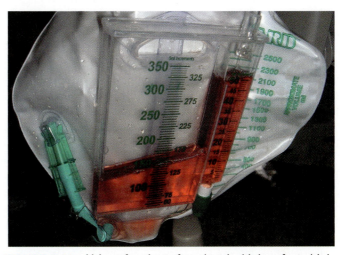

FIGURE 8-17 Urine of patient after electrical injury from high-tension wires. The patient has myoglobinuria after extensive muscle destruction.

twice that seen in patients burned by other mechanisms.[10] The patient's eardrum may rupture, resulting in hearing difficulties. Intense and sustained muscle contraction (tetany) can result in compression fractures of the spine and long bones. Patients with electrical injury should have their spine immobilized. Long-bone fractures should be splinted when detected or suspected. Intracranial bleeds may also occur.

It is important to remember that before approaching a person who has sustained electrical burns, the responder must ensure that the patient is no longer in contact with the source of the electricity. Failing to do so could lead to injury to the responder and yet another patient to be cared for.

Circumferential Burns

Circumferential burns of the trunk or limbs are capable of producing a life- or limb-threatening condition. Circumferential burns create a tourniquet-like effect that can prevent blood flow into an arm or leg and make it pulseless. Circumferential burns of the chest can constrict the chest wall to such a degree that the patient suffocates from the inability to take a breath. Therefore, all circumferential burns should be handled as an emergency and patients transported to a burn center or to the local trauma center if a burn center is not available.

Smoke Inhalation Injuries

The leading cause of death in fires is not burn injury but the inhalation of toxic smoke. Any patient with a history of exposure to smoke in an enclosed space should be considered at risk of having an inhalation injury. Any patient with burns to the face or soot in their sputum is at risk for a smoke inhalation injury; however, the absence of these signs does not exclude the diagnosis of a toxic inhalation. Maintaining a high index of suspicion is vitally important because signs and symptoms of smoke inhalation may not become apparent for several days after the exposure.

There are three components to smoke inhalation: thermal injury, asphyxiation, and delayed toxin-induced lung injury (Figure 8-18). Dry air is a poor conductor of heat; the inhalation of heated air associated with a structure fire rarely causes thermal injury to the airways below the level of the voicebox. The large surface area of the nose and upper pharynx effectively cools the inhaled, heated air to about body temperature by the time the air reaches the level of the vocal cords. When heated dry air at 300° C (572° F) is inhaled, the air is cooled to 50° C (122° F) by the time it is at the level of the trachea.[11] The vocal cords provide additional protection by reflexively closing.[12] The exception to this is the inhalation of steam. Steam has 4000 times the heat-carrying capacity of dry air and is capable of burning the lower airways and bronchioles.[11]

Asphyxiants

Two gaseous products that are clinically important as asphyxiants are carbon monoxide (CO) and cyanide gas (CN). Both of molecules are classified as asphyxiants and thus cause cell death by preventing cells from receiving or using oxygen. Patients with asphyxia from smoke containing one or both of these compounds will have inadequate delivery of oxygen to the tissues of the body. Symptoms of CO inhalation depend on the duration and amount of CO. Symptoms can range from headache to coma and death.

Treatment of CO toxicity is removal of the patient from the source and administration of supplemental oxygen. When breathing room air (21% oxygen), the body will eliminate half of the CO in 250 minutes.[13] When the patient is placed on 100% oxygen, the half-life of the CO-hemoglobin complex is reduced to 40 to 60 minutes.[14]

Cyanide gas is produced from the burning of plastics or polyurethane. Cyanide poisons cellular machinery, preventing the body's cells from using oxygen. The patient can die from asphyxia despite having adequate oxygen in the blood. Symptoms of cyanide toxicity include altered level of con-

---

FIGURE 8-18   Signs and Symptoms of Smoke Inhalation

- Burn in a confined space
- Confusion or agitation
- Burns to face or chest
- Singing of eyebrows or nasal hair
- Soot in the sputum
- Hoarseness, loss of voice, or stridor

---

sciousness, dizziness, headache, and tachycardia or tachypnea. Patients with carbon monoxide toxicity from a structure fire should also be considered to be at risk for CN poisoning. The treatment of cyanide poisoning has traditionally been rapid transport to an emergency center capable of providing the patient with the antidote therapy. However, a commercially available antidote kit widely used in Europe for many years and recently available in the United States allows for field treatment of CN toxicity by advanced level providers.

Toxin-Induced Lung Injury

The thermal and asphyxiant components of an inhalation injury are usually apparent at the time of the rescue. In contrast, the signs and symptoms of toxin-induced lung injury typically do not manifest for several days. The first several days after a smoke inhalation injury are often described as the "honeymoon period." During this period the patient may appear deceptively stable with little or no lung dysfunction. The severity of this lung injury is largely dependent on two factors: the components of the smoke and the duration of exposure.[15]

In simplified terms, smoke is the product of incomplete combustion—that is, chemical dust. The chemicals in the smoke react with the lining of the trachea and lungs and damage the cells lining the airways and lungs.[15–17] Compounds such as ammonia, hydrogen chloride, and sulfur dioxide form corrosive acids and alkalis when inhaled.[18] These poisons cause death of the cells lining the trachea and bronchioles.

Prehospital Management

The initial element of caring for a patient with smoke exposure is to remove the patient from any ongoing exposure to the smoke and that the airway is open. Giving the patient supplemental oxygen will assist in removing carbon monoxide. Continuous reevaluation of the airway is required. Any change in the character of the voice, difficulty handling secretions, or drooling indicates swelling of the airway and impending obstruction.

Patients with smoke inhalation should be transported to burn centers even in the absence of surface burns. Burn centers treat a greater volume of patients with smoke inhalation and offer unique modes of mechanical ventilation.

Child Abuse

Approximately 20% of all child abuse is the result of intentional burning. The majority of the children intentionally burned are 1 to 3 years of age.[19]

The most common form of burn child abuse is forcible immersion. These injuries typically occur when an adult places a child in hot water, often as a punishment related to toilet training. Factors that determine the severity of injury include age of the patient, temperature of the water, and duration of exposure. The child may sustain deep second- or third-degree burns of the hands or feet in a glovelike or stockinglike pattern. This is especially suspicious when the burns are symmetric and lack splash patterns[20] (Figures 8-19 and 8-20). In cases of intentional scalding, the child will tightly flex the arms and legs into a defensive posture because of fear or pain. The resultant burn pattern will spare the flexion creases of the knee, the elbow, and the groin. Sharp lines of demarcation will also be seen between burned and unburned tissue, essentially indicating a dip into hot water[21,22] (Figure 8-21).

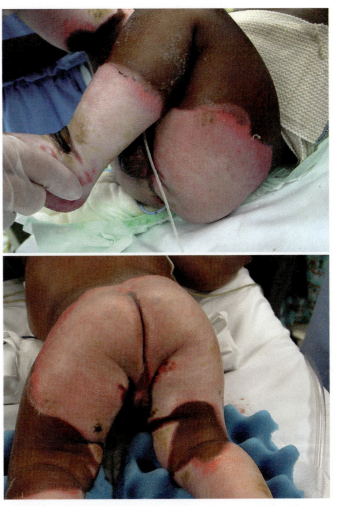

FIGURE 8-20   The straight lines of the burn pattern and absence of splash marks indicate that this burn is the result of abuse.

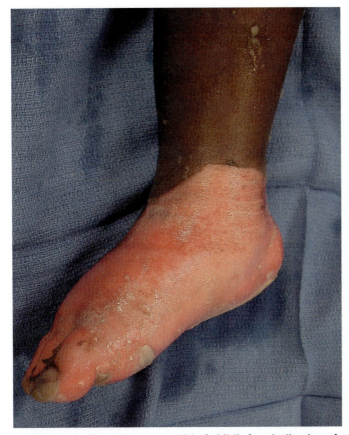

FIGURE 8-19   Stocking-type scald of child's foot indicative of intentional immersion burn injury consistent with child abuse.

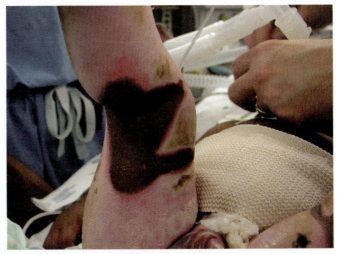

FIGURE 8-21   The sparing of the areas of flexion and the sharp lines of demarcation between burned and unburned skin indicate that this child was in a tightly flexed, defensive position before injury. Such a posture indicates that the scald is not accidental.

In accidental scald injuries, the burns will have variable burn depth, irregular margins, and smaller burns remote from the large burns, indicating splash.[23]

Contact Burns

Contact burns are the second most common mechanism of burn injury in children, whether accidental or intentional. All body surfaces have some degree of curvature. When an accidental contact burn occurs, the burning agent makes contact with the curved body surface area. The burning instrument is deflected off the curved surface, or the victim of the burn withdraws from the hot object. The resultant injury has an irregular burn edge and depth. When a child receives an intentional contact burn, the hot implement is pressed onto the child's skin. The resultant injury has sharp lines of demarcation between burned and unburned tissue and uniform depth.[22]

Many jurisdictions require health care providers to report such cases of suspected child abuse.

Chemical Burns

Injuries from chemicals are the result of exposure to the offending agent. The severity of chemical injury is determined by four factors: nature of the chemical, concentration of the chemical, duration of contact, and mechanism of action of the chemical.

Chemical agents are classified as acid, base (alkali), organic, or inorganic. Acids are chemicals with a pH between 7 (neutral) and 0 (strong acid). Bases are agents with a pH between 7 and 14. Acids and bases injure human tissue by two different mechanism of action. Acids damage tissue by a process called coagulative necrosis; the acid causes proteins to coagulate and the damaged tissue transforms into a barrier that prevents deeper penetration of the acid. In contrast, alkali burns destroy the tissue by liquefaction necrosis; the basic chemical liquefies the tissue, which allows the chemical to penetrate more deeply and cause increasingly deeper damage.

Treatment

The greatest priority in the care of a chemically exposed patient, as in any emergency, is personal and scene safety. Always protect yourself first. If there is any question of a chemical hazard, ensure scene safety and determine if any special garments or breathing apparatus are required. Avoid contamination of your equipment and emergency vehicles; a contaminated vehicle creates a risk of exposure to other, unsuspecting individuals wherever that vehicle travels. Attempt to identify the offending agent as soon as possible.

Remove all clothing from the patient. Clothing will be contaminated with either liquid or powder chemical. The contaminated clothing needs to be discarded with care so as not to pose a hazard to anyone who might inadvertently come into contact with the clothes. If any powder or particulate substance is on the skin, it should be brushed away. Next, wash or shower the patient with copious amounts of water. Water will dilute the chemical and wash away any that has not reacted with exposed skin. The key is to use large amounts of the water. A common error is to rinse 1 or 2 L of water across the patient, then stop the process once the water starts to pool and accumulate on the floor. When washed with only small amounts of fluid, the offending agent is only spread across the patient's body and not flushed away.[24,25] Failure to provide adequate runoff and drainage of lavage (irrigation) fluid may cause injury to previously unexposed and uninjured areas of the body as the contaminated fluid accumulates. One simple way of promoting runoff in the prehospital setting is to place the patient on a backboard and then tilt it with cribbing or other means to elevate an end. At the lower end of the board, tuck a large plastic garbage bag to contain the contaminated runoff.

Attempting to neutralize a chemical should never be done. Often in the neutralizing process, the reaction of the neutralizing agent and the original chemical will give off heat. Therefore, a well-meaning responder may create a thermal burn in addition to the chemical burn. Most commercially available decontamination solutions are made for the purpose of decontaminating equipment, not people.

The trauma first responder may need to treat injuries to the eye caused by exposure to chemicals, especially alkali (bases). A small exposure to the eye can result in a vision-threatening injury. The eyes should be washed out with large amounts of fluid.

Specific Chemical Exposures

Cement is an alkali that may be retained on the clothing or footwear of individuals. The powdered cement will react with the patient's sweat in a reaction that gives off heat and dries out (desiccates) the skin. These injuries typically present with a burn injury hours or the day after contact with the cement.

Fuels such as gasoline and kerosene can cause contact burns after prolonged exposure. These organic hydrocarbons can dissolve cell membranes, resulting in skin necrosis.[26] An exposure of sufficient duration or severity also may result in systemic toxicity. Decontamination of the patient covered with fuel is accomplished by irrigation with large volumes of water.

Hydrofluoric acid is a dangerous substance widely used in domestic, industrial, and military settings. The real danger of this chemical is the fluoride ion, which produces profound alterations in the chemical makeup of the patient's blood serum.[27] Left untreated, hydrofluoric acid will liquefy tissues and draw the calcium out of bones. Initial treatment for hydrofluoric acid exposure is irrigation with water. Patients with hydrofluoric acid burns should be promptly transferred to a burn center for additional treatment.

Sulfur and nitrogen mustards are compounds that are classified as vesicants. These agents have been used as chemical weapons and are recognized as a threat in chemical terrorism. These chemicals will burn and blister skin on exposure. These agents not only are irritants to the skin but also cause irritation to the lungs and the eyes. After exposure, patients will complain of a burning sensation of the throat and eyes. The skin involvement develops several hours later as redness is followed by blistering in the exposed or contaminated areas. After intense exposure, the patients will develop full-thickness burns and respiratory failure.[28–30] The principal treatment required from the prehospital care provider is decontamination. In caring for patients with vesicant exposure, providers must wear appropriate gloves, garments, and breathing equipment. The patients must be decontaminated and showered with water or saline. Additional specialized treatment is required when the patient arrives at a specialty center.

Tear gas and similar chemicals are known as "riot control agents." These agents will rapidly and briefly disable those exposed by causing irritation to the skin, lungs, and eyes. The extent of the injury is determined by the magnitude of exposure to the agent. The duration of the irritation typically is 30 to 60 minutes. Treatment consists of removing those exposed from the source of the exposure, removing contaminated clothing, and washing the skin and eyes.

SUMMARY

- All burns are serious, regardless of their size.
- Potentially life-threatening burns include large thermal burns, electrical injuries, and chemical burns.
- Unlike in mechanical trauma (e.g., penetrating, blunt), the body has little to no adaptive mechanisms to survive a burn injury.
- Burn injuries are not isolated to the skin; these involve the entire body. Patients with major burn injury will have dysfunction of the cardiovascular, pulmonary, GI, renal, and immune systems.
- Dramatic burns may focus the prehospital provider's attention away from other, potentially life-threatening injuries. Performing primary and secondary assessments will reduce the likelihood of missing these injuries.

- Constant vigilance is required to avoid becoming a victim oneself. Often the injuring agent still poses a risk for injuring the providers.
- Even small burns in areas of high function (hands, face, joints, perineum) may result in long-term impairment from scar formation.
- The leading cause of death in burn patients is complications from smoke inhalation: asphyxiation, thermal injury, and delayed toxic-induced lung injury. Often, patients do not develop symptoms of respiratory failure for 48 hours or longer. Even without burns to the skin, patients suffering from smoke inhalation should be transported to burn centers.

SCENARIO SOLUTION

Patient 1: This patient has sustained critical injuries. Given that the patient was found collapsed in a burned building with burns to the face and labored respirations, you must be concerned that the patient has inhaled a large amount of smoke. You need to be sure that the burning process has been stopped, so clothing should be removed and the patient covered with clean sheets.

Evaluate and reevaluate for airway swelling and an inhalation injury. Keeping an open airway needs to be a concern; however, the patient currently is managing his own airway. The patient clearly needs 100% oxygen given the exposure to smoke and concerns about asphyxiants.

Patient 2: This patient is at risk for smoke inhalation based on the historical information provided. He has serious burns to his arm and hand. The patient is spontaneously managing his airway and breathing without any problems. The burns of the entire arm and hand comprise 9% of the total body surface area. You cool the burns with ambient temperature water and then cover the burn with sterile towels. The circumferential nature of these burns makes this a potentially limb-threatening injury that will require hospital evaluation. ■

References

1. Tredget EE, Shankowsky HA, Taerum TV, et al: The role of inhalation injury in burn trauma: a Canadian experience, *Ann Surg* 212:720, 1990.

2. Herndon D, Rutan R, Rutan T: Management of the pediatric patient with burns, *J Burn Care Rehabil* 14(1):3, 1993.

3. Rossignal A, Locke J, Burke J: Pediatric burn injuries in New England, USA, *Burns* 16(1):41, 1990.

4. Mortiz AR, Henrique FC, Jr: Studies of thermal injury: the relative importance of time and surface temperature in the causation of cutaneous burn injury, *Am J Pathol* 23:695, 1947.

5. Robinson MC, Del Becarro EJ: Increasing dermal perfusion after burning by decreasing thromboxane production, *J Trauma* 20:722, 1980.

6. Heggers JP, Ko F, Robson MC, et al: Evaluation of burn blister fluid, *Plast Reconstr Surg* 65:798, 1980.

7. Dunn K, Edwards-Jones VT: The role of Acticoat with nanocrystalline silver in the management of burns, *Burns* 30(suppl):S1, 2004.

8. Wright JB, Lam K, Burrell RE: Wound management in an era of increasing bacterial antibiotic resistance: a role for topical silver treatments, *Am J Infect Control* 26:572, 1998.

9. Yin HQ, Langford R, Burrell RE: Comparative evaluation of the antimicrobial activity of Acticoat antimicrobial dressing, *J Burn Care Rehabil* 20:195, 1999.

10. Layton TR, McMurty JM, McClain EJ, et al: Multiple spine fractures from electrical injuries, *J Burn Care Rehabil* 5:373–375, 1984.

11. Moritz AR, Henriques FC, McClean R: The effects of inhaled heat on the air passages and lungs, *Am J Pathol* 21:311, 1945.

12. Peters WJ: Inhalation injury caused by the products of combustion, *Can Med Assoc J* 125:249, 1981.

13. Forbes WH, Sargent F, Roughton FJW: The rate of carbon monoxide uptake by normal men, *Am J Physiol* 143:594, 1945.

14. Mellins RB, Park S: Respiratory complications of smoke inhalation in victims of fires, *J Pediatr* 87:1, 1975.

15. Crapo R: Smoke inhalation injuries, *JAMA* 246:1694, 1981.

16. Herndon DN, Traber DL, Niehaus GD, et al: The pathophysiology of smoke inhalation in a sheep model, *J Trauma* 24:1044, 1984.

17. Till GO, Johnson KJ, Kunkel R, et al: Intravascular activation of complement and acute lung injury, *J Clin Invest* 69:1126, 1982.

18. Thommasen HV, Martin BA, Wiggs BR, et al: Effect of pulmonary blood flow on leukocyte uptake and release by dog lung, *J Appl Physiol Respir Environ Exerc Physiol* 56:966, 1984.

19. Hight DW, Bakalar HR, Lloyd JR: Inflicted burns in children: recognition and treatment, *JAMA* 242:517, 1979.

20. Chadwick DL: The diagnosis of inflicted injury in infants and young children, *Pediatr Ann* 21:477, 1992.

21. Adronicus M, Oates RK, Peat J, et al: Non-accidental burns in children, *Burns* 24:552, 1998.

22. Purdue GF, Hunt JL, Prescott PR: Child abuse by burning: an index of suspicion, *J Trauma* 28:221, 1988.

23. Lenoski EF, Hunter KA: Specific patterns of inflicted burn injuries, *J Trauma* 17:842, 1977.

24. Bromberg BF, Song IC, Walden RH: Hydrotherapy of chemical burns, *Plast Reconstr Surg* 35:85, 1965.

25. Leonard LG, Scheulen JJ, Munster AM: Chemical burns: effect of prompt first aid, *J Trauma* 22:420, 1982.

26. Mozingo DW, Smith AD, McManus WF, et al: Chemical burns, *J Trauma* 28:642, 1998.

27. Mistry D, Wainwright D: Hydrofluoric acid burns, *Am Fam Physician* 45:1748, 1992.

28. Willems JL. Clinical management of mustard gas casualties, *Ann Med Milit Belg* 3S:1, 1989.

29. Papirmeister B, Feister AJ, Robinson SI, et al: The sulfur mustard injury: description of lesions and resulting incapacitation. In *Medical defense against mustard gas,* Boca Raton, Fla, 1990, CRC Press, p. 13.

30. Sidell FR, Takafuji ET, Franz DR: *Medical aspects of chemical and biological warfare,* Washington, DC, 1997, Office of the Surgeon General.

CHAPTER 9

Environmental and Wilderness Trauma

CHAPTER OBJECTIVES

At the completion of this chapter, the reader will be able to do the following:

✓ Differentiate between heat exhaustion and heatstroke.

✓ Give the reason why heatstroke is considered a life-threatening condition.

✓ List two effective cooling procedures for heat exhaustion and heatstroke.

✓ List the five factors that place prehospital care providers at risk for heat illness.

✓ Explain the fluid hydration guidelines and how they should be used to prevent dehydration in hot or cold environments.

✓ Describe the various ways the body can lose heat to the environment.

✓ Differentiate the management of mild hypothermia from that of severe hypothermia.

✓ List the signs of mild frostbite, and discuss how to prevent its progression.

✓ Discuss the rationale for the statement, "Patients are not dead until they are warm and dead."

✓ List five risk factors for a near-drowning incident.

✓ List three signs or symptoms that can occur in a patient after a near-drowning incident.

✓ List five methods for preventing a drowning incident.

✓ Explain the "30-30" rule in lightning injury prevention.

✓ Differentiate the use of "reverse" triage for multiple lightning casualties from its use for other multiple-casualty scenarios.

✓ List four factors that distinguish the "wilderness" and "street" EMS contexts.

✓ Given a particular patient situation and location, list four factors that affect the decision whether "wilderness" or "street" care is more appropriate.

✓ Describe methods used for improvised wilderness evacuation.

✓ Describe methods for dealing with elimination needs during evacuations, as well as potential medical consequences if this is not addressed.

✓ Explain the reasons for the dictum that "every wilderness patient is cold, has low blood sugar, and is dehydrated until proven otherwise."

✓ Explain the meaning of the term *SPF* (sun protection factor).

✓ Describe standard ways to manage bleeding wounds in the backcountry.

✓ Describe the reasons, specific indications, and technique for wound irrigation.

✓ Explain when, in the wilderness context, an attempt at CPR is appropriate, and when it is not appropriate.

Heat and Cold

SCENARIO 1

At 2:00 AM, your ambulance unit responds to a dispatch on a cold and windy evening (28° F [−2° C]), 25 mph northeast wind) after an 8-hour urban search for a 76-year-old woman who wandered from an assisted care retirement facility. She was recently moved closer to her daughter at this new location from her home in another state. She apparently was reported missing around 6:00 PM and was noted to be agitated most of the day. After a lengthy search, a volunteer search and rescue member found her disorientated and lightly dressed in a windbreaker and pants 400 yards from the facility. She was located on the ground, cold and wet, and stuck in some briars near an icy drainage ditch. The initial assessment shows that she is unresponsive, respirations are shallow, pulse is weak, and skin is cold.

What are possible causes for this patient to wander, and what is her medical condition?

What is the best way to assess this patient for cold-related injuries and other potential medical conditions? Is this a life-threatening situation for the patient?

How would you treat this patient? Should you attempt to rewarm the patient?

If you transport the patient immediately, how do you treat the patient en route to the closest emergency department?

What is the wind chill index during this incident, and how do you best protect the patient from ongoing cold injury?

The most significant morbidity and mortality in the United States from all environmental traumas are caused by thermal trauma.[1–4] Environmental extremes of heat and cold have a common outcome of injuries and potential death that can affect many individuals during the peak summer and winter months. Individuals who are especially susceptible to both highs and lows of temperature are very young persons, the elderly population, urban poor people, individuals who take specific medications, chronically ill patients, and alcoholic persons.[3–7] The majority of EMS responses in the United States for heat and cold injuries are for the *hyperthermic* and *hypothermic* patient in an urban setting. However, interest in recreational and high-risk adventure activities in the wilderness backcountry during periods of environmental extremes places more individuals at risk for heat-related and cold-related injuries and fatalities.[8–11]

Epidemiology

Heat-Related Illness

During a 20-year period (1979–1999) in the United States, 8015 heat-related deaths from all causes were recorded.[2] More deaths were caused by heat stress than by hurricanes, lightning, tornadoes, floods, and earthquakes combined. Of these, 3829 (48%) deaths were related to high ambient temperatures. This averages to about 182 heat-related deaths per year during the 4 warmest months (May through August). The greatest number of deaths (1891, or 45%) occurred in those who were 65 years of age and older. Furthermore, morbidity and mortal-

ity can be extremely high when periodic seasonal heat waves occur (3 or more consecutive days of air temperatures 90° F or higher [≥32.2° C]). From 1999 to 2003, the Centers for Disease Control and Prevention reported a total of 3442 deaths resulting from exposure to extreme heat (annual average: 688). Of the deaths recorded, in 2239 (65%) the underlying cause was exposure to excessive heat, whereas in the remaining 1203 (35%) hyperthermia (increased body temperature) was recorded as a contributing factor. Males accounted for 66% of deaths and outnumbered deaths among females in all age groups. Of the 3401 decedents for whom age information was available, 228 (7%) were younger than 15 years; 1810 (53%) were age 15 to 64 years; and 1363 (40%) were age 65 years or older.[3]

Cold-Related Illness

Mild to severe cold weather conditions caused 13,970 unintentional hypothermia-related deaths in the United States between 1978 and 1998 (an average of 699 deaths per year), and 6857 (49%) of these deaths occurred in persons 65 years of age and older.[4] When adjusted for age, death from hypothermia (decreased body temperature) occurred approximately 2.5 times more often in men than women. The incidence of hypothermia related–deaths progressively increases with age and is three times higher in males than females after age 15 years. In 2003, 599 deaths were reported from exposure to cold weather in the United States; 67% were males and 51% were older than 65 years of age.[7] Major contributing factors for accidental hypothermia are urban poverty, socio-

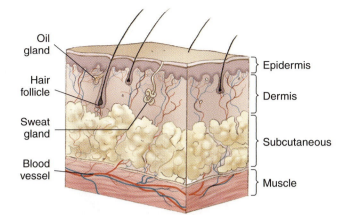

FIGURE 9-1 The skin is composed of three tissue layers—epidermis, dermis, and subcutaneous layer—and associated muscle. Some layers contain structures such as glands, hair follicles, blood vessels, and nerves. All these structures are interrelated to the maintenance, loss, and gain of body temperature.

economic conditions, alcohol intake, malnutrition, and age (the very young and senior citizens).[4,7]

Anatomy

The skin, the largest organ of the body, interfaces with the external environment and serves as a layer of protection. It prevents the invasion of microorganisms, maintains fluid balance, and regulates temperature. Skin is comprised of three tissue layers—the epidermis, dermis, and subcutaneous tissue (Figure 9-1). The outermost layer, called the *epidermis*, is made up entirely of epithelial cells, with no blood vessels. Underlying the epidermis is the thicker dermis. The *dermis,* or deeper layer of skin, is 20 to 30 times thicker than the epidermis. The dermis is made up of a framework of connective tissues that contain blood vessels, blood products, nerves, sebaceous glands, and sweat glands. The innermost layer, the *subcutaneous* layer, is a combination of elastic and fibrous tissue as well as fatty deposits, and below this layer is skeletal muscle. The skin, nerves, blood vessels, and other underlying anatomic structures have major roles in regulating body temperature.

Physiology

Thermoregulation and Temperature Balance

Humans are considered homeotherms, or warm-blooded animals. A key feature of homeotherms is that they are able to regulate their own internal body temperature independent of varying environmental temperatures. The body can essentially be divided into a warmer inner *core* layer (including the brain and the thoracic and abdominal organs) and the skin and subcutaneous outer *shell* layer. *Core temperature* is regulated through a balance of heat production and heat dissipation mechanisms. The temperatures on the skin surface and the thickness of the shell depend on the *environmental temperature,* so the shell becomes thicker in the colder temperatures and thinner in the warmer temperatures based on shunt-

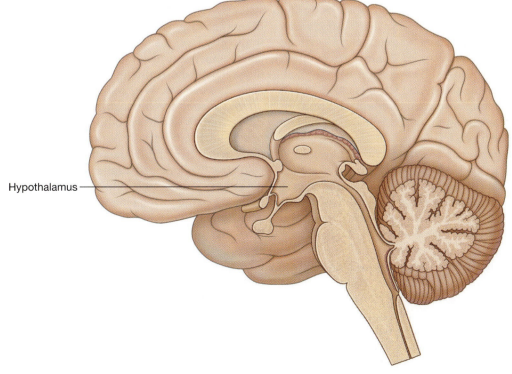

FIGURE 9-2 The hypothalamus.
(From Drake R, Vogl A, Mitchell A: *Gray's anatomy for students,* 2009, New York, Churchill Livingstone.)

ing blood away or to the skin, respectively. This shell or tissue insulation, as induced by vasoconstriction, has been estimated to be about the same outer protection as wearing a light business suit, compared with six to eight times the insulation created when wearing heavy, insulated clothing in cold temperatures.

The body normally functions within a narrow temperature range, known as *steady-state metabolism,* of about 1° on either side of 98.6° F (37° C ± 0.6° C). Normal body temperature is maintained within a narrow range by homeostatic mechanisms regulated in the *hypothalamus,* which is located in the brain (Figure 9-2). The hypothalamus is known as the *thermoregulatory center* and functions as the body's thermostat to control neurologic and hormonal regulation of body temperature. As noted in preceding chapters, trauma to the brain can disrupt the hypothalamus, which in turn causes an imbalance in the regulation of the body temperature.

Humans have two systems to regulate body temperature: *behavioral regulation* and *physiologic thermoregulation.* Behavioral regulation is governed by the individual thermal sensation and comfort, and the distinguishing feature is the conscious effort to reduce thermal discomfort (e.g., adding additional clothing, seeking shelter in cold environments). The processing of sensory feedback to the brain of thermal information in behavioral thermoregulation is not well understood, but the feedback of thermal sensation and comfort responds more quickly than physiologic responses to changes in environmental temperature.[12]

Heat Production and Thermal Balance. Basal metabolic rate is the heat produced primarily as a by-product of metabolism, principally from the large organs of the core of the body and from skeletal muscle contraction. The heat generated is transferred throughout the body by blood in the circulatory system. Shivering increases the metabolic rate. There are some individual differences, but typically shivering starts when the core temperature drops to between 94° and 97° F (34.4° C–36° C) and continues until the core temperature is 88°F [31° C].[13] With maximal shivering, heat production is increased by five to six times the resting level.[13,14]

When body temperature rises, the normal physiologic response is to increase skin blood flow and to begin sweating. The majority of body heat is transferred to the environment at the skin surface by conduction, convection, radiation, and evaporation, as defined next. Because heat is transferred from greater temperature to lower temperature, the human body can gain heat by radiation and conduction during hot weather conditions. Methods to maintain and dissipate body heat are important concepts for prehospital care providers. They must understand how both heat and cold are transferred to and from the body so that they can effectively manage a patient who has hyperthermia or hypothermia (Figure 9-3).

Radiation is the loss or gain of heat in the form of electromagnetic energy; it is the transfer of energy from a warm object to a cooler one. Radiation does not use an intermediary

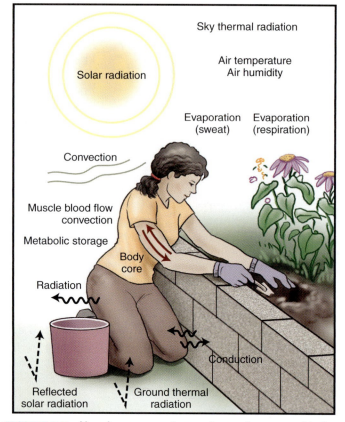

FIGURE 9-3   How humans exchange thermal energy with the environment.

source such as air or water. The sun warms the earth through space by this method of energy transfer. A patient with heat illness can acquire additional body heat from the hot ground or directly from the sun. These sources of heat will increase body temperature and impede efforts to cool the patient until the prehospital care provider eliminates these sources of radiant heat when assessing and treating the patient.

Conduction is the transfer of heat between two objects in direct contact with each other, as with a patient lying on a frozen lawn after a fall. A patient will generally lose heat faster when lying on the cold ground than when exposed to cold air. Therefore, prehospital care providers need to lift the patient off the ground in cold temperatures rather than merely cover the patient with a blanket.

Convection is the transfer of heat from a solid object to a medium that moves across that solid object. Air or water currents are the two mediums generally considered in convective heat loss because they come into contact with the human body. The movement of cool air or water across the warmer skin provides for the continuous elimination of heat from the warmer skin. Furthermore, a patient will lose body heat 25 times faster in water than in air of the same temperature, so it is important to keep a patient dry and to remove wet clothing in mild to cold temperatures. When prehospital care providers are effectively managing a heat illness patient, they use the principle of convective heat loss by moistening and fanning their patient to dissipate body heat quickly.

Evaporation of sweat from a liquid to a vapor is an extremely effective method of heat loss from the body, depending on the relative humidity or moisture in the air. Evaporative heat loss increases in cool, dry, and windy conditions (e.g., southwestern U.S. deserts). Collectively, convection and evaporation are more important than other methods of heat transfer because they are regulated by the body to control core temperature.[5]

Increases *(hyperthermia)* and decreases *(hypothermia)* in body temperature beyond the steady-state range (98.6°F ± 1° F [37° C ± 0.6° C]) can result from different internal and external causes and return to steady-state temperature without complications.[15] Hyperthermia occurs primarily in one of three ways: (1) as a normal response to sustained exercise, in which the heat produced elevates core temperature and is the stimulus for heat-dissipating responses (e.g., sweating, increased blood flow in skin); (2) when the sum of heat production and heat gained from the environment is greater than the body's ability to dissipate it; and (3) from a fever. Unlike the first two ways, fever usually occurs in response to inflammation because of a change in the thermoregulatory set point, and the body responds by elevating body temperature to a higher value (100° F–106° F [38°–41° C]). Heat production increases only temporarily to achieve a new set-point temperature in an attempt to make the environment less hospitable for the invading infection.[15]

Injuries Produced By Heat

Risk Factors in Heat Illness

Many studies on humans have demonstrated large individual differences in their tolerance to hot environments.[16] These differences can be partially explained by both physical characteristics and medical conditions that are associated with an increased risk for heat illness (Figure 9-4). It is important to realize that any situation in which heat production exceeds the body's ability to dissipate heat may result in heat injury. Key risk factors that contribute to the onset of heat illness are alcohol consumption, medications, dehydration, higher body mass index, obesity, inadequate diet, improper clothing, low fitness, sleep loss, extremes of age, cardiovascular disease, skin injuries, previous heat-related illness, sickle cell trait, sunburn, viral illness, and exercise during the hottest hours of day.[17,18] Transient conditions include those affecting individuals who travel from cooler climates and are not heat-acclimatized to warmer climates on arrival. Other transient factors that place individuals at risk for heat illness are common illnesses, including colds and other conditions that cause fever, vomiting, and diarrhea, along with poor dietary and fluid intake.[19,20]

FIGURE 9-4	Heat Illness Risk Factors
CONDITIONS	**TOXINS/DRUGS**
Cardiovascular disease	**Increase Heat Production**
Dehydration	Thyroid hormone
Autonomic neuropathies	Cyclic antidepressants
Parkinsonism	Hallucinogens (e.g., LSD)
Dystonias	Cocaine
Skin disorders: psoriasis, sunburn, burns	Amphetamines
Endocrine disorders	**Decrease Thirst**
Fever	Haloperidol
Delirium tremens	Angiotensin-converting
Psychosis	enzyme (ACE) inhibitors
Neonates, elderly persons	
History of heatstroke	**Decrease Sweating**
Obesity	Antihistamines
Low fitness	Anticholinergics
	Phenothiazines
BEHAVIOR	Glutethimide
Injudicious exertion	Beta blockers
Inappropriate clothing	
Poor acclimatization	**Increase Water Loss**
Poor fluid intake	Diuretics
Poor supervision	Ethanol
High motivation	Nicotine
Athletic profile	
Military recruit profile	

(Modified from Tek D, Olshaker JS: Heat illness. *Emerg Med Clin North Am* 10(2):299, 1992.)

Factors considered to be *chronic* conditions that place individuals at greater risk for heat illness are fitness, body size, age, medical condition, and medications.

Fitness and Body Mass Index

Low levels of physical fitness caused by genetic factors or a sedentary lifestyle with inadequate daily physical activity will reduce tolerance to heat exposure. Being physically fit provides a cardiovascular reserve to maintain cardiac output as needed to sustain thermoregulation. Overweight individuals have a normal response to heat exposure of vasodilatation of skin blood vessels and increased sweating, but the combination of low fitness, lack of heat acclimatization, and excessive body weight (higher body mass index) increases the energy cost of movement, placing them at greater risk for heat illness.

Age

Thermoregulatory capacity and tolerance to heat diminish with age. However, this state can be improved by maintaining a low body weight and a high level of physical fitness.

Gender

Recent studies indicate that women demonstrate equal work tolerance in heat and, in some studies, are more tolerant of heat than men.

Medical Conditions

Medical conditions that can increase the risk for heat intolerance and heat illness are diabetes mellitus, thyroid disorders, and renal disease. Cardiovascular disease and circulatory problems that increase cutaneous blood flow and circulatory demand are aggravated by heat exposure.

Medications

The use of specific prescription or over-the-counter medications can place individuals at a greater risk for heat illness (see Figure 9-4). Certain medications can increase metabolic heat production, suppress body cooling, reduce cardiac reserve, and alter renal electrolyte and fluid balance. Sedative and narcotic drugs will affect mental status and can affect logical reasoning and judgment, suppressing decision-making ability, when the individual is exposed to heat.

Dehydration

Body water is the largest component of the human body, representing 45% to 70% of body weight; for example, a 165-pound (75-kg) man contains approximately 45 L of water, representing 60% of body weight. Excessive changes in the normal body water balance *(euhydration)* resulting from either overconsumption of water *(hyperhydration)* or fluid loss (causing acute dehydration) alter homeostasis, producing specific signs and symptoms. Acute dehydration can be a serious outcome of both heat and cold exposure, but it is also seen as a dangerous side effect of diarrhea, vomiting, and fever.

Heat-Related Disorders

Heat-related disorders can range from minor to severe in patients with heat illness.[9,18,21] It is important to note that prehospital care providers may or may not see a progression of signs and symptoms, starting with minor syndromes (e.g., heat cramps) and then advancing to major heat-related illness (e.g., classic heatstroke). In the majority of heat exposures, the patient is able to dissipate core body heat adequately and maintain core temperature within the normal range. However, when heat-related conditions do result in a call for EMS assistance, the minor heat-related conditions may be apparent to the prehospital care provider during patient assessment, along with signs and symptoms of a major heat illness (Figure 9-5).

Minor Heat-Related Disorders

The minor heat-related disorders include heat rash, heat edema, heat tetany, muscle (heat) cramps, and heat syncope.

Heat Rash. Heat rash, also known as "prickly heat" and miliaria rubra, is a red, itchy (pruritic), papular rash normally seen on the skin in areas of restrictive clothing and heavy sweating. This condition is caused by inflammation of the sweat glands that results in blockage of the sweat ducts. As a result, affected areas cannot sweat, putting individuals at increased risk of heat illness, depending on the amount of skin surface involved.

Management. Treatment is by cooling and drying the affected area and by preventing further conditions that cause sweat in these areas.

Heat Edema. Heat edema is a mild, dependent swelling in the hands, feet, and ankles seen during early stages of heat acclimatization while plasma volume is expanding to compensate for the increased need for thermoregulatory blood flow. This form of edema does not indicate excessive fluid intake or cardiac, renal, or hepatic disease. In the absence of other diseases, this condition is of no clinical significance and is self-limited. Heat edema is observed more often in females.

Management. Treatment consists of loosening any constricting clothes and elevating the legs. Diuretics (medication to promote fluid excretions in the urine) are not indicated and may increase risk of heat illness.

Heat Tetany. Heat tetany is a rare and self-limited condition that may occur in patients acutely exposed to short, intense heat conditions. The hyperventilation that results from these conditions is considered to be the principal cause. Paresthesias (numbness and tingling), carpopedal (hand and foot) spasm, and tetany may develop.

Management. Treatment consists of removal from the source of heat and controlling hyperventilation. Dehydration is not a common occurrence with these short heat exposures. Heat tetany may be seen along with signs and symptoms of heat exhaustion and heatstroke.

Muscle (Heat) Cramps. Heat cramps are manifested by short-term, painful muscle contractions commonly seen in the calf (gastrocnemius) muscles but also in the voluntary muscles of the abdomen and extremities and are commonly observed after prolonged physical activity, often in warm to hot temperatures. This occurs in individuals during exercise that produces profuse sweating or during the exercise recovery period. Muscle (heat) cramps can occur alone or in association with heat exhaustion. The cause is unknown, but it is believed to be a function of muscle fatigue, body water loss, and large sodium loss. Salt supplementation in the diet has been shown to reduce the incidence of heat cramps.

Management. Treatment consists of rest in a cool environment, prolonged stretching of the affected muscle, and consumption

FIGURE 9-5 Common Heat-Related Disorders

Disorder	Cause/Problem	Signs/Symptoms	Treatment
Muscle (heat) cramps	Failure to replace sodium lost through sweating Electrolyte and muscle problems	Painful muscle cramps, usually in legs or abdomen	Move to cool place Massage/stretch muscles Hydrate with athletic drinks or fluids with sodium (e.g., tomato juice) Transport those with signs or symptoms listed below
Dehydration	Failure to replace sweat loss with fluids	Thirst, nausea Excessive fatigue Headache Hypovolemia Decreased thermoregulation Reduced physical and mental capacity	Replace sweat loss with lightly salted fluids Rest in cool place until body weight and water losses are restored In some patients, IV rehydration by ALS
Heat exhaustion	Excessive heat strain with inadequate water intake Cardiovascular problems with venous pooling, decreased cardiac filling time, reduced cardiac output Untreated, may progress to heatstroke	Low urine output Tachycardia Weakness Unstable gait Extreme fatigue Wet, clammy skin Headache Dizziness Nausea Collapse	Remove from heat source and place in cooler location Cool body with water and fanning Drink lightly salty fluids (e.g., athletic drinks) Administer IV 0.9 % by ALS
Heatstroke	High core temperatures: >105° F (40.6° C) Cellular disruption Commonly, dysfunction of multiple organ systems Neurologic disorder with thermoregulatory center failure	Mental status changes; irrational behavior or delirium Possible shivering Tachycardia initially, then bradycardia late Hypotension Rapid and shallow breathing Dry or wet, hot skin Loss of consciousness Seizures and coma	*Emergency:* Rapid, immediate cooling by water immersion, or wet patient or wrap in cool, wet sheets and fan vigorously until core temperature <102° F (39° C) Treat for shock if necessary once core temperature is lowered Immediate transport to emergency department

ABC, airway, breathing, circulation; *IV,* intravenous; *NRM,* non-breather mask.

of oral fluids and food containing salt (sodium chloride—e.g., ⅛–¼ teaspoon table salt added to 300–500 mL fluids or sport drinks; 1–2 salt tablets with 300–500 mL fluid; boullion broth; or salty snacks). Avoid the use of salt tablets by themselves because these can cause gastrointestinal (GI) distress.

Heat Syncope. Heat syncope is seen with prolonged standing in warm environments and is caused by low blood pressure that results in fainting or feeling faint or lightheaded. Heat causes vasodilation, and venous blood pools in the legs, causing low blood pressure.

Management. After removal to a cool environment, patients rest in a recumbent position and are provided oral rehydration. If a fall occurred, patients should be thoroughly evalu-

ated for any injury that might have been sustained as a result. Patients with a significant history of cardiac or neurologic disorders need further evaluation for the cause of their syncopal episode. Monitoring of vital signs during transport is essential.

Major Heat-Related Disorders
The major heat-related disorders include exertion-associated collapse, heat exhaustion, and heatstroke (classic and exertional forms).

Exertion-Associated Collapse. This disorder occurs when an individual collapses after strenuous exercise.[22,23] During exercise, contraction of the muscles of the lower extremities assists in maintaining venous blood return to the heart. When exercise stops, such as at the end of a jog, the muscle contraction that assisted blood return to the heart slows significantly. This, in turn, causes venous blood return to the heart to decrease, resulting in a decreased cardiac output to the brain.

Assessment. Signs and symptoms include nausea, light-headedness, collapse, and syncope. Patients may feel better while lying down but become lightheaded when they attempt to stand or sit *(orthostatic hypotension)*. Profuse sweating is not unusual. Ventilations and pulse rates may be rapid. The patient's core body temperature may be normal or slightly elevated. It is difficult to rule out dehydration, but this type of post-exercise collapse is not from hypovolemia. In contrast, collapse that occurs during exercise needs immediate evaluation for other causes (e.g., cardiovascular).

Management. The patient is removed to a cool environment and rests in a recumbent position. Oral rehydration is provided as needed. As with any form of collapse, further evaluation at a hospital is necessary to rule out other disorders (e.g., blood chemistry abnormalities, cardiac or neurologic causes). Monitoring of vital signs during transport is essential to detect cardiac arrhythmias.

Heat Exhaustion. Heat exhaustion is the most common heat-related disorder seen by prehospital care providers. This condition can develop over days of exposure, as in elderly persons living in poorly ventilated homes or apartments, or acutely, as in athletes. This condition results from cardiac output that is insufficient to meet the competing demands of thermoregulatory heat dissipation, increased skin blood flow, reduced plasma volume, reduced venous return to the heart from vasodilation, and sweat-induced depletion of salt and water.[20] Patients with heat exhaustion normally present with a rectal temperature less than 104° F (<40° C), but this is a guide and not always a reliable finding.[23]

Another form of heat exhaustion is known as exertional heat exhaustion. This occurs with physical exercise or heavy exertion in all temperatures and is defined as the inability to continue the exercise or exertion; it may or may not be associated with physical collapse.[18] The key predisposing factors are dehydration and high body mass index that place one at greater risk for exertional heat exhaustion.

Distinguishing severe heat exhaustion from heatstroke often may be difficult, but a quick mental status assessment will determine the level of neurologic involvement. If heat exhaustion is not effectively treated, it may lead to heatstroke, a life-threatening form of heat illness. Heat exhaustion is a diagnosis of exclusion when there is no evidence of heatstroke. These patients will need further physical and laboratory evaluation in the emergency department.

Assessment. Signs and symptoms of heat exhaustion are neither specific nor sensitive. They include low fluid intake, frontal headache, drowsiness, euphoria, nausea, vomiting, light-headedness, anxiety, fatigue, irritability, decreased coordination, heat sensation on head and neck, chills, and apathy. Patients may feel better while lying down but may become lightheaded when they attempt to stand or sit (orthostatic hypotension). During the acute stage of heat exhaustion, the blood pressure is low; pulse and respiratory rates are rapid. The radial pulse may feel thready. The patient generally appears sweaty, pale, and ashen. The patient's core body temperature may be either normal or slightly elevated but is generally below 104° F (40° C). It is important to obtain a good history of prior heat illness and the current heat exposure incident because these patients may display signs and symptoms of other conditions of fluid and sodium loss. Ongoing assessment is critical. Continuously look for any changes in mentation and personality (i.e., confusion, disorientation, irrational or unusual behavior). Any such change should be taken as a progressive sign of hyperthermia indicating heatstroke—*a life-threatening condition.*

Management. Immediately remove the patient from the hot environment to a cooler location either in the shade or an air-conditioned space (i.e., ambulance). Place the patient in a supine resting position. Remove clothing and anything that restricts heat dissipation, such as a hat. Assess the patient's heart rate, blood pressure, respiratory rate, and rectal temperature (if a thermometer is available and conditions permit) and particularly for mental status changes as an early indicator of life-threatening heatstroke. Oral rehydration should be considered for any patient who can take fluids by mouth and who is not at risk of aspirating using sport electrolyte fluids diluted to half strength. Large amounts of oral fluids may increase bloating, nausea, and vomiting. In exertional heat exhaustion, most exercising patients recover with recumbent rest and oral fluids.

Because heat exhaustion may be difficult to distinguish from heatstroke, and because heatstroke patients should be cooled rapidly, the best course of action is to provide some active cooling procedures to all heat exhaustion patients. Active cooling can be done simply and quickly by wetting the head and upper torso with water and fanning the patient to increase *convective* body heat dissipation. Body cooling procedures will also improve mental status. Transport all patients who are unconscious, who do not recover rapidly, or who have a significant medical history. Proper environmental temperature control and monitoring of vital signs and mental status are essential during transport.

Heatstroke. Heatstroke is considered the most emergent and life-threatening form of heat illness. Heatstroke is a form of hyperthermia resulting in failure of the thermoregulatory system—a failure of the body's physiologic systems to dissipate heat and cool down. Heatstroke is characterized by an elevated core temperature of 104° F (40° C) or greater and central nervous system (CNS) dysfunction, resulting in delirium, convulsions, or coma.[21,24]

The most significant difference in heatstroke compared with heat exhaustion is *neurologic disability,* which presents to the prehospital care provider as mental status changes. Pathophysiologic changes often result in multiple organ failure.[21,25] These pathophysiologic changes occur when organ tissue temperatures rise above a critical level.[18] The degree of complications in patients with heatstroke is not entirely related to the magnitude of core temperature elevation. This pathophysiologic dysfunction is the underlying reason for early heatstroke recognition by prehospital care providers, who can quickly provide aggressive whole-body cooling in effort to rapidly reduce core temperature and decrease the associated heatstroke morbidity and mortality too frequently seen in the emergency departments.

Morbidity and mortality are directly associated with the duration of elevated core temperature. Even with aggressive prehospital intervention and in-hospital management, heatstroke can be fatal, and many patients who survive have permanent neurologic disability.

Heatstroke has two different clinical presentations: classic heatstroke and exertional heatstroke (Figure 9-6).

Classic heatstroke is a disorder of infants, febrile children, poor people, the elderly population, alcoholic persons, and sick patients that may be compounded by the risk factors listed in Figure 9-4 (e.g., medications). A classic presentation is a patient who is exposed to elevated humidity and high room temperatures over several days without air conditioning, leading to dehydration and high core temperature. Often their sweating mechanism has stopped, known as *anhidrosis.* This is especially common in large cities during summer heat waves, when effective home ventilation is either not possible or not used.[26] Scene assessment will provide information helpful in the identification of classic heatstroke.

Exertional heatstroke (EHS) is a preventable disorder often seen in those individuals with poor physical fitness or lack of heat acclimatization who are involved in short-term, strenuous physical activity (e.g., industrial workers, athletes, military recruits, firefighters, and other public safety personnel) in a hot and humid environment. These conditions can rapidly elevate internal heat production and limit the body's ability to dissipate heat. Almost all EHS patients exhibit sweat-soaked and pale skin at time of collapse, as compared with dry, hot, and flushed skin in the classic heatstroke patient.[27] Even though drinking fluids can slow the rate of dehydration during strenuous activity and reduces the rate at which core temperature rises, hyperthermia and EHS may still occur in the absence of significant dehydration.

Assessment. The appearance of signs and symptoms depends on the degree and duration of hyperthermia.[28] Heatstroke patients typically present with hot, flushed skin. They may or may not be sweating, depending on where they are found and whether they have classic or exertional heat stroke. Blood pressure may be elevated or diminished, and the radial pulse is usually fast (tachycardic) and thready; 25% of these patients

FIGURE 9-6 Classic versus Exertional Heat Stroke

	Classic	Exertional
Patient characteristics	Elderly	Men (15–45 yrs)
Health status	Chronically ill	Healthy
Concurrent activity	Sedentary	Strenuous exercise
Drug use	Diuretics, antidepressants, antihypertensives, anticholinergics, antipsychotics	Usually none
Sweating	May be absent	Usually present
Hypoglycemia	Uncommon	Common

(Modified from Knochel JP, Reed G: Disorders of heat regulation. In Kleeman CR, Maxwell MH, Narin RG, editors: *Clinical disorders of fluid and electrolyte metabolism,* New York, 1987, McGraw-Hill.)

have low blood pressure (hypotensive). The patient's level of consciousness (LOC) can range from confused to unconscious, and seizure activity may also be present, particularly during cooling.[24] As measured usually in hospitals, rectal temperature may range from 104° to 116° F (40° C–47° C).[21,24]

The keys to distinguishing heatstroke from one of the other heat-related conditions are the elevation in body temperature and altered mental status. Any patient who is warm to the touch with an altered mental status (confused, disoriented, combative, or unconscious) should be suspected of having heatstroke and managed immediately and aggressively.

Management. Heatstroke is a true emergency. Immediately remove the patient from the source of heat. Cooling the patient should begin immediately in the field by one prehospital care provider as another provider assesses and stabilizes the patient's airway, breathing, and circulation (ABCs). Cool the patient with whatever means are available (e.g., garden hose, fire hose, bottled water), even before removing clothing. Ideally, ice water immersion is the fastest method of cooling, but this is generally limited in the prehospital setting.[27,29,30] The next most effective method is application of ice-water towels or sheets combined with ice packs on the head, trunk, and extremities.[18] If cold water and ice are not immediately available, remove excess clothing, wet down the patient head to toe, and provide fanning of the skin. This is the next most effective technique causing evaporation and convective heat loss when humidity is low.[29] Since the late 1950s it has been thought that cold- or ice-water immersion will cause vasoconstriction sufficient to decrease heat loss from the body and cause the onset of shivering so that internal heat is produced. However, recent research has shown that this does not interfere with the critical lowering of the elevated core temperature.[29,30] Individuals who rapidly become lucid during whole-body cooling usually have the best prognosis. The most important intervention prehospital care providers can deliver to a heatstroke patient (along with ABCs) is immediate and rapid whole-body cooling to reduce core temperature.

During transport, the patient should be placed in a prepared air-conditioned ambulance. It is an error to place a heatstroke patient in a hot internal cabin of the ambulance even if it is a short transfer time to the hospital. Remove any additional clothing, cover the patient with a sheet, and wet down the sheet with irrigation fluids along with continuous fanning. Ice packs, if available, should be placed in the groin area, in the axillae, and around the anterior lateral neck because blood vessels are closest to the skin surface in these areas. However, ice packs alone are insufficient to lower core body temperature rapidly and should be considered only as an extra cooling method.[4] Active cooling should stop when the rectal temperature reaches 102.2° F (39° C).[4,30] Provide high-flow oxygen and support ventilations with a bag-mask device as needed.

Transport the patient in a right or left lateral recumbent position to maintain an open airway and to avoid aspiration. Rendezvous with an advanced-life support ambulance should be considered for additional interventions such as cardiac monitoring.

Prevention of Heat-Related Illness

Because heat stress is a significant public health factor in the United States, methods for preventing heat illness are vital to any community, particularly for those individuals who must work in high-heat occupational settings. For example, in 2006 there were a total of 106 firefighter deaths in the United States for all causes, and of these deaths, 54 (50.9%) occurred at the scene due to stress/overexertion, which included heat illness as a cause of death in this category.[31] As with the general public, it may not be possible to prevent all forms of heat-related illness in prehospital care providers; therefore, EMS and other public safety personnel need to use prevention strategies and prepare for exposure to high ambient temperature and high occupational exposures. These strategies, which include administrative policies, procedures, engineering controls, use of equipment, and medical surveillance programs, are designed to help minimize the overall impact from acute or chronic heat exposure. The implementation of simple preventive procedures can have a dramatic impact on lowering the incidence of heat illness, but individuals in an organization often do not consider these strategies. Figure 9-7 provides an overview of heat stress prevention strategies for EMS providers, firefighters, and other public safety personnel.[32]

FIGURE 9-7 **Prevention of Heat-Related Disorders in Prehospital Care Providers**

You can prevent the serious consequences of heat disorders by improving your level of fitness and becoming acclimated to the heat.

Maintaining a high level of aerobic fitness is one of the best ways to protect yourself against heat stress. The fit worker has a well-developed circulatory system and increased blood volume. Both are important to regulate body temperature. Fit workers start to sweat sooner, so they work with a lower heart rate and body temperature. They adjust to the heat twice as fast as the unfit worker. They lose acclimatization more slowly and regain it quickly.

Heat acclimatization occurs in 5 to 10 days of heat exposure as the body:

- Increases sweat production
- Improves blood distribution
- Decreases the heart rate and lowers the skin and body temperatures

You can acclimatize by gradually increasing work time in the heat, taking care to replace fluids and resting as needed. You maintain acclimatization with periodic work or exercise in a hot environment.

(Modified from U.S. Department of Agriculture, U.S. Forest Service: *Heat stress*, www.fs.usda.gov/fire/safety/fitness/heat_stress/hs_pg1.html.)

Injuries Produced By Cold

Dehydration

Dehydration occurs very easily in the cold, particularly with increased physical activity. This occurs for three primary reasons: (1) evaporation of sweat, (2) increased respiratory heat and fluid losses caused by the dryness of cold air, and (3) cold-induced diuresis.

Cold-induced diuresis (urination) is a normal physiologic response resulting from skin vasoconstriction from prolonged cold exposure. This is the body's method to reduce body heat loss by shunting blood away from the colder periphery to deeper veins of the body and thus maintain body heat. This response causes a central blood volume expansion, which results in a rise in the mean arterial pressure (MAP), stroke volume, and cardiac output.[33] The expanded blood volume can produce a diuresis, manifested by frequent urination. Cold-induced diuresis can reduce plasma volume by 7% to 15%, resulting in acute dehydration from almost a twofold fluid loss over normal.

FIGURE 9-8   Hydration Guidelines to Minimize Dehydration

1. Start exercise well-hydrated.
Drink 2 to 3 cups (16–24 ounces) of fluid 2 to 3 hours before physical activity to allow excess fluid to be lost as urine. About one half hour before physical activity, drink 5 to 10 ounces. There is no benefit to overconsumption of fluids (hyperhydration), so do not drink excessively.

2. Weigh yourself.
The best way to determine if you have replaced sweat loss during heavy work or exercise is to check to see how much weight you have lost. Determine your body weight before and after physical activity. Minimal weight loss means that you have done a good job staying hydrated. Remember that weight loss during exercise or work is water loss, not fat loss, and must be replaced.

3. Drink during physical activity.
Drink 5 to 10 oz of water or sports electrolyte drink every 10 to 20 minutes during a workout. Heavy sweaters can benefit from drinking more often (e.g., every 10 minutes) and light sweaters should drink less often (every 20+ minutes).

4. Ingest sodium during physical activity.
The best time to begin replacing the sodium lost in sweat is during exercise. That is one reason why a good sports electrolyte drink is better than plain water.

5. Follow your own plan.
Everybody sweats differently, so everybody needs a drinking plan tailored to his or her individual needs.

6. Drink plenty during meals.
If you were not able to drink enough during heavy work or exercise to keep from losing weight, be sure to drink enough before the next practice or returning to work. Mealtime is the best time to do that because of the ease of drinking and the sodium that comes along with food.

7. Do not rely solely on water.
Drinking only water keeps you from replacing the electrolytes lost in sweat and from ingesting carbohydrates that help you work or exercise longer and stronger. Excessive water drinking can lead to dangerous electrolyte disturbances (hyponatremia).

8. Do not overdrink.
Water is definitely a good thing, but you can get too much of a good thing. Drinking large amounts of fluid not only is unnecessary but also can be dangerous (hyponatremia). Bloated stomach, puffy fingers and ankles, a bad headache, and confusion are warning signs of hyponatremia.

9. Do not gain weight during exercise.
A sure sign of drinking too much is weight gain during heavy work or exercise. If you weigh more after work or exercise than you did before, that means that you drank more than you needed. Be sure to cut back the next time so that you do not gain weight.

10. Do not restrict salt in your diet.
Ample salt (sodium chloride) in the diet is essential to replace the salt lost in sweat. Because athletes sweat a lot, their need for salt is much greater than for nonathletes. (This principle holds true for those who work and sweat heavily each day in occupations conducted in moderate to hot environments.)

11. Do not use dehydration to lose weight.
Restricting fluid intake during work or exercise impairs physical performance and increases the risk of heat-related problems. Dehydration should be kept to a minimum by following a wise fluid replacement plan.

12. Do not delay drinking during exercise or work.
Stick to a drinking schedule so that you avoid dehydration early in exercise or work. Once dehydrated, it is almost impossible to catch up to what your body needs because dehydration actually slows the speed at which fluid exits the stomach.

(Modified from Murray B, Eichner ER, Stofan J: Hyponatremia in athletes. *Sports Sci Exchange* 16(1):88, 2003, www.gssiweb.com.)

As with exposure to heat, adherence to fluid hydration guidelines (Figure 9-8) while working in cold environments is necessary to minimize dehydration and the associated fatigue and physical and cognitive changes. Because thirst is suppressed in cold environments, dehydration is a significant risk.

Cold-Related Disorders

Minor Cold-Related Disorders

Contact Freeze Injury. When cold material comes into contact with unprotected skin, it can produce local frostbite immediately. Do not touch any metal surface, alcohol, gasoline, anti-

freeze, ice, or snow with the hands. (See the frostbite section for assessment and management.)

Frostnip. Frostnip is a precursor to *frostbite* and produces reversible signs of skin blanching and numbness in localized tissue. It is typically seen on the face, nose, and ears.[10] Frostnip is a self-limited tissue injury as long as cold exposure does not continue; it does not require prehospital care provider intervention and transport.

Solar Keratitis (Snow Blindness). Without protection from dry air and from exposure to bright reflections on snow, the risk of ultraviolet burns to the skin and eyes increases. This risk is greatly enhanced at higher altitudes. Solar keratitis is insidious during the exposure phase, with corneal burns occurring within 1 hour but not becoming apparent until 6 to 12 hours after exposure.

Management of snow blindness is based on symptoms, which include excessive tearing, pain, redness, swollen eyelids, pain when looking at light, headache, a gritty sensation in the eyes, and decreased (hazy) vision. Prehospital care providers need to consider patching affected eyes if there is no other method to prevent further ultraviolet exposure (e.g., sunglasses), then transport the patient. Medical attention is required to determine the level of severity and the need for antibiotics and analgesics.

Major Cold-Related Disorders

Localized Cutaneous Cold Injury. Cold injuries occur at peripheral sites on the body such as the fingers, toes, ears, and nose and are classified as either freezing (e.g., frostbite) or nonfreezing (e.g., immersion foot) injuries. Localized cold injuries are preventable with proper preparation for cold exposure, early recognition of cold injury, and effective medical care.

It is imperative to recognize, manage, and prevent further tissue freezing in mild to severe forms of freezing injury. Nicotine, alcohol intoxication, homelessness, and major psychiatric disorders remain important predisposing factors.[34] Tight or constricting clothes, too many socks, and tight-fitting footwear are predictable factors in the onset of frostbite. With an increase in adventure sports and other recreational activities conducted in the winter season, localized cold injuries are now seen more often. Prehospital care providers need to prevent body heat loss and protect exposed skin from frostbite in patients during prolonged exposure to cold conditions. For example, in patients needing vehicular extrication, in scenarios resulting in the inability to move the patient, and in patients in cold environments with soft tissue swelling, impaired circulation can lead to an increased incidence of localized cold injury.

Nonfreezing Cold Injury. Nonfreezing cold injury (NFCI), a syndrome also called immersion foot and trench foot, results from damage to peripheral tissues caused by prolonged (hours to days) wet/cold exposure.[35–37] NFCI may coexist with freezing injury such as frostbite. This syndrome primarily involves the feet and is reflected in two types of NFCI. *Trench foot* occurs primarily in military personnel during infantry operations and is related to the combined effects of prolonged cold exposure and restricted circulation in the feet without immersion in water.[35] *Immersion foot* is caused by prolonged immersion of extremities to wet and cool to cold temperatures. Prehospital care providers may see immersion foot in homeless, alcoholic, or elderly persons; hikers and hunters; multiday adventure sport athletes; and ocean survivors.[35,38,39] Often this syndrome goes unrecognized during assessment of individuals who have been exposed to cold or wet conditions because of the lack of formal medical training in NFCI.[35]

This syndrome occurs as a result of many hours of cooling of the lower extremities in temperatures ranging from 32° F to 65° F (0° C–18° C). Soft tissue injury occurs to the skin of the feet, known as *maceration*. The breakdown of the skin will predispose individuals to infection as well. The greatest injury is seen to the peripheral nerves and blood vessels, caused by secondary ischemic injury. Mild NFCI is self-limited initially, but with continued prolonged cold exposure, it becomes irreversible. When the feet are wet and cold, this increases the risk and accelerates the injury because wet socks insulate poorly, and water cools more effectively than air at the same temperature. Any factors that reduce circulation to the extremities also contribute to the injury, such as constrictive clothing, boots, prolonged immobility, hypothermia, and crouched posture.

Assessment. Because the patient has experienced mild or moderate cold exposure, it is essential to rule out hypothermia and assess for dehydration. Even though this is not a freezing injury, NCFI still is an insidious and potentially disabling injury; the common finding with these two localized cold injuries is that the extremity is cooled to the point of anesthesia or numbness while the injury is occurring.

The key to management of NFCI is detection and recognition during assessment. During the initial assessment, injured tissue appears macerated, edematous, pale, anesthetized, pulseless, and immobile, but not frozen. Patients complain of clumsiness and stumbling when attempting to walk. After removal from cold, and during or after rewarming, peripheral blood flow increases as reperfusion of ischemic tissue begins. Extremities change color from white to mottled pale blue while remaining cold and numb. The diagnosis of trench foot or immersion foot is generally made when these signs have not changed after passive rewarming of the feet. From 24 to 36 hours after rewarming, a marked hyperemia (increase in blood flow) develops, along with severe burning pain and reappearance of sensation proximally, but not distally. This is caused by venous vasodilation. Edema and blisters develop in the injured areas as perfusion increases. Skin will remain poorly perfused after hyperemia appears, and the skin is likely to slough as the injury evolves. Any pulselessness in the injured extremity after 48 hours suggests severe, deep injury and a greater chance of substantial tissue loss.

Management. Once a possible NFCI is detected, the priorities are to eliminate any further cooling, prevent further trauma to the extremity, and transport the patient. Do not allow the patient to walk on an injured extremity. Carefully remove the footwear and socks. Cover the injured part or extremity with a loose, dry, sterile dressing; protect it from the cold; and begin passive rewarming of injured tissue during transport. The affected area may be aggravated by the weight of a blanket. No active rewarming is necessary. Do not massage the affected area because this may cause further tissue damage. As needed, treat the patient for dehydration and reassess.

Freezing Cold Injury. On the continuum of further peripheral cold tissue exposure beginning with frostnip, *frostbite* ranges from mild to severe tissue destruction and possibly the loss of tissue.[6,10] The most susceptible body parts for frostbite are those tissues with large surface-to-mass ratios, such as the ears and nose or areas farthest from the body's core, such as the hands, fingers, feet, toes, and male genitalia. The body's normal response to lower-than-desirable temperatures is to reduce blood flow to the skin surface to reduce heat exchange with the environment. The body accomplishes this by vasoconstriction of peripheral blood vessels in an attempt to shunt warm blood to the body's core to maintain a normal body temperature. Reduction of this blood flow greatly reduces the amount of heat delivered to the distal extremities.

The longer the period of exposure to the cold, the more the blood flow is reduced to the periphery. The body conserves core temperature at the expense of extremity and skin temperature. The heat loss from the tissue becomes greater than the heat supplied to that area.

Tissue does not freeze at 32° F (0° C) because cells contain electrolytes and other solutes that prevent tissue from freezing until skin temperature reaches approximately 28° F (−2° C). In cases of below-freezing temperatures when the extremities are left unprotected, the intracellular and extracellular fluids can freeze. This results in the formation of ice crystals. As the ice crystals form, they expand and cause damage to involved cells and tissues. Blood clots may also form, further impairing circulation to the injured area.

The type and duration of cold exposure are the two most important factors in determining the extent of freezing injury. Frostbite is classified by depth of injury and clinical presentation.[10] The degree of injury in many cases will not be known for at least 24 to 72 hours after thawing, except in very minor or severe exposures. Skin exposure to cold that is short in duration but very intense will create a superficial injury, whereas severe frostbite to a whole extremity can occur during prolonged exposures. Direct cold injury is usually reversible, but permanent tissue damage occurs during rewarming. In more severe cases, even with appropriate rewarming of tissue, small blood clots can develop, leading to early signs of gangrene and necrosis. If the injured site freezes, thaws, and then refreezes, the second freezing causes a greater amount of clotting and vascular damage and tissue loss. For this reason, prehospital care providers need to prevent any frozen tissue that thaws during initial field treatment from being subjected to refreezing.

Traditional methods of frostbite classification present four degrees of injury (similar to burns) based on initial physical findings after freezing and rewarming[9] (Figures 9-9 and 9-10).

Although traditional classification of frostbite is by the four degrees of injury, it is easiest for EMS providers in the prehospital setting to classify as either superficial or deep.[40–42] *Superficial frostbite* (first and second degrees) affects the skin and subcutaneous tissues, resulting in clear blisters when

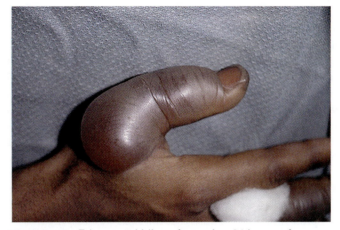

FIGURE 9-9 Edema and blister formation 24 hours after frostbite injury.
(From McCauley RL, Killyon GW, Smith DJ, et al: Frostbite. In Auerbach PS: *Wilderness medicine,* ed 5, St Louis, 2007, Mosby Elsevier. Photograph courtesy Cameron Bangs, MD.)

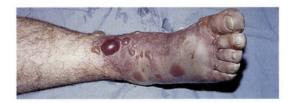

FIGURE 9-10 Deep second-degree and third-degree frostbite with hemorrhagic blebs, 1 day after thawing.
(From McCauley RL, Killyon GW, Smith DJ, et al: Frostbite. In Auerbach PS: *Wilderness medicine,* ed 5, St Louis, 2007, Mosby Elsevier. Photograph courtesy Murray P. Hamlet, DVM.)

rewarmed. *Deep frostbite* (third and fourth degrees) affects skin, muscle, and bone, and the skin has hemorrhagic blisters when rewarmed.

Assessment. On arrival, assess scene safety and then the patient for ABCs. Remove the patient from the cold, and place in an area protected from moisture, cold, and wind. Many frostbite victims may have additional associated medical conditions, such as dehydration, hypovolemia, hypothermia, hypoglycemia, and traumatic injury. Remove any wet clothing to minimize further body heat loss. When in doubt, treat hypothermia first. Superficial frostbite is usually assessed through a combination of recognizing the environmental conditions, locating the patient's chief complaint of pain or numbness, and observing discolored skin in the same area. The environmental conditions during exposure must be below freezing.

Frostbite injuries are insidious because the patient may have no pain at the injury site when skin is frozen and covered by a glove or footwear. Detection of the affected area requires direct visual inspection of highly suspect body regions, as previously listed. Gentle palpation of the area can determine if the underlying tissue is compliant or hard. Ensure that the patient or prehospital care provider does not rub or massage the affected skin, because this will cause further cellular damage to frozen tissues. The patient with superficial freezing will usually complain of discomfort during the manipulation of the frostbitten area. In patients with deep frostbite the frozen tissue will be hard and usually is not painful when touched. After inspection of the affected area, a decision is necessary about the method of rewarming, which is usually based on transport time to the emergency department. The State of Alaska EMS protocol for frostbite rewarming in the prehospital phase states the following:[43]

1. If transport time is short (1–2 hours at most) then the risks posed by improper rewarming or refreezing in the prehospital phase outweigh the risks for delaying treatment for deep frostbite.
2. If transport time will be prolonged (more than 1–2 hours) frostbite will often thaw spontaneously. It is more important to prevent hypothermia than to rewarm frostbite rapidly in warm water. This does not mean that a frostbitten extremity should be kept in the cold to prevent spontaneous rewarming. Anticipate that frostbitten areas will rewarm as a consequence of keeping the patient warm and protect them from refreezing at all costs.

Management. Patients with superficial frostnip or frostbite should be placed with the affected area against a warm body surface, such as covering the patient's ears with warm hands or placing affected fingers into armpits (axillae) or groin regions. Superficial frostbite only needs to be warmed at normal body temperatures. Management of deep frostbite in the prehospital setting includes the following:

1. Assess and treat the patient for hypothermia, if present.
2. Provide supportive care and appropriate shelter for the patient and the affected part to minimize heat loss.
3. Assess frostbite area, remove any clothing and jewelry from the affected area, and check for loss of sensation.
4. If there is frostbite distal to a fracture, attempt to align the limb unless there is resistance. Splint the fracture in a manner that does not compromise distal circulation.
5. Cover with a loose, dry, sterile dressing that is noncompressive and nonadherent.
6. Do not allow the patient to walk on affected feet.
7. Fingers and toes should be separated by and protected with sterile cotton gauze.
8. Do not drain blisters.
9. Hands and feet should be splinted and elevated to reduce edema.
10. Protect fragile tissues from further trauma during patient movement.
11. *Attempts to begin rewarming of deep frostbite patients in the field can be hazardous to the patient's eventual recovery and are not recommended unless prolonged transport times are involved.* If prolonged transport is involved, thaw in warm water bath at a temperature no

greater than 102° F (>39° C) on the affected area (if refreezing is a concern, do not thaw).
12. Do not allow the thawed part to thaw and refreeze.
13. Ensure early transport to an appropriate facility.

The patient can drink something warm (and nonalcoholic) if it is available, depending on the patient's LOC and other injuries. Tobacco use (smoking, chewing, using nicotine patches) should be discouraged because nicotine causes further vasoconstriction.

Accidental Hypothermia. Hypothermia is defined as the condition in which the core body temperature is below 95° F (35° C), as measured by a rectal thermometer placed at least 6 inches (15 cm) into the rectum.[11] Hypothermia can be viewed as a decrease in core temperature that renders a victim unable to generate sufficient heat production to return to homeostasis or normal bodily functions. Hypothermia can occur in many different situations, resulting from cold ambient air, cold-water immersion, or cold-water submersion (cold-water near-drowning), and can be intentionally induced during surgery.[11,43,44] Immersion ("head out") hypothermia typically occurs when an individual is accidentally placed into a cold environment without preparation or planning. For example, a person who has fallen into ice water is immediately in danger of becoming a submersion casualty, resulting from "cold shock" gasp reflex, loss of motor skills, hypothermia, and drowning. These unique aspects of submersion incidents can lead to hypoxia and hypothermia (see later discussion).

Unlike frostbite, hypothermia can occur in environments with temperatures well above freezing. *Primary hypothermia* generally occurs when healthy individuals are in adverse weather conditions and are unprepared for overwhelming acute or chronic cold exposure. Deaths by primary hypothermia are a direct result of cold exposure and are documented by the medical examiner as accidental, homicides, or suicides.[11]

Secondary hypothermia is considered a normal consequence of a patient's systemic disorders, including hypothyroidism, hypoadrenalism, trauma, carcinoma, and sepsis. If unrecognized or improperly treated, hypothermia can be fatal, in some cases within 2 hours. Mortality is greater than 50% in cases of secondary hypothermia caused by complications of other injuries and in severe cases in which the core body temperature is below 89.6° F (32° C).[11]

Rapid attention by the prehospital care provider to preventing further body heat loss in the traumatic patient is needed because mild hypothermia is very common after injury in all weather conditions. Therefore, the trauma patient should be moved off of cold ground as soon as possible and placed in a warm ambulance. The temperature in the ambulance should be adjusted to minimize heat loss from the patient and not for the comfort of the provider. Warmed IV fluids provided by ALS personnel will also help to maintain the patient's body temperature.

Immersion Hypothermia. When immersion occurs in cold water (temperature < 91° F [33° C]), the immediate physiologic changes are a rapid decline in skin temperature; peripheral vasoconstriction resulting in shivering; and increased metabolism, ventilation, heart rate, cardiac output, and blood pressure. To offset any heat loss in water, heat production must occur by increasing physical activity, shivering, or both. If not, core temperature continues to fall and shivering ceases, and these physiologic responses decrease proportionally with the fall in core temperature.[44]

The greatest risk of immersion hypothermia usually begins in water temperature colder than 77° F (25 °C).[45] Because the heat dissipation capacity of water is 24 times greater than that of air, individuals are at risk for more rapid hypothermia in water. However, continued physical activity, such as swimming to keep warm, in cold water will eventually become a detriment by increasing convective heat loss to the colder water surrounding the body, resulting in a faster onset of hypothermia. This understanding has lead to the recommendation for individuals to minimize heat loss during cold-water immersion by using the *heat escape lessening posture* (HELP) or the *huddle position* when multiple immersion victims are together[45] (Figure 9-11).

The lowest recorded core temperature for an infant with an intact neurologic recovery from accidental hypothermia is 59° F (15° C).[46] In an adult, 56.8° F (13.7° C) is the lowest recorded core temperature for a survivor of accidental hypothermia. This occurred in a 29-year-old female who struggled to self-rescue for more than 40 minutes before symptoms of severe hypothermia affected muscular contraction.[47] She was immersed for more than 80 minutes before a rescue team arrived, and cardiopulmonary resuscitation (CPR) was initiated during transport to a local hospital. After 3 hours of continuous rewarming, her core temperature returned to normal, and she survived with normal physiologic function.

This case of accidental hypothermia illustrates why all prehospital care providers managing hypothermic patients should not stop treatment interventions and declare the patient dead until they have been rewarmed to over 95° F (>35° C) and still have no evidence of cardiorespiratory and neurologic function. The lessons from this case and others with a similar outcome are that the initial impression of these patients as likely being dead is not sufficient justification to withhold basic or advanced life support. This is the reason the following phrase was coined: **"Patients are not dead until they are warm and dead."**

Pathophysiologic Effects of Hypothermia on the Body. Whether from exposure to a cold environment or immersion, the influence of hypothermia on the body affects all major organ systems, particularly the cardiac, renal, and central nervous systems. As the body's core temperature decreases to 95° F (35° C), maximal vasoconstriction, shivering, and metabolic rate occurs, with increases in heart rate, respiration, and blood pressure. Cerebral metabolism oxygen demand decreases and

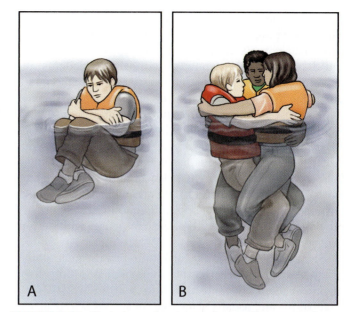

FIGURE 9-11 Techniques for decreasing cooling rates of survivors in cold water. **A,** Heat escape lessening posture (HELP). **B,** Huddle technique.

cerebral metabolism is preserved. When core temperature falls to between 86° F (30° C) and 95° F (35° C), cognitive function, cardiac function, metabolic rate, respiratory rate, and shivering rate are all significantly decreased or completely inhibited. At this point, the limited physiologic defensive mechanisms to prevent heat loss from the body are overwhelmed and core temperature falls rapidly. At a core temperature of 85° F (29.5° C), cardiac output and metabolic rate are reduced approximately 50%. Ventilation and perfusion are inadequate and do not keep up with the metabolic demand, causing cellular hypoxia, increased lactic acid, and an eventual metabolic and respiratory acidosis. Oxygenation and blood flow are maintained in the core and brain.

Bradycardia (slow heart rate) occurs in a large percentage of patients as a direct effect of cold on the heart.

When the core temperature reaches 80° F to 82° F (26.7° C–28° C), any physical stimulation of the heart can cause ventricular fibrillation (VF) or cardiac arrest. CPR or rough handling (patient assessment and movement) of the patient could be sufficient to cause VF. At these extremely low core temperatures, pulse and blood pressure are not detectable and the joints are stiff. The pupils become fixed and dilated at extremely low core temperatures. Again, a patient should not be assumed to be dead until he or she is rewarmed and still has no signs of life (as determined by electrocardiogram [ECG], pulse, ventilation, and CNS function).

Assessment. It is imperative to assess scene safety on arrival. All responders need to ensure their own safety and protection from cold exposure while working in this environment. There should be a high suspicion for hypothermia even when the environmental conditions are not highly suggestive (e.g., wind, moisture, temperature). Some patients may present with vague complaints of fatigue, lethargy, nausea, vomiting, and dizziness. With trauma and critically ill patients, it is important to begin assessment and assume hypothermia by protecting the patient from the cold environment; assessment starts with the ABCs. Neurologic function is assessed and monitored frequently. Severely hypothermic patients generally present with slow breathing (bradypnea), stupor, and coma. Rectal temperatures are not usually assessed in the field or widely used as a vital sign in most prehospital systems. To accurately measure hypothermic temperatures, a low-range rectal thermometer is often necessary. Figure 9-12 provides the anticipated physiologic responses with decreasing core temperature.

Signs of shivering and mental status change are important in the assessment of suspected hypothermia. Mildly hypothermic patients (core temperature > 90° F [32° C]) will be shivering and usually show signs of altered LOC (e.g., confusion, slurred speech, altered gait, clumsiness). They will be slow in their actions and are usually found in a non-ambulatory state, sitting or lying. Law enforcement personnel and prehospital care providers may misinterpret this condition as drug or alcohol intoxication or as cerebrovascular accident (CVA, stroke) in elderly patients. However, a patient's LOC is not a reliable indicator of the degree of hypothermia; some patients have remained conscious at core temperature below 80° F (27° C).

When the patient's core temperature falls below 90° F (32° C), moderate hypothermia is present, and the patient will probably not complain of feeling cold. Shivering will be absent, and the patient's LOC will be greatly decreased, possibly to the point of unconsciousness and coma. The patient's pupils will react slowly or may be dilated and fixed. The patient's palpable pulses may be diminished or absent, and systolic blood pressure may be low or indeterminate. The patient's ventilations may have slowed to as few as 2 breaths/minute. As the heart becomes progressively colder and more irritable at about 82° F (28° C), cardiac arrest is observed more often. Because of the changes in cerebral metabolism, evidence of "paradoxical undressing" may be observed before the patient loses consciousness. This is an attempt by the patient to remove clothing while in the cold environment, and it is thought to represent a response to an impending thermoregulatory failure.

Management. Prehospital care of the hypothermic patient consists of preventing further heat loss, gentle handling, initiating rapid transport, and rewarming. This includes moving the patient away from any cold source to a warm ambulance or to a warm shelter if transportation is not immediately available (see Prolonged Transport section). Wet clothing should be removed by cutting with trauma shears to avoid unnecessary movement and agitation of the patient. Concern for initiating cardiac arrest based on the handling of the patient should not delay any critical interventions. This concern becomes more

realistic in severe hypothermic patients (<86° F [30° C]). The patient's head and body should be covered with warm blankets or sleeping bags, followed by an outer windproof layer to prevent convective and evaporative heat loss.

If the patient is conscious and alert, the patient should avoid alcohol and caffeine drinks. Hypothermic patients need high-flow oxygen because they have decreased oxygen delivery to the tissues. High-flow oxygen should be delivered using a non-rebreather mask or bag-mask device. Ideally, the patient may benefit more if the oxygen can be warmed and humidified (108° F–115° F [42° C–46° C]). Hot packs or massaging of the patient's extremities are not recommended. Typically, active external rewarming occurs only to the thoracic region, with no active rewarming of the extremities. This will prevent increased peripheral circulation, causing an increased amount of colder blood returning from the extremities to the thorax before central core rewarming. Increased return of peripheral blood can actually decrease the core temperature ("afterdrop"). This complicates resuscitation and may precipitate cardiac arrest.

National Guidelines for Treatment of Cold-Related Disorders

Emergency Cardiovascular Care: Basic Lifesaving Guidelines for Management of Hypothermia

Guidelines for resuscitation of the hypothermic patient have evolved over many decades. The most recent revision of the Emergency Cardiovascular Care (ECC) guidelines published in 2010 by the American Heart Association (AHA) represents the latest findings.[48]

Basic Life Support Guidelines for Treatment of Mild to Severe Hypothermia

Hypothermic patients should be kept in a horizontal position at all times to avoid aggravating hypotension because these patients are often dehydrated. It may be difficult to feel or detect respiration and a pulse in the hypothermic patient. Therefore, it is recommended initially to assess for breathing and then a pulse to confirm one of the following:

- Respiratory arrest
- Pulseless cardiac arrest
- Bradycardia (requiring CPR)

If the patient is not breathing, start rescue breathing immediately. Start chest compressions immediately in any hypothermic patient who is pulseless and has no detectable signs of circulation.[48] If there is a doubt about detecting a pulse, begin compressions. Never withhold basic life support (BLS) interventions until the patient is rewarmed. If the patient is determined to be in cardiac arrest, use the current BLS guidelines, as outlined elsewhere.

An automated external defibrillator (AED) should be used to determine if pulseless ventricular tachycardia or VF is

FIGURE 9-12   Physiologic Characteristics of Hypothermia

°C	°F	Characteristics	°C	°F	Characteristics
37.6	99.6 ±1	Normal rectal temperature	28.0	82.4	Decreased ventricular fibrillation threshold; 50% decrease in oxygen consumption and pulse Hypoventilation
37.0	98.6 ±1	Normal oral temperature	27.0	80.6	Loss of reflexes and voluntary motion
36.0	96.8	Increase in metabolic rate and blood pressure and preshivering muscle tone	26.0	78.8	Major acid–base disturbances No reflexes or response to pain
35.0	95.0	Urine temperature 34.8° C; maximum shivering thermogenesis	25.0	77.0	Cerebral blood flow one third of normal Loss of cerebrovascular autoregulation Cardiac output 45% of normal Pulmonary edema may develop
34.0	93.2	Amnesia, difficulty speaking, poor judgment, and maladaptive behavior develop Normal blood pressure; maximum respiratory stimulation Tachycardia, then progressive bradycardia	24.0	75.2	Significant hypotension and bradycardia
33.3	91.4	Ataxia and apathy develop Linear depression of cerebral metabolism Tachypnea, then progressive decrease in respiratory minute volume Cold diuresis	23.0	73.4	No corneal or oculocephalic reflexes; areflexia
			22.0	71.6	Maximum risk of ventricular fibrillation; 75% decrease in oxygen consumption
32.0	89.6	Stupor; 25% decrease in oxygen consumption	20.0	68.0	Lowest resumption of cardiac electromechanical activity; pulse 20% of normal
31.0	87.8	Extinguished shivering thermogenesis	19.0	66.2	Electroencephalographic silencing
30.0	86.0	Atrial fibrillation and other arrhythmias develop Pupils and cardiac output two thirds of normal Insulin ineffective	18.0	64.4	Asystole
			15.0	59.0	Lowest infant accidental hypothermia survival
29.0	84.2	Progressive decrease in level of consciousness, pulse, and respiration Pupils dilated; paradoxical undressing	13.7	56.8	Lowest adult accidental hypothermia survival
			10.0	50.0	92% decrease in oxygen consumption
			9.0	48.2	Lowest therapeutic hypothermia survival

(Modified from Danzl DF: Accidental hypothermia. In Auerbach PS: *Wilderness medicine,* ed 5, St Louis, 2007, Mosby Elsevier.)

present. If a shockable rhythm is determined, give one shock, then continue CPR. If the hypothermic patient does not respond to one shock with a detectable pulse, further attempts to defibrillate the patient may or may not be successful. Efforts directed toward effective CPR with an emphasis on rewarming the patient should be undertaken. Repeat attempts at defibrillation may be attempted as per BLS protocols though they may not be effective until body temperature rises to more than 86° F (>30° C).[49] When performing chest compression in a hypothermic patient, a greater force is required because the chest wall is stiff when cold.[50] The importance of not declaring a patient dead until he or she has been rewarmed and remains unresponsive is even greater today, with new evidence from studies of hypothermic patients indicating that cold exerts a protective effect on the vital organs.[50,51]

Finally, BLS procedures performed in the field should be withheld only in patients with injuries incompatible with life, if the body is frozen such that chest compressions are impossible, or if the mouth and nose are blocked with ice.[11,48]

Prolonged Transport

At times, the location of a patient will result in a delay in transport or a prolonged transport to an appropriate facility, necessitating extended prehospital care. Consequently, EMS providers may need to consider management options beyond what would be used with a rapid transport. How the patient is managed will depend on the time to definitive care, approved medical protocols, equipment and supplies on hand, additional personnel and resources, and location of the patient and severity of the injuries.

As with all patient care, it is understood that the first priorities are scene safety, ABCDEs, and the use of standard assessment and management procedures appropriate to these environments. If medical control is available, always obtain a consult early, and communicate routinely throughout the extended care period. Any of the procedures listed that fall outside the scope of practice are to be used by other, credentialed medical providers.

Also, it is important to know that all agencies have established guidelines for discontinuation of CPR. The Wilderness Medical Society recommends that once CPR is initiated, it should be continued until resuscitation is successful with an awake patient, rescuers are exhausted, rescuers are placed in danger, the patient is turned over to more definitive care, or the patient does not respond to prolonged (30 minutes) resuscitative efforts.[52] The National Association of EMS Physicians also provides guidelines for the termination of CPR in the prehospital environment (see Chapter 3).[53] If medical control is available, begin patient consult early, if possible, for consideration of CPR termination after a total time of 20 minutes, depending on special patient circumstances (e.g., cold-water submersion, lightning strike) in which CPR may be extended longer than 20 to 30 minutes.[52]

Heat-Related Illness

Heatstroke

Guidelines for prolonged transport of a patient with heatstroke are as follows:

- Provide whole-body cooling as quickly as possible. Think about using any available access to water. Immersion of the body to neck level in cool water (maintain body control and protect the airway) is the fastest way to lower temperature but is not practical in the field; therefore, field management involves spraying the whole body with water (e.g., IV fluids, saline, water bottles, water from hydration backpacks). In addition, provide a source of continuous wind current (e.g., natural wind current, fanning with towel, fire ventilation fans).
- When possible, maintain communication to keep medical control informed of patient status and to receive further medical directions.
- Stop body cooling when the rectal temperature reaches 102° F (39° C). Then protect the patient from shivering and hypothermia.
- As you are cooling the patient, manage the airway in unresponsive patients and initiate good ventilation with the bag-mask device with high-flow oxygen. Patients should have vital signs assessed at regular intervals. Place the patient in the recovery position, and continue assessment to include level of consciousness and vital signs. Provide supportive care and basic bodily needs throughout the remaining extended care period.

Cold-Related Illness

Frostbite

Guidelines for prolonged transport of a patient with frostbite are as follows:

- In a situation of significant transport delay, active rewarming should be considered. Rapid, active rewarming can

reverse the direct injury of ice crystals in tissues, but it may not change the injury severity.[10] It is critical to keep the thawed tissue from refreezing because this significantly worsens the outcome compared with passive thawing. Thus, when and where to begin active rewarming becomes critical in the decision making, if it is to be done at all.

- A standard rewarming procedure is to immerse the affected extremity in circulating water warmed to between 99° F and 102° F (37° C–39° C) in a container large enough to accommodate the frostbitten tissues without them touching the sides or bottom of the container.[54] Water should feel warm, but not hot, to the normal hand. (Note that this new temperature range is lower than previously recommended because this temperature range decreases pain for the patient while only slightly slowing the rewarming phase). If available, an oral or rectal thermometer should be used to measure water temperature. A temperature below that recommended will thaw tissue but is less beneficial for rapid thawing and for tissue survival. Any greater temperature will cause greater pain and may cause a burn injury.[10] Avoid active rewarming with intense sources of dry heat (e.g., placing near campfire). Continue immersion until tissue is soft and pliable, which may take up to 30 minutes. Active motion of the extremity during immersion is beneficial, without directed rubbing or massaging of the affected part.
- Extreme pain is experienced during rapid thawing. Provide ibuprofen, 400 mg orally every 12 hours. Aspirin may be given if ibuprofen is not available, although the optimal dosage regimen has not been determined. (Aspirin is contraindicated in pediatric patients because of the risk of Reye's syndrome.)
- The return of normal skin color, warmth, and sensation in the affected part are all favorable signs. Dry all affected parts with warm air (do not towel dry affected parts) and, ideally, apply topical aloe vera on skin; place sterile gauze between toes or fingers; and bandage, splint, and elevate extremity. Cover any extremity with insulating material, and wrap a windproof and waterproof material (e.g., trash bag) as the outer layer, particularly if continuing patient extraction outdoors to a transport location.

Hypothermia

Guidelines for prolonged transport of a patient with hypothermia are as follows:

- Start active rewarming procedures. The key point is to prevent further heat loss.
- Shivering is the single best way for rewarming mildly hypothermic patients in the prehospital setting compared with external methods for rewarming. Hypothermic patients who are able to shiver maximally can increase core temperature by up to 6° to 8° F ($\approx$3° C–4° C) per hour. External heat sources are often used but

may provide only minimal benefit.[44] For the moderately to severely hypothermic patient, these remain important considerations in the extended-care situation when used in combination with the hypothermia insulation wrap.

- External heat sources include the following:
  1. Warmed (maximum 108° F (42° C)), humidified oxygen by mask can prevent heat loss during ventilation and provide some heat transfer to the chest from the respiratory tract.
  2. Body-to-body contact has merit for heat transfer, but many studies fail to show any advantage except in mildly hypothermic patients.
  3. Electric and portable heating pads provide no additional advantage.
  4. Forced-air warming has some benefit in minimizing post-cooling core temperature ("afterdrop"); it provides an effective warming rate comparable to shivering for mildly hypothermic patients.

- Insulate all hypothermic patients in the remote setting to minimize heat loss. Prepare a multilayer hypothermia wrap. Place a large, waterproof plastic sheet on the floor or ground. Add an insulation layer of blankets or a sleeping bag on top of the waterproof layer. Lay the patient on top of the insulation layer along with any external heat sources. Add a second insulating layer on top of the patient. The left side of the hypothermia wrap is folded over the patient first, then the right side. The patient's head is covered to prevent heat loss, keeping an opening at the face to allow patient assessment.

On the Job

Exposure to heat is a concern not only for the patient populations already mentioned, but also for field providers who will be working in elevated temperatures. The heat stress index

(Figure 9-13) illustrates how temperature and humidity combine to create moderate-heat or high-heat stress conditions.

Be alert for heat stress when radiant heat from the sun or nearby flames is high, when the air is still, or when you are working hard, creating large amounts of metabolic heat.

Some organizations use the WBGT heat stress index (Figure 9-14). The index, which is often available locally from the National Weather Service, uses dry bulb, wet bulb, and black globe temperatures. The temperatures are weighted to indicate the impact of each measure on the worker:

- *Wet bulb* (humidity) accounts for 70%
- *Black globe* (radiant heat and air movement) accounts for 20%
- *Dry bulb* (air temperature) accounts for 10%

Heat stress indexes do not take into account the effects of long hours of hard work and dehydration, or the impact of personal protective clothing and equipment.

When heat stress conditions exist, you must modify the way you work or exercise. Pace yourself. There are individual differences in fitness, acclimatization, and heat tolerance. Push too hard and you will be a candidate for a heat disorder.

When possible:

- Avoid working close to heat sources
- Do harder work during cooler morning and evening hours
- Change tools or tasks to minimize fatigue
- Take frequent rest breaks
- Most important, maintain hydration by replacing lost fluids.

Hydration

Maintaining body fluids is essential for sweating and the removal of internal heat generated during physical activities. To minimize dehydration and the risk of heat illness,

Temperature (°F) versus Relative Humidity (%)						
°F	90%	80%	70%	60%	50%	40%
80	85	84	82	81	80	79
85	101	96	92	90	86	84
90	121	113	105	99	94	90
95		133	122	113	105	98
100			142	129	118	109
105				148	133	121
110						135

High	Possible Heat Disorder
80°F - 90°F	Fatigue possible with prolonged exposure and physical activity.
90°F - 105°F	Sunstroke, heat cramps, and heat exhaustion possible.
105°F - 130°F	Sunstroke, heat cramps, and heat exhaustion likely, and heatstroke possible.
130°F or greater	Heatstroke highly likely with continued exposure.

Due to the nature of the heat index calculation, the values in the tables have an error +/– 1.3° F

FIGURE 9-13 Heat stress index.
(Courtesy National Weather Service, Pueblo, CO, www.crh.noaa.gov/pub/heat.htm.)

FIGURE 9-14   Fluid Replacement Guidelines for Warm Weather Training

Heat Category	WBGT Index (° F)	Easy Work		Moderate Work		Hard Work	
		Work/Rest (min)	Water Intake (qt/hr)	Work/Rest (min)	Water Intake (qt/hr)	Work/Rest (min)	Water Intake (qt/hr)
1	78–81.9	NL	½	NL	¾	40/20	¾
2	82–84.9	NL	½	50/10	¾	30/30	1
3	85–87.9	NL	¾	40/20	¾	30/30	1
4	88–89.9	NL	¾	30/30	¾	20/40	1
5	>90	50/10	1	20/40	1	10/50	1

NL, No limit to work time per hour. *Rest* means minimal physical activity (sitting or standing), accomplished in shade if possible.
The work/rest times and fluid replacement volumes will sustain performance and hydration for at least 4 hours of work in the specified heat category. Individual water needs will vary ± 1 quart per hour.
Caution: Hourly fluid intake should not exceed 1.5 quarts. Daily fluid intake should not exceed 12 quarts.
Wearing body armor: add 5° F to WBGT index in humid climates.
Wearing personal protective equipment (PPE) over garment: add 10° F to WBGT index for easy work and 20° F for moderate and hard work.

Easy Work	Moderate Work	Hard Work
Walking on hard surface at 2.5 mph, less than 31-pound load	Walking on hard surface at 3.5 mph, less than 41-pound load Walking in loose sand at 2.5 mph, no load Calisthenics	Walking on hard surface at 3.5 mph, more than 40-pound load Walking in loose sand at 2.5 mph with load

(Current version of WBGT, hydration, and work/rest guidelines as updated by U.S. Army Research Institute for Environmental Medicine [USARIEM] and published by Montain SJ, Latzka WA, Sawka MN: *Mil Med* 164:502, 1999.)

you must hydrate before, during, and after exercise or physical work. Individual characteristics (e.g., body weight, genetic predisposition, heat acclimatization state, and metabolic state) will influence sweat rate for a given activity. These factors will result in large individual sweat rates and total sweat loss. For example, long distance running is known to cause an average sweat rate of 1.8 liters per hour (1.0–2.6 L/hour) in summer months, where football players (large body mass and wearing protective gear) are known to sweat on average 2.1 liters per hour (1.1–3.2 L/hour) and up to 8.8 L/day.[55] There needs to be a commitment to frequent hydration breaks to ensure dehydration does not exceed greater than 2% of body weight (based on preactivity nude body weight) throughout the duration of physical activity.

Before work, you should take extra fluids to prepare for the heat. Drink 1 to 2 cups of water, juice, or a sport drink before work. Avoid excess caffeine. It hastens fluid loss in the urine. There is no physiologic advantage to consume excessively large amounts of fluid prior to physical activity. The American College of Sports Medicine (ACSM) now recommends to prehydrate slowly several hours before a physical activity and consume approximately 5 to 7 mL/kg of body weight. The goal is to produce urine output that is clear to straw colored in appearance and prevent starting an activity in a dehydrated state.

While working, take several fluid breaks every hour, drinking approximately 1 quart of fluid per hour. Individual sweat rates will vary as will the amount of water needed to consume per hour. Caution should be used to prevent consumption of excessive fluids greater than 1.5 L/hour for prolonged periods unless you have determined your individualized sweat loss rate per hour. ACSM now recommends a starting point of 0.4 to 0.8 L on average per hour for exercise activities (e.g., marathon running); adjust the amount consumed based on individual lower or higher sweat rates for activities in cool or warm temperature conditions, and for lighter or heavier individuals.[55] Water is your greatest need during work in the heat. Studies show that workers drink more when lightly flavored beverages are available. Providing a portion of fluid replacement with a carbohydrate/electrolyte sport beverage will help you retain fluids and maintain energy and electrolyte levels. Unfortunately, many sports drinks contain large amounts of sugar, which can actually slow absorption of ingested fluid.

After work, you need to continue drinking to replace fluid losses. To achieve rapid and complete recovery from activities resulting in large sweat loss, such as firefighting, drink approximately 1.5 L of fluids for each kilogram of body weight loss.[55] *Thirst always underestimates fluid needs,* so you should drink more than you think you need. Rehydration is enhanced when fluids contain sodium and potassium, or when foods with these electrolytes are consumed along with the fluid.

Sodium lost in sweat is easily replaced at meals with liberal use of the salt shaker. Unacclimatized workers lose more salt in the heat, so they need to pay particular attention to salt replacement. Do not overdo salt intake; too much salt impairs temperature regulation. Excessive salt can cause stomach distress, fatigue, and other problems.

Make potassium-rich foods such as bananas and citrus fruits a regular part of your diet, and drink lots of lemonade, orange juice, or tomato juice. Limit the amount of caffeine drinks such as coffee and colas because caffeine increases fluid loss in the urine. Avoid alcoholic drinks. They also cause dehydration. Avoid sharing water bottles except in emergencies.

You can reassess your hydration by observing the volume, color, and concentration of your urine; low volumes of dark, concentrated urine and painful urination indicate a serious need for rehydration. Other signs of dehydration include a rapid heart rate, weakness, excessive fatigue, and dizziness. Rapid loss of several pounds of body weight is a certain sign of dehydration. Rehydrate before returning to work. Continuing to work in a dehydrated state can lead to serious consequences, including heatstroke, muscle breakdown, and kidney failure.

Clothing

Personal protective clothing strikes a balance between protection and worker comfort. Australian researchers have concluded that *the task for personnel wearing personal protection equipment is not to keep heat out, but to let it out.* About 70% of the heat load comes from within, from metabolic heat generated during hard work. Only 30% comes from the environment and the fire. Wear loose-fitting garments to enhance air movement. Wear cotton T-shirts and underwear to help sweat evaporate. Avoid extra layers of clothing that insulate, restrict air movement, and contribute to heat stress.

Individual Differences

Individuals differ in their response to heat. Some workers are at greater risk for heat disorders. The reasons include inherited differences in heat tolerance and sweat rate. Excess body weight raises metabolic heat production. Illness, drugs, and medications can also influence your body's response to work in a hot environment. Check with your physician or pharmacist if you are using prescription or over-the-counter medications, or if you have a medical condition.

You should always train and work with a partner who can help in the event of a problem. Remind each other to drink lots of fluids, and watch each other. If your partner develops a heat disorder, start treatment immediately.

SUMMARY

Prevention
- Improve or maintain aerobic fitness.
- Acclimate to the heat.

On the Job
- Be aware of conditions (temperature, humidity, air movement).
- Take frequent rest breaks.
- Avoid extra layers of clothing.
- Pace yourself.

Hydrate
- The hydration goal is to prevent dehydration (sweat loss) of greater than 2% of nude body weight.
- Before work, drink several cups of water, juice, or a sport drink.

- During work, take frequent fluid breaks.
- After work, keep drinking to ensure rehydration.
- Remember, only you can prevent dehydration.

Partners
- Always work and train with a partner.

Drinks
- Sport drinks with carbohydrates (no more than 6%–8%; approximately 30–60 grams/hour) and electrolytes (e.g., sodium 20–50 mEq/L) encourage fluid intake, provide energy, and diminish urinary water loss. The carbohydrates also help maintain immune function and mental performance during prolonged arduous work. Drinks with caffeine and alcohol interfere with rehydration by increasing urine production.[32]

SCENARIO 1 SOLUTION

This 76-year-old female patient has mild to moderate Alzheimer's disease. Individuals with this disease are subject to wandering and may experience bouts of hallucination and psychosis. If not found within 24 hours, these patients have a high mortality rate caused by dehydration and hypothermia, or drowning. There is a greater rate of fatality when these patients are exposed to high temperature or in cold and rainy climates. These patients can have narrowing of their vision resulting in poor peripheral field of view that corresponds with a trademark behavior of moving straight forward until they reach some form of barrier, such as a fence, bushes, briars, drainage, or sources of water. It is not uncommon for these patients who have been recently relocated to attempt to return to their previous residence even though they are not sure of the direction. Approach these patients from the front with good eye contact and move slowly to their side. Speak to them in slow and simple terms. Use of forceful directions and arguing will be not beneficial and may lead to an undesirable patient reaction. After initial rapid ABCs and assessing for all primary and secondary illness or injury, think about "E," or environment, early because this patient has been exposed for many hours in approximately 16° F (−9° C) wind chill temperature, which accelerates convective body heat loss along with conductive heat loss when lying or sitting on a cold surface such as a bench, a rock, or the ground. A quick decision is necessary to get some protective material under and on top of the patient to slow down body heat transfer if there are any delays getting the victim onto a stretcher and into a heated ambulance. Do not delay transport waiting for a paramedic unit to arrive on scene since you can rendezvous en route to the hospital unless it is a very short transport time. Furthermore, do not delay patient transport to the hospital in the attempt to provide any means of active rewarming, because these attempts will have limited benefit to rewarm the patient. In regions with prolonged transport, if available, provide warm humidified oxygen (maximum 108° F [42° C]) and thoroughly surround the victim in a hypothermia wrap—that is, multiple blankets surrounding the patient with a vapor-barrier tarp (wind-water–proof outer layer) from head to toe. Gently handle all hypothermic patients; aggressive movement can trigger cardiac arrest because the heart is irritable when cold. Provide supportive care with high flow. Remember that all hypothermic victims are not considered dead until they have been rewarmed and declared dead at the hospital. ■

Drowning and Lightning

SCENARIO 2

At 4:15 PM on a hot and humid summer afternoon, you are called to assist an unconscious male on the 18th hole at the city country club. A fast-moving thunderstorm passed through the country club less than 15 minutes ago with rain, hail, and lightning. As you arrive on the 18th hole, you observe one golfer lying on the fairway and another golfer sitting against a nearby tree, along with a number of bystanders in the area. The scene now appears safe, with one downed large tree branch and dark thunderclouds moving fast eastward. As you prepare to assess the victims, an uninjured golfer from the foursome states that a thunderstorm approached the area rapidly with high winds, heavy rain, and severe lightning and thunder. The two injured golfers ran for cover at the base of a large tree and two others ran to the clubhouse nearby. Apparently, lightning struck the tree, traveled down the trunk, and hit the ground near the two huddled golfers. He initially thought they both were hit by lightning; one looked dead, the other looked injured and dazed.

Is the scene safe?

How would you begin to immediately assess these two patients?

What are your priorities for triage? How would you assess and manage lightning injuries?

What is the underlying medical concern for lightning strike victims?

Are there other primary or secondary injuries to consider in this scenario?

ach year in the United States, significant injury and death are caused by a variety of environmental conditions, including drowning or near-drowning, lightning, recreational scuba diving, and high altitude. This section will address the most common of these—drowning and near-drowning and lightning.

Drowning or Near-Drowning

Submersion incidents in water that lead to injury are all too common in the United States and the world. Drowning remains a leading cause of preventable death across all age groups[56] but is an epidemic in children.[57] The World Health Organization estimates that there are more than 400,000 deaths annually from unintentional submersion incidents, not including deaths from drowning resulting from floods, suicide, or homicide.[58] Submersion injuries have a substantial cost to society; an estimated $450 to $650 million or more is spent on these patients each year in the United States alone.[59]

The definitions for drowning and near-drowning are as follows [60–63]:

- **Drowning:** death within 24 hours of the submersion incident.
- **Near-drowning:** surviving for at least 24 hours after the submersion.

Because resuscitative care at the scene is initiated for all water-related casualties, it may be more practical to avoid using these two terms and instead use the term *submersion incident*, which encompasses drowning *and* near-drowning. Furthermore, the term *submersion incident* implies no particular outcome of the patient at the scene, en route to the hospital, or later at the hospital. This should help prevent providers of all types from making any judgment on withholding resuscitative efforts based on the mechanism of injury, length of submersion, water temperature, or the patient who presents without vital signs.[64] This last point is critical because there are numerous reports of those who have survived prolonged periods (>30 minutes) of cold-water submersion.[47,65–66] Immediate and effective delivery of CPR and the activation of EMS by bystanders are two important factors that influence the survival of a submersion patient.[67]

Prevention strategies are vital in the effort to lower the rates of submersion incidents in the United States. Many education programs are emphasizing the reduction of unintentional water entry of infants and children by encouraging the installation of various types of barriers around pools (e.g., isolation fences, pool covers, alarms, etc.) and the use of personal flotation devices such as life vests. Furthermore, CPR initiated by a bystander before the arrival of prehospital care personnel is associated with improved patient prognosis.[68]

Epidemiology

Death by unintentional drowning is the seventh leading cause of death for all ages, the second leading cause of death for ages 1 to 14 years, and the fifth leading cause of death of infants (<1 year of age).[56] Infants are at risk from drowning in bathtubs, buckets, and toilets.[67] The incidence of near-drowning may be 500 to 600 times the rate of drowning.[68] In 2000, there were 3281 cases of unintentional drowning in the United States, and for every child who drowned, three others survived and required emergency care for their submersion incident. Each week, approximately 40 children die from drowning, 115 are hospitalized, and 12 have irreversible brain injury.[57]

The Centers for Disease Control and Prevention (CDC) reported a total of 7546 submersion casualties (fatal and nonfatal) in 2001 and 2002[56] (Figure 9-15). Of these, 3372 persons experienced unintentional drowning in various recreational settings, such as pools, oceans, and rivers. In comparison, 4174 unintentional nonfatal submersion incidents were treated in emergency departments in the United States. The nonfatal and fatal injury rates were the highest for children

FIGURE 9-15 Unintentional Drowning/Near-Drowning—United States, 2001–2002

Characteristic	Nonfatal*	Fatal*
AGE (YR)		
0–4	2168	442
5–14	1058	333
≥15	948	2563
Unknown	—	34
GENDER		
Male	2721	2789
Female	1452	583
LOCATION		
Pool	2571	596
Natural water (ocean, lakes, rivers)	909	1467
Other	513	1309
DISPOSITION		
Treated/released	1925	—
Hospitalized	2233	—
Other	16	—
TOTAL	4174	3372

(Data from Centers for Disease Control and Prevention: Nonfatal and fatal drownings in recreational water settings—United States, 2001–2002. *MMWR* 53(21):447, 2004.)
*Estimated number.

age 4 years or younger and for males of all ages. The nonfatal rate for males was almost twice that of females, whereas the fatal rate for males was almost five times that of females. Nonfatal submersion injuries in pools accounted for 75%, whereas 70% of the fatal submersions occurred in natural settings, such as oceans, lakes, and rivers.

Mechanism of Injury

A common scenario of *head-out immersion* in water or a whole-body submersion incident begins with a situation that creates a panic response, leading to breath-holding, air hunger, and increased physical activity in effort to stay or get above the water surface. As the submersion incident continues, a reflex inspiratory effort draws water into the pharynx and larynx, causing a choking response and laryngospasm (spasm of the vocal cords). The onset of laryngospasm represents the first step in suffocation, which in turn causes the victim to lose consciousness and submerge underwater even farther.

Approximately 15% of drownings are termed "dry drowning" because the severe laryngospasm prevents the aspiration of fluid into the lungs. The remaining 85% of submersion incidents are considered "wet drownings," in which the laryngospasm relaxes, the glottis opens, and the victim aspirates water into the lungs.[69] For prehospital care providers, the common denominator in these submersion scenarios is hypoxia caused by either laryngospasm or water aspiration. Management at the scene should be aimed at reversing any hypoxia in these patients, thereby preventing cardiac arrest.

Surviving Cold-Water Submersion. In numerous cases of prolonged submersion, in one case for as long as 66 minutes, patients have presented to the hospital with severe hypothermia and recovered with either partial or full neurologic function.[70] In these submersion incidents, the lowest recorded core temperature of a survivor is 56.6° F (13.7° C) in an adult female.[47] In another case, a child survived fully intact after being submerged in ice water for 40 minutes, with a core temperature of 75° F (24° C). After 1 hour of resuscitation, spontaneous circulation returned.[71] No explanation exists for such cases, but hypothermia is thought to be protective. Every submersion patient should receive full resuscitation efforts. The factors described next appear to influence the outcome of a cold-water submersion patient.

Age. Many successful infant and child resuscitations have been well documented in the United States and Europe. The smaller mass of a child's body cools faster than an adult's body, thus permitting fewer harmful by-products of anaerobic metabolism to form and causing less irreversible damage.

Submersion Time. The shorter the duration of submersion, the lower is the risk for cellular damage caused by hypoxia. Accurate information concerning submersion time needs to be obtained. Immersion longer than 66 minutes is probably fatal.

Therefore, a reasonable approach to resuscitation of a submersion victim is that efforts should be initiated if the duration of submersion is less than 1 hour.

Water Temperature. Water temperatures of 70° F (21° C) and below are capable of inducing hypothermia. The colder the water, the better is the chance of survival, probably because of the rapid decrease in brain temperature and metabolism when the body is quickly chilled.

Quality of CPR and Resuscitative Efforts. Patients who receive adequate and effective CPR, combined with proper rewarming and advanced life support (ALS) measures, generally do better than patients receiving one or more substandard measures. Immediate initiation of CPR is a key factor for submersion hypothermia patients. Past and current studies reveal that poor CPR technique is directly related to poor resuscitation outcome.[72,73]

Associated Injuries or Illness. Patients with an existing injury or illness, or who become ill or injured in combination with the submersion, do not fare as well as otherwise healthy individuals.

Assessment

The initial priorities for any submersion patient include the following:

1. Prevent injuries to the patient and emergency responders.
2. Initiate plans early for water extraction and rapid transport to ED.
3. Conduct a safe water rescue (consider a possible diving-related cause and the need for spine immobilization).
4. Assess for ABCs (airway, breathing, circulation).
5. Reverse hypoxia and acidosis.
6. Restore or maintain a stable heartbeat.
7. Prevent further loss of body heat and initiate rewarming efforts in hypothermic patients.

Initially, it is safest to presume the submersion patient is hypoxic and hypothermic until proved otherwise. Consequently, all efforts should be made to establish effective respirations during water rescue and to remove the patient from water and other sources of cold to minimize further body heat loss. Quickly assess the patient for any life threats, and assess for head trauma and cervical spine injuries, particularly if there is suspicion of trauma associated with the submersion incident (e.g., falls, boat accidents, diving into water with underwater hazards). However, it has been shown that the typical submersion casualty has a low chance of traumatic injury, unless the victim dove into the water.[74]

Assess for altered mental status and neurologic function of all extremities because many submersion victims develop sustained neurologic damage. Acquire a baseline Glasgow Coma Scale (GCS) score and continue to assess for trends.

Remove all wet clothing and assess rectal temperature (if appropriate thermometers are available and the situation permits) to determine the level of hypothermia, and initiate steps to minimize further heat loss.

Management

A patient who has experienced some form of submersion incident but who is not presenting with any signs or symptoms at the time of the initial assessment still needs follow-up care in a hospital after being assessed at the scene due to the potential for delayed onset of symptoms. Many asymptomatic patients are released in 6 to 8 hours, depending on clinical findings in the hospital. In one study of 52 swimmers who experienced a submersion incident and were all initially asymptomatic immediately after the incident, 21 (40%) went on to develop shortness of breath and respiratory distress due to hypoxemia within 4 hours.[78] In general, all symptomatic patients are admitted to the hospital for at least 24 hours for support care and observation because the initial clinical assessment can be misleading. It is critical to obtain a good history of the incident detailing the estimate of submersion time and any medical history.

All suspected submersion patients should receive high-flow oxygen (12–15 L/minute) independent of their initial breathing status, based on the concern for delayed pulmonary distress, particularly if the patient develops shortness of breath. Transport to the ED for evaluation. Because many near-drowning patients are asymptomatic, some may refuse transport because they have no immediate chief complaint. If so, take the time necessary to provide good patient education about the delayed signs and symptoms in a near-drowning incident and that many victims develop secondary complications from pulmonary injury. Firm and persistent persuasion is needed for them to agree to be transported or for them to report to the closest ED for further evaluation and observation. If the patient is adamant about refusing care, the patient must be informed of the potential ramifications of refusing care and a signed refusal of care against medical advice obtained.

A symptomatic patient with a history of submersion who presents with signs of distress (e.g., anxiety, rapid respirations, trouble breathing, coughing) is considered to have a submersion pulmonary injury until hospital evaluation has proved otherwise. Provide cervical spine immobilization in all patients with suspicion of trauma. In unresponsive patients, use suction to clear the airway and keep the airway open with an airway adjunct. Hypoxia and acidosis can be corrected with effective ventilation support. Apneic patients should be supported with bag-mask ventilation. Provide transport to local ED.

Patient Resuscitation. Rapid initiation of effective CPR and calling for ALS responders for submersion patients in cardiopulmonary arrest is associated with the best chance of survival.[61]

Routine stabilization of the cervical spine during in-water rescue is not necessary unless the reasons leading to the sub-

mersion indicate that trauma is likely (e.g., diving, use of water slide, signs of injury, alcohol use).[76] When these indicators are not present, spinal injury is unlikely. Cervical stabilization and other means to immobilize the spine during a water rescue can cause delays in opening the airway so that rescue breathing can begin.

The use of CPR during in-water rescue is not recommended because compressions of the chest are usually ineffective in water. Besides delaying effective CPR out of water, attempting to provide CPR in water puts rescuers at risk from fatigue, cold-water, wave, surge, and current dangers. Place a greater emphasis on establishing an open airway and providing rescue breathing for apneic patients as soon as possible, depending on the patient's in-water position, number of rescuers, and rescue equipment (e.g., in-water backboard).

When a beach rescue (or any location) involves sloping terrain, it is no longer recommended to place a patient in a head-down (or head-up) position in an effort to drain the airway. Resuscitation efforts are shown to be more successful when the patient is placed level on the ground, parallel to the water, with effective ventilation and chest compressions. Furthermore, no evidence suggests that lung drainage is effective with any particular maneuver.

The Heimlich maneuver has been previously suggested for use in drowning victims. However, the Heimlich maneuver is designed for airway obstruction and does not remove water from the airway or lungs. Rather, it may induce vomiting in drowning victims and place them at greater risk for aspiration. Currently, the AHA and the Institute of Medicine advise against the Heimlich maneuver except when the airway is blocked with foreign material.[77] If the patient recovers with spontaneous breathing, the patient should be placed in a lateral recumbent position with head slightly lower than the trunk to reduce the risk of aspiration if the patient vomits.

Use the regional EMS medical protocol for established guidelines that determine the criteria for an obviously dead individual. Acceptable guidelines for an obviously dead victim are a normal rectal temperature in a patient who presents with asystole, apnea, postmortem lividity, rigor mortis, or other injuries incompatible with life. A patient who has been recovered from warm water without vital signs or resuscitative efforts lasting 30 minutes may be considered dead on the scene.[60,63] Consult local medical control early for any individual recovered from cold-water submersion. As stated previously, many individuals have fully recovered from more than 60 minutes of cold-water submersion. These patients should be managed as hypothermic based on the rectal temperature.

Figure 9-16 summarizes assessment and management of a submersion patient.

Water Rescue

Many water safety organizations recommend the use of highly skilled professionals who regularly train for water rescue, retrieval, and resuscitation. If no professional water rescue

FIGURE 9-16   Submersion Patient: Summary of Assessment and Management

History	Examination	Intervention
ASYSMPTOMATIC PATIENT		
Time submerged	Appearance	Administer oxygen by facemask at 8–10 L/minute
Description of incident	Vital signs	Initiate IV line at KVO rate (ALS responders)
Complaints	Head and neck trauma Chest examination: lung fields	Reexamine patient as needed
Medical history	ECG monitor	Transport patient to ED
SYMPTOMATIC PATIENT		
Description of incident	General appearance	Administer oxygen by non–rebreathing mask at 12–15 L/minute
Time submerged Water temperature, water contamination Vomiting Type of rescue	Level of consciousness (AVPU)	
Symptoms	Vital signs; monitor ECG	Transport patient to ED
On-scene field resuscitation	Assess ABCDEs Vital signs AED or ECG monitor	Initiate CPR early; 100% oxygen at 12–15 L/minute via bag-valve mask

(Modified from Schoene RB, Nachat A, Gravatt AR, Newman AB: Submersion incidents. In Auerbach PS: *Wilderness medicine*, ed 5, St Louis, 2007, Mosby Elsevier.)
ABCDEs, airway, breathing, circulation, disability, expose/environment; *ACLS,* advanced cardiac life support; *AED,* automatic external defibrillator; *AVPU,* alert, responds to verbal stimulus, responds to painful stimulus, unresponsive; *CPR,* cardiopulmonary resuscitation; *ECG,* electrocardiogram; *ED,* emergency department; *IV,* intravenous; *KVO,* keep vein open; *NG,* nasogastric; *VF,* ventricular fibrillation.

teams are available, however, first responders must consider their own safety and the safety of all responders before attempting an in-water rescue. The following guidelines are recommended to safely rescue a victim out of the water[60]:

REACH Attempt to perform the water rescue by reaching out with a pole, stick, paddle, or anything so that the rescuer stays on land or on a boat. Use caution to avoid being inadvertently pulled into the water.
THROW When reaching is not possible, throw something to a victim, such as a life preserver or rope, so that it floats to the victim.
TOW Once the victim has a rescue line, tow him or her to safety.
ROW If a water entry is necessary, it is preferable to use a boat or paddleboard to reach the victim; wear a personal floatation device (PFD) if entering the water in a boat or to swim.

Swimming rescues are not recommended unless the responder has been trained appropriately to manage a patient who can rapidly turn violent from panic, creating a potential double drowning. Too many well-intentioned first responders have become additional victims because their own safety was

not the priority. See Figure 9-17 for a few options for in-water rescue systems equipment for a submersion or trauma patient (C-spine precaution) and movement while in deep water.

Lightning

Lightning is the most widespread threat to people and property during the thunderstorm season and has been second only to floods in causing storm-related death in the United States since 1959.[78] The National Weather Service estimates that 100,000 thunderstorms occur each year in the United States and that lightning is present in all storms. Lightning is reported to start approximately 75,000 forest fires annually and starts 40% of all fires.[79] The most destructive form of lightning is the cloud-to-ground strike (Figure 9-18). Based on real-time lightning detection systems, it is estimated that cloud-to-ground lightning strikes occur approximately 20 million times per year, with as many as 50,000 flashes per hour during a summer afternoon.[80,81] Central Florida is the region with the highest number of lightning ground strikes each year (see Figure 9-19 for distribution of lightning flashes in the United States). Lightning occurs most frequently from June through August but occurs in Florida and along the southeastern coast of the Gulf of Mexico throughout the year.[82]

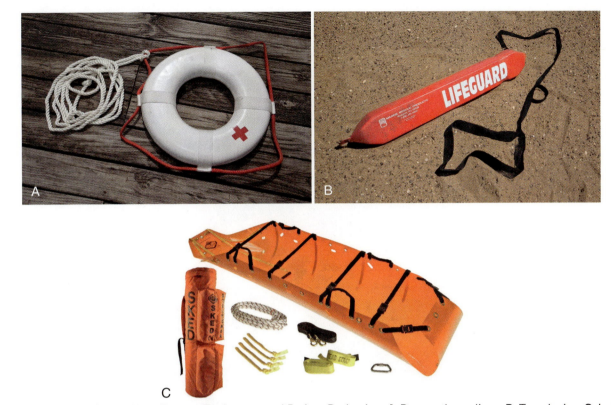

FIGURE 9-17 Options for In-Water Rescue Equipment and Patient Packaging: **A,** Rescue throw lines; **B,** Tow device; **C,** In-Water Patient Packing Equipment.

It is now reported that lightning kills 50 to 300 individuals each year and injures about 1000.[78,83] The greatest life threats from lightning strikes are neurologic and cardiopulmonary injuries.

Clearly, prevention of lightning strike is optimal. This can be accomplished by using the 30-30 rule. If one hears thunder less than 30 seconds after a lightning flash, shelter should immediately be sought because the storm is dangerously close. Then, one should stay in that shelter for 30 minutes after the last thunderclap is heard.

Epidemiology

Based on the National Oceanic and Atmospheric Administration (NOAA) publication called *Storm Data,* 3529 deaths (average 98 deaths per year), 9818 injuries, and 19,814 property damage reports occurred during the 36-year period from 1959 to 1994.[78] This report showed that the top four states for casualties (death and injuries) from lightning are Florida (523), Michigan (732), Pennsylvania (644), and North Carolina (629). The highest number of deaths occurred in Florida (345), North Carolina (165), Texas (164), and New York (128). Figure 9-20 shows the ranking of lightning injuries and deaths by state from 1959 to 1994.

There were 1318 lightning deaths between 1980 and 1995 in the United States, on review of medical examiners' death certificates listing lightning as the cause of death.[84] Of those who died during this 16-year period, 1125 (85%) were male and 896 (68%) were age 15 to 44 years. The highest death rate from lightning occurred among those age 15 to 19 years (6 deaths per 10,000,000). Analysis shows that about 30% die and 74% of the survivors have permanent disabilities. Furthermore, victims with cranial or leg burns are at a greater risk for death.[85] Of the individuals who died from a lightning strike, 52% were outside (25% of whom were at work). Death occurred within 1 hour in 63% of the lightning victims.[83]

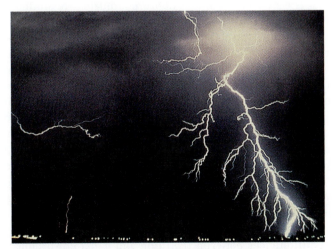

FIGURE 9-18 A cloud-to-ground lightning strike, with streak lightning pattern.
(From Cooper MA, Andrews CJ, Holle RL, Lopez RE: Lightning injuries. In Auerbach PS: *Wilderness medicine,* ed 5, St Louis, 2007, Mosby Elsevier.)

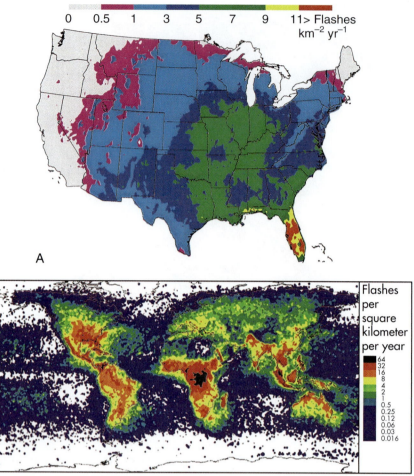

FIGURE 9-19 **A,** Distribution of lightning ground strikes in the United States, with the heaviest concentration in the southeast region. **B,** Distribution of lightning ground strikes worldwide.

(From Huffines GR, Orville RE: Lightning ground flash density and thunderstorm duration in the continental United States, 1989–1996, *J Appl Meteorol* 38:1013, 1999.)

Mechanism of Injury

Injury from lightning can result from the following five mechanisms[79,86,87]:

- *Direct strike* occurs when a person is in the open environment and unable to find shelter.
- *Side flash* or *splash contact* occurs when lightning hits an object (e.g., ground, building, tree) and splashes onto a victim or multiple victims. Splashes occur from person to person, tree to person, and even indoors from telephone wire to a person talking on the phone.
- *Contact* occurs when a person is in direct contact with an object that is struck directly or by a splash.
- *Step voltage,* also known as *stride voltage* or *ground current,* occurs when lightning hits the ground or a nearby object. The current will spread outward and will travel, for example, up one leg and down the other in the path of least resistance.
- *Indirectly.* Blunt trauma can occur from a shock wave produced by lightning, which can move a person up to

10 yards. Injuries can result from lightning that causes forest fires, building fires, and explosions.

It is easy to assume that lightning injuries are similar to high-voltage electrical injuries. However, significant differences exist between the two mechanisms of injury. A lightning strike is direct current (DC) as opposed to the alternating current (AC) that is responsible for industrial and household electrical injures. Lightning produces millions of volts of current, 30,000 to 50,000 amps, and the duration of exposure to the body is extremely short (10–100 milliseconds). The temperature of lightning varies with the diameter, but the average temperature is approximately 14,430° F (8000° C).[86] In comparison, high-voltage electrical exposure tends to be a much lower voltage than lightning. However, the key factor that distinguishes lightning from high-voltage electrical injury and the different patterns of injury is the duration of current exposure within the body.[86] Figure 9-21 lists differences between lightning and generator-produced high-voltage electrical injuries.

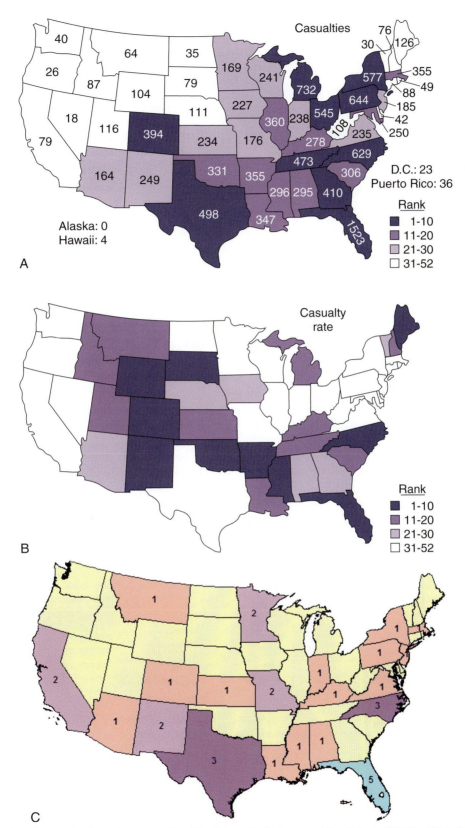

FIGURE 9-20   Rank of each state in lightning casualties (deaths and injuries combined) from 1959 to 1994. **A,** Casualties per state. **B,** Casualties weighted by state population. **C,** The year 2008 had the lowest number of lightning fatalities ever recorded. (Data from Curran EB, Holle RL, Lopez RE: Lightning fatalities, injuries, and damage reports in the United States from 1959–1994, *NOAA Tech Memo NWS SW-193*, 1997.)

5e

FIGURE 9-21 Comparison of Lightning and High-Voltage Electrical Injuries

Factor	Lightning	High Voltage
Energy level	30 million volts; 50,000 amperes	Usually much lower
Time of exposure	Brief, instantaneous	Prolonged
Pathway	Flashover, orifice	Deep, internal
Burns	Superficial, minor	Deep, internal
Cardiac	Primary and secondary arrest, asystole	Fibrillation
Renal	Renal failure rare	Renal failure common
Blunt injury	Explosive thunder effect	Falls, being thrown

(Modified from Cooper MA, Andrews CJ, Holle RL, Lopez RE: Lightning injuries. In Auerbach PS: *Wilderness medicine*, ed 5, St Louis, 2007, Mosby Elsevier.)

At times, lightning can show injury patterns similar to those seen with high-voltage electricity because of a rare lightning pattern that produces a prolonged strike lasting up to 0.5 second. This type of lightning, called "hot lightning," is capable of causing deep burns, exploding trees, and setting fires. Lightning can show entry and exit wounds on the body, but a more common pathway of lightning, once it strikes a victim, is to pass over the body. This is referred to as a "flashover" current. A flashover current can also enter the eyes, ears, nose, and mouth. It is theorized that the flashover current flow is the rea-son why many victims survive lightning strikes. It is also known that a flashover current may vaporize moisture on skin or blast a part of clothing or shoes off a victim. The immense flashover current generates large magnetic fields, which in turn can induce secondary electric currents within the body and are thought to cause cardiac arrest and other internal injuries.[88,89]

Injuries from Lightning

Lightning injuries range from minor superficial wounds to major multisystem trauma and death. Figure 9-22 lists common signs and symptoms of lightning injury.

Minor Injury. Patients with minor injury are awake and report an unpleasant and abnormal sensation (dysesthesias) in the affected extremity. In a more serious lightning strike, victims report they have been hit in the head or state that an explosion hit them, because they are unsure of the source. A patient may present at the scene with the following:

- Confusion (short term or hours to days)
- Amnesia (short term or hours to days)
- Eardrum (tympanic membrane) rupture
- Temporary deafness
- Blindness
- Temporary unconsciousness
- Temporary numbness and tingling (paresthesias)
- Muscular pain
- Cutaneous burns (rare)
- Transient paralysis

Victims present with normal vital signs or with mild, transient hypertension, and recovery is usually gradual and complete.[88]

FIGURE 9-22 Lightning Injury: Common Signs, Symptoms, and Treatment

Injuries	Signs/Symptoms	Treatment
Minor	Feeling of strange sensation in extremity Confusion Amnesia Temporary unconsciousness, deafness, or blindness Tympanic membrane rupture	Scene safety ABCDEs Medical history and secondary exam Give oxygen and transport all patients with mild injuries
Moderate	Disoriented, combative Paralysis, fractures, blunt trauma, absent pulses in lower extremities Spinal shock Seizures Temporary cardiorespiratory arrest Comatose	Scene safety ABCDEs Medical history and secondary exam CPR early when needed Give oxygen and transport all patients
Severe	Any minor-moderate symptoms, plus otorrhea in ear canal, cardiac fibrillation or cardiac asystole	CPR and advanced lifesaving procedures Use "reverse" triage with multiple patients

(Data from O'Keefe GM, Zane RD: Lightning injuries, *Emerg Med Clin North Am* 22:369, 2004; and Cooper MA, Andrews CJ, Holle RL, Lopez RE: Lightning injuries. In Auerbach PS: *Wilderness medicine*, ed 5, St Louis, 2007, Mosby Elsevier.)
ABCDEs, airway, breathing, circulation, disability, expose/environment; *CPR*, cardiopulmonary resuscitation.

Moderate Injury. Victims with moderate injury have progressive, single or multisystem injuries, some of which are life threatening. Some patients in this category also have a permanent disability. Patients may present at the scene with the following[88]:

Immediate Effects
- Neurologic signs
- Seizures
- Cardiac arrest
- Confusion, amnesia
- Blindness
- Dizziness
- Contusion from shockwave
- Blunt trauma (e.g., fractures)
- Chest pain, muscle aches
- Tympanic membrane rupture
- Headache, nausea, post-concussion syndrome
- Tympanic membrane rupture (common)

Delayed Effects
- Memory deficits
- Neuropsychological changes
- Coding and retrieval problems
- Distractibility
- Personality changes
- Irritability
- Chronic pain
- Seizures

A strike affecting the respiratory center of the brain can result in prolonged respiratory arrest that may lead to secondary cardiac arrest as a result of hypoxia.[88] Victims in this category may experience immediate cardiopulmonary arrest, although the internal pacemaker of the heart may produce a spontaneous return to normal sinus rhythm.[85] Because immediate cardiopulmonary arrest is the greatest threat, prehospital care providers need to assess the ABCs quickly in all lightning-strike patients and continuously monitor the ECG for secondary cardiac events.

Severe Injury. Victims with severe injury from a direct lightning strike (cardiovascular or neurologic injuries) or delays in CPR have a poor prognosis. On arrival at the scene, the prehospital care provider may find the patient in cardiac arrest. Lightning causes a massive DC countershock, which simultaneously depolarizes the entire heart.[89] The American Heart Association recommends vigorous resuscitation measures for those who appear dead on initial evaluation. This is based on many reports of excellent recovery after lightning-induced cardiac arrest, and that victims in this category are mostly young and without heart disease.[89]

Other common findings are tympanic membrane rupture with cerebrospinal fluid (CSF) and blood in the ear canal, ocular injuries, and various forms of blunt trauma from falls, including soft tissue contusions and fractures of the skull, ribs, extremities, and spine. Many patients in this category have no evidence of burns. In those patients presenting with cutaneous burns caused by lightning, it is generally reported to be less than 20% of total body surface area.[88]

Assessment
On arrival at the scene, as with any other call, the priority is the safety of the prehospital care providers and other public safety personnel. Know whether or not there is still the chance of lightning in the area, because lightning remains a very real threat as far as 10 miles away.[86] The mechanism of injury may be unclear without a witness because lightning can strike during a perceived sunny day. When in doubt about the mechanism of injury, immediately assess for ABCDEs and any life-threatening conditions, as for any emergency. These patients do not carry an electrical charge, and touching them poses no risk in providing patient care. Assess for the presence of absence of a pulse and respirations.

If the patient is stable, a detailed head-to-toe assessment is necessary to identify the wide range of injuries that can occur with this type of trauma. Assess the patient's situational awareness and the neurologic function of all extremities because the upper and lower extremities may experience transient paralysis (known as keraunoparalysis). Assess the eyes because 55% of victims have some form of ocular injury. Lightning victims are known to have a dysfunction causing dilated pupils, which will mimic head trauma.[90] Look for blood and cerebrospinal fluid in the ear canals; 50% of these victims will have one or two ruptured tympanic membranes. All victims of lightning injury have a high probability of blunt trauma from being thrown against a solid object or from objects falling on the patient. Cervical spine precautions are needed during the assessment to minimize further injury. Assess the skin for signs of any burns, ranging from first degree to full thickness. It is common to see a reddish feathering appearance in the skin, known as "Lichtenberg's figures," but these patterns are not burns and resolve in 24 hours. It is more common to see burns secondary to igniting of clothes and heating of jewelry or other objects.

Management
The priorities for managing a lightning victim are to ensure scene safety, then stabilize the patient's airway, breathing, and circulation. If spontaneous respiration or circulation is absent, initiate effective CPR up to 5 cycles (2 minutes) and evaluate the heart rhythm with an AED.[80] Evaluate and treat for shock and hypothermia. Apply high-flow oxygen for all moderately and severely injured patients. Stabilize any fractures, and package the blunt trauma patient for cervical spine immobilization. Lightning-strike patients with minor to severe injuries need to be transported to an ED for further evaluation and observation. Transport the patient by either ground or air based on availability, distance, and time to the hospital and overall risk to the flight crew and benefit to patient.

As mentioned previously, lightning victims have a higher probability of a positive outcome from early and effective resuscitation. However, there is little evidence to suggest that these patients can regain a pulse from BLS or ALS procedures lasting longer than 20 to 30 minutes.[79] Before terminating resuscitation, all efforts should be made to stabilize the patient by establishing an airway, along with high-flow oxygen and supported ventilation, and to correct hypothermia and acidosis.

If the incident involves multiple victims, principles of triage should be implemented immediately. The normal rules of triage are to focus limited personnel and resources on patients with moderate and severe injuries and quickly bypass those patients without respiration and circulation. However, with multiple lightning-strike patients, the rule changes to use "reverse" triage and "resuscitate the dead," because these patients are either in respiratory arrest or cardiac arrest and have a high probability of recovery if managed expeditiously.[86,91] In contrast, other patients who have survived a lightning strike have little likelihood of deteriorating unless there is associated trauma and occult hemorrhage.

Prolonged Transport

Near-Drowning

Guidelines for prolonged transport of near-drowning patients are as follows:

- Asymptomatic patients can become symptomatic in an extended-care situation with a delay of 4 hours before pulmonary symptoms.

- Provide high-flow oxygen via a nonrebreather mask at 12 to 15 L/minute.
- Any patient with altered mental status, apnea, or coma may require early active airway management to protect from aspiration. Liberal use of suction is necessary to remove pulmonary secretions and water aspirated during submersion.
- Determine the GCS score and assess routinely for trends because it is predictive of patient outcome.
- Monitor for hypothermia.

Lightning Injury

Guidelines for prolonged transport of patients with lightning injury are as follows:

- Initiate CPR quickly.
- When in the extended-care situation with multiple patients, use "reverse triage" and first resuscitate those who appear dead. However, prolonged (multiple hours) CPR on these patients has a poor outcome, and there is little benefit from CPR or ACLS procedures lasting longer than 20 to 30 minutes. All measures to stabilize the patient to correct for hypoxia, hypovolemia, hypothermia, and acidosis should be attempted before terminating resuscitative efforts.[77]
- Establish a baseline GCS score, and reassess every 10 minutes as an indicator of progressive cerebral edema and increased ICP.

SCENARIO 2 SOLUTION

As you respond at the country club, you anticipate a single unconscious male on the 18th fairway, but you should be thinking about additional injured players because golfers normally play in a group of four. It has been frequently reported that when a lightning ground strike occurs the electrical energy splashes in many directions, hitting multiple golfers standing near each other. Therefore, it is important to conduct a remote assessment and look for multiple victims; note where they are located, whether or not they are moving around or unconscious, and if there are any potential threats to the victims, bystanders, or your medical team. Even though you do not hear thunder or see lightning, the lead provider should communicate that there is still a threat environment and to be continually aware for lightning because there are dark thunder clouds in the area. With multiple lightning strike casualties, rapid assessment of the ABCs is paramount, but use reverse triage on the patients. Resuscitate the "dead" first because these victims are usually in respiratory or cardiac arrest and have a high probability of recovery if

appropriately selected rescue breathing, CPR, or cardiac defibrillation is performed soonest after a lightning strike. Then conduct a thorough head-to-toe assessment with specific emphasis on eyes, ear canals, and signs of blunt trauma. Perform a rapid neurologic exam because many victims experience transient paralysis in the upper or lower extremities. Your exam should also identify any lightning entry or exit wounds on the body. Direct contact burns from lightning are rare but can occur from burning clothes, shoes, or hot metal objects, such as belt buckles, touching the skin; these should be removed from the body. Once all patients have been assessed, all severely injured patients receive high-flow oxygen. Splint any fractures and backboard all patients with blunt trauma. Think early on about the onset of hypothermia if the patient is wet from rain and lying on a cool surface. All patients, both minor and severely injured, need to be transported to the emergency department for evaluation and treatment for any neurologic, cardiopulmonary, or metabolic complications from lightning strike. ■

Wilderness Trauma Care

SCENARIO 3

It is 9 AM and you are working as a member of the local search and rescue team that has been looking for a lost hunter since 6 PM last night. The hunter is found a short distance from your location by a K9 team. On your arrival you find that the hunter, although cold, is alert and oriented and is complaining of a broken right lower leg and a cut to the back of his head. The temperature overnight dropped to 38° F (3° C). He explains that late yesterday afternoon he was trying to make his way back to the road and slipped on a wet rock, catching his leg between two rocks. He has fashioned a splint of sorts using some sticks and torn cloth from his shirt. He is approximately 2 miles from the nearest access point over rocky terrain. On examination you find an alert and oriented 40-year-old male with a GCS of 15. Secondary examination reveals only an angulated open right lower leg fracture with no active bleeding and a 5 cm laceration of the occipital scalp.

How would you manage this patient in the field?

Proper Care Depends on Context

Although our medical knowledge, understanding, and technology change from month to month, the *principles* of medical care change little over the years. "The critically injured patient must be transported as quickly as possible, without detailed examination and treatment of noncritical conditions."[1] Proper care is still somewhat context dependent, however, and the definitions of "detailed examination" and "noncritical conditions" may be different on an urban street than deep within a cave (Figure 9-23). This concept was introduced in Chapter 3 showing how situation, knowledge level, scene conditions, and available equipment may alter management of the trauma patient.

Consider a patient with a complex fracture-dislocation of the shoulder. What is the proper care in the operating room (OR)? In many cases it involves surgery to perform an open reduction to align the bones. However, proper care in the OR may not be proper care in the emergency department (ED). It would *not* be proper care to attempt an open reduction in the ED. In the ED the patient will have x-ray films taken to evaluate the fracture-dislocation; be given a short-acting pain medication; and undergo a *closed* reduction of the dislocation to reduce pain and swelling, to realign the bones grossly, and to decrease pressure on nerves and blood vessels. However, the definitive surgery will occur later, in the OR.

Furthermore, proper care in the ED may not be proper care on the street. The prehospital providers may not have the advantage of a large, warm, dry area. They may be working where it is raining or snowing, where the patient is hanging upside down inside a crushed vehicle, or where a rescue crew

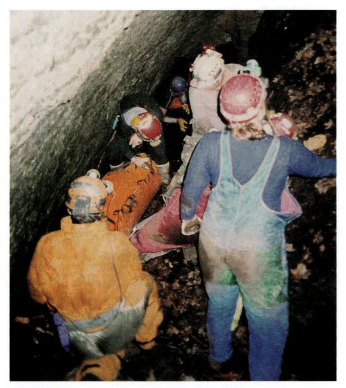

FIGURE 9-23 Trauma care in the wilderness is often hampered by adverse environmental conditions, mud, underbrush, and confined spaces.

is using power tools to cut and crush metal all around them. On the street, the patient will have an assessment for scene safety, rescue from immediate dangers, an assessment for other injuries, a check of distal neurovascular status in the arm, immobilization of the shoulder, possibly some pain medication, and rapid transport to the ED. On the street, it would *not* be proper care to attempt an open reduction to reduce the fracture-dislocation.

Finally, proper care on the street may not be proper care in the backcountry. What if, instead of being in a crushed vehicle, the patient had fallen off a rope while a half mile into a limestone cave in the mountains, facing a multi-hour evacuation through the cave passages, followed by a several hour drive to the nearest hospital? For most conditions, proper care is proper care whether it is done in the OR, in the ED, on the street, or in the backcountry, limited only by equipment and training.

For a small but significant number of common conditions, however, great differences exist between proper "street" emergency medical services (EMS) care and proper backcountry EMS care. This brings up the following important questions, as discussed later in this chapter:

- Is "street" EMS care always optimal in the backcountry?
- If "street" EMS care is not optimal, how do you know *what* the optimal care is? Where is this written down?
- How do you deal with situations where, in the field, you are not sure precisely what the injury might be? For example, in the previous case, how do you determine a fracture-dislocation is present when you are examining the patient who is hanging upside down, whether in a crushed vehicle or from a rope dangling down a pit deep within a cave?
- How do you decide, for a particular patient in a particular situation, which is *more* proper, street or backcountry care?
- What makes a situation "backcountry" or "street"? What about all the "in-between" cases?

Definitive answers to all the questions cannot be provided—often the answer is, "It depends"—but at least good background information can be provided so that providers may, as needed and in a particular patient care situation, answer the question. The prehospital trauma life support (PHTLS) philosophy has always been that, given a good fund of knowledge and key principles, prehospital care providers such as emergency medical technicians (EMTs) are capable of making reasoned decisions regarding patient care.

This section provides an overview of the many issues involved in wilderness-related medical emergencies. Prehospital care providers who will be functioning in a formal capacity in the wilderness setting should obtain specific training in managing these patients. In addition, medical direction by a knowledgeable physician should be an integral component of wilderness medicine activities.

The "Wilderness EMS" Context

Many terms are used for areas far from civilization: backcountry, remote, wilderness, isolated. EMS personnel tend to lump these together under the rubric "wilderness" and to speak of

"wilderness EMS." The dictionary definition of "wilderness" follows[92]:

1. a (1): a tract or region uncultivated and uninhabited by human beings; (2): an area essentially undisturbed by human activity together with its naturally developed life community; b: an empty or pathless area or region; c: a part of a garden devoted to wild growth;
2. wild or uncultivated state;
3. a: a confusing multitude or mass: an indefinitely great number or quantity; b: a bewildering situation.

Our use of "wilderness" differs from the dictionary definition, however, because we are thinking about *patient care*. Our definition is really the answer to a question: "When should we think about wilderness EMS?" That is, "When should we think and work differently from what we do on the street?"

The answer to this question goes beyond simple geography and involves the following considerations:

- Access to the scene
- Weather
- Daylight
- Terrain
- Special transport and handling needs
- Access and transport times
- Available personnel
- Communications
- Hazards present
- Medical and rescue equipment available
- Injury patterns for the specific environment

In a city after an earthquake, it may be very difficult to access those who are injured or trapped, there may be no road for transport, and local EMS systems may be out of action. In this situation, patients are likely to remain in their location for a considerable time. They will have the same care requirements as a hiker who has fallen in the mountains and is hours—or days—away from a hospital.

A person who has fallen into a suburban landfill site, late in the evening, during an ice storm, is at risk from the same factors as in the wilderness. The patient may need a rescue team with ropes, ice axes and crampons, and trauma care providers who can anticipate and cope with issues such as hypothermia, toileting needs, prevention of pressure sores, wound management, and food and fluid requirements.

We often talk of "wilderness EMS," but in reality, *all* EMS lies on a spectrum. At one extreme is a scene half a block from a level I trauma center, and at the other extreme are scenes such as the summit of Mount Everest or the deepest part of the Mammoth–Flint Ridge cave system in Kentucky.

Therefore, in the final analysis, where does "the street" end and "the wilderness" begin? The answer is, "It depends." It depends on the distance from the ambulance (and the ED). It depends on the weather. It depends on the terrain.

Even more importantly, it depends on the nature of the injury or illness and the capabilities of the EMS and rescue personnel on-scene. We return to this topic at the end of the section.

Backcountry Injury Patterns

As mentioned in Chapter 1, death from trauma has a trimodal (three-peaked) distribution. The *first peak of death* is within seconds to minutes of injury. Deaths occurring during this period are usually caused by lacerations of the brain, brainstem, high spinal cord, heart, aorta, or other large vessels and can best be managed by preventive measures such as helmets and seat belts. Only a few of these patients can be saved, and then only in large urban areas where rapid emergency transport is available. The *second death peak* occurs within minutes to a few hours after injury. **Rapid assessment and resuscitation are carried out to reduce this second peak of trauma deaths.** Deaths occurring during this period are usually caused by intracranial hematomas, hemopneumothorax, ruptured spleen, lacerations of the liver, pelvic fractures, or multiple injuries associated with significant blood loss. The fundamental principles of trauma care learned in this course can best be applied to these patients. The *third death peak* occurs several days or weeks after the initial injury and is almost always caused by sepsis and organ failure.

The PHTLS course focuses mostly on saving patients from the second "peak" of the trimodal death distribution. In the backcountry, most of those who survive to be rescued have already weathered the first and usually most of the second "peak" of the trimodal death graph; however the presence of medically trained individuals on the rescue team may also help to prevent deaths related to this second peak. More often, backcountry care focuses on the question "What can we do *now* that will keep the patient from dying later?" We need to make sure the patient does not develop problems such as kidney failure from dehydration, overwhelming infection from poor resistance due to starvation, pulmonary embolism from deep venous thrombosis (blood clots in the legs breaking off and going to the lungs), and infections from decubiti (bedsores).

Safety. In the backcountry, even more so than on the street, scene safety is paramount. An injured or dead rescuer never did anyone any good. "Street" scene safety considerations still apply—even in the backcountry—but there are other considerations as well. In the backcountry, scene dangers are usually much less obvious than on the street; they tend to slowly "sneak up" on unwary rescuers.

The provider and patient will be exposed to the weather, and changes in weather, such as an incoming cold front with freezing rain, may complicate the operation or even injure or kill the provider and patient. If a rescue lasts for hours, the lack of food and water may cause debilitation. The terrain is often rugged, and poisonous plants and wildlife may complicate patient care (Figure 9-24). Providers need to be aware of

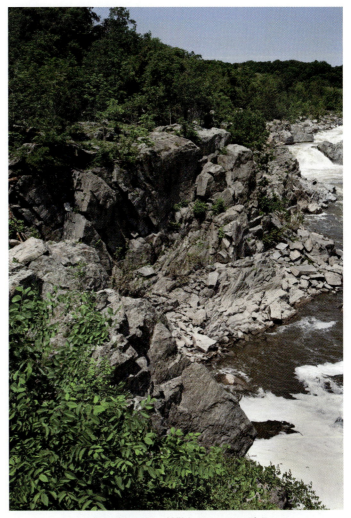

FIGURE 9-24 Wilderness terrain.

dangers specific to the environment, such as rockfall, avalanche risk, rising water, bad air or altitude exposure, and recirculating eddies at the base of waterfalls (Figure 9-25).

The Wilderness Is Everywhere

In the rest of this section, we talk about "wilderness EMS" and "in the wilderness" and "wilderness patients." Remember, however, that "the wilderness" might be a short distance from the road, if it is dark and the weather is bad, or even *on* the road if a disaster has made roads impassable or made nearby hospitals unable to accept patients.

EMS Decision Making: Balancing Risks and Benefits

Experienced EMTs and paramedics (and even doctors nurses) know that procedures such as airway management and wound management are the easy part of medicine. The difficult part is knowing *when* to do *what*: critical thinking. Even more often than on the street, in the wilderness one risk needs to be

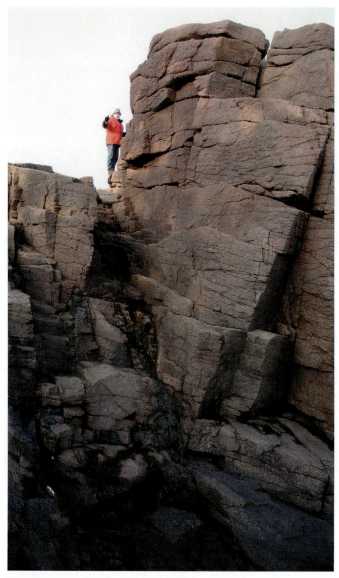

FIGURE 9-25 Steep slopes and uneven footing are a danger in wilderness rescue.

weighed carefully against another and against the potential benefits.

For this particular patient, in this particular setting, with these particular resources, and with this particular likelihood of this particular help arriving at this particular time in the future, what are the potential risks? What are the potential benefits? Wilderness EMS is largely the art of compromise: balancing the particular risks and benefits for each patient.

To illustrate wilderness EMS decision making, we will use the example of a potential spinal injury.

"Clearing" the Cervical Spine in the Wilderness. A healthy 24-year-old woman was rock climbing along a river gorge when she fell 65 feet. All her chocks (anchors placed in cracks in the cliff) came out one by one, so she fell all the way to the ground, but was slowed by each anchor as it failed. She was

wearing a helmet but hit her head and had a brief loss of consciousness. When you and your partner arrive, after an hour-long hike up the river gorge from where you parked the ambulance at the end of the road, she is alert and conscious, with no complaints, a normal neurologic examination, and a normal physical examination. It is late fall, it is getting dark, the nearest helicopter landing zone is back at the road an hour away, and the forecast is for a blizzard to start tonight. Does she need to be immobilized? Do you have to call for a team with a Stokes litter and a long backboard? Or can you walk her out?

"Street" Cervical Spine Management History

Spinal immobilization for severely injured trauma patients became the standard of care decades ago. As EMT training became more and more widely used by backcountry search and rescue teams, the practice of strapping everyone to a board after an accident did not seem to make sense, especially if the patient was on the side of a mountain in a snowstorm and the nearest board was 10 miles away and 10,000 feet down. So search and rescue teams and the physicians working with them developed guidelines, based on the available literature, for when *not* to immobilize trauma patients in the backcountry.[93]

A large and important multi-center study called "NEXUS" showed that many patients can be "cleared" without x-ray films if the following selection criteria are used:

- Absence of tenderness at the posterior midline of the cervical spine
- Absence of a focal neurologic deficit
- Normal level of alertness
- No evidence of intoxication
- Absence of clinically apparent pain that might distract the patient from the pain of a cervical spine injury

Variants of these criteria have been used by many EMS systems. A few studies suggest some problems with using these criteria in the field. The wording of some EMS "selective spinal immobilization protocols" deviate significantly from the NEXUS wording, raising concerns about whether they really reflect the NEXUS criteria. However, it is generally accepted that the NEXUS criteria, properly applied, are a good guide to patients who do not need to be strapped to a board, whether on the street or in the backcountry. Although NEXUS may be useful for inference, one should remember that NEXUS was not designed as a prehospital spinal immobilization trial, but rather a study of the need for cervical spine x-rays in-hospital.

The problem in the backcountry, however, is not as simple. What if a patient doesn't quite meet these criteria? Does that mean that the patient *has* to be immobilized?

As discussed earlier, wilderness EMS is the art of compromise, and nowhere is this more apparent than in making decisions about spinal immobilization.

What if the patient has a potential spine injury and it is a 2-hour walk from the nearest road, and no spinal immobilization equipment is at hand? Is it necessary to send someone on the 4-hour round-trip hike back to the ambulance for it? What if the patient is in a cave, with the water level rising? Could the patient and rescuers be cut off from an escape route and drown if the team delays? What if the patient is in the mountains, far from the ambulance, and a storm is moving in? What are the risks if the patient and rescuers are forced to spend the night on the mountain?

In each of these situations, prehospital care providers at the scene are faced with the following two options:

- Staying and waiting for the spinal immobilization to arrive
- Starting an improvised evacuation without spinal immobilization

Neither option is ideal, and prehospital care providers need to choose. To make this choice intelligently, the following questions must be asked and answered:

- What are the risks of an improvised evacuation without spinal immobilization, and what are the risks of waiting for spinal immobilization equipment to arrive *for this particular patient in this particular situation*?
- What are the benefits of moving without waiting for spinal immobilization and for waiting for spinal immobilization equipment to arrive *for this particular patient in this particular situation*?

The benefits of spinal immobilization depend on the likelihood that this particular patient has an unstable spinal injury.

- In the NEXUS study, those who did *not* meet the NEXUS criteria and who could not be "cleared" still had a very low risk of unstable spinal fracture: Approximately 2% of those who *failed* the NEXUS clearing protocol had "clinically significant" fractures.
- Of that 2%, only a small fraction likely required specific treatment.
- Of *that* small fraction, only a small fraction likely had injuries that might endanger the spinal cord if not immobilized, and most of those were in patients with multiple major fractures and multiple life-threatening injuries.

Therefore, it seems likely that for backcountry trauma patients who have survived long enough to be rescued, the incidence of unstable spine injury will be less than 1%. Prehospital care providers at the scene need to assess these potential risks and benefits to make an informed decision.

Improvised Evacuations

When discussing spinal injury in the wilderness context, we mentioned the idea of starting an improvised evacuation

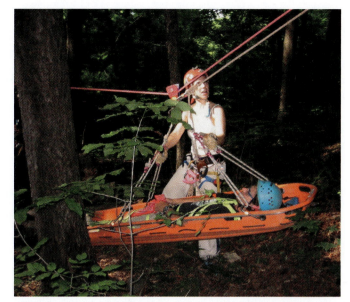

FIGURE 9-26 Because of uneven terrain, creativity and technical rescue skills may be needed to evacuate patients safely out of the backcountry.

rather than waiting for a litter and spinal immobilization equipment (Figure 9-26).

Carrying patients in the backcountry is an extremely difficult, time-consuming, and somewhat dangerous activity for both the patient and those doing the carrying. Those with no search and rescue (SAR) experience generally underestimate the time and difficulty of a backcountry evacuation by at least half, or sometimes up to a factor of five for more difficult evacuations, especially cave rescues.

If someone without SAR experience says, "It'll take us about 2 hours to get the patient out of here," triple this, and expect it to take 6 hours—or longer if the patient is in a cave, if the team is short on people, if the terrain is particularly difficult, or if the weather is bad. This is especially important to remember if darkness is approaching or the weather is deteriorating.

Walking a patient out, even with a couple of people helping, is almost always *much* faster. Certainly if the patient starts moving *now*, rather than waiting for a litter or spinal immobilization, the evacuation will be much, much faster. If the patient cannot walk (e.g., because of an ankle fracture), it is possible to do a piggyback carry or to make an improvised stretcher out of sticks and rope.

Patient Care in the Wilderness

Elimination Needs. The truth described in a popular children's book called *Everyone Poops*[94] applies to backcountry patients as well. Given the relatively short transport times in an urban setting, most patients do not have an elimination need. If you are caring for a patient who has been in the backcountry for a day, however, and it takes you several hours to get to the patient, it is *much* more likely the patient will need to urinate or defecate.

Having patient care supplies that include "blue pads" for under the patient, having some toilet paper, and even stopping to let the patient urinate or defecate are all reasonable measures (Figure 9-27).

It is possible for men and women to urinate even while immobilized in a Stokes litter (Figure 9-28) with a full body vacuum splint if packaging is planned carefully and the litter is up on an end. For women, a small funnel device commonly carried by women when backpacking will be needed.

However, people who are lying on their backsides for a long time tend to develop decubiti (bedsores). These may end up requiring surgery, resulting in a longer hospital admission. Some patients even die from infection and other complications from bedsores.

Lying in one's own urine and feces for a long time (just hours, not even days) may make bedsores more likely. If patient care is only for a few minutes during an urban transport, urine and feces are not a major issue. However, if a provider has been taking care of a patient for several hours and then delivers the patient to the ED lying in his own feces, the nurses might (legitimately) complain about the level of care.

Food and Water Needs. Every backcountry patient is cold, hungry, and thirsty; that is, hypothermic, starved, and dehydrated, or if you prefer a good mnemonic at a slight expense of accuracy, *hypothermic, hypoglycemic,* and *hypovolemic.*

Starvation is much more than just hypoglycemia (low blood sugar), and not all starving patients are significantly hypoglycemic. Dehydration is more than just hypovolemia, which refers only to intravascular volume within the blood vascular system. Patients who are dehydrated have also lost water out of their cells and the interstitial spaces between the cells.

On the street, water or food are *not* generally given to patients. There are good reasons not to feed patients on the street. A patient will not starve or dehydrate in a few min-

utes. If the patient might need to go to the OR, having food or fluid in the stomach is harmful; it increases the likelihood of vomiting or, more likely, passive regurgitation when under anesthesia.

However, the stomach only needs to be empty for a few hours before anesthesia. If a patient rescued from the back-

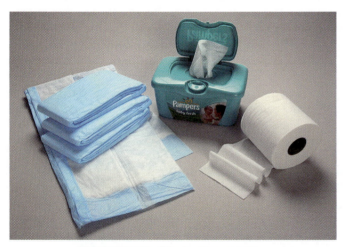

FIGURE 9-27 Elimination supplies.

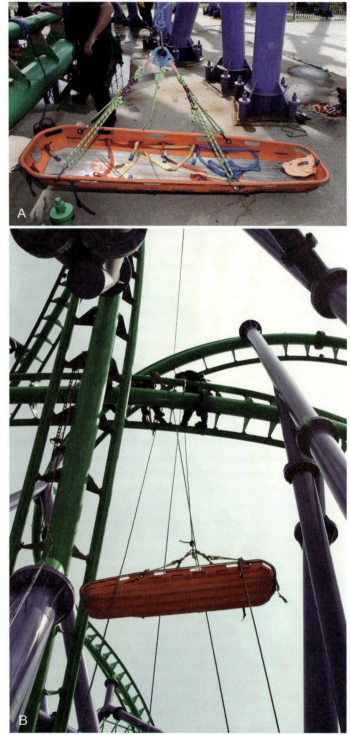

FIGURE 9-28 Stokes litter.

country needs to go the OR, it will almost always take a few hours for the patient to get prepared for the OR in any event.

As noted earlier, with wilderness patients the focus is to ensure that the patient does not die sometime after hospital admission. Starving people is seldom good for them. Feeding the patient today will make the patient better tomorrow. Therefore, provide food and water to any reasonably alert backcountry patient.

Vomiting and aspiration are always a danger, and careful attention to the patient's airway is always important (e.g., positioning on the side for long transports, even if the patient needs spinal immobilization). However, rescuers should still attempt to provide food and water for backcountry patients, even though they have vomited once or twice, as long as their airway is protected.

Long Backboards Hurt Patients

Other important preventive measures for backcountry patients, especially those who face prolonged evacuation, include prevention of decubiti (bedsores), as follows:

- Allow (and assist) the patient to turn from side to side in the litter.
- Keep the patient's sacrum (buttocks) clean and dry.

If the patient truly needs spinal immobilization, prevention of decubiti is even more important, although correspondingly more difficult. Techniques to avoid decubiti during spinal immobilization include the following:

- Put the patient in a full-body vacuum splint rather than on a long backboard. Vacuum mattresses provide excellent spinal immobilization and are much less likely to cause decubiti.[95–98]
- If no full-body vacuum splint is available, pad the long backboard well and add support under the lumbar spine, knees, and neck. Studies show that immobilization on an unpadded long backboard causes even uninjured people to experience excruciating pain in about 45 minutes and skin necrosis (cell death) in about 90 minutes.[99–103]
- Carry the litter first on one side, then the other, so that pressure alternates between the two hips rather than always on the sacrum.

To prevent deep venous thrombosis and pulmonary embolism, do the following:

- Package patients so that they can move their legs; do not tie them down tight.
- Consider rest stops to allow patients out of the litter to stretch their legs.

If there is mild suspicion of a cervical spine injury but not a lumbar spine injury, it might even be appropriate to allow an alert patient out of the litter, still wearing a cervical collar, and, with many trained hands to help, allow the patient to stretch the legs and urinate. Speaking with a physician conversant with wilderness EMS might be reassuring if this is contemplated.

Sun Protection. One hazard worth discussing in more detail is sun protection. The ultraviolet (UV) rays of the sun can damage the skin, sometimes severely. Second-degree and third-degree sunburns are seen in some victims of exposure, and such severe sunburn can cause shock or death. Sunburn also makes skin cancer more likely.

Sun protection is measured by the *sun protection factor* (SPF) (Figure 9-29). The SPF is a numeric measure of how much the clothing or cream increases the minimum dose of UV light to make the skin red. For example, a sunscreen lotion with a rating of SPF 45 provides protection from sunburn for about 45 times longer than without the sunscreen.

To check clothing for SPF, hold a piece of clothing up against a light bulb. If an image of the light bulb is seen through it, the SPF is slightly below 15. If light is seen through it but not the image of the light bulb, the SPF is in the range of 15 to 60 SPF.

Protective lotions with a minimum SPF of 15 should be applied to exposed skin to minimize the potential injury from sun exposure. With profuse sweating, lotion should be reapplied frequently.

Sunburn is treated as any other burn, and the care is essentially the same in the wilderness as on the street. The only major difference is that in the backcountry, the prehospital care provider needs to be aware of and treat the potential fluid loss, dehydration, or sometimes even shock, and to recognize that patients with sunburn are at higher risk for hypothermia.

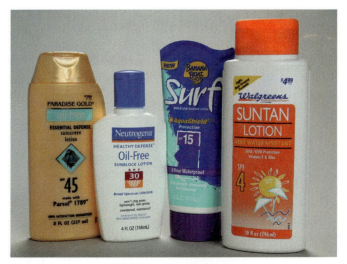

FIGURE 9-29 Sunscreen.

Specifics of Backcountry EMS

This section reviews a few of the most important situations in which proper backcountry trauma care differs from that on the street.

Wound Management

Wound management encompasses the following:

■ Hemostasis (stopping bleeding)
■ Antisepsis (prevention of infection)
■ Restoration of function (returning the skin to its protective function, and restoring a limb or other body part to normal function)
■ Cosmesis (pleasant appearance)

In the backcountry, prevention of infection and restoration of function assume great importance.

Hemostasis. Control of bleeding is part of the primary survey. On the street, arterial bleeding can kill. In the backcountry, however, even venous bleeding can kill if it continues for a sufficient time; *every red blood cell counts.* Therefore, bleeding control, using standard measures such as direct pressure, is as important or more important in the wilderness. Unless the medical personal are part of the actual injured party's group, severe bleeding that is not stopped by someone else or the patients themselves will probably result in the patients' demise before the rescue party's arrival. Educational programs for those venturing into wilderness situations should address these lifesaving skills.

At times, however, finding a bleeding site to provide direct digital (finger) pressure over the "bleeder" (bleeding blood vessel) is not that easy. If manpower and circumstances allow, direct digital pressure for 10 to 15 minutes is probably superior to a pressure bandage at controlling bleeders.

Therefore, some wilderness EMS protocols suggest using a proximal blood pressure (BP) cuff as a tourniquet for 1 or 2 minutes to control the bleeding initially. Then, after letting the BP cuff down carefully, the location of the bleeder usually becomes obvious, and a gloved finger covered with a gauze pad (to prevent slipping) can be carefully placed over the bleeder for 10 to 15 minutes. If the bleeder starts bleeding again, direct digital pressure for another 10 to 15 minutes almost always stops it.

Note that we are suggesting using a BP cuff tourniquet for only a few minutes. It is important to remember to *let the BP cuff down* and not use it by itself to stop bleeding; otherwise, the patient might develop permanent damage in the limb. A commercially manufactured arterial tourniquet could also be utilized in this manner.

Topical hemostatic agents may have a useful purpose in wilderness care in the control of severe bleeding. Wilderness responders may encounter injured patients who have had such agents already applied by others in their group. Some of these agents are available for sale to the general public through many outdoor recreational supply companies. The efficacy of some of these over-the-counter agents may be questionable. (See Chapter 5, Circulation and Shock.)

Prevention of Infection

After injury in the backcountry, it may be a long time until the wound receives definitive treatment in an ED. Routine wound care in the ED includes appropriate cleaning to prevent infection. Wounds contaminated by dirt or caused by penetration from a dirty object are cleaned with high-pressure irrigation. Noncontaminated wounds are cleaned with low-pressure irrigation.

High-pressure irrigation causes swelling of wounds, but in the case of contaminated wounds full of dirt and bacteria, the benefit of removing bacteria outweighs the risks from wound swelling.[104,105] Infections may set in quickly. After a wound has been open for about 8 hours, bacteria have spread from the skin deep into the wound. After 8 hours, sewing up a wound is likely to create a deep wound infection. Deep wound infections develop pressure, which keeps out white blood cells, the body's normal defense mechanism against infection.

Routine wound care on the "street" does not include cleansing the wound because it makes sense to delay cleansing for a few minutes until the patient reaches the ED, which is better suited for wound cleansing and evaluating the patient. The ED can determine if the patient has a tendon or nerve laceration, an associated fracture, a spleen laceration, or a subdural hematoma in the head.

Delaying wound care does *not* make sense in the backcountry. If it will take hours to get to the ED, the wound should be cleaned. In remote areas the wound could become infected before the patient arrives at the ED several days later.

Studies have shown that early irrigation is essential to removing bacteria and reducing wound infections.[106–108] It is not necessary or practical to carry sterile solutions for wound irrigation. There is no need to add antiseptics to the water.[108] Water that is good enough to drink is good enough to irrigate a wound. Water from streams or melted snow can be treated with any standard backcountry drinking water treatment.[49,104,110–113]

When cleaning an uncontaminated wound, such as a laceration sustained from banging the forehead against a teammate's helmet, it is only necessary to "slosh a bit of water through the wound." Some recommendations call for using a blue bulb syringe, usually available in the ED, but sloshing some water from a drinking-water bottle will do as well.

If the wound is contaminated, it must be irrigated with enough pressure to clean out bacteria. The original studies showed that a 35-mL syringe with an 18-gauge needle provided an appropriate amount of pressure (5–15 psi).[114–116] Squirt the water, at high pressure, throughout the wound. However, this is a major bloodborne pathogen risk; protection from the spray of blood when irrigating is necessary. Eye protection and gloves are essential.

Sometimes it is necessary to use a gauze pad or clean cloth with gloved fingers to clean out some gross dirt or foreign material. The patient's pain may need to be treated before cleaning the wound. Once done, dress and bandage the wound. Reapply a clean dressing at least daily.

If the wound is gaping open, a wet dressing will prevent tissue damage from drying out; change or at least rewet the dressing with clean water several times a day. In most cases, however, because the wound will be mostly closed by bandaging, apply a dry dressing.

Restoration of Function and Cosmesis: Closing Backcountry Wounds

Because of the lack of good lighting, x-ray films, and a warm dry place to work, it does not make sense to perform definitive wound closure in the backcountry. However, it is possible simply to cleanse the wound, dress and bandage, do good wound care for 4 days, and then do a *delayed primary closure*. Four days later, as long as the wound is not infected, it is safe to close the wound as if it had just occurred. Although bacteria move into the wound soon after injury, eventually enough of the body's defenses (e.g., white blood cells) have entered the wound and make it safe to close. This occurs about 4 days after the initial injury.

Because delayed primary closure is available, there is no pressing reason to close wounds in the backcountry. If a surgeon or someone else experienced at wound closure is present, the wound may be closed at the scene. However, it is still reasonable to only cleanse, dress, and bandage the wound and allow closure to occur later.

Dislocations. A healthy 20-year-old man was kayaking along a whitewater stream when the top of his kayak paddle hit a low-hanging tree branch. Now his right shoulder is swollen and deformed and painful. He cannot bring his right arm across his chest. Distal pulses, capillary refill, sensation, and movement are intact. From the ambulance, you and your partner hiked a mile through the woods to get to the stream. Should you "splint it as it lies"? Or try to reduce what looks like an anterior shoulder dislocation?

The standard of care for fractures and dislocations on the street is to "splint it as it lies" and transport for definitive treatment. The only exception is the patient whose pulse is not palpable.

Although "splint it as it lies" is a good general rule for the street, "make it look normal" is a better general rule for the wilderness context. It is certainly appropriate for both fractures and dislocations when transport is delayed.

There are many types of dislocations—finger, toe, shoulder, patella, knee, elbow, hip, ankle, and jaw—and all have been successfully reduced in the backcountry, some more easily than others. It is usually very easy to reduce dislocations of the ankle (which are almost always fracture-dislocations), patella, toe, or finger, except the proximal interphalangeal joint of the index finger in some cases. Elbow, knee, and hip dislocations are usually quite difficult. All are much easier with training and practice; in particular, it takes training or experience to know without a

radiograph *when* a joint is likely dislocated, and to attempt reduction.

EMT and paramedic courses seldom provide training in dislocation reduction. Because backcountry dislocations are so common, however, dislocation reduction is covered in almost all wilderness first-aid, wilderness first-responder, and wilderness EMT training. Those who might provide EMS in the backcountry or who regularly travel in the backcountry are advised to take one of these courses.

Cardiopulmonary Resuscitation in the Backcountry

Backcountry Traumatic Arrest. A few signs can be uniformly equated with nonsurvivability:

- Decapitation
- Transection of the torso
- Patient frozen so that the chest cannot be compressed
- Very cold rectal temperature that is the same as the environment
- Well-progressed decomposition (see later discussion)

The following presumptive signs of death may be of use to prehospital care providers, although no one sign by itself is reliable:

- *Rigor mortis.* Postmortem rigidity is well known but not always present, and similar rigidity is often observed in hypothermic but semiconscious patients.
- *Dependent lividity.* This is common in corpses but also is found along with pressure necrosis and frostbite in some patients exposed to the elements for a long time.
- *Decomposition.* This is usually self-evident.
- *Lack of presumptive signs of life.* Hypothermia can mimic death, in that pulses may not be palpable and respirations may be undetectable, with dilated unreactive pupils and no signs of consciousness. However, such severely hypothermic patients have occasionally been resuscitated, with full neurologic recovery.

We know that traumatic cardiac arrest "on the street" has a poor prognosis, even if the scene is within minutes of a level I trauma center. No person survives more than a few minutes of CPR after traumatic arrest.[117,120] This fact is recognized in many EMS protocols:

- For traumatic cardiac arrest, initiate CPR with cervical spine stabilization if:
  1. Cardiac arrest occurs in the presence of EMS personnel
  2. Victim of penetrating trauma had signs of life within 15 minutes before the arrival of EMS personnel

Therefore, in the wilderness context, CPR is inappropriate for traumatic arrest. It would be appropriate for prehospital care providers and the mountain rescue team members to examine the patient, then gently but firmly tell the companions that the victim is dead and there is no reason to initiate resuscitation. The prehospital care providers and mountain rescue team members should then deal appropriately with the expected denial and grief reactions, with a check of scene safety, especially if oncoming darkness may make exiting the area hazardous to the victim's mentally and physically exhausted companions.

Backcountry Medical Arrest

A medical arrest applies to a patient who has chest pain and then sustains a cardiac arrest. Again, in the wilderness context, the chances of survival are poor or nonexistent when the patient is more than a few minutes of CPR from defibrillation.[121–126] It is possible that a rescue team might be carrying out a patient with chest pain when the patient sustains a cardiac arrest. However, the usefulness-to-weight ratio of defibrillators is so poor that they are seldom carried by wilderness rescue teams.

There are a variety of other causes of cardiac arrest in the backcountry, and in the previous example, ventricular fibrillation cardiac arrest secondary to hypothermia or cardiac arrest secondary to pulmonary embolism is likely. For such cardiac arrests, however, survival is even less likely than with a cardiac arrest secondary to a myocardial infarction.

However, "nontraumatic" backcountry cardiac arrest might be survivable in the following situations:

- Hypothermia[127]
- Cold-water near-drowning[67,128–130]
- Lightning strike[131]
- Electrocution
- Drug overdose
- Avalanche burial[132]

In all these cases, a patient may appear to be in cardiac arrest but still might be resuscitated by basic CPR. For hypothermia in particular, remember the saying, "Nobody's dead until they're warm and dead." A significant minority of those who appear dead from the mechanisms listed can be resuscitated. There are special considerations for each of these situations; for example, scene safety for those who have been electrocuted and are still attached to a backcountry power line, or knowing that external cardiac compression can actually induce a VF cardiac arrest in a hypothermic patient whose heart is beating just enough to keep the patient alive.[133–136] Although appropriate in a wilderness EMT course, detailed discussion of these topics is beyond the scope of this chapter.

However, two standard wilderness CPR rules are as follows[123]:

- If the patient appears to be in cardiac arrest from causes other than trauma, attempt CPR for 15 to 30 minutes; if this does not resuscitate the patient, stop CPR and consider the patient dead.
- However, do *not* start CPR if it will put rescuers at risk and decrease their chances of retreating from the scene

safely, given concerns about daylight, terrain, weather, and available nearby shelter.

Bites and Stings. Bites and stings are common backcountry problems. The exact type of bite or sting likely in a backcountry area depends on the locale.

Bee Stings. The most widespread, common, and deadly sting is that of the common honeybee, at least to those who are allergic. Most reactions to bee stings are severe (although brief) local pain and in some cases local swelling and redness for 1 or 2 days; these latter reactions are likely directly related to injected toxins and not an indication of allergy.

Some who are stung will progress within a few minutes to a generalized allergic reaction. This may range from urticaria to a full-blown anaphylactic reaction. Although the exact spectrum of generalized allergic reaction depends on the contents of the injected toxin (which varies among the many species of bees and wasps) and the allergic history of the patient, one or more of the following are usually seen:

- Urticaria (hives) (Figure 9-30)
- Lip swelling
- Hoarseness or stridor
- Wheezing and/or shortness of breath
- Abdominal cramping, vomiting, or diarrhea
- Tachycardia *or* bradycardia
- Low blood pressure
- Syncope
- Shock

Those with a history of a generalized allergic reaction to a sting are more likely to have another generalized reaction to the next sting. However, venom among different species varies enough that, despite a history of generalized allergy in the past, a patient might have no generalized reaction to the next sting.

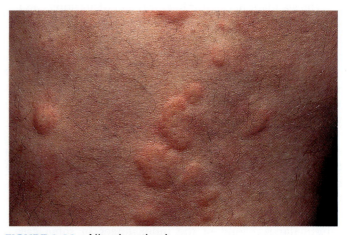

FIGURE 9-30 Allergic urticaria.
(From Forbes CD, Jackson WF: *World atlas and text of clinical medicine*, ed 3, London, 1993, Mosby–Year Book Europe Limited.)

A patient with mild urticaria after a sting probably will do well. If a patient with hives after a sting progresses to "real" anaphylaxis, however, the best early sign is hoarseness. The major cause of death after bee sting allergy is airway obstruction from hives in the airway, and hoarseness is usually the first sign of airway swelling. Any patient with a generalized reaction to a bee sting needs treatment immediately.

Basic life support (BLS) interventions involve keeping the patient flat or with the legs somewhat elevated, performing standard airway management, and providing oxygen.

One simple but useful intervention is to remove an embedded stinger properly. Although only a small fraction of bee stings still have an embedded stinger, it often requires good eyes and bright light or a magnifying glass to see the stinger, and improper removal could be deadly. Squeezing an embedded stinger with a pair of forceps, clamps, or tweezers can squeeze more venom into the skin. Instead, using a credit card or *carefully* scraping with a knife blade can remove the stinger without squeezing additional venom into the skin.

It is important to remove embedded stingers as soon as possible; the venom sac continues to squeeze in venom even after the bee has flown away.

The main medications to treat bee stings include the following:

1. *Epinephrine (adrenalin).* Although epinephrine only acts for a few minutes, it can be lifesaving.
2. *Antihistamines (e.g., diphenhydramine [Benadryl]).* Anyone who requires epinephrine for a bee sting allergy should receive an antihistamine.
3. *Steroids (e.g., prednisone).* Most people who require epinephrine also require steroids.

Some wilderness SAR teams carry drugs for bee sting allergy in their medical kits; the team's wilderness EMTs have special training in their use. Also, some people with a history of bee-sting allergy carry these medications in their personal first-aid kits.

The most important drug is epinephrine. Epinephrine is available as a pen-sized autoinjector (e.g., Epi-Pen), which is often prescribed to any patient who has had a generalized allergy to bee stings. These autoinjectors are found in many wilderness first-aid kits.

Snakebite. There are many species of poisonous snakes. Few are found in northern latitudes. Most occur in tropical areas, and many are deadly. Although many snakes have venom glands, in North America there are only two types of snakes with venom strong enough to cause more than minor irritation to humans.

Coral snakes are small snakes found in the southern parts of North America that have a venom that is neurotoxic—that is, causes paralysis (Figure 9-31). However, the snakes are small, have small fangs, cannot open their mouths very far

compared with larger snakes, and have to chew to allow the venom to penetrate.

Pit vipers are found throughout large portions of North America and include *rattlesnakes* of various types (Figure 9-32), *copperheads* (Figure 9-33), and *water moccasins* or *cottonmouths* (Figure 9-34). The majority of pit viper bites do not occur in the backcountry but rather in rural, suburban, and even urban areas. A classic example is the intoxicated

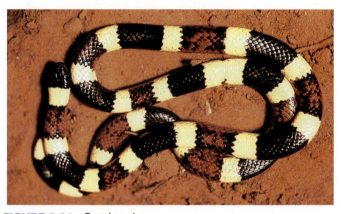

FIGURE 9-31 Coral snake.
(From Sanders M: *Mosby's paramedic textbook,* ed 3, St Louis, 2006, Mosby.)

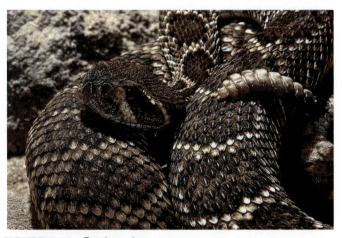

FIGURE 9-32 Rattlesnake.
(From Sanders M: *Mosby's paramedic textbook,* ed 3, St Louis, 2006, Mosby.)

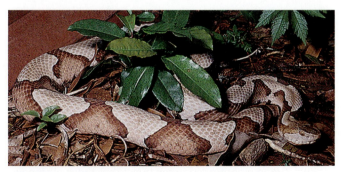

FIGURE 9-33 Copperhead snake.
(From Auerbach PS: *Wilderness medicine: management of wilderness and environmental emergencies,* ed 4, St Louis, 2001, Mosby.)

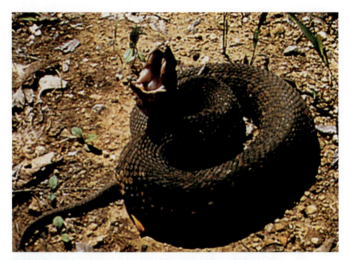

FIGURE 9-34 Water moccasin (cottonmouth) snake.
(From Auerbach PS: *Wilderness medicine: management of wilderness and environmental emergencies,* ed 4, St Louis, 2001, Mosby.)

man who was kissing his pet rattlesnake when he was bitten on the tongue or lips.

Snakebites are not as rare as one might think. This is further complicated by the variety of prehospital treatments attempted by patients, bystanders, and sometimes EMS personnel. The only treatment shown to be effective for envenomated pit viper bites is antivenin (antivenom), which is very expensive (thousands of dollars for a single treatment) and thus not routinely carried in first-aid kits. Indeed, the only "street" care proven to be helpful is transportation to the hospital.

The first thing to do to treat snakebite is to *watch for signs of envenomation.* Only a fraction of bites by pit vipers actually result in envenomation (venom was injected), and the signs of envenomation are fairly distinct. Although signs and symptoms of envenomation usually develop in a few minutes, sometimes they are delayed by 6 to 8 hours or perhaps even longer, so starting to the hospital after a suspected poisonous snakebite is appropriate. Signs of envenomation include the following:

1. Severe local swelling, bruising, and pain
2. Continued bleeding from the bite
3. Paresthesias in the fingers and toes (paresthesias are unusual sensations, usually caused by damage to nerves or biochemical abnormalities; a feeling of "pins and needles" is a common paresthesia)
4. Metallic taste in the mouth
5. Feeling of severe anxiety ("impending doom")
6. Nausea, vomiting, and abdominal pain

The following are treatments that have been recommended in the past but are not supported by the literature:

1. *Rest.* Some recommendations insist that those who have been bitten should always avoid exertion. Deaths from North American snakebite are very rare,[137] and it is highly unlikely that the exertion of hiking out from a backcountry area will make a snakebite victim significantly more ill. If the victim can be carried out, that is ideal. However, if waiting for a carryout will delay the victim's arrival at a hospital, the victim should walk out with whatever assistance can be given.
2. *Catch the snake and bring it to the hospital.* There are numerous reports of bystanders who tried to catch a suspected poisonous snake and were bitten during the attempt. A single antivenin is used for all domestic pit viper venoms, and treatment is based on clinical degree of envenomation, relying on the previous signs and symptoms. Therefore, identifying a domestic snake is of minor importance compared with the dangers of attempting to catch the snake. A digital photograph of the snake might be useful, but identification is not worth the risk of an additional bite.
3. *Suction.* Suction, with or without cutting, has been shown to be useless for poisonous snakebite. Snakebite kits consisting of suction devices should be left out of all first-aid kits and should never be used.[138,139]
4. *Electric shock.* Electric shock, whether applied to the snake or to the snakebite, has been shown to be totally ineffective and should never be used.[140,141]
5. *Cold packs.* Cold packs have been shown to increase tissue damage from North American pit viper bites and should not be used.[142]
6. *Splinting, arterial or venous tourniquets, lymph constrictors, or elastic bandages.* Although widely recommended, none of these treatments has been shown to be effective and they may worsen local damage to the bite area.[143,144]

The "Wilderness EMS" Context Revisited

At the beginning of this section, we asked *when* EMS is "wilderness EMS": "When should we think about wilderness EMS; that is, when should we think and work differently from what we do on the street?"

From the bulk of the section, the reader can probably provide the short answer: "It depends."

Time, distance, weather, and terrain all enter into the decision. The decision that a particular patient, in a particular situation, with a particular set of injuries, needs "wilderness" care rather than "street" care is a medical decision and one best made by the prehospital care provider directly attending the patient. If the provider at the scene can contact a knowledgeable EMS physician, especially one with wilderness EMS experience or training, the advice is definitely worth seeking. Ultimately, the decision is up to the prehospital care provider at the scene.

PHTLS has always held that, given a good fund of knowledge and key principles, prehospital care providers, other EMS personnel, and EMTs are capable of making reasoned decisions regarding patient care.

SCENARIO 3 SOLUTION

You, as the team's wilderness EMT, briefly examine the patient and find a open fractured tibia and fibula. Although the fall also caused a laceration to the scalp, a cervical spinal exam does not reveal any necessity for spinal immobilization. You are also concerned that the patient has been in low temperatures overnight but are somewhat relieved that the patient's level of consciousness is normal, suggesting only mild hyperthermia. You decide to treat this finding using passive rewarming techniques. You radio for the incoming extraction team to bring a lower leg splint along with a Stokes basket. While waiting for extrication crew to arrive, you realign and dress the lower leg and begin to rehydrate the hunter because he did not have any water with him overnight. You also give him some high-carbohydrate energy bars because he has not eaten since noon yesterday. You then examine the head wound and find that it is contaminated with dirt and debris. You irrigate the wound and dress it. It takes the extraction team 90 minutes to reach your location. You splint the lower leg with the commercial splint. Because you have determined by examination that no cervical immobilization is needed, you place the patient directly into the Stokes basket for transport. At this point you have 12 rescuers available and begin to transport the patient toward the extraction point. After an hour you have only made it a half mile from the site. Additional rescuers are called to help with the extraction. As the team medic, besides providing care for the patient, you are also responsible for the team's health and safety. You make sure team members have sunscreen available because it is reaching the middle of the day. You monitor the hydration status of not only the patient but also the team members, reminding them to take breaks and drink plenty of fluid. Finally after 2½ hours you reach the ambulance and turn the patient over to the awaiting crew for transport to the local hospital 17 miles away. ■

SUMMARY

- Prehospital care providers will inevitably be faced with environmental encounters such as those described in this chapter.
- Basic knowledge of common environmental emergencies is necessary to provide rapid assessment and treatment in the prehospital setting.
- It is not easy to remember this type of information because these problems are infrequently encountered, so remember the general principles involved.
- For heat-related illness, treat heatstroke patients with effective, rapid, whole-body cooling to reduce core temperature quickly.
- For cold-related illness, manage all moderately to severely hypothermic patients gently, taking the time to remove them from the cold environment and begin passive rewarming while monitoring core temperature—the key is to prevent further body heat loss.
- Patients are not dead until they are warm and dead.
- Remember that you must maintain your own safety. There are too many cases in which prehospital care providers have lost their lives as a result of attempting a rescue.

- Prehospital care providers will inevitably be faced with unpredictable environmental encounters such as those described in this chapter. Basic knowledge of common environmental emergencies is necessary so that rapid assessment and treatment in the prehospital setting can be provided. It is not easy to remember this type of information because these problems are not frequently encountered. Therefore, remember the general principles involved, as follows:
- *Drowning or near-drowning.* Assume all near-drowning patients have pulmonary distress until proved otherwise; correct hypoxia and hypothermia as indicated.
- *Lightning.* Patients with severe lightning injury need rapid assessment of cardiopulmonary status. Use the "reverse triage" principle for multiple victims. Initiating CPR early is the key to survival.
- In every case, remember that personal safety must be maintained. There are too many cases in which EMS and other prehospital care providers have lost their lives as a result of attempting a rescue.
- Although many of the principles of wilderness EMS are the same as "street" EMS, preferences and practice may change because of the unique circumstances.

- Wilderness patients seldom need more or different procedures; they do usually need prehospital care providers with keen critical thinking skills.
- Clinical situations in which wilderness care is different include clearing the cervical spine, irrigating wounds, reducing dislocations, and terminating CPR.

- When managing patients in the wilderness, the prehospital care providers have to also consider food and water requirements and elimination needs.
- A basic principle of wilderness care is that all patients are hypothermic, hypoglycemic, and hypovolemic.

References

1. National Center for Health Statistics: *Compressed mortality file,* Hyattsville, MD, 2002, U.S. Department of Health and Human Services, Centers for Disease Control and Prevention.
2. Center for Disease Control and Prevention: Heat-related deaths—Chicago, Illinois, 1996-2001, and United States, 1979–1999. *MMWR* 52(26):610, 2003.
3. Centers for Disease Control and Prevention: Heat-Related Deaths—United States, 1999—2003. *MMWR* 55(29):796, 2006.
4. Center for Disease Control and Prevention: Hypothermia-related deaths—Utah, 2000, and United States, 1979–1998. *MMWR* 51(4):76, 2002.
5. Lugo-Amador NM, Rothenhaus T, Moyer P: Heat-related illness. *Emerg Med Clin North Am* 22:315, 2004.
6. Ulrich AS, Rathlev NK: Hypothermia and localized injuries. *Emerg Med Clin North Am* 22:281, 2004.
7. Center for Disease Control and Prevention: Hypothermia-related deaths—United States, 2003. *MMWR* 53(8):172, 2004.
8. Speedy DB, Noakes TD: Exercise-associated hyponatremia: a review. *Emerg Med* 13:17, 2001.
9. Moran DS, Gaffen SL: Clinical management of heat-related illnesses. In Auerbach PS: *Wilderness medicine,* ed 5, St Louis, 2007, Mosby Elsevier.
10. McCauley RL, Killyon GW, Smith DJ, et al: Frostbite. In Auerbach PS: *Wilderness medicine,* ed 5, St Louis, 2007, Mosby Elsevier.
11. Danzl DF: Accidental hypothermia. In Auerbach PS: *Wilderness medicine,* ed 5, St Louis, 2007, Mosby Elsevier.
12. Hardy JD: Thermal comfort: skin temperature and physiological thermoregulation. In Hardy JD, Gagge AP, Stolwijk JAJ, editors: *Physiological and behavioral temperature regulation,* Springfield, IL, 1970, Charles C Thomas.
13. Pozos RS, Danzl DF: Human physiological responses to cold stress and hypothermia. In Pandolf KB, Burr RE, editors: *Medical aspects of harsh environments,* vol 1, Washington, DC, 2001, Office of The Surgeon General, Borden Institute/TMM Publications.
14. Stocks JM, Taylor NAS, Tipton MJ, Greenleaf JE: Human physiological responses to cold exposure. *Aviat Space Environ Med* 75:444, 2004.
15. Wenger CB: The regulation of body temperature. In Rhoades RA, Tanner GA, editors: *Medical physiology,* Boston, 1995, Little, Brown.
16. Nunnelely SA, Reardon MJ: Prevention of heat illness. In Pandolf KB, Burr RE, editors: *Medical aspects of harsh environments,* vol 1, Washington, DC, 2001, Office of the Surgeon General, Borden Institute/TMM Publications.
17. Yeo T. Heat Stroke: a comprehensive review. *AACN Clin Issues* 15:280, 2004.
18. Wenger CB: Section I: Hot environments. In Pandolf KB, Burr RE, editors: *Medical aspects of harsh environments,* vol 1, Washington, DC, 2001, Office of the Surgeon General, Borden Institute/TMM Publications.
19. Sonna LA: Practical medical aspects of military operations in the heat. In Pandolf KB, Burr RE, editors: *Medical aspects of harsh environments,* vol 1, Washington, DC, 2001, Office of the Surgeon General, Borden Institute/TMM Publications.
20. Tek D, Olshaker JS: Heat illness. *Emerg Med Clin North Am* 10(2):299, 1992.
21. Bouchama A, Knochel JP: Medical progress: heat stroke. *N Engl J Med* 346(25):1978, 2002.
22. Holtzhausen LM, Noakes TD: Collapsed ultraendurance athlete: proposed mechanisms and an approach to management. *Clin J Sport Med* 7(4):292, 1997.
23. Gardner JW, Kark JA: Clinical diagnosis, management and surveillance of exertional heat illness. In Pandolf KB, Burr RE, editors: *Medical aspects of harsh environments,* vol 1, Washington, DC, 2001, Office of the Surgeon General, Borden Institute/TMM Publications.
24. Knochel JP, Reed G: Disorders of heat regulation. In Narins RE, editor: *Maxwell & Kleenman's clinical disorders of fluid and electrolyte metabolism,* ed 5, New York, 1994, McGraw-Hill.
25. Gaffin SL, Hubbard RW: Pathophysiology of heatstroke. In Pandolf KB, Burr RE, editors: *Medical aspects of harsh environments,* vol 1, Washington, DC, 2001, Office of the Surgeon General, Borden Institute/TMM Publications.
26. Semenza JC, Rubin CH, Flater KH, et al: Heat-related deaths during the July 1995 heat wave in Chicago. *N Engl J Med* 335(2):84, 1996.
27. Costrini A: Emergency treatment of exertional heatstroke and comparison of whole body cooling techniques. *Med Sci Sports Exerc* 22:15, 1984.
28. Neufer PD, Young AJ, Sawka MN: Gastric emptying during exercise: effects of heat stress and hypohydration. *Eur J Appl Physiol* 58:433, 1989.
29. Armstrong LE, Crago AE, Adams R, et al: Whole-body cooling of hyperthermic runners: comparison of two field therapies. *Am J Emerg Med* 14:335, 1996.
30. Gaffin SL, Gardner J, Flinn S: Current cooling method for exertional heatstroke. *Ann Intern Med* 132:678, 2000.
31. U.S. Fire Administration: *Firefighter fatalities in the United States in 2006,* www.usfa.dhs.gov/downloads/pdf/publications/ff_fat06.pdf, FEMA, July 2007.

32. U.S. Department of Agriculture, U.S. Forest Service: *Heat stress,* www.fs.fed.us/fire/safety/fitness/heat_stress/hs_pg1.html.

33. Stocks JM, Taylor NAS, Tipton MJ, Greenleaf JE: Human physiological responses to cold exposure. *Aviat Space Environ Med* 75:444, 2004.

34. Ulrich AS, Rathlev NK: Hypothermia and localized injuries. *Emerg Med Clin North Am* 22:281, 2004.

35. Thomas JR, Oakley EHN: Nonfreezing cold injury. In Pandolf KB, Burr RE, editors: *Medical aspects of harsh environments,* vol 1, Washington, DC, 2001, Office of the Surgeon General, Borden Institute/TMM Publications.

36. Montgomery H: Experimental immersion foot: review of the physiopathology. *Physiol Rev* 34:127, 1954.

37. Francis TJR: Non-freezing cold injury: a historical review. *J R Nav Med Serv* 70:134, 1984.

38. Wrenn K: Immersion foot: a problem of the homeless in the 1990s. *Arch Intern Med* 151:785, 1991.

39. Ramstead KD, Hughes RB, Webb AJ: Recent cases of trench foot. *Postgrad Med J* 56:879, 1980.

40. Biem J, Koehncke N, Classen D, Dosman J: Out of cold: management of hypothermia and frostbite. *Can Med Assoc J* 168(3):305, 2003.

41. Vogel JE, Dellon AL: Frostbite injuries of the hand. *Clin Plast Surg* 16:565, 1989.

42. Mills WJ: Clinical aspects of freezing injury. In Pandolf KB, Burr RE, editors: *Medical aspects of harsh environments,* vol 1, Washington, DC, 2001, Office of the Surgeon General, Borden Institute/TMM Publications.

43. Sessler DI: Mild preoperative hypothermia. *N Engl J Med* 336:1730, 1997.

44. Giesbrecht GG: Cold stress, near drowning and accidental hypothermia: a review. *Aviat Space Environ Med* 71:733, 2000.

45. Giesbrecht GG, Steinman AM: Immersion into cold water. In Auerbach PS: *Wilderness medicine,* ed 5, St Louis, 2007, Mosby Elsevier.

46. Nozaki R, Ishibashi K, Adachi N, et al: Accidental profound hypothermia. *N Eng J Med* 315:1680, 1986 (letter).

47. Gilbert M, Busund R, Skagseth A, et al: Resuscitation from accidental hypothermia of 13.7° C with circulatory arrest. *Lancet* 355:375, 2000.

48. American Heart Association, 2010 Guidelines for cardiopulmonary resuscitation and emergency cardiovascular care science. *Circulation* 12; Suppl 639–946, 2010.

49. Moscati R, Mayrose J, Fincher L, Jehle D: Comparison of normal saline with tap water for wound irrigation. *Am J Emerg Med* 16(4):379, 1998.

50. Southwick FS, Dalglish PH: Recovery after prolonged asystolic cardiac arrest in profound hypothermia: a case report and literature review. *JAMA* 243:1250, 1980.

51. Bernard MB, Gray TW, Buist MD, et al: Treatment of comatose survivors of out-of-hospital cardiac arrest with induced hypothermia. *N Engl J Med* 346(8):557, 2002.

52. Wilderness Medical Society: Myocardial infarction, acute coronary syndromes, and CPR. In Forgey WW, editor: *Practice guidelines for wilderness emergency care,* ed 5, Guilford, 2006, Globe Pequot Press.

53. Bailey DE, Wydro GC, Cone DC: Position paper of the National Association of EMS Physicians: Termination of resuscitation in the prehospital setting for adult patients suffering nontraumatic cardiac arrest. *Prehosp Emerg Care* 4:190, 2000.

54. Gilbertson J, Mandsager R: *State of Alaska cold injuries guidelines.* Department of Health and Social Services, Juneau, Alaska, 2005 (revision). www.chems.alaska.gov/EMS/documents/AKCold Inj2005.pdf.

55. Kizer KW: Dysbaric cerebral air embolism in Hawaii. *Ann Emerg Med* 16:535, 1987.

56. Centers for Disease Control and Prevention: Nonfatal and fatal drowning in recreational water settings—United States, 2001-2002. *MMWR* 53(21):447, 2004.

57. Zuckerman GB, Conway EE Jr: Drowning and near drowning. *Pediatr Ann* 29:6, 2000.

58. Facts about injuries: drowning. www.who.int/violence_injury_prevention/publications/other_injury/en/drowning_factsheet.pdf. Accessed November 25, 2009.

59. Zamula WW: In *Social costs of drowning and near drowning from submersion accidents occurring to children under five in residential swimming pools,* Washington, DC, 1987, US Consumer Product Safety Commission.

60. Schoene RB, Nachat A, Gravatt AR, Newman AB: Submersion incidents. In Auerbach PS: *Wilderness medicine,* ed 5, St Louis, 2007, Mosby Elsevier.

61. DeNicola LK, Falk JL, Swanson ME, Kissoon N: Submersion injuries in children and adults. *Crit Care Clin* 13(3):477, 1997.

62. American Heart Association: 2005 American Heart Association guidelines for cardiopulmonary resuscitation and emergency cardiovascular care: Part 10.3: Drowning. *Circulation* 112:IV–133, 2005.

63. Wilderness Medical Society: Submersion injuries. In Forgey WW: *Practive guidelines for wilderness emergency care,* ed 5, Helena, Mont, 2006, Globe Pequot Press.

64. Orlowski JP, Szppilman D: Drowning. *Pediatr Clin North Am* 48(3):627, 2001.

65. Bolte RG, Black PG, Bowers RS: The use of extracorporeal rewarming in a child submerged for 66 minutes. *JAMA* 260:377, 1988.

66. Lloyd EL: Accidental hypothermia. *Resuscitation* 32:111, 1996.

67. Olshaker JS: Submersion. *Emerg Med Clin North Am* 22:357, 2004.

68. Kyriacou DN, Arcinue EL, Peek C, Kraus JF: Effect of immediate resuscitation on children with submersion injury. *Pediatrics* 94:137, 1994.

69. Karch KB: Pathology of the lung in near-drowning. *Am J Emerg Med* 4(1):4, 1986.

70. Bolte RG, Black PG, Bowers RS: The use of extracorporeal rewarming in a child submerged for 66 minutes. *JAMA* 260:377, 1988.

71. Siebke H, et al: Survival after 40 minutes submersion without cerebral sequelae, *Lancet* 1:1275, 1975.

72. Abella BS, Alvarado JP, Myklebust H, et al: Quality of cardiopulmonary resuscitation during in-hospital cardiac arrest. *JAMA* 293(3):305, 2005.

73. Wik L, Kramer-Johansen J, Myklebust H, et al: Quality of cardiopulmonary resuscitation during out-of-hospital cardiac arrest. *JAMA* 293(3):299, 2005.

74. V. Hwang, S. Frances, D. Durbin, and J. Baren. Prevalence of Traumatic Injuries in Drowning and Near Drowning in Children and Adolescents. *Arch Pediatr Adolesc Med.* 2003; 157(1):50–53).

75. Pratt FD, Haynes BE. Incidence of "secondary drowning" after saltwater submersion. *Ann Emerg Med* 15(9):1084, 1986.

76. Olshaker JS: Near drowning. *Emerg Med Clin North Am* 10(2):339, 1992.

77. Rosen P, Stoto M, Harley J: The use of the Heimlich maneuver in near drowning: Institute of Medicine report. *J Emerg Med* 13:397, 1995.

78. Curran EB, Holle RL, Lopez RE: Lightning fatalities, injuries and damage reports in the United States, 1959-1994. *NOAA Tech Memo NWS SR-193*, 1997, www.nssl.noaa.gov/papers/techmemos/NWS-SR-193/techmemo-sr193.html.

79. Gatewood MO, Zane RD: Lightning injuries. *Emerg Med Clin North Am* 22:369, 2004.

80. Huffins GR, Orville RE: Lightning ground flash density and thunderstorm duration in the contiguous United States. *J Appl Meteorol* 38:1013, 1999.

81. Cummins KL, Krider EP, Malone MD: A combined TOA/MDF technology upgrade of the US National Lightning Detection Network. *J Geophys Res* 103:9035, 1998.

82. MacGorman, DR, Rust WD: Lightning strike density for the contiguous United States from thunderstorm duration records, Pub No NUREG/CR03759, Washington, DC, 1984, Office of Nuclear Regulatory Research.

83. Dulcos PJ, Sanderson LM, Klontz KC: Lightning-related mortality and morbidity in Florida. *Pub Health Rep* 105:276, 1990.

84. Centers for Disease Control and Prevention: Lightning associated deaths—1980-1995, *MMWR* 47(19):391, 1998.

85. Cooper MA: Lightning injuries: prognostic signs of death. *Ann Emerg Med* 9:134, 1980.

86. Andrews CJ, Darveniza M, Mackerras D. Lightning injury: a review of the clinical aspects, pathophysiology and treatment. *Adv Trauma* 4:241, 1989.

87. American Heart Association: 2005 American Heart Association guidelines for cardiopulmonary resuscitation and emergency cardiovascular care. Part 10.9: electric shock and lightning strike. *Circulation* 112:IV–154, 2005.

88. Cooper MA, Andrews CJ, Holle RL, Lopez RE: Lightning injuries. In Auerbach PS: *Wilderness medicine*, ed 5, St Louis, 2007, Mosby Elsevier.

89. Ritenour AE, Morton MJ, McManus JG, et al: Lightning injury: a review. *Burns* 34:585, 2008.

90. Casten JA, Kytilla J: Eye symptoms caused by lightning. *Acta Ophthalmol* 41:139, 1963.

91. Taussig HB: Death from lightning and the possibility of living again. *Ann Intern Med* 68:1345, 1968.

92. *Merriam-Webster's collegiate dictionary*, ed 10, Springfield, MA, 1996, Merriam-Webster, Inc.

93. Conover K: EMTs should be able to clear the cervical spine in the wilderness. *J Wild Med* 3(4):339, 1992 (editorial).

94. Gomi T: *Everyone poops*, New York, 1993, Kane/Miller Book Publishers.

95. Goldberg R, Chan D, Mason J, Chan L: Backboard versus mattress splint immobilization: a comparison of symptoms generated. *J Emerg Med* 14(3):293, 1996.

96. Hamilton RS, Pons PT: The efficacy and comfort of full-body vacuum splints for cervical-spine immobilization. *J Emerg Med* 14(5):553, 1996.

97. Johnson DR, Hauswald M, Stockhoff C: Comparison of a vacuum splint device to a rigid backboard for spinal immobilization. *Am J Emerg Med* 14(4):369, 1996.

98. Lovell ME, Evans JH: A comparison of the spinal board and the vacuum stretcher, spinal stability and interface pressure. *Injury* 25(3):179, 1994.

99. Chan D, Goldberg R, Tascone A, et al: The effect of spinal immobilization on healthy volunteers, *Ann Emerg Med* 23(1):48, 1994.

100. Cordell WH, Hollingsworth JC, Olinger ML, et al: Pain and tissue-interface pressures during spine-board immobilization. *Ann Emerg Med* 26(1):31, 1995.

101. Delbridge TR, Auble TE, Garrison HG, Menengazzi JJ: Discomfort in healthy volunteers immobilized on wooden backboards and vacuum mattress splints. *Prehosp Disaster Med* 8(suppl 2), 1993.

102. Linares HA, Mawson AR, Suarez E: Association between pressure sores and immobilization in the immediate post-injury period. *Orthopedics* 10:571, 1987.

103. Mawson AR, Bundo JJ, Neville P: Risk factors for early occurring pressure ulcers following spinal cord injury. *Am J Phys Med Rehab* 67:123, 1988.

104. Edlich RF, Rodeheaver GT, Morgan RF, et al: Principles of emergency wound management. *Ann Emerg Med* 17(12):1284, 1988.

105. Edlich RF, Thacker JG, Buchanan L, Rodeheaver GT: Modern concepts of treatment of traumatic wounds. *Adv Surg* 13:169, 1979.

106. Bhandari M, Thompson K, Adili A, Shaughnessy SG: High and low pressure irrigation in contaminated wounds with exposed bone. *Int J Surg Invest* 2(3):179, 2000.

107. Bhandari M, Adili A, Lachowski RJ: High pressure pulsatile lavage of contaminated human tibiae: an in vitro study. *J Orthop Trauma* 12(7):479, 1998.

108. Bhandari M, Schemitsch EH, Adili A, et al: High and low pressure pulsatile lavage of contaminated tibial fractures: an in vitro study of bacterial adherence and bone damage. *J Orthop Trauma* 13(8):526, 1999.

109. Anglen JO: Wound irrigation in musculoskeletal injury. *J Am Acad Orthop Surg* 9(4):219, 2001.

110. Valente JH, Forti RJ, Freundlich LF, et al: Wound irrigation in children: saline solution or tap water? *Ann Emerg Med* 41(5):609, 2003.

111. Backer HD: Field water disinfection. In Auerbach PS, Geehr EC, editors: *Wilderness medicine: management of wilderness and environmental emergencies,* ed 2, St Louis, 1989, Mosby.

112. Griffiths RD, Fernandez RS, Ussia CA: Is tap water a safe alternative to normal saline for wound irrigation in the community setting? *J Wound Care* 10(10):407, 2001.

113. Moscati RM, Reardon RF, Lerner EB, Mayrose J: Wound irrigation with tap water. *Acad Emerg Med* 5(11):1076, 1998.

114. Rodeheaver GT, Pettry D, Thacker JG, et al: Wound cleansing by high pressure irrigation. *Surg Gynecol Obstet* 141(3):357, 1975.

115. Edlich RF, Reddy VR: Revolutionary advances in wound repair in emergency medicine during the last three decades: a view toward the new millennium—5th Annual David R. Boyd, MD, Lecture. *J Emerg Med* 20(2):167, 2001.

116. Singer AJ, Hollander JE, Subramanian S, et al: Pressure dynamics of various irrigation techniques commonly used in the emergency department. *Ann Emerg Med* 24(1):36, 1994.

117. Fulton RL, Voigt WJ, Hilakos AS: Confusion surrounding the treatment of traumatic cardiac arrest, *J Am Coll Surg* 181:209, 1995.

118. Pasquale MD, Rhodes M, Cipolle MD, et al: Defining "dead on arrival": impact on a Level I trauma center. *J Trauma* 41:726, 1996.

119. Mattox KL, Feliciano DV: Role of external cardiac compression in truncal trauma. *J Trauma* 22:934, 1982.

120. Shimazu S, Shatney CH: Outcomes of trauma patients with no vital signs on admission. *J Trauma* 23(3):213, 1983.

121. Forgey WW, Wilderness Medical Society: *Practice guidelines for wilderness emergency care,* ed 2, Guilford, Conn, 2001, Globe Pequot Press.
122. Goth P, Garnett G, Rural Affairs Committee, National Association of EMS Physicians: Clinical guidelines for delayed/prolonged transport. I. Cardiorespiratory arrest. *Prehosp Disaster Med* 6(3):335, 1991.
123. Bowman WD: CPR and wilderness rescue: when and when not to use it, *Response,* 1987.
124. Eisenberg MS, Bergner L, Hallstrom AP: Cardiac resuscitation in the community: importance of rapid provision and implications of program planning. *JAMA* 241:1905, 1979.
125. Kellermann AL, Hackman BB, Somes G: Predicting the outcome of unsuccessful prehospital advanced cardiac life support. *JAMA* 270(12):1433, 1993.
126. Bonnin MJ, Pepe PE, Kimball KT, Clark PS: Distinct criteria for termination of resuscitation in the out-of-hospital setting. *JAMA* 270(12):1457, 1993.
127. Leavitt M, Podgorny G: Prehospital CPR and the pulseless hypothermic patient. *Ann Emerg Med* 13:492, 1984.
128. Keatinge WR: Accidental immersion hypothermia and drowning, *Practitioner* 219:183, 1977.
129. Olshaker JS: Near drowning. *Emerg Med Clin North Am* 10(2):339, 1992.
130. Orlowski JP: Drowning, near-drowning, and ice-water drowning. *JAMA* 260(3):390, 1988 (editorial).
131. Cooper MA: Lightning injuries. In Auerbach PS, Geehr EC, editors: *Wilderness medicine: management of wilderness and environmental emergencies,* ed 2, St Louis, 1989, Mosby.
132. Durrer B, Brugger H: Recent advances in avalanche survival. Presented at the Second World Congress on Wilderness Medicine, Aspen, Colo, 1995.
133. Steinman AM: Cardiopulmonary resuscitation and hypothermia, *Circulation* 74(6, pt 2):29, 1986.
134. Zell SC: Epidemiology of wilderness-acquired diarrhea: implications for prevention and treatment, *J Wild Med* 3(3):241, 1992.
135. Lloyd EL: *Hypothermia and cold stress,* Rockville, Md, 1986, Aspen Systems.
136. Maningas PA, DeGuzman LR, Hollenbach SJ, et al: Regional blood flow during hypothermic arrest, *Ann Emerg Med* 15(4):390, 1986.
137. Curry SC, Kunkel DB: Death from a rattlesnake bite. *Am J Emerg Med* 3(3):227, 1985.
138. Bush SP: Snakebite suction devices don't remove venom: they just suck, *Ann Emerg Med* 43(2):187, 2004.
139. Alberts MB, Shalit M, LoGalbo F: Suction for venomous snakebite: a study of "mock venom" extraction in a human model, *Ann Emerg Med* 43(2):181, 2004.
140. Davis D, Branch K, Egen NB, et al: The effect of an electrical current on snake venom toxicity. *J Wild Med* 3(1):48, 1992.
141. Howe NR, Meisenheimer JL Jr: Electric shock does not save snakebitten rats. *Ann Emerg Med* 17(3):254, 1988.
142. Gill KA Jr: The evaluation of cryotherapy in the treatment of snake envenomation. *South Med J* 63:552, 1968.
143. Norris RL: A call for snakebite research. *Wilderness Environ Med* 11(3):149, 2000.
144. Stewart ME, Greenland S, Hoffman JR: First-aid treatment of poisonous snakebite: are currently recommended procedures justified? *Ann Emerg Med* 10(6):331, 1981.

Suggested Reading

Auerbach PS, editor: *Wilderness medicine,* ed 5, St Louis, 2007, Mosby.

Bennett P, Elliott D: *The physiology and medicine of diving,* ed 4, Philadelphia, 1993, Saunders.

Bove AA: *Bove and Davis' diving medicine,* ed 5, Philadelphia, 2003, Saunders.

Fregly MJ, Blatteis CM: *Environmental physiology,* vols I & II, New York, 1996, Oxford University Press.

Goth P, Garnett G: Clinical guidelines for delayed or prolonged transport: II. Dislocations. Rural Affairs Committee, National Association of Emergency Medical Services Physicians. *Prehosp Disaster Med* 8(1):77, 1993.

Goth P, Garnett G: Clinical guidelines for delayed or prolonged transport: IV. Wounds. Rural Affairs Committee, Nation Association of Emergency Medical Services Physicians. *Prehosp Disaster Med* 8(3):253, 1993.

Pandolf KB, Burr RE, editors: *Medical aspects of harsh environments,* vol 1, Washington, DC, 2001, Office of the Surgeon General, Borden Institute/TMM Publications.

Sutton JR, Coates G, Remmers JE, editors: *Hypoxia: the adaptations,* Philadelphia, 1990, BC Decker.

CHAPTER 10

Pediatric and Geriatric Trauma

CHAPTER OBJECTIVES

At the completion of this chapter, the reader will be able to do the following:

✓ Discuss the unique anatomy, physiology, and pathophysiology considerations of the pediatric trauma patient.

✓ Discuss the common mechanisms of injury associated with pediatric trauma.

✓ Demonstrate an understanding of the special importance of managing the airway and restoring adequate tissue oxygenation in pediatric patients.

✓ Identify the quantitative vital signs for children.

✓ Demonstrate an understanding of management techniques for the various injuries found in pediatric patients.

✓ Identify the signs of pediatric trauma suggestive of nonaccidental trauma.

✓ Discuss the common mechanisms of injury in the elderly population.

✓ Discuss the anatomic and physiologic effects of aging as a factor in causes of geriatric trauma and as a factor in the pathophysiology of trauma.

✓ Explain the interaction of various preexisting medical problems with traumatic injuries in elderly patients to produce differences in the pathophysiology and manifestations of trauma.

✓ Explain the physiologic effects of specific common classes of medications on the pathophysiology and manifestations of geriatric trauma.

✓ Compare and contrast the assessment techniques and considerations used in the elderly population with those used in younger populations.

✓ Demonstrate modifications in spinal immobilization techniques for safe and effective spinal immobilization of the elderly patient with the highest degree of comfort possible.

✓ Compare and contrast the management of the elderly trauma patient with that of the younger trauma patient.

✓ Assess the scene and elderly patients for signs and symptoms of abuse and neglect.

SCENARIO 1

You are called to the scene of a motor vehicle crash on a heavily traveled highway. Two vehicles have been involved in a frontal offset collision. One of the vehicle's occupants was a child who had been placed in, but not properly restrained in, a child car seat. No weather-related factors are involved on this average spring afternoon.

On arrival at the scene, you see that the police have secured and blocked traffic from the area around the crash. As your partner is assessing the other patients, you approach the child; you see a young boy, approximately 2 years of age, sitting in the car seat slightly turned at an angle, there is blood on the back of the headrest of the seat in front of him. You also note that despite numerous abrasions, and minor bleeding from the head, face, and neck; the child appears very calm.

Your primary and secondary surveys reveal a 2-year-old boy who repeats weakly "ma-ma, ma-ma." He has central and distal pulses at a rate of 180 beats/min, with the radial pulse weaker than the carotid; his blood pressure is 50 mm Hg by palpation; and his ventilatory rate is 18 breaths/minute, slightly irregular, but without abnormal sounds. As you continue to assess him, you note that he has stopped saying "ma-ma" and seems to just stare into space. You also note that his pupils are slightly dilated, and his skin is pale and sweaty. A woman who identifies herself as the family's nanny tells you that the mother is en route and that you should wait for her.

What are the management priorities for this patient?

What are the most likely injuries in this child?

Where is the most appropriate destination for this child?

Pediatric Trauma

Annual data reporting from the Centers for Disease Control and Prevention shows that although the leading cause of death continues to vary by age group, injury is the most common cause of death for children in the United States. More than 8.7 million children are injured annually, and approximately every 30 minutes a child dies as a result of injuries.[1,2] Tragically, as many as 80% of these deaths may be avoidable, either by effective injury prevention strategies or by ensuring proper care in the acute injury phase.[3]

As with all aspects of pediatric care, proper assessment and management of an injured child requires a thorough understanding of not only the unique characteristics of childhood growth and development (including their immature anatomy and developing physiology) but also their unique mechanisms of injury.

Thus, the adage holds true that "children are not just little adults." Children have distinct, reproducible patterns of injury, different physiologic responses, and special treatment needs, based on their physical and psychosocial development at the time of injury.

This chapter describes the special characteristics of the pediatric trauma patient and reviews optimal trauma management and its rationale. Although the unique characteristics of pediatric injury are important to understand, the fundamental treatment approach using the primary and secondary surveys are the same for every patient, regardless of age or size.

The Child as Trauma Patient

Demographics of Pediatric Trauma

The incidence of blunt (vs. penetrating) trauma is highest in the pediatric population (Figure 10-1). The consequences of penetrating trauma are relatively predictable, but blunt trauma mechanisms have a greater potential for multisystem injury. Falls, pedestrians struck by auto, and occupant injury

FIGURE 10-1 Common Causes of Unintentional Pediatric Death and Injury

Unintentional Injury—Fatal	Unintentional Injury—Nonfatal
1. Transportation related	1. Falls
2. Drowning	2. Struck by
3. Suffocation	3. Overexertion
4. Other	4. Motor vehicle occupant
5. Poisoning	5. Lacerations
6. Fires/burns	6. Bites/stings
7. Falls	7. Bicycle related

(From Borse NN, Gilchrist J, Dellinger AM, et al: *CDC Childhood Injury Report: Patterns of Unintentional Injuries among 0–19 Year Olds in the United States, 2000–2006*, Atlanta, 2008, National Center for Injury Prevention and Control.)

as a result of motor vehicle crashes are the most common causes of pediatric injury in the United States, with falls alone accounting for more than 2.5 million injuries a year.[2] According to statistics, injury is "unintentional" in 87% of cases, sports related in 4%, and the result of assault in 5%. For a variety of reasons, to be discussed throughout this chapter, multisystem involvement is the rule rather than the exception in major pediatric trauma. Although there may only be minimal external evidence of injury present, potentially life-threatening internal injury may still exist and must be evaluated for at a definitive treatment center.

Kinematics of Pediatric Trauma

A child's size produces a smaller target to which the forces and energy from fenders, bumpers, and falls are applied. Because of minimal cushioning body fat, increased elasticity of connective tissue, and proximity of the organs to the surface of the body, these forces are not as easily dissipated as they are in the adult and therefore energy is more readily transmitted to underlying organs. Additionally, the skeleton of a child is incompletely calcified, contains multiple active growth centers, and is more resilient than that of an adult. Consequently, the skeleton of a child is less able to absorb the kinetic forces applied to it during a traumatic event, allowing significant force to be transmitted to underlying organs. As a result, there may be significant internal injuries without obvious evidence of external trauma. For example, in a pediatric patient with blunt thoracic trauma, the chest wall might appear intact without evidence of rib fractures, though significant underlying pulmonary contusion might still exist.

Common Patterns of Injury

The unique anatomic and physiologic characteristics of the pediatric patient, combined with the age-specific common mechanisms of injury, produce distinct but predictable patterns of injury (Figure 10-2). Improper seat belt usage or placement in the vehicle with resulting impact with airbags can lead to significant injury in the pediatric patient (Figure 10-3). Trauma is often a time of critical illness, and being familiar with these patterns will assist the prehospital provider in optimizing management decisions for the injured child in an expeditious manner. For example, blunt pediatric trauma involving closed head injury results in apnea, hypoventilation, and hypoxia much more commonly than hypovolemia and hypotension. Therefore, clinical care guidelines for pediatric trauma patients should include greater emphasis on aggressive management of the airway and breathing.

Body Heat and Temperature Maintenance

The ratio between a child's body surface area (BSA) and body mass is highest at birth and diminishes throughout infancy and childhood. Consequently, more surface area exists through which heat can quickly be lost, not only providing additional stress to the child but also complicating the child's physiologic responses to concomitantly occurring metabolic

FIGURE 10-2 **Common Patterns of Injury Associated with Pediatric Trauma**

Type of Trauma	Patterns of Injury
Motor vehicle crash (child is passenger)	*Unrestrained:* Multiple trauma, head and neck injuries, scalp and facial lacerations *Restrained:* Chest and abdomen injuries, lower spine fractures *Side impact:* Head, neck, and chest injuries; extremity fracture *Deployed air bag:* Head, face, chest injuries; upper extremity fractures
Motor vehicle crash (child is pedestrian)	*Low speed:* Lower extremity fractures *High speed:* Multiple trauma, head and neck injuries, lower extremity fractures
Fall from a height	*Low:* Upper extremity fractures *Medium:* Head and neck injuries, upper and lower extremity fractures *High:* Multiple trauma, head and neck injuries, upper and lower extremity fractures
Fall from bicycle	*Without helmet:* Head and neck lacerations, scalp and facial lacerations, upper extremity fractures *With helmet:* Upper extremity fractures *Striking handlebar:* Internal abdominal injuries

(Modified from American College of Surgeons Committee on Trauma: Extremes of age: pediatric trauma. In *Advanced trauma life support for doctors, student course manual,* ed 7, Chicago, 2004, ACS.)

derangements and shock. Severe hypothermia can result in coagulopathy and potentially irreversible cardiovascular collapse. In addition, many of the clinical signs of hypothermia are similar to those of impending uncompensated shock, thereby potentially complicating the prehospital provider's clinical assessment.

Psychosocial Issues

The psychological ramifications of caring for an injured child also present a major challenge. Particularly with a very young child, regressive psychological behavior may result when stress, pain, or other perceived threats impair the child's ability to compensate for the surrounding events. A child's ability to interact with unfamiliar individuals in strange surroundings is usually limited and makes history taking, examination, and treatment an arduous task. An understanding of these characteristics and a willingness to soothe and comfort an injured child are often the most effective means of

Pediatric Injuries Associated with Seat Belts and Air Bags

Despite laws in all 50 states requiring the use of car safety seats or child restraint devices for young children, in almost half of motor vehicle crashes (MVCs) the child is not restrained or is improperly restrained.[25] Furthermore, if a child is the front-seat occupant in a vehicle with a passenger-side air bag, the child is just as likely to sustain serious injury whether appropriately restrained or not.[26] A child exposed to a passenger-side air bag is twice as likely to sustain significant injury as a front-seat passenger without an air bag.[27]

Children with lap belt or inappropriate seat belt placement are thought to be at increased risk for bowel injury in MVCs. The incidence is difficult to determine. In one study, 20% of injured children had a visible seat belt bruise, and 50% of those had significant intraabdominal injuries; almost 25% of those had intestinal perforation.[31] Others have shown an increased risk, but not to this extent, with only 5% of injured children having an abdominal wall bruise from the seat belt, and only 13% of those with bruising having intestinal injury.[32] It is reasonable to assume that any child found restrained by a lap belt with abdominal wall bruising after a motor vehicle crash has an intraabdominal injury until proved otherwise.

Approximately 1% of all MVCs involving children also resulted in exposure of the child to a deployed passenger air bag. Of these children, 14% suffered serious injury, compared with 7.5% of restrained front-seat passengers not exposed to an airbag. Overall risk of any injury was 86% versus 55% in the control (non–airbag-exposed) group of patients.[27] Minor air bag injury included minor upper torso and facial burns and lacerations. Major air bag injury consisted of significant chest, neck, face, and upper extremity injury.[33] There has been a documented decapitation of a child by a passenger air bag.[2]

achieving good rapport and obtaining a comprehensive assessment of the child's physiologic state.

The child's parents, or caregivers, also commonly have unique needs and issues that if addressed may assist the prehospital care provider in caring for the child successfully, though if ignored can present significant obstacles to effective care. Whenever a child is sick or injured, the caregivers are also affected and should be considered your patients as well. The treatment of all patients begins with effective communication, but this become even more important when dealing with these "parent-patients." It may consist only of simple words of compassion, or it may require great lengths of patience, but you cannot be an effective provider for a pediatric patient if you are ignorant of the parents/caregivers needs. When you include

the parents/caregivers in the process, they can often act as functional members of their child's emergency care team.

Recovery and Rehabilitation

Another problem unique to the pediatric trauma patient is the effect that even minor injury may have on subsequent growth and development. Unlike an anatomically mature adult, a child must not only recover from the injury but also continue his or her normal growth. The effect of injury on this process, especially in terms of permanent disability, growth deformity, or subsequent abnormal development, cannot be overestimated. Children sustaining even minor traumatic brain injury may have prolonged disability in cerebral function, psychological adjustment, or other regulated organ systems. As many as 60% of children who have suffered severe multiple trauma have personality changes, and 50% are left with subtle cognitive or physical handicaps. The reach of these injuries does not stop there, because these disabilities can have a substantial effect on siblings and parents, resulting in a high incidence of family dysfunction, including divorce. The direct and indirect costs of correcting these problems are staggering and lifelong.

The effects of inadequate or suboptimal care in the acute injury phase may have far reaching consequences not only on the child's immediate survival but also, perhaps more importantly, on the long-term quality of the child's life.

Pathophysiology

The final outcome for the injured child may be determined by the quality of care rendered in the first moments following an injury. During this critical period, a coordinated, systematic primary survey is the best strategy to avoid overlooking a potentially fatal injury or one that may cause unnecessary morbidity. As in the adult patient, the three most common causes of immediate death in the child are hypoxia, massive hemorrhage, and overwhelming central nervous system (CNS) trauma. Lack of expedient triage, stabilizing emergency medical treatment and transport to the most appropriate center for treatment can compound these problems or even eliminate the potential for a meaningful recovery.

Hypoxia. The first priority in prehospital care is always to maintain a clear and open airway. Confirming that a child has an open and functioning airway does not preclude the need for supplemental oxygen and assisted ventilation, especially when CNS injury, hypoventilation, or hypoperfusion is present. Well-appearing injured children can rapidly deteriorate from mild tachypnea to a state of total exhaustion and apnea. Once an airway is established, the rate and depth of ventilation should be carefully evaluated to confirm adequate ventilation. If ventilation is inadequate, merely providing an excessive concentration of oxygen will not prevent ongoing or worsening hypoxia; instead, ventilations must be assisted with a bag-mask device.

The effects of even transient hypoxia on the traumatically injured brain can be particularly devastating and hence deserve special attention. A child may have significant alteration in level of consciousness (LOC) but retain an excellent potential for a complete functional recovery if cerebral hypoxia is avoided. Many children can be adequately ventilated and oxygenated using good basic life support skills, such as bag-mask ventilation.

Hemorrhage

Most pediatric injuries do not cause immediate exsanguination. Unfortunately, however, children who sustain injuries that result in major blood loss often die within moments of the injury or shortly after arrival at a receiving facility. These fatalities often have multiple internal organs injured and have at least one significant injury associated with acute blood loss.

As in adults, the injured child compensates for hemorrhage by constricting blood vessels; this is, however, at the expense of peripheral circulation. In fact, children are physiologically more adept at this response because their ability to vasoconstrict is not limited by preexisting peripheral vascular disease. Therefore, utilizing blood pressure measurements alone is an inadequate strategy to identify the early signs of shock. Tachycardia, although it may be the result of fear or pain, should be considered to be secondary to hemorrhage or hypovolemia until proven otherwise. An increasing tachycardia may be the first subtle sign of impending shock. Furthermore, the prehospital provider must pay close attention to signs of ineffective organ perfusion as evidenced by a decreased level of consciousness and diminished skin perfusion (decreased temperature and poor color). Unlike the adult, these early signs of hemorrhage in the child may be subtle and difficult to identify, leading to a deceptive presentation of shock. If the prehospital care provider misses these early signs, a child may lose enough circulating blood volume that compensatory mechanisms fail. When this happens, cardiac output plummets, organ perfusion decreases, and the child can rapidly decompensate, often leading to irreversible, fatal hypotension and shock. Therefore, every child who sustains blunt trauma should be carefully monitored to detect these subtle signs that might signal ongoing hemorrhage long before there are vital sign abnormalities.

Central Nervous System Injury. The pathophysiologic changes after CNS trauma begin within minutes. Early and adequate resuscitation is the key to increased survival of children with CNS trauma. Although a subset of CNS injuries are instantaneous and overwhelmingly fatal, many children may present with the appearance of a devastating neurologic injury only to go on to a complete and functional recovery, but only if there is a coordinated and deliberate effort to prevent secondary injury. This is achieved through the prevention of subsequent episodes of hypoperfusion, hypoventilation, hyperventilation, and ischemia. Adequate ventilation and oxygenation (while avoiding hyperventilation) are as critical in the management of TBIs as the avoidance of hypotension.[6] Thus, in traumatic brain injury, care must be taken with every child to prevent secondary brain injury from hypotension, hypoxia, and other insults.

Children with TBI often present with an alteration in consciousness, and they may have sustained a period of unconsciousness not recorded during the initial evaluation. A history of loss of consciousness is one of the most important prognostic indicators of potential CNS injury, and should be investigated and recorded for every case. In the event that the injury was unwitnessed, amnesia to the event is commonly used as a surrogate for a loss of consciousness. Similarly, complete documentation of baseline neurologic status is important, including the following:

1. Glasgow Coma Scale score (modified for pediatrics)
2. Pupillary reaction
3. Response to sensory stimulation
4. Motor function

These are essential steps in the initial pediatric trauma assessment for neurologic injury. The absence of an adequate baseline assessment makes ongoing follow-up and evaluation of the effectiveness of any interventions extremely imprecise and difficult.

ASSESSMENT

Primary Survey

The small and variable size of the pediatric patient (Figure 10-4), the diminished caliber and size of the blood vessels and circulating volume, and the unique anatomic characteristics of the airway often make the standard procedures used in basic life support extremely challenging and technically difficult. Effective pediatric trauma resuscitation mandates the availability of appropriately sized blood pressure cuffs, oxygen masks, bag-mask devices, and associated equipment. Attempting to place an overly large device can do more harm than good, not only because of the potential physical damage to the patient but also because it may delay transport to the appropriate facility.

FIGURE 10-4 **Height and Weight Range for Pediatric Patients**

| | | Range of Mean Norms | |
		Average Height (cm/in)	Average Weight (kg/lbs)
Group	Age		
Newborn	Birth–6 wk	51–63/20–25	4–5/8–11
Infant	7 wk–1 yr	56–80/22–32	4–11/8–24
Toddler	1–2 yr	77–91/30–36	11–14/24–30
Preschool	2–6 yr	91–122/36–48	14–25/30–55
School age	6–13 yr	122–165/48–66	25–63/55–138
Adolescent	13–16 yr	165–182/66–72	62–80/138–176

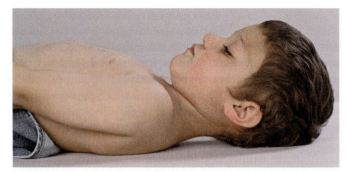

FIGURE 10-5 Compared with an adult, a child has a larger occiput and more shoulder musculature. When placed on a flat surface, these factors result in flexion of the neck.

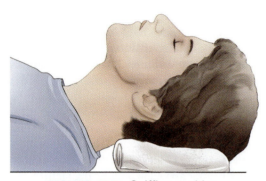

FIGURE 10-6 Sniffing position.

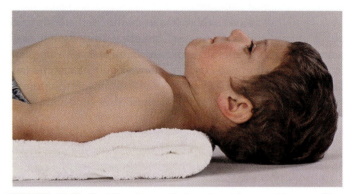

FIGURE 10-7 Padding beneath the shoulders and torso will prevent this hyperflexion.

Airway. As in the adult, the immediate priority and focus in the acutely injured child is on airway management. However, there are several anatomic differences that complicate the care of the injured child. Children have a relatively large occiput, tongue and anterior position of the airway. Additionally, the smaller the child, the greater the discrepancy in size between the cranium and the face. Therefore, the relatively large occiput forces passive flexion of the cervical spine (Figure 10-5). These factors all predispose children to a higher risk of anatomic airway obstruction than adults. In the absence of trauma, the pediatric patient's airway is best protected by a slightly superior-anterior position of the face, known as the *sniffing position* (Figure 10-6). In the presence of trauma, however, the *neutral position* best protects the cervical spine while ensuring adequate airway opening. Thus, in the pediatric trauma patient, the neck should be kept immobilized to prevent movement that occurs to place the head in the sniffing position. Placing a pad or blanket of 2 to 3 cm in thickness under the child's chest and shoulders will lessen the acute flexion of the neck and help keep the airway patent (Figure 10-7). Manual stabilization of the cervical spine is done during airway management and maintained until the child is immobilized on a long backboard with an appropriate cervical immobilization device, whether it is commercially purchased or a simple solution such as towel rolls.

Bag-mask ventilation with high flow (at least 15 L/minute) 100% oxygen probably represents the best choice when the injured child requires assisted ventilation, whether for failure to ventilate, failure to oxygenate, or anticipated course.[4] If the child is unconscious, an oropharyngeal airway (OPA) may sometimes be safely placed, but it is likely to cause vomiting in the child with an intact gag reflex.

Breathing. As in all trauma patients, a significantly traumatized child typically needs an oxygen concentration of 85% to 100%. This is accomplished by the use of supplemental oxygen and an appropriately sized, *clear plastic* pediatric mask. When hypoxia occurs in the small child, the body compensates by increasing the ventilatory rate (tachypnea) and by a strenuous increase in ventilatory effort, including increased thoracic excursion efforts and the use of accessory muscles in the neck and abdomen. This increased metabolic demand can produce severe fatigue and result in ventilatory failure, as an increasing percentage of the patient's cardiac output is being devoted to maintaining this respiratory effort. Ventilatory distress can rapidly progress from a compensated ventilatory effort to ventilatory failure, then respiratory arrest, and ultimately a hypoxic cardiac arrest. Cyanosis is a fairly late and often inconsistent sign of respiratory failure and should not be depended on to recognize developing respiratory failure.

Evaluation of the child's ventilatory status with early recognition of the signs of distress and the provision of ventilatory assistance are key elements in the management of the pediatric trauma patient. The normal ventilatory rate of infants and children younger than 4 years is typically two to three times that of adults (Figure 10-8).

Tachypnea with signs of increased effort or difficulty may be the first manifestation of respiratory distress and shock. As distress increases, additional signs and symptoms include shallow breathing or minimal chest movement. Breath sounds may be weak or infrequent, and air exchange at the nose or mouth may be reduced or minimal. Ventilatory effort becomes more labored and may include the following:

- Head bobbing with each breath
- Gasping or grunting

FIGURE 10-8 **Ventilatory Rates for Pediatric Patients**

Group	Age	Ventilatory Rate (breaths/min)	Ventilatory Rate (breaths/min) That Indicates Possible Need for Ventilatory Assistance with Bag-Valve-Mask
Newborn	Birth–6 wk	30–50	< 30 or > 50
Infant	7 wk–1 yr	20–30	< 20 or > 30
Toddler	1–2 yr	20–30	< 20 or > 30
Preschool	2–6 yr	20–30	< 20 or > 30
School age	6–13 yr	(12–20)–30	< 20 or > 30
Adolescent	13–16 yr	12–20	< 12 or > 20

- Flared nostrils
- Stridor or snoring respirations
- Suprasternal, supraclavicular, subcostal, or intercostal retractions
- Use of accessory muscles of neck and abdominal wall muscles
- Distension of the abdomen when the chest falls (seesaw effect between the chest and abdomen)

The effectiveness of a child's ventilation should be evaluated using the following indicators:

- Rate and depth (minute volume) and effort indicate adequacy of ventilation.
- Pink skin may indicate adequate ventilation.
- Dusky, gray, cyanotic, or mottled skin indicates insufficient oxygenation and perfusion.
- Anxiety, restlessness, and combativeness can be early signs of hypoxia.
- Lethargy, depressed LOC, and unconsciousness are probably advanced signs of hypoxia.

In the child initially presenting with tachypnea and increased ventilatory effort, normalization of the ventilatory rate and apparent lessening of the respiratory effort should not be immediately interpreted as a sign of improvement as it may indicate exhaustion or impending failure. As with any change in the patient's clinical status, frequent reassessment is necessary to determine if this is an improvement or deterioration in physiologic status. Ventilatory assistance should be given to those children in acute ventilatory distress. Because the main problem is one of inspired volume rather than concentration of oxygen, assisted ventilation is best given by use of a bag-mask device, supplemented with an oxygen reservoir attached to high-concentration oxygen. Because a child's airway is so small, it is prone to obstruction from increased secretions, blood/body fluids, and foreign materials; therefore, early and periodic suctioning may be necessary. In infants, who are obligate nose breathers, the nostrils should also be suctioned.

When obtaining a mask seal in infants, caution should be exercised to avoid compressing the soft tissues underneath the chin because this pushes the tongue against the soft palate and increases the risk of occluding the airway. Pressure on the uncalcified, soft trachea should also be avoided. One or two hands can be used to obtain a mask seal, depending on the size and age of the child.

Use of the correct size bag-mask device is essential for obtaining a proper mask seal, providing the proper size breath, and ensuring that the risks of hyperinflation and barotrauma are minimized. Ventilating a child too forcefully or with too large a volume can lead to gastric distension. In turn, *gastric distension* can result in regurgitation, aspiration, and can prevent adequate ventilation by limiting diaphragmatic excursion. Changes in a child's ventilatory status can be subtle, but ventilatory effort can rapidly deteriorate until ventilation is inadequate and hypoxia ensues. The patient's breathing should be evaluated as part of the primary survey and carefully and periodically reassessed to ensure its continued adequacy. Whenever a child is being manually ventilated, it is important to carefully control the rate at which ventilations are being administered. It is relatively easy to inadvertently hyperventilate the patient, which will decrease the CO_2 level in the blood and cause cerebral vasoconstriction. This can lead to poorer outcomes in patients with traumatic brain injury.

Circulation. The survival rate from immediate exsanguinating injury is low in the pediatric population. Fortunately, the incidence of this type of injury is also low. External hemorrhage should be quickly identified and controlled by direct manual pressure during the primary survey. Injured children usually present with at least some circulating blood volume. As in the assessment of the airway, a single measurement of heart rate (HR) or blood pressure (BP) does not equate with physiologic stability. Serial measurements and changing trends of vital signs are critical in gauging a child's evolving hemodynamic state in the acute injury phase. Close monitoring of vital signs is absolutely essential to recognizing the signs of impending shock, so that the appropriate interventions can be performed to prevent clinical deterioration. Figures 10-9 and 10-10 provide the normal ranges for pulse rate and BP, respectively, for different pediatric age groups.

If the primary survey suggests hypotension, the most likely cause is blood loss through a major external wound that is readily observable (large scalp laceration, open femur fracture), an intrathoracic wound (identifiable by diminished ventilatory mechanics and auscultatory findings), or a major intraabdominal injury. Blood loss from a major intraabdominal injury can produce abdominal distension and increasing abdominal girth. However, increased abdominal girth in the young pediatric trauma patient can also commonly be caused by gastric distension from crying and air swallowing. It is best to assume that a distended abdomen is a sign of potentially significant abdominal injury.

A major consideration in the assessment of a pediatric patient is compensated shock. Because of their increased physiologic reserve, children with hemorrhagic injury frequently present with only slightly abnormal vital signs. Initial tachycardia may be not only the result of hypovolemia but also the effect of psychological stress, pain, and fear. All injured children should have their heat rate, ventilatory rate,

FIGURE 10-9 Pulse Rate for Pediatric Patients

Group	Age	Pulse Rate (beats/min)	Pulse Rate (Beats/Min) That Indicates a Possible Serious Problem*
Newborn	Birth–6 wk	120–160	< 100 or > 160
Infant	7 wk–1 yr	80–140	< 80 or > 150
Toddler	1–2 yr	80–130	< 60 or > 140
Preschool	2–6 yr	80–120	< 60 or > 130
School age	6–13 yr	(60–80)–100	< 60 or > 120
Adolescent	13–16 yr	60–100	< 60 or > 100

*Bradycardia or tachycardia.

FIGURE 10-10 Blood Pressure (BP) for Pediatric Patients

Group	Age	Expected BP Range (mm Hg)	Lower Limit of Systolic BP (mm Hg)
Newborn	Birth–6 wk	74–100 50–68	>60
Infant	7 wk–1 yr	84–106 56–70	>70
Toddler	1–2 yr	98–106 50–70	>70
Preschool	2–6 yr	98–112 64–70	>75
School age	6–13 yr	104–124 64–80	>80
Adolescent	13–16 yr	118–132 70–82	>90

Top numbers represent systolic range; bottom numbers represent diastolic range.

and overall CNS status monitored closely. An accurate BP reading may be difficult to obtain in the prehospital setting, and focus should be placed on other signs of perfusion. If measured, a small patient may have a systolic BP that, although considered alarmingly low for an adult, may be within the normal range for a healthy child.

A child with hemorrhagic injury can maintain adequate circulating volume by constricting their blood vessels to maintain blood pressure. Clinical evidence of this compensatory mechanism includes peripheral pallor or mottling, cool peripheral skin temperature, and decreased intensity of the peripheral pulses. In the child, signs of significant hypotension develop with the loss of approximately 30% of the circulating volume. If initial resuscitation is inadequate, circulating volume will eventually diminish to a point below which the vasoconstriction cannot maintain arterial pressure. The concept of evolving shock must be of paramount concern in the initial management of an injured child and is a major indication for transport to an appropriate facility for expeditious evaluation and treatment.

Disability. After assessment of airway, breating, and circulation, the primary survey must include an assessment of neurologic status. Although the *AVPU scale* (**A**lert, responds to **V**erbal stimulus, responds to **P**ainful stimulus, **U**nresponsive) remains a simple, rapid assessment tool for the child's neurological status, it remains less informative than the Glasgow Coma Scale (Figure 6-8, page 139). It should be combined with a careful examination of the pupils to determine whether they are equal, round, and reactive to light. As in adults, the GCS provides a more thorough assessment of neurologic status and should be calculated for each pediatric trauma victim. The scoring for the verbal section for children under 4 years of age must be modified because of developing communication skills in this age group, and the child's behavior should be observed carefully (Figure 10-11).

The GCS score should be repeated frequently and used to document progression or improvement of neurologic status during the post-injury period. A more thorough assessment of motor and sensory function should be performed in the secondary survey if time permits.

FIGURE 10-11 Pediatric Verbal Score

Verbal Response	Verbal Score
Appropriate words or social smile; fixes and follows	5
Crying but consolable	4
Persistently irritable	3
Restless, agitated	2
No response	1

Expose/Environment. Children should be examined for other potentially life-threatening injuries; however, they may be frightened at attempts to remove their clothes. In addition, because of children's high BSA, they are more prone to developing hypothermia. Therefore, once the examination to identify other injuries is complete, the patient should be covered to preserve body heat and prevent further heat loss.

Secondary Survey (Detailed Physical Examination)

The secondary survey of the child should follow the primary survey only after life-threatening conditions have been identified and managed. Although the exam will be discussed in a head-to-toe fashion, in the pediatric patient, it is often less anxiety-producing for the child if the examiner begins at the toes and works their way up to the head. The head and neck should be examined for obvious deformities, contusions, abrasions, punctures, burns, tenderness, lacerations, or swellings. The thorax should be re-examined.

Examination of the abdomen should focus on distension, tenderness, discoloration, ecchymoses, and presence of a mass. Careful palpation of the iliac crests may suggest an unstable pelvic fracture and increase the suspicion for possible retroperitoneal or urogenital injury as well as increased risk for hidden blood loss. An unstable pelvis should be noted, but repeated examinations of the pelvis should not be performed, because this may result in further injury and increased blood loss. The patient should be appropriately immobilized on a long board and prepared for transfer to a pediatric trauma facility.

Each extremity should be inspected and palpated to rule out tenderness, deformity, diminished vascular supply, and neurologic deficit. A child's incompletely calcified skeleton with its multiple growth centers increases the possibility of epiphyseal (growth plate) disruption. Accordingly, any area of swelling, pain, tenderness, or diminished range of motion should be treated as if it were fractured until evaluated by radiographic examination. In children, as in adults, a missed orthopedic injury in an extremity may have little effect on mortality but may lead to long-term deformity and disability.

Management. The keys to pediatric trauma survival are rapid cardiopulmonary assessment, age-appropriate aggressive management, and transport to a facility capable of managing pediatric trauma. Most prehospital systems have a guideline for selecting appropriate destination facilities for pediatric trauma patients.

Airway. Ventilation, oxygenation, and perfusion are as essential to an injured child as an adult, if not more so. Thus, the primary goal of the initial resuscitation of an injured child is restoration of adequate tissue oxygenation as quickly as possible. The first priority of assessment and resuscitation is the establishment of a patent airway.

A patent airway should be ensured and maintained with suctioning, manual maneuvers, and airway adjuncts. As in

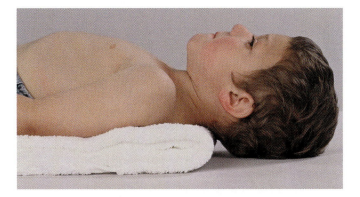

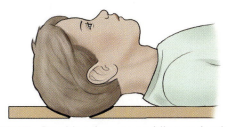

FIGURE 10-12 Provide adequate padding under the child's torso or use a pediatric spine board that has a depression to accommodate the child's head.

the adult, initial management includes in-line cervical spine stabilization. Unless a specialized pediatric spine board that has a depression at the head is being used, adequate padding (2–3 cm) should be placed under the torso of the small child so that the cervical spine is maintained in a straight line rather than forced into slight flexion because of the disproportionately large occiput (Figure 10-12). When adjusting and maintaining airway positioning, compressing the soft tissues of the neck and trachea should be avoided. Once manual control of the airway is achieved, an oropharyngeal airway can be placed if no gag reflex is present. The device should be inserted carefully and gently, parallel to the course of the tongue rather than turned 90 or 180 degrees in the posterior oropharynx as in the adult. Use of a tongue blade to depress the tongue can be helpful.

Breathing. The patient's ventilatory effort should be evaluated carefully. Because of the potential for rapid deterioration from mild hypoxia to ventilatory arrest, ventilation should be assisted if dyspnea and increased ventilatory effort are observed. A properly sized bag-mask device with a reservoir and high-flow oxygen to provide an oxygen concentration of between 85% and 100% should be used.

Circulation. Once the patient's external hemorrhage is controlled, perfusion should be evaluated. Controlling external hemorrhage involves applying direct manual pressure on the bleeding point, the use of hemostatic dressings, and the selective use of tourniquets in extreme cases where other measures have failed, not just covering the bleeding site with layer after layer of absorbent dressing. If the initial dressing does become saturated in blood, it is best to add an additional dressing rather than to replace it, because the removal may dislodge any clot that has begun to form, while at the same time performing additional interventions to stop the ongoing hemorrhage. The pediatric vascular system is usually able to maintain a normal BP until severe collapse occurs, at which point it is often unresponsive to resuscitation.

Transport. Because timely arrival at the most appropriate facility may be the key element in the patient's survival, *triage* is an important consideration of management.

The tragedy of preventable pediatric traumatic death has been documented in multiple studies reported over the past three decades. It is estimated that as many as 80% of pediatric trauma deaths can be classified as preventable or potentially preventable. These statistics have been one of the primary motivations for the development of regionalized pediatric trauma centers, where continuous, coordinated, high-quality, sophisticated care can be provided.

Many urban areas have both pediatric trauma centers and adult trauma centers. Ideally, the pediatric multisystem trauma patient will benefit from the initial resuscitation capability and definitive care available at a pediatric trauma center because of its specialization in treating traumatized children. Thus, bypassing an adult trauma center in favor of transport to a pediatric trauma canter is justifiable. For many communities, however, the nearest specialized pediatric trauma center may be hours away. In these cases the seriously traumatized child should be transported to the nearest adult trauma center, because early resuscitation and evaluation before transport to a pediatric facility may improve survival.[13] In areas where no specialized pediatric trauma center is nearby, personnel working in adult trauma centers should be experienced in the resuscitation and treatment of both adult and pediatric trauma patients. In areas where neither facility is readily close, the seriously injured child should be transported to the nearest appropriate hospital capable of caring for pediatric trauma victims, according to local prehospital triage guidelines. Aeromedical transport may be considered in rural areas to expedite transport. There is little evidence that aeromedical transport provides any benefit in urban areas where ground transport to a pediatric trauma center is almost as quick.[14] It is becoming increasingly evident that utilizing aeromedical transport exposes both the patient and the crew to a significant amount of risk. These concerns must be carefully weighed when deciding whether to utilize this resource.

Review of more than 15,000 records in the National Pediatric Trauma Registry (NPTR) indicates that 25% of injured children are injured severely enough to require triage to a designated pediatric trauma center. Many emergency medical services (EMS) and trauma systems use other pediatric triage criteria, which may be dictated by state, regional, or local guidelines. All prehospital care providers need to be familiar with the triage protocols in place within their own systems.

Specific Injuries

Traumatic Brain Injury. Traumatic brain injury (TBI) is the most common cause of death in the pediatric population. Of the fatalities included in the first 40,000 patients in the NPTR, 89% had a CNS injury as either the primary or the secondary contributor to mortality. Although many of the most severe injuries are treatable only by prevention, initial resuscitative measures may minimize secondary brain injury, and consequently the severity of the child's injury. Adequate ventilation, oxygenation, and perfusion are needed to prevent secondary morbidity. The outcome of children sustaining severe TBI is typically better than in adults, except in the subset of children younger than 3 years, in whom it is worse than that of older children.

The results of the initial neurologic assessment are useful for prognosis. Even with a normal initial neurologic evaluation, however, any child who sustains a head injury may be susceptible to cerebral edema, hypoperfusion and secondary insults. These conditions can result even from a mechanism that appears minor.

A baseline GCS score should be assessed and frequently repeated during transport. Supplemental oxygen should be administered. Although vomiting is common after a concussion, persistent or forceful projectile vomiting is of concern and requires further evaluation.

As with hypoxia, hypovolemia may dramatically worsen the original TBI. External hemorrhage must be controlled and the patient's fractured extremities immobilized to limit internal blood loss associated with these injuries. On rare occasions, infants less than about 6 months of age may become hypovolemic as a result of intracranial bleeding because they have open cranial sutures and fontanelles (soft spot of the head). The infant with an open fontanelle may better tolerate an expanding intracranial hematoma but may not become symptomatic until rapid decompensation occurs. An infant with a bulging fontanelle should be considered to have a more severe TBI.

A child with signs and symptoms of intracranial hypertension, or increased intracranial pressure (ICP), such as a sluggishly reactive or nonreactive pupil, systemic hypertension, bradycardia, and abnormal breathing patterns, may benefit from temporary mild hyperventilation to lower ICP. A ventilation rate of 30 breaths/minute for children and 35 breaths/minute for infants should be used.[5] However, this effect of hyperventilation is transient and also decreases overall oxygen delivery to the CNS, actually causing additional secondary brain injury.[7] It is strongly recommended that this strategy not be used unless the child is exhibiting signs of active herniation or lateralizing signs.

Spinal Trauma. The indication for spinal immobilization in a pediatric patient is based on the mechanism of injury and physical findings; the presence of other injuries that suggest violent or sudden movement of the head, neck, or torso; or the presence of specific signs of spine injury, such as deformity, pain, or a neurologic deficit. As with adult patients, the correct prehospital management of a suspected spine injury is inline manual stabilization followed by the use of a properly fitting cervical collar and immobilization of the patient to a long backboard so that the head, neck, torso, pelvis, and legs are maintained in a neutral inline position. This should be achieved without impairing the patient's ventilation, ability to open the mouth, or any other resuscitative efforts. The threshold for performing spinal immobilization is lower in young children because of their inability to communicate or otherwise participate in their own assessment.

When most small children are placed on a rigid surface, the relatively larger size of the child's occiput will result in passive neck flexion. Unless you are using a specialized pediatric spine board that has a depression at the head to accommodate the occiput, sufficient padding (2–3 cm) should be placed under the patient's torso to elevate it and allow the head to be in a neutral position. The padding should be continuous and flat from the shoulders to the pelvis and extend to the lateral margins of the torso to ensure that the thoracic, lumbar, and sacral spine are on a flat, stable platform without the possibility of anterior-posterior movement. Padding should also be placed between the lateral sides of the child and the edges of the board to ensure that no lateral movement occurs when the board is moved or if the patient and board need to be rotated to the side to avoid aspiration during vomiting episodes.

Thoracic Injuries. The extremely resilient rib cage of a child often results in less injury to the bony structure of the thorax, but more risk for lung injury, such as pulmonary contusion, pneumothorax, or hemothorax. Although rib fractures are rare in childhood, when present they are associated with a high risk of intrathoracic injury. Crepitance may be appreciated on examination and may be a sign of pneumothorax. The risk of mortality increases with the number of ribs fractured. A high index of suspicion is the key to identifying these injuries. Every child who sustains trauma to the chest and torso should be carefully monitored for signs of respiratory distress and shock. Abrasions or contusions over the child's torso after blunt force trauma may be the only clues to the provider that the child has suffered thoracic trauma. In all cases, the key items in managing thoracic trauma involve careful attention to ventilation, oxygenation, and timely transport to an appropriate facility.

Abdominal Injuries. The presence of blunt trauma to the abdomen; an unstable pelvis; post-traumatic abdominal distension, rigidity, or tenderness; or otherwise unexplained shock can be associated with possible intraabdominal hemorrhage. A "seat belt sign" or bruise across the abdomen of a child is often an indicator of serious internal injuries (Figure 10-13). The key prehospital elements in management of abdominal injuries include supplemental high-concentration oxygen and rapid transport to an appropriate facility with continued careful monitoring en route. There are really no definitive interventions that prehospital providers can offer to patients with intraabdominal injuries, and as such there should be

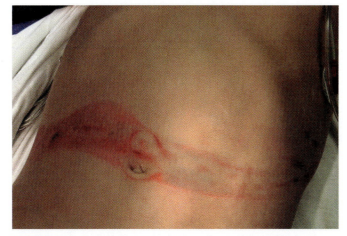

FIGURE 10-13 "Seat belt sign" in a 6-year-old patient who was found to have a ruptured spleen. Seat belt signs are often associated with serious intraabdominal injuries.

every effort to transport these patients rapidly to the closest, most appropriate facility.

Extremity Trauma. Compared with the adult skeleton, the child's skeleton is actively growing and consists of a large proportion of cartilaginous tissue and metabolically active growth plates. The ligamentous structures that hold the skeleton together are often stronger and better able to withstand mechanical disruption than the bones to which they are attached. As a result, children with skeletal trauma often sustain major traumatic forces before developing long-bone fractures, dislocations, or deformities. Incomplete ("greenstick") fractures are common and may be indicated only by bony tenderness and pain on use of the affected extremity.

The association of neurovascular injuries with orthopedic injuries in children should always be considered, and the distal vascular and neurologic exam should be carefully evaluated. Often the presence of a potentially debilitating injury can be determined only by radiologic study or, when the slightest suggestion of a decrease in distal perfusion exists, by arteriography.

The apparent gross deformity sometimes associated with extremity injury should not distract focus from dealing with potentially life-threatening injuries. Uncontrolled hemorrhage represents the sole life-threatening condition associated with extremity trauma. In multisystem pediatric and adult trauma patients alike, the initiation of transport to an appropriate facility without delay after completion of the primary survey, resuscitation, and rapid packaging remains paramount in reducing mortality. If basic splinting can be provided en route without detracting from the child's resuscitation, it will help to minimize bleeding and pain from long-bone fractures, but attention to life-threatening injuries should remain the primary focus.

Thermal Injuries. Following motor vehicle crashes and drowning, burns rate third as the cause of pediatric trauma deaths.[8] Caring for an injured child always poses significant physical and emotional challenges to the prehospital care provider and these difficulties are only amplified when caring for the burned child. (See Chapter 8, Burn Trauma, for more details.)

The primary survey should be followed, as in other causes of pediatric trauma, but every step of the primary assessment may be more complicated than in a non–thermally injured child. Most deaths related to structure fires are not directly related to soft tissue burns but are secondary to smoke inhalation. When children are trapped in a structure fire, they often hide from the fire under beds or in closets. These children often die, and their recovered bodies generally have no burns; they die from carbon monoxide or hydrogen cyanide toxicity and hypoxia. More than 50% of children less than 9 years old in structure fires have some degree of smoke inhalation injury.

Thermally induced swelling of the airway is always a concern in burn patients, but especially in children. The smaller diameter of the pediatric trachea means that 1 mm of edema will produce a greater magnitude of airway obstruction than in an adult with a larger-diameter airway. A child with an edematous airway may be sitting forward and drooling or complaining of hoarseness or voice changes. Early involvement of advanced life support providers should be done before the child develops signs or symptoms of respiratory compromise.

Each year approximately 1.5 million children are abused by burning, accounting for 20% of all child abuse.[9,10] Approximately 20% to 25% of children admitted to a pediatric burn center are victims of child abuse.[11,12] An increased awareness of this problem among prehospital providers can improve detection of this cause of pediatric trauma. Careful documentation of the situation surrounding the injury, as well as of the injury patterns themselves can aid officials in the prosecution of the offenders.

The two most common mechanisms by which these children receive burns are scalds and contact burns. Scalds are the most common source of nonaccidental burns. Scalding injuries typically are inflicted on children of toilet-training age. The usual scenario is that children soil themselves, and are subsequently immersed in a tub of scalding water. These scald burns are characterized by a pattern of sharp demarcation between burned and unburned tissue and sparing of flexion creases, as the child will often draw their legs up to avoid the scalding water.

Contact burns are the second most common mechanism of abuse burns. Common items used to inflict contact burns are curling irons, clothing irons, and cigarettes. Cigarette burns appear as round wounds measuring slightly larger than 1 cm in diameter (typically 1.3 cm). To conceal these injuries, the abuser may place these in areas usually covered by clothing, above the hairline in the scalp, or even in the axillae. All the surfaces of the human body have some degree of curvature. Therefore, a hot item that falls onto any body surface will have an initial point of contact, and then the hot item will deflect from the point of contact. Therefore, the resultant accidental contact burns will have irregular borders and a uneven depth. In contrast, when a hot item is deliberately used to burn someone, the item is pressed onto the region of the body. The burn will then have a pattern with a sharp regular outline and uniform burn depth (see Chapter 8).

A high index of suspicion for abuse is important, and *all* cases of suspected abuse should be reported. Make meticulous observations of the surroundings, such as the position of various pieces of furniture, curling irons, and depth of bath water. Record the names of individuals present at the scene. Any child suspected of being abused by burns, regardless of the size of the burns, needs to be cared for at a center experienced in pediatric burn care.

The Abused and Neglected Child. Child abuse (maltreatment or nonaccidental trauma) is a significant cause of childhood injury. Prehospital care providers must always consider the possibility of child abuse when circumstances warrant.

Prehospital care providers should suspect abuse or neglect if they note any of the following scenarios:

- Discrepancy between the history and the degree of physical injury, or a history that changes often
- Inappropriate response from the family
- Prolonged interval between time of injury and call for medical care
- History of the injury inconsistent with the developmental level of the child; for example, a history indicating that a newborn rolled off a bed would be suspect because newborns are developmentally unable to roll over

Certain injury types also suggest abuse, such as the following (Figure 10-14):

- Multiple bruises in varying stages of healing (excluding the palms, forearms, tibial areas, and the forehead, in ambulatory children, which are often injured in normal falls); accidental bruises usually occur over bony prominences
- Bizarre injuries such as bites, cigarette burns, rope marks, or any pattern injury
- Sharply demarcated burns or scald injuries in unusual areas (see Chapter 8)

In many jurisdictions, prehospital care providers are legally mandated reporters if they identify potential child abuse. Generally, prehospital providers who act in good faith and in the best interests of the child are protected from legal action. Reporting procedures vary, so prehospital providers should be familiar with the appropriate agencies that handle child abuse cases in their location. The need to report abuse is emphasized by data suggesting that up to 50% of maltreated children are released back to their abusers because abuse was not suspected or reported (Figure 10-15).

Prolonged Transport. Occasionally a situation arises, as a result of patient location, triage decisions, or environmental considerations, in which transport will be prolonged or delayed and prehospital personnel need to manage the initial resuscita-

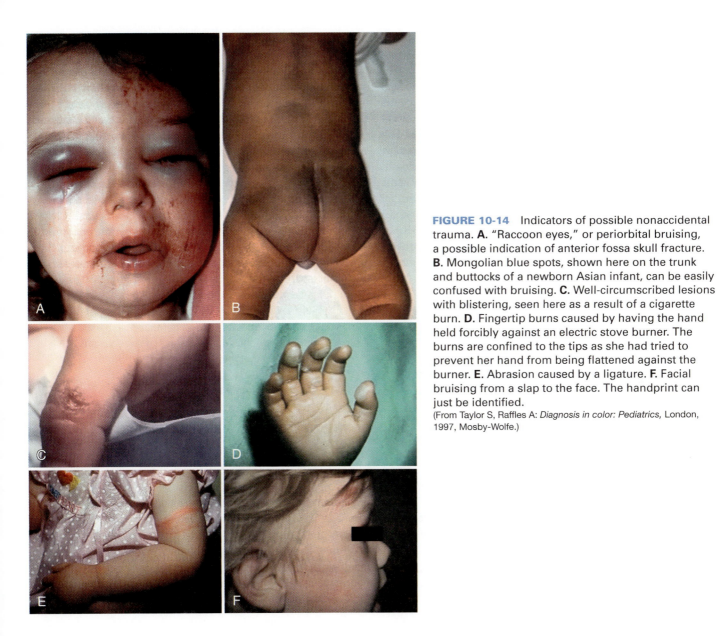

FIGURE 10-14 Indicators of possible nonaccidental trauma. **A.** "Raccoon eyes," or periorbital bruising, a possible indication of anterior fossa skull fracture. **B.** Mongolian blue spots, shown here on the trunk and buttocks of a newborn Asian infant, can be easily confused with bruising. **C.** Well-circumscribed lesions with blistering, seen here as a result of a cigarette burn. **D.** Fingertip burns caused by having the hand held forcibly against an electric stove burner. The burns are confined to the tips as she had tried to prevent her hand from being flattened against the burner. **E.** Abrasion caused by a ligature. **F.** Facial bruising from a slap to the face. The handprint can just be identified.
(From Taylor S, Raffles A: *Diagnosis in color: Pediatrics,* London, 1997, Mosby-Wolfe.)

tion of an injured child. By applying the principles discussed in this chapter in an organized fashion, the child can be safely managed until arrival at a trauma center. If radio or cellular contact with the receiving facility is possible, constant communication and feedback are crucial for both prehospital and hospital-based members of the trauma team.

Management consists of continued serial evaluation of the components of the primary survey. The child should be securely stabilized on a backboard with spine precautions. The board should be padded as well as possible to prevent pressure sores. If the airway is tenuous and the crew is well trained in pediatric airway management, then airway management should be performed. Conscientious bag-mask ventilation is an acceptable management strategy, assuming it provides adequate oxygenation and ventilation. The GCS should be calculated early and followed serially. Assessment for other injuries should continue, and all efforts to keep the child normothermic should be standard practice. Fractures

should be splinted and stabilized with serial neurovascular assessments. This cycle of continued assessment of the primary survey should be repeated until the child can be safely transported or transferred to definitive care.

Any change or decompensation in the child's clinical exam requires immediate reassessment of the primary survey. Perhaps there is a hidden source of bleeding, such as intraabdominal injury or missed scalp laceration? Has the GCS changed? Are there now lateralizing signs suggesting progressive head injury and requiring more aggressive treatments? Is the circulation and neurologic status of the extremities still intact? Is the child maintaining body heat or is hypothermia developing? If radio contact is available, continued advice and guidance from medical control should be sought throughout the resuscitation and transport.

By paying attention to the basics and continually reassessing your patient, adequate resuscitation can be performed until the child can be transferred to a definitive care.

FIGURE 10-15   Documenting Nonaccidental Trauma in Children

Emergency medical technicians (EMTs) may be the only medical responders to a potential crime scene involving nonaccidental (abuse) trauma. While recognizing that EMTs are under intense pressure at an emergency scene, they are in a unique position to collect items of evidentiary importance that may assist in determining the mechanism of injury and the identification of the abuser. EMTs should ideally document 10 fundamental items when responding to a "child in need of assistance" call:

1. Document all adults and children present.
2. Document all statements and the demeanor of all persons present. As recorders of "scene" statements, EMTs must be familiar with the general requirements that allow certain statements to be used in court.
   a. Identify and document the maker of the statement.
   b. Record all statements in the official report.
   c. Record verbatim content, using quotes where appropriate.
   d. Document the time when the statement was made.
   e. Record the speaker's demeanor.
   f. Explain your job.
   g. Ask probing follow-up questions, though do not expose yourself to risk if you encounter aggression at this further questioning.
   h. Record the question. The content of an answer can often be understood only by knowing the question that was asked.
   i. List all persons present who heard the statement.
3. Document the environment. EMTs may arrive before caregivers clean up, modify, or destroy evidence.

4. Collect significant items. Preserving the potential mechanism of injury is vital to verifying a suspect history.
5. Identify and record the child's age and developmental stage.
6. Know the signs of abuse and neglect.
   a. Signs of physical abuse: unexplained fractures, bruises, black eyes, cuts, burns, and welts; pattern injuries and bite marks; antisocial behavior; fear of adults; signs of apathy, depression, hostility, or stress; eating disorders.
   b. Signs of sexual abuse: difficulty walking or sitting, overcompliance, excessive aggressiveness, nightmares, bed-wetting, drastic change in appetite, inappropriate interest or knowledge of sexual acts, fear of a particular person.
   c. Signs of neglect: unsuitable clothing; unbathed/dirty; severe body odor; severe diaper rash; underweight; lack of food, formula, or toys; parent or child use of drugs or alcohol; apparent lack of supervision; unsuitable living conditions.
7. Assess children present at unrelated calls.
8. Evaluate children and adults with disabilities.
9. Adhere to mandatory reporting requirements and procedures.
10. Interact with the multidisciplinary team (MDT).

Nonaccidental pediatric trauma and neglect cases are wrought with difficult issues. Holding abusers responsible for their acts requires meticulous documentation; thorough, coordinated investigations; and teamwork. EMTs are uniquely positioned to observe and document vital information when assessing the possibility of child abuse.

(Modified from Rogers LL: Emergency medical professionals: Assisting in identifying and documenting child abuse and neglect. *NCPCA Update Newslett* 17[7]:1, 2004.)

SUMMARY

- The initial assessment and management of the injured child in the prehospital setting requires application of standard trauma life support principles modified to account for the unique characteristics of children.
- Traumatic brain injury is the leading cause of death from trauma, as well as the most common injury for which the child requires airway management.
- Children have the ability to compensate for volume loss longer than adults, but when they decompensate they deteriorate suddenly and severely.
- Significant underlying organ and vascular injury can occur with few or no obvious signs of external injury.

- Injured children with the following signs are unstable and should be transported without delay to an appropriate facility, ideally a pediatric trauma center:
  - Respiratory compromise
  - Signs of shock or circulatory instability
  - Any period of post-injury unconsciousness
  - Significant blunt trauma to the head, thorax, or abdomen
  - Fractured ribs
  - Pelvic fracture

SCENARIO 1 SOLUTION

You correctly identify this child as a victim of multisystem trauma who is in shock and critically injured. Because of the probable traumatic brain injury combined with the change in mentation, you have to determine the greatest threat to his survivability: the brain injury and other injuries not yet identified. You correctly identify hypotension and tachycardia, which you assume are related to hypovolemic shock, probably the result of an unrecognized intraabdominal injury. Initially, his breathing is supported with high-concentration oxygen through a non-rebreather mask. You realize that his respiratory rate is low for a child of his age and are prepared to provide more aggressive airway control if his condition deteriorates. As you consider options for airway management, you ask your partner to hold manual stabilization of the head and neck.

Because of the nature of the child's injuries, you consult with online medical control, who agrees that helicopter transport to the closest pediatric trauma center is more appropriate than ground transport to a nearby community hospital that has no pediatric critical care, neurosurgical, or orthopedic resources. The patient's mother arrives just as you are transferring care to the helicopter crew. ■

Geriatric Trauma

SCENARIO 2

You are dispatched to the scene of a single-car motor vehicle crash into a tree. On your initial scene assessment, police and fire personnel have secured the scene. The vehicle is an older model car without seat belts or air bags. The driver appears to be an elderly male who is unresponsive. Bystanders report he was driving erratically moments before the crash. While maintaining inline stabilization of the spine, you note that the patient is unresponsive to your commands. He has a visible laceration of the forehead where he apparently impacted the windshield. He is wearing a Medic-Alert bracelet that indicates that he is diabetic.

Was the injury the primary event or secondary to a medical event?

Did the crash cause the significant injuries, or was there an antecedent event?

How does the information that the patient is diabetic affect your level of suspicion for traumatic brain injury?

How do the patient's age, medical history, and medications interact with the injuries received to make the pathophysiology and manifestations different from those in younger patients?

How will you modify your approach to the management of this patient, especially in terms of stabilizing his airway?

Should advanced age alone be used as an additional criterion for transport to a trauma center?

The elderly population represents the fastest-growing age group in the United States. Gerontologists (medical specialists who study and care for elderly patients) divide the term *elderly* into three specific categories, as follows:

- *Middle age:* 50 to 64 years of age
- *Late age:* 65 to 79 years of age
- *Older age:* 80 years of age and older

It is important to recognize that the physiologic changes of aging occur along the entire age spectrum and vary among individuals. Recovery from closed head injury starts to decline beginning in the mid-20s, and overall survival from trauma starts to decline in the late 30s. In addition, increasing age is often associated with multiple preexisting medical conditions. The approach to the elderly patient includes recognition of this fact, although younger patients with comorbidities may share similar attributes.

Almost 39 million Americans (13% of the U.S. population) are 65 years of age or older, and the size of this group has risen dramatically during the last 100 years.[15] By the year 2050, nearly 25% of Americans will be eligible for Medicare, and the population over 85 years of age will have grown from 4 million to 19 million people.[16]

The injured elderly present unique challenges in prehospital care management, second only to those encountered with infants. Data from more than 3800 patients age 65 and older were compared with almost 43,000 patients younger than age 65.[17] Mortality increased over ages 45 to 55 and doubled by age 75 years. The age-adjusted risk occurs across the spectrum of injury severity, suggesting that injuries that could be easily tolerated by younger patients may result in mortality in those of advanced age.

Because older persons are more susceptible to critical illness and trauma than the rest of the population, a wider range of complications in patient assessment and management needs to be considered. The range of disabilities experienced by elderly patients is enormous, and field assessment may take longer than with younger patients. Difficulties in assessment can be expected as a result of sensory deficits in hearing and vision, senility, and physiologic changes.

Although trauma occurs most frequently in young people and geriatric emergencies are most often medical problems, a growing number of geriatric calls result from or include trauma. Trauma is the sixth leading cause of death in persons age 55 to 64, and is the ninth leading cause of death in those age 65 and older.[19] Approximately 15% of injury-related deaths in elderly patients are classified as homicide. Trauma deaths in this age group account for 25% of all trauma deaths nationwide.[19]

Specific patterns of injury are also unique to the geriatric population.[20] Although MVCs are the leading cause of death from trauma overall, falls are the predominant cause of traumatic death in patients older than age 75. As with small children (<5 years), scald injuries account for a greater percentage of burns in those older than 65.

Social changes have increased the number of older people living in independent housing, retirement communities, and other assisted-living facilities compared with those in nursing homes or other, more guarded and limited environments. This suggests an increase in the incidence of simple household trauma, such as falls, in elderly persons. The past few years have also seen an increase in geriatric victims of crime in the home and on the streets. Older people are often singled out as "easy marks" and can sustain substantial trauma from crimes of seemingly limited violence, such as purse snatching, when they are struck, are knocked down, or fall.

With the growing awareness of this expanding population at risk, the prehospital care provider must understand the unique needs of an elderly trauma patient. The special considerations outlined in this section should be included in the assessment and management of any trauma patient who is 65 years of age or older, physically appears elderly, or is middle-aged and has any of the significant medical problems typically associated with the elderly population.

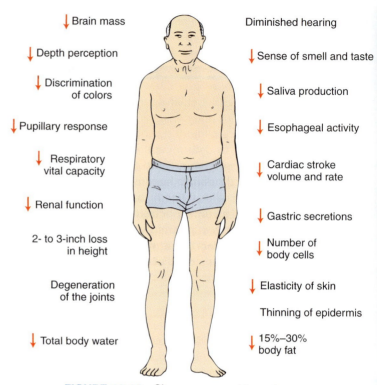

FIGURE 10-16   Changes caused by aging.

Anatomy and Physiology of Aging

The aging process causes changes in physical structure, body composition, and organ function, and it can create unique problems during prehospital care. Aging, or senescence, is a natural biologic process and is sometimes referred to as a process of "biologic reversal" that begins during the years of early adulthood. At this time, organ systems have achieved maturation, and a turning point in physiologic growth has been reached. The body gradually loses its ability to maintain homeostasis (the state of relative constancy of the body's internal environment), and viability declines over a period of years until death occurs.

The fundamental process of aging occurs at the cellular level and is reflected in both anatomic structure and physiologic function. The period of "old age" is generally characterized by frailty, slower cognitive processes, impairment of psychological functions, diminished energy, the appearance of chronic and degenerative diseases, and a decline in sensory acuity. Functional abilities are lessened, and the well-known external signs and symptoms of older age appear, such as skin wrinkling, changes in hair color and quantity, osteoarthritis, and slowness in reaction time and reflexes (Figure 10-16).

Influence of Chronic Medical Problems

Although some individuals can reach an advanced age without any serious medical problems, statistically an older person is more likely to have one or more significant medical conditions. Usually, proper medical care can control these conditions, helping to avoid or minimize exacerbations from becoming repeated acute and often life-threatening episodes.

A medical problem can result in chronic residual effects on the body. A patient who has previously had an acute myocardial infarction sustains permanent heart damage. The resultant reduced cardiac capacity continues for the rest of the patient's life, affecting the heart and, because of the ensuing chronic impairment of circulation, other organs as well.

Regardless of whether the patient is pediatric, middle-aged, or elderly, the priorities, intervention needs, and life-threatening conditions that usually result from serious trauma are the same. However, because of these preexisting physical conditions, elderly patients often die from less severe injuries and die sooner than younger patients. Data show that preexisting conditions play a role in the survival of an elderly trauma patient (Figure 10-17) and that the more conditions a trauma patient has, the higher his or her mortality rate (Figure 10-18). Certain conditions are associated with a higher mortality rate because of the way in which they interfere with an elderly patient's ability to respond to trauma (Figure 10-19).[21]

Ears, Nose, and Throat

Tooth decay, gum disease, and injury to teeth result in the need for various dental prostheses. The brittle nature of capped teeth, fixed bridges, or loose, removable bridges and dentures poses a special problem of foreign bodies that can be easily broken, aspirated, and obstruct the airway.

FIGURE 10-17   Percentage of Patients with Preexisting Disease (PED)[21]

Age (years)	PED (%)
13–39	3.5
40–64	11.6
65–74	29.4
75–84	34.7
85+	37.3

FIGURE 10-18   Number of Preexisting Diseases (PEDs) and Patient Outcome[21]

Number of PEDs	Survived	Died	Mortality rate (%)
0	6341	211	3.2
1	868	56	6.1
2	197	36	15.5
3 or more	67	22	24.7

FIGURE 10-19   Prevalence of Preexisting Diseases (PEDs) and Associated Mortality Rates

PED	Number of Patients	PED Present (%)	Total (%)	Mortality Rate (%)
Hypertension	597	47.9	7.7	10.2
Pulmonary disease	286	23	3.7	8.4
Cardiac disease	223	17.9	2.9	18.4
Diabetes	198	15.9	2.5	12.1
Obesity	167	13.4	2.1	4.8
Malignancy	80	6.4	1	20
Neurologic disorder	45	3.6	0.6	13.3
Renal disease	40	3.2	0.5	37.5
Hepatic disease	41	3.3	0.5	12.2

Changes in the contours of the face result from resorption of the mandible, in part because of absence of teeth (edentulism). The characteristic look is an infolding and shrinking of the mouth. These changes can adversely affect the ability to create an effective seal with a bag-mask device and sufficiently visualize the airway during endotracheal intubation.

Respiratory System

Ventilatory function declines in the elderly person partly as a result of the inability of the chest cage to expand and contract and partly from stiffening of the airway. As a result of these changes, the chest cage is less pliable. With declines in the efficiency of the respiratory system, the elderly person requires more exertion to carry out daily activities.

The alveolar surface area in the lungs decreases with age; it is estimated to decrease by 4% for each decade after 30 years of age. A 70-year-old person, for example, would have a 16% reduction in alveolar surface area. Any alteration of the already-reduced alveolar surface decreases oxygen uptake. Additionally, as the body ages, its ability to saturate hemoglobin with oxygen decreases, leading to lower baseline oxygen saturation as a normal finding and less reserve available.[22] Because of impaired mechanical ventilation and diminished surface for gas exchange, the elderly trauma patient is less capable of compensating for physiologic losses associated with trauma.

Changes in the airway and lungs of elderly persons may not always be related to aging alone. Cumulative chronic exposure to environmental toxins over the course of their lives may be caused by occupational hazards or tobacco smoke. Impaired cough and gag reflexes, along with poor cough strength and diminished esophageal sphincter tone, result in an increased risk of aspiration pneumonitis. A reduction in the number of *cilia* (hair-like projections that propel foreign particles and mucus from the bronchi) predisposes the elderly person to problems caused by inhaled particulate matter.

Another factor that affects the respiratory system is a change in the spinal curvature. Curvature changes accompanied by an anteroposterior hump (as seen in osteoporosis patients) often lead to additional ventilatory difficulty (Figure 10-20). Changes that affect the diaphragm can also contribute to ventilatory problems. Stiffening of the rib cage can cause more reliance on diaphragmatic activity to breathe. This increased reliance on the diaphragm makes an older person especially sensitive to changes in intraabdominal pressure. Thus, a supine position or a full stomach from a large meal can provoke ventilatory insufficiency. Obesity can also play a part in diaphragm restriction, especially when fat distribution tends to be central.

Cardiovascular System

Diseases of the cardiovascular system are the primary cause of death in the elderly population and account for more than 3000 deaths per 100,000 persons older than 65 years. In 2002, myocardial infarction accounted for 29% of deaths in the United States, with an additional 7% caused by stroke.[22]

The myocardium and blood vessels rely on their elastic, contractile, and distensible properties to function properly. With aging, these properties decline, and the cardiovascular system becomes less efficient at moving circulatory fluids around the body. The cardiac output diminishes by approximately 50% from 20 to 80 years of age. As many as 10% of those older than 75 years will have some degree of congestive heart failure.

Atherosclerosis is a narrowing of the blood vessels as fatty deposits build up within the artery. These deposits, called *plaque,* protrude above the surface of the inner layer and decrease the diameter of the internal channel of the vessel. The same luminal narrowing occurs in the coronary vessels. Almost 50% of the U.S. population have coronary artery stenosis by age 65 years.[23]

One result of this narrowing is *hypertension,* a condition that affects one of six adults in the United States. Of particular concern is that the baseline normal blood pressure of the elderly trauma patient may be higher than in younger patients. What would otherwise be accepted as normotension may indicate profound hypovolemic shock in the patient with pre-existing hypertension.[24]

With age, the heart itself shows an increase in fibrous tissue and size *(myocardial hypertrophy)* as well as an increased incidence of cardiac dysrhythmias. In particular, the normal reflexes in the heart that respond to hypotension diminish with age, resulting in the inability of elderly patients to increase their heart rate appropriately. Patients with a permanent pacemaker have a fixed heart rate, and cardiac output cannot meet the demands accompanying the stress of trauma. Patients with hypertension taking beta-blocker medications may also not have an increase in heart rate to compensate for hypovolemia.

In the elderly trauma patient, this reduced circulation contributes to cellular hypoxia. In addition, total circulating blood volume decreases, creating less physiologic reserve for blood loss from trauma. The reduced circulation and circulatory defense responses, coupled with increasing cardiac failure, produce a significant problem in managing shock in the elderly trauma patient.

Nervous System

As individuals age, brain weight and the number of neurons (nerve cells) decrease. The weight of the brain reaches its peak (1.4 kg, or 3 pounds) at approximately 20 years of age.

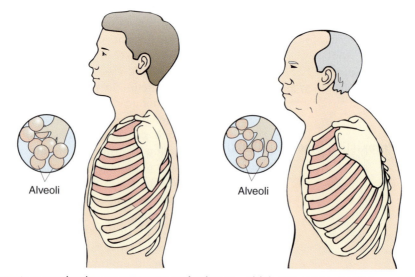

FIGURE 10-20 Spinal curvature can lead to an anteroposterior hump, which can cause ventilatory difficulties. Reduction in the alveolar surface area can also reduce the amount of oxygen that is exchanged in the lungs.

By 80 years of age, the brain loses about 10% of weight, with progressive cerebral atrophy.[25] The body compensates for the loss of space with increased cerebrospinal fluid. Although this additional space around the brain can protect it from contusion, it also allows for more brain movement in response to acceleration/deceleration injuries. The increased space in the cranial vault also explains why the elderly patient may have significant volumes of blood accumulate around the brain with minimal symptomatology.

The speed with which nerve impulses are conducted along certain nerves also decreases. These decreases result in only small effects on behavior and thinking. Reflexes are slower, but not to a significant degree. Compensatory functions can be impaired resulting in an increased incidence of falls. The peripheral nervous system is also affected by the slowing of nerve impulses, resulting in tremors and an unsteady gait.

General information and vocabulary abilities increase or are maintained, whereas skills requiring mental and muscular activity (psychomotor ability) may decline. The intellectual functions that involve verbal comprehension, arithmetic ability, fluency of ideas, experiential evaluation, and general knowledge tend to increase after 60 years of age in those who continue learning activities. Exceptions are those who develop senile dementia and other disorders such as Alzheimer's disease.

As changes occur in the brain, memory can be affected, and personality changes and other reductions in brain function can occur. These changes may involve the need for some form of mental health service. About 10% to 15% of elderly persons require professional mental health services. However, when assessing an elderly trauma patient, any impairment in mentation should be assumed to be the result of an acute traumatic insult, such as shock, hypoxia, or brain injury and not the effect of age, until proven otherwise.

Sensory Changes

Vision and Hearing

Overall, approximately 28% of elderly persons have hearing impairment, and approximately 13% have visual impairment. Men tend to be more likely to have hearing difficulties, whereas both genders have a similar incidence of eye-related impairment.

As a result of changes to the various structures of the eye, elderly persons have more difficulty seeing in dimly lit environments. Decreased tear production leads to dry eyes and itching, burning, and the inability to keep the eyes open for long periods. The lens of the eye begins to become cloudy and impenetrable to light. This gradual process results in a *cataract,* or a milky lens that blocks and distorts light that enters the eye and blurs vision. Some degree of cataract formation is present in 95% of elderly persons. This deterioration of vision increases the risk of an MVC, particularly while driving at night.[26]

A gradual decline in hearing *(presbycusis)* is also characteristic of aging. Presbycusis is usually caused by loss of conduction of sound into the inner ear; the use of hearing aids can compensate for this loss to some degree. This hearing loss is most pronounced when the person attempts to discriminate complex sounds, such as when many people are speaking at once, or with loud ambient noise present, such as the wailing of sirens.

Pain Perception

Because of the aging process and the presence of diseases such as diabetes, elderly persons may not perceive pain normally, placing them at increased risk of injury from excesses in heat and cold exposure. Conditions such as arthritis result in chronic pain. Living with daily pain can cause an increased tolerance to pain, which may result in a patient's failure to identify areas of injury. In evaluating patients, especially those who usually "hurt all over" or who appear to have a high tolerance to pain, areas where the pain has increased or where the painful area has enlarged should be located. Also, it is also important to note whether the pain's characteristics or exacerbating factors have changed since the trauma occurred.

Renal System

Changes common with aging include reduced levels of filtration by the kidneys and a reduced excretory capacity. Chronic renal inhibition contributes to a reduction in a patient's overall health status and ability to withstand trauma. For example, renal dysfunction may be one cause of chronic anemia, which would lower a patient's physiologic reserve.

Musculoskeletal System

Bone loses mineral as it ages. The loss of bone *(osteoporosis)* is unequal among the genders. During young adulthood, bone mass is greater in women than in men. However, bone loss is more rapid in women and accelerates after menopause. With this higher incidence of osteoporosis, older women have a greater probability of fractures, particularly of the neck of the femur (hip), as well as compression fractures of the vertebral bodies.

Kyphosis (curvature of the spine) in the thoracic region can lead to height loss and is often caused by osteoporosis (Figure 10-21). As the bones become more porous and fragile, erosion occurs anteriorly, and compression fractures of the vertebrae may develop. If chronic obstructive pulmonary disease (COPD), particularly emphysema, is present, the kyphosis may be more pronounced because of the increased development of the accessory muscles of breathing.

After age 25, there is a reduction in muscle mass of about 4% per decade until age 50, when the process accelerates to

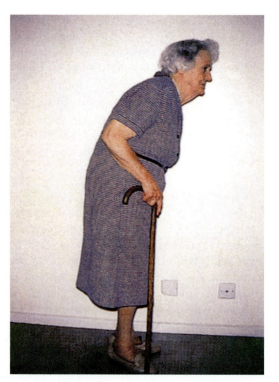

FIGURE 10-21 Kyphosis, typically caused by osteoporosis. Because of the elderly person's tendency to flex the legs, the arms appear longer. As the thoracic spine becomes more curved, the head and shoulders appear to be pushed forward.

between 10% and 35% per decade. Deficits that relate to the musculoskeletal system (e.g., inability to flex the hip or knee adequately with changes in terrain) predispose the elderly person to falls. Muscle fatigue can cause many problems that affect movement, especially falls.

Some degree of osteoporosis is universal with aging. Because of this, the bones become less pliant, more brittle, and more easily broken. The decrease in bone strength, coupled with reduced muscle strength caused by less active exercise, can result in multiple fractures with only mild or moderate force. The most common sites of long-bone fracture in elderly persons include the proximal femur, hip, humerus, and wrist.

The entire vertebral column changes with age, primarily because of the effects of both osteoporosis and calcification (*osteophysis*) of the supporting ligaments. This calcification results in decreased range of motion and narrowing of the spinal canal. The narrowed canal and progressive osteophytic disease put these patients at high risk for spinal cord injury with even minor trauma. The narrowing of the spinal canal is called *spinal stenosis* and increases the likelihood of cord compression without any actual break in the bony cervical spine. A high level of suspicion for spinal injury is needed during patient assessment because more than 50% of vertebral compression fractures are asymptomatic.[27]

Skin

Cell numbers decrease, tissue strength is lost, and the skin has impaired functional status. As the skin ages, sweat and sebaceous glands are lost. Loss of sweat glands reduces the body's ability to regulate temperature. Loss of sebaceous glands, which produce oil, makes the skin dry and flaky. Production of melanin, the pigment that gives color to skin and hair, declines, causing an aging pallor. The skin thins and appears translucent, primarily because of changes in connective tissue. The thinning and drying of the skin also reduce its resistance to minor injury and microorganisms, resulting in an increased infection rate from open wounds. As elasticity is lost, the skin stretches and falls into wrinkles and folds, especially in areas of heavy use, such as those overlying the facial muscles of expression.

Loss of fatty tissue can predispose the elderly person to *hypothermia*. The loss of up to 20% of dermal thickness with advanced aged and an associated loss in vascularity are also responsible for impaired thermoregulatory dysfunction. This loss of fatty tissue also leads to less padding over bony prominences, such as the head, shoulders, spine, buttocks, hips, and heels. Prolonged immobilization without additional padding can result in tissue necrosis and ulceration as well as increased pain and discomfort during treatment and transport. Thinning of the skin also results in the potential for significant tissue loss and injury in response to relatively low energy transfers.

The Immune System

As the immune system ages, its ability to function decreases. Grossly, organs associated with the immune response (thymus, liver, and spleen) all decrease in size. A decrease in cell-mediated and humoral responses also results. Coupled with any preexisting nutritional problems common in the elderly population, there is an increased susceptibility to infection. *Sepsis* is a common cause of late death after severe or even insignificant trauma in the elderly patient.

Assessment

Prehospital assessment of the elderly patient is based on the same method used for all trauma patients. Although the methodology is unchanged, the process may be altered in elderly patients. As with all trauma patients, however, the mechanism of injury should be considered first. This section discusses some special considerations in assessing an elderly trauma patient.

Kinematics
Falls

Falls are the leading cause of trauma death and disability in those older than 75 years of age. Approximately one third of community-dwelling people older than 65 years fall each year, increasing to 50% by 80 years of age. Men and women fall with equal frequency, but women are more than twice as likely to sustain a serious injury because of more pronounced osteoporosis.

Long-bone fractures account for the majority of injuries, with fractures of the hip resulting in the greatest mortality and morbidity rates. The mortality rate from hip fractures is 20% at 1 year after the injury and rises to 33% at 2 years.

Vehicular Trauma

MVCs are the leading cause of trauma death in the geriatric population between 65 and 74 years of age. An elderly patient is five times more likely to be fatally injured in an MVC than a younger driver, even though excessive speed is rarely a causative factor in the older age group.[28] For many reasons, elderly persons are often involved in collisions during daylight hours, during good weather, and close to their domicile.

Alcohol is rarely involved, unlike with MVCs in younger persons. Only 6% of fatally injured elderly persons are intoxicated, compared with 23% for all other age categories.[28]

Elderly pedestrians represent more than 20% of all pedestrian fatalities. Because of slower walking speeds, the time allowed by traffic signals may be too short for the elderly person to traverse the crosswalk safely. This may explain the observation that more than 45% of all elderly pedestrian fatalities occur near a crosswalk.

Assault and Domestic Abuse

Abuse is defined as willful infliction of injury, unreasonable confinement, intimidation, or cruel punishment resulting in physical or psychological harm or pain, or the withholding of services that would prevent these. The elderly are highly vulnerable to crime. Violent assaults have been estimated to account for more than 10% of trauma admissions in elderly patients. The need for chronic care because of debilitation may predispose an elderly person to abuse or neglect from his or her caregivers. It is estimated that only about 15% of cases are reported to the proper authorities.[29,30]

Burns

Elderly patients represent 20% of burn unit admissions, with an estimated 1500 fire-related deaths per year. Burn fatalities in elderly patients occur from burns of smaller size and severity compared with other age groups. Fatality rates are seven times those of younger burn victims.

Decreased pain perception can result in more significant burns. Thinning of dermal elements may result in a deeper thickness of burns.

The presence of preexisting medical conditions, such as cardiovascular disease and diabetes, results in poor tolerance to the resuscitative care of burns. Vascular collapse and infection are the most common causes of death from burns in elderly patients.

Traumatic Brain Injury

The brain has undergone a 10% reduction in mass by 70 years of age. The dura mater adheres more closely to the skull, resulting in a loss of some brain volume. The dural bridging veins become more stretched and thus susceptible to tearing. This results in a lower frequency of epidural hemorrhage and a higher frequency of subdural hemorrhage. Because of brain atrophy, a fairly large subdural hemorrhage can exist with minimal clinical findings. The combination of head trauma and hypovolemic shock yields a greater fatality rate. Preexisting medical conditions or their treatment may be a cause of altered mentation in elderly patients. When in doubt as to whether confusion represents an acute or chronic process, the injured patient should be preferentially transported to a trauma center for evaluation when possible.

Airway

Physical evaluation of the elderly patient begins with assessment of the airway. Changes in mentation may be associated with the tongue blocking the airway. The oral cavity should be examined for foreign bodies, such as dentures, that have become dislodged.

Breathing

Elderly patients who breathe at a rate of less than 10 or greater than 30 breaths/minute will not have adequate breathing and will require positive-pressure assisted ventilations, similar to any other adult. In most adults a ventilatory rate between 12 and 20 breaths/ minute is normal and confirms that an adequate minute volume is present. However, in an elderly patient, reduced pulmonary function may result in inadequate respirations, even at rates of 12 to 20 breaths/ minute; therefore, careful assessment of the patient is required.

Hypoxia is much more likely to be a consequence of shock than in younger patients. Elderly patients also have a decreased ability for chest excursions. Reductions in capillary oxygen and carbon dioxide exchange are significant. Hypoxemia tends to be progressive.

Circulation

Some findings can only be interpreted properly by knowing the individual patient's pre-event, or "baseline," status. Expected ranges of vital signs and other findings usually accepted as normal are not "normal" in every individual, and deviation is much more common in the elderly patient. Medication may contribute to these changes. For example, in the average adult, a systolic blood pressure (SBP) of 120 mm Hg is considered normal and generally unimpressive. However, in the chronically hypertensive patient who normally has an SBP of 150 mm Hg, a pressure of 120 mm Hg would be a concern, suggestive of hidden bleeding (or some other mechanism causing hypotension) of such a degree that decompensation has occurred. Likewise, heart rate is a poor indicator of trauma in elderly patients because of the effects of medications and the heart's poor response to the stress of trauma. Failing to recognize that such a change occurred, or that it is a serious pathologic finding in a particular patient, can produce a poor outcome for the patient.

Disability

Wide differences in mentation, memory, and orientation (to the past and present) can exist in elderly persons. Significant neurologic trauma should be identified in light of the individual's normal pre-injury status. Unless someone on the scene can describe this status, it should be assumed that the patient has a neurologic injury, hypoxia, or both. The ability to distinguish between a patient's chronic status and acute changes is an essential factor to prevent under-reaction or overreaction to the patient's present neurologic status when evaluating his or her overall condition. However, unconsciousness remains a serious sign in all cases.

The elderly patient's orientation to time and place should be assessed by careful and complete questioning. People who work 5 days a week with weekends off usually know the day of the week. If they do not, it can be assumed that they have some level of disorientation. For those who no longer work a traditional job and who are often surrounded by others who do not, a lack of distinction between days of the week or even months of the year may not indicate disorientation but only of a lack of "calendar" importance in the structure of their lives. Similarly, people who no longer drive pay less attention to roads, town borders, locations, and maps. Although normally oriented, they may not be able to identify their present location. Confusion or the inability to recall events and details long past may be more indicative of how long ago the events occurred rather than how forgetful the individual is.

Expose/Environment

Elderly persons are more susceptible to ambient environmental changes. They have a decreased ability to respond to temperature changes, decreased heat production, and a decreased ability to rid the body of excessive heat. Therefore, it is essential to appropriately protect the patient from the extremes of the environment upon completion of the physical examination.

Secondary Survey (Detailed History and Physical Examination)

The secondary survey of the elderly trauma victim is performed in the same manner as for younger patients and after urgent life-threatening conditions have been addressed. However, a number of factors may complicate assessment of the geriatric patient. Because of this, more than the average time may need to be taken while assessing elderly patients.

Communication Challenges

- *Additional patience may be needed because of the elderly patient's hearing or visual deficits.* Empathy and compassion are essential. A patient's intelligence should not be underestimated merely because communication may be difficult or absent. If the patient has close associates or relatives, they may participate in giving information or may stay nearby to help validate information. However, not all elderly patients have sig-

nificant deficits. Speaking in a louder tone or slower cadence to the elderly patient may be unnecessary and insulting.

- *A significant other may need to be involved.* With the patient's permission, involving the caregiver or spouse may be necessary to gather valid information. It is important, however, to not approach elderly patients as if they were small children. A common mistake by health care professionals in both prehospital and emergency department settings is to treat the elderly in this way. Often, well-meaning relatives are so aggressive in reporting the events for an elderly loved one that they take over as the respondent to all inquiries. In such a situation, the provider can easily overlook that the clinical impression and history are from someone other than the patient and may not be correct. Not only does this increase the danger of obtaining incomplete or inaccurate information through a third party's impressions and translation, but it also discounts the patient as a mature adult. Some elderly patients may be reluctant to give information without the assistance of a relative or support person. However, the elderly patient may not want any other person present for many reasons, including abuse problems. Also, some problems may embarrass the elderly patient, and the person may not want any family members to know about them.
- *Pay attention to impaired hearing, sight, comprehension, and mobility capabilities.* Eye contact should be made with the patient. The patient may be hearing impaired and depend on watching your lips and other facial movements. Noise, distractions, and interruptions should be minimized. Fluency in speech, an involuntary movement, cranial nerve dysfunction, or difficulty breathing should be noted. Is the patient's movement easy, unsteady, or unbalanced?
- *Address the patient by his or her last name, unless otherwise told by the patient.*

Physiologic Changes

- *Altered comprehension or neurologic disorders are a significant problem for many elderly patients.* These impairments can range from confusion to senile dementia of the type associated with Alzheimer's disease. Not only may these patients have difficulty in communicating, but they may also be unable to comprehend or help in the assessment. They may be restless and sometimes combative.
- *Shake the patient's hand to feel for grip strength, skin turgor, and body temperature. Look at the patient's state of nourishment.* Does the patient appear to be well, thin, or emaciated? Elderly patients have a decreased thirst response and a decreased amount of body fat (15%–30%) and total body water.
- *Elderly patients have a decrease in skeletal muscle weight, widening and weakening of bones, degeneration of joints, and osteoporosis.* They have an increased prob-

ability of fractures with minor injuries and a greatly increased risk of fractures to the vertebrae, hip, and ribs.

Environmental Factors

■ *Look for behavioral problems or manifestations that do not fit the scene.* Look at grooming. Are the patient's attire and grooming appropriate for where and how the patient was found? The ease of rising or sitting should be observed. Is there the potential for elder abuse or neglect?

Medications

Knowledge of a patient's medications can provide key information in determining prehospital and hospital care. Preexisting disease in the elderly trauma patient is a significant finding. It is important to look about the scene for the presence of medications that the patient is taking and provide them to ALS providers and hospital staff. The following classes of drugs are of particular interest because of their frequent use by elderly persons and their potential to affect care of the trauma patient:

■ Beta blockers (e.g., propranolol, metoprolol) may account for a patient's slow heart rate. In this situation, an increasing tachycardia as a sign of developing shock may not occur. Such patients can rapidly decompensate, seemingly without warning.
■ Calcium channel blockers (e.g., verapamil) may prevent periph eral vasoconstriction and accelerate hypovolemic shock.
■ Nonsteroidal anti-inflammatory agents (e.g., ibuprofen) may increase bleeding.
■ Anticoagulants (e.g., clopidogrel, aspirin, warfarin) may increase blood loss. Data suggest that use of warfarin increases the risk of isolated head injury and adverse outcome. Any bleeding from trauma will be more brisk and difficult to control when a patient is taking an anticoagulant. More importantly, internal bleeding can progress rapidly, leading to shock and death.
■ Hypoglycemic agents (e.g., insulin, metformin, rosiglitazone) may be the cause of the events that lead to the injury.
■ Over-the-counter (OTC) medications, including herbal preparations and supplements, are commonly used by elderly persons. Their inclusion in the list of medications is often omitted by patients, who should be specifically questioned about their use. These preparations are unregulated and thus have unpredictable dose effects and possible drug-drug interactions. Complications of these agents include bleeding (e.g., garlic) and myocardial infarction (e.g., ephedrine/Ma-Huang).

The difficulty in assessing the elderly trauma patient's medication list may include loss of consciousness and an extensive list of medications with difficult names. In some communities, Emergency Medical Services (EMS) agencies have promoted programs such as the File of Life Project. In this program, the patient's detailed medical history is placed in a common location in any house, the refrigerator door. The patient completes a medical history form that is then placed into a magnetic holder that is applied to the refrigerator, alerting the prehospital team to the File of Life (Figure 10-22).

Medical Conditions

Numerous medical conditions may predispose individuals to traumatic events, especially those that result in an alteration in the level of consciousness or other neurologic deficit. Common examples include seizure disorders, insulin shock from diabetes mellitus, syncopal episodes from antihypertensive medication, cardiac dysrhythmias from an acute coronary syndrome, and strokes (cerebrovascular accidents or CVAs). Because the incidence of chronic medical conditions increases with age, geriatric patients are more prone to sustaining trauma as the result of such a medical problem than are younger victims. For example:

■ Bystanders may note that a victim appeared unconscious before a crash
■ A Medic-Alert bracelet indicates the patient has diabetes
■ An irregular heartbeat is noted on examination

This key information is passed on to the receiving facility.

Management

Airway. The presence of dentures, common in the elderly population, may affect airway management. Ordinarily, dentures should be left in place to maintain a better seal around the mouth with a mask. However, partial dentures (plates) may become dislodged during an emergency and may completely or partially block the airway; these should be removed.

Thin, easily damaged nasopharyngeal mucosal tissues and the possible use of anticoagulants put the elderly trauma patient at increased risk of bleeding from placement of a nasopharyngeal airway. This hemorrhage may further compromise the patient's airway and result in aspiration. Arthritis may affect the temporomandibular joints and cervical spine. The decreased flexibility of these areas may make airway management more difficult.

The objective of airway management is primarily to ensure a clear and open airway for the delivery of adequate tissue oxygenation. Early assisted ventilation by bag-mask device should be considered in elderly trauma patients because of their greatly limited physiologic reserve.[32]

Breathing. In all trauma patients, supplemental oxygen should be administered as soon as possible. The increased stiffness of the chest wall, reduced chest wall muscle power and stiffening of the cartilage make the entire chest less flexible. These and other changes are responsible for reductions in lung volumes. The elderly patient may need ventilatory support by assisted ventilations with a bag-mask device earlier than younger trauma patients. The mechanical force applied to the

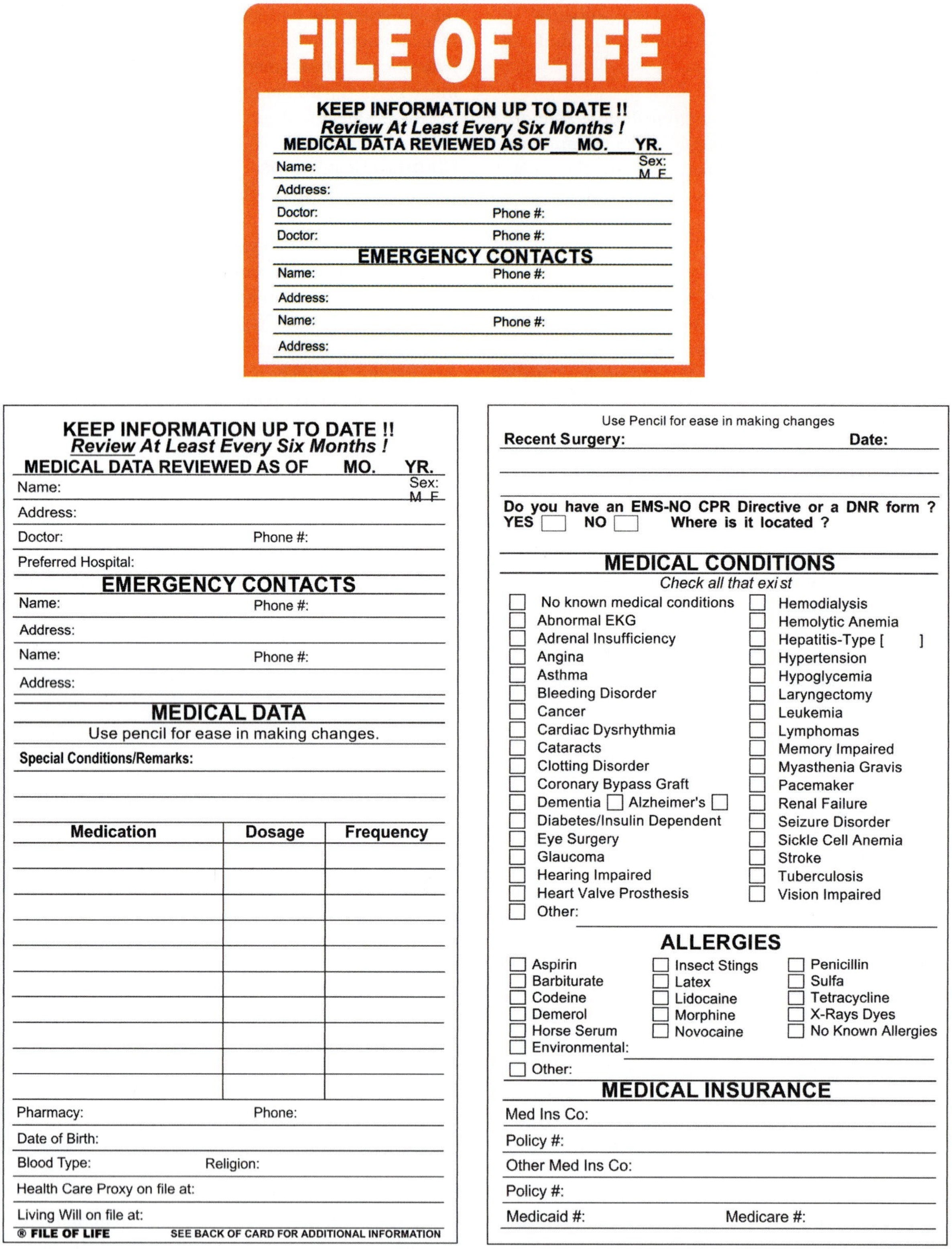

FILE OF LIFE

KEEP INFORMATION UP TO DATE !!
Review At Least Every Six Months !
MEDICAL DATA REVIEWED AS OF ___ MO. ___ YR.

Name: _____ Sex: M F

Address: _____

Doctor: _____ Phone #: _____

Doctor: _____ Phone #: _____

EMERGENCY CONTACTS

Name: _____ Phone #: _____

Address: _____

Name: _____ Phone #: _____

Address: _____

KEEP INFORMATION UP TO DATE !!
Review At Least Every Six Months !
MEDICAL DATA REVIEWED AS OF ___ MO. ___ YR.

Name: _____ Sex: M F

Address: _____

Doctor: _____ Phone #: _____

Preferred Hospital: _____

EMERGENCY CONTACTS

Name: _____ Phone #: _____

Address: _____

Name: _____ Phone #: _____

Address: _____

MEDICAL DATA
Use pencil for ease in making changes.

Special Conditions/Remarks: _____

Medication	Dosage	Frequency

Pharmacy: _____ Phone: _____

Date of Birth: _____

Blood Type: _____ Religion: _____

Health Care Proxy on file at: _____

Living Will on file at: _____

® FILE OF LIFE   SEE BACK OF CARD FOR ADDITIONAL INFORMATION

Use Pencil for ease in making changes

Recent Surgery: _____ Date: _____

_____

Do you have an EMS-NO CPR Directive or a DNR form ?
YES ☐   NO ☐   Where is it located ?

MEDICAL CONDITIONS
Check all that exist

☐ No known medical conditions   ☐ Hemodialysis
☐ Abnormal EKG   ☐ Hemolytic Anemia
☐ Adrenal Insufficiency   ☐ Hepatitis-Type [   ]
☐ Angina   ☐ Hypertension
☐ Asthma   ☐ Hypoglycemia
☐ Bleeding Disorder   ☐ Laryngectomy
☐ Cancer   ☐ Leukemia
☐ Cardiac Dysrhythmia   ☐ Lymphomas
☐ Cataracts   ☐ Memory Impaired
☐ Clotting Disorder   ☐ Myasthenia Gravis
☐ Coronary Bypass Graft   ☐ Pacemaker
☐ Dementia ☐ Alzheimer's ☐   ☐ Renal Failure
☐ Diabetes/Insulin Dependent   ☐ Seizure Disorder
☐ Eye Surgery   ☐ Sickle Cell Anemia
☐ Glaucoma   ☐ Stroke
☐ Hearing Impaired   ☐ Tuberculosis
☐ Heart Valve Prosthesis   ☐ Vision Impaired
☐ Other:

ALLERGIES

☐ Aspirin   ☐ Insect Stings   ☐ Penicillin
☐ Barbiturate   ☐ Latex   ☐ Sulfa
☐ Codeine   ☐ Lidocaine   ☐ Tetracycline
☐ Demerol   ☐ Morphine   ☐ X-Rays Dyes
☐ Horse Serum   ☐ Novocaine   ☐ No Known Allergies
☐ Environmental:
☐ Other:

MEDICAL INSURANCE

Med Ins Co: _____

Policy #: _____

Other Med Ins Co: _____

Policy #: _____

Medicaid #: _____ Medicare #: _____

FIGURE 10-22 File of Life.

resuscitation bag may need to be increased to overcome the increased chest wall resistance.

Circulation

Elderly persons may have poor cardiovascular reserve. Vital signs are a poor indicator of shock in the elderly patient because the patient who is normally hypertensive may be in shock with a blood pressure that is considered "normal" for a younger patient. Reduced circulating blood volume, possible chronic anemia, and preexisting myocardial and coronary disease leave the patient with very little tolerance for even modest amounts of blood loss. Because of the laxity of skin or use of anticoagulant agents, geriatric patients are prone to the development of larger hematomas and potentially more significant internal hemorrhage. Early control of hemorrhage through direct pressure on open wounds, stabilization or immobilization of fractures, and rapid transport to a trauma center are essential.

Immobilization

Protection of the cervical spine, particularly in trauma patients who have sustained multisystem injury, is an expected standard of care. Degenerative arthritis of the cervical spine may subject the elderly patient to spinal cord injury from positioning and manipulating the neck, even if the patient has no injury to the bony spine. Another consideration with improper movement of the cervical spine is the possibility of occlusion of the arteries to the brain, which can result in unconsciousness and even stroke.

A cervical collar applied to an elderly patient with severe kyphosis should not compress the airway or carotid arteries. Less traditional means of immobilization, such as a rolled towel and head block, can be considered if standard collars are inappropriate.

Padding may need to be placed under the patient's head and between the shoulders when immobilizing the supine elderly patient. Because of the thin skin and lack of adipose tissue in frail elderly patients, they are more likely to develop pressure (decubitus) ulcers from lying on their back; therefore, additional padding will be required when these patients are immobilized to a long backboard. It is always a good idea to check for pressure points where the patient is resting on the board and pad appropriately. When applying the straps to secure the patient, the elderly patient may not be able to straighten the legs fully because of decreased range of motion of the hips and knees. This may require the placement of padding under the legs for comfort and security of the patient during transport.[33]

Temperature Control

The elderly patient should be monitored closely for hypothermia and hyperthermia during treatment and transportation. Although it is appropriate to expose the patient to facilitate a thorough examination, elderly persons are especially prone to heat loss. On the other hand, the effects of various medications may mean that a patient is more prone to overheating; therefore, some means of cooling the patient should be considered if the patient is unable to be moved quickly to a controlled environment. Prolonged extrication in the extremes of heat and cold may also place the elderly patient at risk and should be rapidly addressed. External methods of heating or cooling the elderly trauma patient should be balanced by the possibility of direct thermal injury to the site of application with the patient's attenuated skin structure.

Elder Maltreatment

Elder abuse is defined as any action by an elderly person's family member (any relative), associated persons who have daily household contact (housekeeper, roommate), anyone on whom the elderly person is reliant for daily needs of food, clothing, and shelter, or a professional caregiver who takes advantage of the elderly person's property or emotional state.

Reports and complaints of abuse, neglect, and other related problems among the elderly population are increasing. The exact extent of elder abuse is not known for the following reasons:

1. Elder abuse has been largely hidden from society.
2. Abuse and neglect of elderly persons have varying definitions.
3. Elders are uneasy or fearful of reporting the problem to law enforcement agencies or human and social welfare personnel. A typical victim of elder abuse may be a parent who feels ashamed or guilty because he or she raised the abuser. The abused may also feel traumatized by the situation or fear continued reprisal by the abuser.
4. Some jurisdictions lack formal reporting mechanisms. Some areas do not even have a statutory provision requiring the reporting of elder abuse.

The physical and emotional signs of abuse, such as rape, beating, or nutritional deprivation, are often overlooked or perhaps are not accurately identified. Older women in particular are not likely to report incidents of sexual assault to law enforcement agencies. Sensory deficits, senility, and other forms of altered mental status (e.g., drug-induced depression) may make it impossible or extremely difficult for the elderly patient to report the maltreatment.

Profile of the Abused. The elderly adult most likely to be abused fits into the following profile:

- Older than 65 years of age, especially women older than 75 years
- Frail
- Multiple chronic medical conditions
- Demented
- Impaired sleep cycle, sleepwalking, or loud shouting at night

- Incontinent of feces, urine, or both
- Dependent on others for activities of daily living or incapable of independent living

Profile of the Abuser. Because many elderly people live in a family environment and are typically women older than 75 years of age, that environment may provide clues. Most abusers are untrained in the particular care required by the elderly and have little relief time from the constant care demands of their family.

Abuse is not restricted to the home. Other environments such as nursing, convalescent, and continuing care centers are sites where the elderly may sustain physical, chemical, or pharmacologic harm. Care providers in these environments may consider elderly persons to represent management problems or categorize them as obstinate or undesirable patients.

The usual profile of the abuser includes the following signs:

- Existence of household conflict
- Marked fatigue
- Unemployment
- Financial difficulties
- Substance abuse
- Previous history of being abused

Categories of Maltreatment. Abuse can be categorized in the following ways:

1. *Physical abuse:* Includes assault, neglect, malnutrition, poor maintenance of the living environment, and poor personal care. The signs of physical abuse or neglect may be obvious, such as the imprint left by an item (e.g., fireplace poker), or may be subtle (e.g., malnutrition). The signs of elder abuse are similar to those of child abuse (Figure 10-23).
2. *Psychological abuse:* Can take on the forms of neglect, verbal abuse, infantilization, or deprivation of sensory stimulation.
3. *Financial abuse:* Can include theft of valuables or embezzlement.
4. *Sexual assault /abuse*
5. *Self-abuse*

Important Points. Many abused patients are terrorized into making false statements for fear of retribution. In the case of elder abuse by family members, fear of removal from the home environment can cause the elderly patient to lie about the origin of the abuse. In other cases of elder abuse, sensory deprivation or dementia may deter adequate explanation. The prehospital care provider should identify abuse and uncover any pathology reported by the patient. Any history of maltreatment or findings consistent with it should be documented on the patient care report.

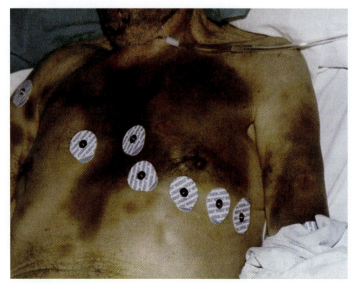

FIGURE 10-23 A 70-year-old man was brought from his caregiver's home to the emergency department by police after his daughter found him severely bruised. He had multiple contusions at varying stages of healing on his chest and arms, as well as a linear patterned injury across his left anterior chest. The central and bilateral locations of the contusions, varying colors, and linear pattern of the bruise on his left chest are highly suggestive of physical abuse.
(From Marx J: *Rosen's emergency medicine,* ed 7, St Louis, 2010, Mosby. Courtesy Dr. D.C. Schneider.)

Further trauma to a patient may be reduced by identifying an abusive situation. Reporting a high index of suspicion for abuse can allow for referral and protective services from human, social, and public safety agencies (Figure 10-24).

Disposition

One of the greatest challenges with prehospital care of the injured patient is defining which patients are most likely to benefit from the surgeons and advanced treatment options available at a trauma center. For many of the reasons mentioned previously, triage criteria may be less reliable in the elderly patient because of physiologic or pharmacologic effects. A major recommendation in the *Guidelines for Geriatric Trauma* of the Eastern Association for the Surgery of Trauma is that prehospital providers treating trauma patients of advanced age should have a lower threshold to triage these victims directly to a trauma center.[34] Data from several states demonstrate that a disproportionate number of elderly trauma patients are receiving care at trauma centers. Furthermore, potentially preventable mortality in the geriatric trauma population is lower at trauma centers.

Prolonged Transport

The majority of care of the elderly trauma patient follows general guidelines for prehospital care of the injured patient.

FIGURE 10-24   Reporting Elder Abuse and Neglect

In many states, EMS personnel are legally considered to be mandated reporters of suspected elder (or *adult*) abuse, neglect, and exploitation. *Abuse* is considered the deliberate infliction of pain, injury, mental anguish, unreasonable confinement, or nonconsensual sexual contact. *Neglect* involves living in conditions in which the adult or responsible caretaker is not providing care required to maintain the elderly person's physical and mental health and well-being. *Exploitation* is the illegal use of an adult's resources for another's gain or advantage. In recent years, elder abuse has been increasingly recognized. However, younger adults who have incapacitating conditions such as mental illness, mental retardation, and physical disability are also at risk for abuse and neglect.

Signs of abuse and neglect include unexplained or unusual injuries; conflicting accounts of how an injury occurred; a caregiver who prevents the adult from speaking with others; dehydration or malnutrition; depression; lack of access to medications, eyeglasses, dentures, or other aids; lack of personal hygiene; unkempt environment; and lack of adequate heating and cooling.

Mandated reporters must report directly to the social services agency responsible for investigating adult abuse, rather than relying on intermediaries such as hospital personnel. If the individual is in immediate danger or has been sexually assaulted, law enforcement must be notified as well. In the event that a death appears to have been caused by abuse or neglect, mandatory reporters generally must notify the office of the medical examiner or coroner and law enforcement. Mandatory reporters are liable for failing to report suspected abuse, neglect, and exploitation. However, they are protected against civil and criminal liability associated with reporting, may be able to keep their identity confidential, and are allowed to share medical information that is related to the case, although this information would be protected under the Health Insurance Portability and Accountability Act (HIPAA) in normal circumstances. Laws governing the mandatory reporting of elder abuse are enacted at the state level. All EMS providers must be aware of the laws in the state in which they work.

However, several special circumstances exist in prolonged transport scenarios. These concerns are particularly important for the recommendations to triage patients with less significant anatomic injuries directly to trauma centers.

Immobilization on a long backboard places these patients at increased risk for pressure-related skin breakdown over extended transports. Before a long transport, consideration should be given to clearing the spine or log rolling a patient onto an appropriately padded long backboard to protect the patient's skin. Agencies in remote regions should consider purchasing a specially designed, low-pressure backboard that immobilizes the patient while limiting the potential for skin breakdown.

Environmental control is essential in geriatric patients with a lengthy transport. Limiting body exposure and controlling ambient temperature of the vehicle may limit hypothermia.

Finally, transport of the geriatric trauma patient from remote regions may be a valid use of aeromedical transport. Transport via helicopter may limit the duration of environmental exposure, reduce the duration of shock, and ensure earlier access to hospital-based care, including early surgery and blood transfusion.

SUMMARY

- Although general guidelines for care of the injured patient remain the same, several specific approaches are unique to care of the injured geriatric patient.
- Anatomic and physiologic changes associated with aging, chronic disease, and medications can make certain types of trauma more likely, complicate traumatic injuries, and cause a decreased ability to compensate for shock. Older patients have less physiologic reserve and tolerate physical insult poorly.

- Knowledge of the elderly trauma patient's medical history and medications is an essential component of care.
- Many factors in elderly trauma patients can mask early signs of deterioration, increasing the possibility of sudden, rapid decompensation without apparent warning.
- With an elderly trauma patient, more serious injury may have occurred than indicated by the initial presentation.
- A lower threshold for direct triage of these patients to trauma centers is important.

SCENARIO 2 SOLUTION

When dealing with trauma in the elderly patient, you cannot always determine immediately whether the trauma was the primary event or whether it was secondary to a medical event, such as a stroke, myocardial infarction, or syncopal episode. However, you always need to consider the possibility that a significant medical event preceded the trauma. Your primary assessment reveals that the patient is maintaining a patent airway and is breathing at 16 times per minute. There is no major external hemorrhage and the bleeding from the forehead laceration is easily controlled with pressure. His heart rate is 84. You immobilize the patient to a longboard and provide appropriate padding underneath. Given his age, the apparent head trauma, and the magnitude of the crash, you transport him emergently to the closest trauma center. ■

References

1. Centers for Disease Control and Prevention National Center for Injury Prevention and Control: *WISQARS ten leading causes of death reports, 2005.* Atlanta, CDC. Available at http://wepappa.cdc.gov/sasweb/ncipc/leadcaus10.html. Accessed February 10, 2009.

2. Centers for Disease Control and Prevention National Center for Injury Prevention and Control: *WISQARS leading causes of nonfatal injuries reports, 2005.* Atlanta, CDC. Available at http://wepappa.cdc.gov/sasweb/ncipc/nfilead2001.html. Accessed February 10, 2009.

3. Gaines BA, Ford HR: Abdominal and pelvic trauma in children. *Crit Care Med* 30(11 suppl):S416, 2002.

4. Gausche M, Lewis RJ, Stratton SJ, et al: Effect of out-of-hospital pediatric endotracheal intubation on survival and neurological outcome: A controlled clinical trial. *JAMA* 283(6):783, 2000.

5. Adelson PD, Bratton SL, Carney NA, et al: Guidelines for the acute medical management of severe traumatic brain injury in infants, children, and adolescents. Chapter 4. Resuscitation of blood pressure and oxygenation and prehospital brain-specific therapies for the severe pediatric traumatic brain injury patient. *Pediatr Crit Care Med* 4(3 suppl):S12, 2003.

6. Manley G, Knudson MM, Morabito D, et al: Hypotension, hypoxia, and head injury: Frequency, duration, and consequences. *Arch Surg* 136(10):1118, 2001.

7. Carmona Suazo JA, Maas AI, van den Brink WA, et al: CO_2 reactivity and brain oxygen pressure monitoring in severe head injury. *Crit Care Med* 28(9):3268, 2000.

8. Centers for Disease Control and Prevention, National Vital Statistics System: Deaths: Final data for 1997. *MMWR* 47(19):1, 1999.

9. Heins M: The "battered child" revisited. *JAMA* 251:3295, 1984.

10. Weimer CL, Goldfarb IW, Slater H: Multidisciplinary approach to working with burn victims of child abuse. *J Burn Care Rehabil* 9:79, 1988.

11. Feldman KW, Schaller RT, Feldman JA, McMillon M: Tap water scald burns in children. *Pediatrics* 62:1, 1978.

12. Montrey JS, Barcia PJ: Nonaccidental burns in child abuse. *South Med J* 78:1324, 1985.

13. Larson JT, Dietrich AM, Abdessalam SF, Werman HA: Effective use of the air ambulance for pediatric trauma. *J Trauma Injury Infect Crit Care* 56(1):89, 2004.

14. Eckstein M, Jantos T, Kelly N, Cardillo A: Helicopter transport of pediatric trauma patients in an urban emergency medical services system: A critical analysis. *J Trauma Injury Infect Crit Care* 53(2):340, 2002.

15. www.census.gov/Press-Release/www/releases/archives/population/013733.html. Accessed August 30, 2009.

16. Scommegna P: *US growing bigger, older, and more diverse.* Population Reference Bureau, 2005. Available at www.prb.org.

17. Champion H et al: The Major Trauma Outcome Study: Establishing national norms for trauma care. *J Trauma* 30(11):1356, 1990.

18. Centers for Disease Control and Prevention National Center for Injury Prevention and Control: *WISQARS leading causes of death, 1999–2004.* Atlanta, CDC. Available at http://webappa.cdc.gov/sasweb/ncipc/leadcaus10.html.

19. Weigelt J: Trauma. Advanced trauma life support for doctors. In *Advanced trauma life support,* ed 6, Chicago, 1997, ACS.

20. Jacobs D: Special considerations in geriatric injury. *Curr Opin Crit Care* 9(6):535, 2003.

21. Milzman DP, Boulanger BR, Rodriguez A, et al: Preexisting disease in trauma patients: a predictor of fate independent of age and injury severity score. *J Trauma* 32:236, 1992.

22. Smith T: Respiratory system: Aging, adversity, and anesthesia. In McCleskey CH, editor: *Geriatric anesthesiology,* Baltimore, 1997, Williams & Wilkins.

23. Centers for Disease Control and Prevention, National Center for Health Statistics: *Stroke and cerebrovascular diseases,* Hyattsville, MD, 2005, National Center for Health Statistics. Available at www.cdc.gov/nchs.

24. Centers for Disease Control and Prevention, National Center for Health Statistics: *Hypertension,* Hyattsville, MD, 2005, National Center for Health Statistics. Available at www.cdc.gov/nchs/.

25. Carey J: *Brain facts: A primer on the brain and nervous system,* Washington, DC, 2002, Society for Neuroscience. Available at www.sfn.org.

26. National Institutes of Health, National Eye Institute: *Cataract: what you should know,* Bethesda, MD, 2005, National Eye Institute. Available at www.nei.nih.gov/health/cataract/cataract_facts.asp.

27. Blackmore C: Cervical spine injury in patients 65 years old and older: Epidemiologic analysis regarding the effects of age and injury mechanism on distribution, type, and stability of injuries. *Am J Roentgenol* 178:573, 2002.

28. Centers for Disease Control and Prevention, National Center for Health Statistics: *Older adult drivers: Fact sheet,* 2005. Hyattsville, MD, National Center for Health Statistics. Available at www.cdc.gov/nchs.

29. U.S. Administration on Aging, National Center on Elder Abuse, 2005. Available at www.elderabusecenter.org/.

30. U.S. Administration on Aging: *Elder rights and resources,* Washington, DC, AOA. Available at www.aoa.gov/eldfam/Elder_Rights/Elder_Rights.asp.

31. *Vial of life,* 2005. Available at www.vialoflife.com/index_old.html.

32. Heffner J, Reynolds S: Airway management of the critically ill patient. *Chest* 127:1397, 2005.

33. American Geriatric Society: *Geriatric education for emergency medical services (GEMS),* Sudbury, MA, 2003, Jones & Bartlett.

34. Eastern Association for the Surgery of Trauma: Guidelines for geriatric trauma. In *Practice management guidelines.* Available at www.east.org/tpg/geriatric.pdf.

Suggested Reading

EMSC Partnership for Children/National Association of EMS Physicians model pediatric protocols: 2003 revision. *Prehosp Emerg Care* 8(4):343, 2004.

American College of Surgeons Committee on Trauma: Extremes of age: Geriatric trauma. In *Advanced trauma life support for doctors, student course manual,* ed 8, Chicago, 2008, ACS.

Callaway D, Wolfe R: Geriatric trauma. *Emerg Med Clin North Am* 25(3):837–860, 2007.

Lavoie A, Ratte S, Clas D, et al: Preinjury warfarin use among elderly patients with closed head injuries in a trauma center. *J Trauma* 56:802, 2004.

Tepas JJ 3rd, Veldenz HC, Lottenberg L, et al: Elderly trauma: A profile of trauma experience in the sunshine (retirement) state. *J Trauma* 48:581, 2000.

Victorino GP, Chong TJ, Pal JD: Trauma in the elderly patient. *Arch Surg* 138:1093–1097.

CHAPTER 11

Disaster Management and Weapons of Mass Destruction

CHAPTER OBJECTIVES

At the completion of this chapter, the reader will be able to do the following:

✓ Describe the components of the disaster cycle.

✓ Discuss common pitfalls encountered during disaster response.

✓ Understand and discuss the components that comprise the medical response to a disaster.

✓ Recognize how disaster response may affect the psychological well-being of prehospital care providers.

✓ Understand the essential considerations regarding mitigation of a weapon of mass destruction (WMD) event:

> Scene assessment
> Incident command
> Personal protective equipment
> Patient triage
> Principle of decontamination

✓ Define *weapon of mass destruction*.

✓ Understand the mechanisms of injury, evaluation and management, and transport considerations associated with the five main categories of WMD agents:

> Explosive agents
> Incendiary agents
> Chemical agents
> Biologic agents
> Radiologic agents

✓ Know how to access and utilize resources for further study.

SCENARIO 1

You are dispatched to a report of an explosion at an apartment building. The dispatcher says that the local gas company was called for an odor of gas leaking at an apartment, but before anyone arrived the explosion occurred. The force of the explosion was enormous. It heavily damaged the apartment building and left an enormous crater on one side with partial collapse of the structure. The blast was felt for several blocks around the area.

What safety and security concerns would first responders encounter?

What triage system should be utilized? Who should be selected as incident commander?

What level of personal protection should first responders utilize?

What are important features of the casualty collection station?

Disaster Management

Unlike the trauma patient who has a finite period of time for presentation, treatment, and recovery, the response to and recovery from a disaster are time consuming, encompass multiple agencies, and include not only medical and psychosocial issues but also the rebuilding of public health, physical safety, and sociologic resources and infrastructures.

The World Health Organization (WHO) has defined a disaster as a sudden ecologic phenomenon of sufficient magnitude to require external assistance. This broad definition does not provide specific reference to the medical response but is inclusive of the overall community response and sociopolitical response to any disaster of significant magnitude.

From a medical perspective, the definition can be more focused. A disaster is when the number of patients presenting for medical assistance within a given time is such that the medical providers cannot provide care for them with the usual resources at hand and require additional, and sometimes external, assistance.[1] This is commonly referred to as a mass casualty incident (MCI). The acronym MCI has also been used to refer to "multiple casualty incidents," which are events that involve more than one casualty but which can be handled with the usual resources available to respond. In this text, MCI will be used to refer to mass casualty incidents that overwhelm the available resources.

In short, these definitions identify two key concepts: (1) A disaster is independent of a specific number of victims, and (2) the impact exceeds the available resources of the medical response. Simply stated, all mass casualty incidents are disasters, but not all disasters are mass casualty incidents.

Disasters are often thought to follow no rules because no one can predict the time, location, or complexity of the next disaster. Traditionally, medical providers have thought that all disasters are different, especially those involving terrorism. However, all disasters, regardless of etiology, have similar medical and public health consequences. Disasters differ in the degree to which these consequences occur and the degree to which they disrupt the medical and public health infrastructure of the disaster scene.

The key principle of disaster medical care is to do the greatest good for the greatest number of patients with the resources available, whereas the objective of "conventional" non–disaster-related medical care is to do the greatest good for the individual patient.

Natural disasters, manmade disasters, and terrorism encompass the spectrum of possible disaster threats. Weapons of mass destruction, creating huge numbers of casualties and "contaminated environments," may be the greatest challenge of all.

A consistent approach to disasters, based on an understanding of their common features and the response expertise required to deal with the incident, is becoming the accepted practice throughout the world. This strategy forms the framework for *mass casualty incident response.* MCI response has the primary objective of reducing the morbidity (injury, disease) and mortality (death) caused by the disaster. All medical responders need to incorporate the key principles of the MCI response in their training, given the complexity of current disasters (Figure 11-1).

The Disaster Cycle

A framework has been developed to describe the sequence of events in a disaster.[1] This description provides an overview of the natural history of an event and also provides the basis for the development of the response process.[2,3] Five phases have been identified, as follows:

1. The *quiescence phase,* or the interdisaster period, represents the time during which risk assessment and prevention activities should be undertaken and when plans for the response to likely events are developed, tested, and implemented.

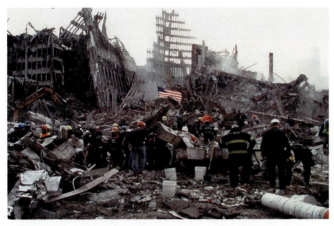

FIGURE 11-1   Mass casualty management at Ground Zero, World Trade Center, New York, 2001.

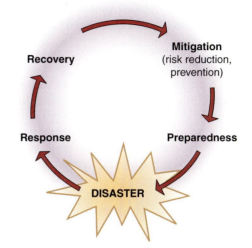

FIGURE 11-2   The life cycle of a disaster. The quiescence phase is represented by the mitigation, risk reduction, prevention, and preparedness arrows. The warning phase comes just before the impact of the event. This is followed by the response and recovery periods.

2. The next phase is the *prodrome phase*, or warning phase. At this point, a specific event has been identified as inevitably going to occur. This could reflect a natural weather condition (e.g., impending landfall of a hurricane) or the active unfolding of a hostile and potentially violent situation. During this period, specific steps may be taken to lessen the effects of the ensuing events. These defensive maneuvers may include such actions as fortifying physical structures, initiating evacuation plans, and mobilizing public health resources to mount a post-event response.

3. The third phase is the *impact phase,* or the occurrence of the actual event. During this period, there is often little that can be done to alter the actual impact or outcome of what is occurring.

4. The fourth phase is the *rescue phase,* which is the time period immediately following the impact during which response occurs and appropriate management and intervention can save lives. The skills of the first responders, rescue teams, and medical support services will be brought to bear to maximize survival from the event.

5. The fifth phase is the *recovery phase,* or reconstruction phase, which addresses the community's resources to endure and emerge from the effects of the disaster through the coordinated efforts of the medical, public health, and community infrastructure (physical and political). This period is by far the longest, lasting months, and perhaps years, before a community fully recovers.

Understanding the disaster cycle (Figure 11-2) allows prehospital care providers to evaluate the preparations that have been made in anticipation of the likely hazards and events that may be encountered in their community. After an incident has occurred, it allows for critical evaluation of the after-action report and assessment of the provider's individual area of responsibility and response, as well as the response of others, to determine the efficiency and efficacy of the response process and identify areas for future improvement. These concepts apply to all disasters, regardless of size.

The duration of each component of the disaster life cycle will vary depending on the frequency with which incidents occur in a given community, the nature of the incident, and the degree to which the community is prepared. For example, the quiescent period in some locations can be extremely long (measured in years) whereas in other communities it may be measured in months. A specific example is that of hurricanes. The southeastern states of the United States prepare for hurricanes annually with a quiescent period between events of approximately 6 to 8 months. In contrast, while the New England states have been the victims of hurricanes, it is a rare event with a quiescent period of years in between hurricane strikes. The response and recovery phases from something like a refinery explosion will be measured in hours or at most a few days. The response and recovery from a major flood may take weeks to months.

Comprehensive Emergency Management

Knowledge of the life cycle or natural history of disasters can be used to implement the steps needed to manage an incident. This is accomplished using a process referred to as "comprehensive emergency management." Comprehensive emergency management consists of four components: mitigation, preparation, response, and recovery.

Mitigation: This component of emergency management generally occurs during the "quiescence" phase. Potential hazards or likely etiologies of mass casualty incidents are identified and assessed. Steps are then taken to prevent these hazards from causing an incident or to minimize their effect should something untoward occur.

FIGURE 11-3 Emergency Supply List

All Americans should have some basic supplies on hand in order to survive for at least 3 days if an emergency occurs. Following is a listing of some basic items that every emergency supply kit should include. However, it is important that individuals review this list and consider where they live and the unique needs of their family in order to create an emergency supply kit that will meet these needs. Individuals should also consider having at least two emergency supply kits, one full kit at home and smaller portable kits in their workplace, vehicle, or other places they spend time.

- Water—3 gallons for each person who would use the kit and an additional 4 gallons per person or pet for use if you are confined to your home
- Food—3-day supply in the kit and at least an additional 4-day supply per person or pet for use at home. *(You may want to consider stocking a 2-week supply of food and water in your home; see Figure 11-4.)*
- Battery-powered or hand-crank radio and a NOAA Weather Radio with tone alert and extra batteries for both
- Flashlight and extra batteries
- First aid kit (see Figure 11-5)
- Whistle to signal for help
- Dust mask, to help filter contaminated air, and plastic sheeting and duct tape to shelter-in-place
- Moist towelettes, garbage bags, and plastic ties for personal sanitation

- Wrench or pliers to turn off utilities
- Can opener for food (if kit contains canned food)
- Local maps

Additional items to consider adding to an emergency supply kit:

- Items for infants—including formula, diapers, bottles, pacifiers, powdered milk, and medications not requiring refrigeration
- Items for seniors, disabled persons or anyone with serious allergies—including special foods, denture items, extra eyeglasses, hearing aid batteries, prescription and nonprescription medications that are regularly used, inhalers, and other essential equipment
- Prescription medications and glasses
- Pet food and extra water for your pet
- Important family documents such as copies of insurance policies, identification, and bank account records in a waterproof, portable container
- Cash or traveler's checks and change
- Emergency reference material such as a first aid book or information from www.ready.gov
- Sleeping bag or warm blanket for each person; consider additional bedding if you live in a cold-weather climate

(Adapted from FEMA: *Ready America* [www.ready.gov] and the Centers for Disease Control and Prevention: *Emergency preparedness and response* [www.bt.cdc.gov/planning].)

Preparedness: This step of comprehensive emergency management involves identification, in advance of the incident, of the specific supplies, equipment, and personnel that would be needed as well as the specific action plan that would be taken if an incident occurred.

Response: This phase involves the activation and deployment of the various resources identified in the preparedness phase in order to manage an incident that has now occurred.

Recovery: This component of emergency management addresses the actions necessary to return the community back to its pre-incident status.

Although this process is typically applied to the management of a disaster, these same steps may also be utilized for the emergency preparedness of each responder.

Responder Personal Preparedness

Just as it is vital that each community and each agency undertake a comprehensive planning process in order to be prepared to meet the challenges of dealing with a disaster, so too is it important that each responder be ready to face the many issues that a disaster may present.

The prehospital provider must have a complete understanding of the many potential hazards that may accompany a disaster response in advance of the actual incident and be prepared to take the necessary steps to protect himself or herself from these dangers. Gaps in knowledge about such issues as building collapse, hazardous materials and situations, weapons of mass destruction and their effects and treatment, and overall incident management should be identified in advance and addressed.

Many disasters will go on for a long time, and responders must have discussed their roles, responsibilities, and potentially prolonged absence with their family. This includes preparing the family, in advance, for what they should do and where they should go during such an event to ensure their safety as well. In similar fashion to the procurement of supplies and equipment that occurs for the medical response, the provider should ensure that adequate supplies are available at home to meet family needs (Figures 11-3, 11-4, and 11-5).

All of these actions will help reassure providers that their family is safely dealing with their needs during the incident, provide comfort to families knowing that the provider is as prepared as possible for his or her role in disaster response, and allow providers to continue to provide care to those requiring medical assistance.

- Complete change of clothing, including a long-sleeved shirt, long pants, and sturdy shoes; consider additional clothing if you live in a cold-weather climate
- Household chlorine bleach and medicine dropper—when diluted 9 parts water to 1 part bleach, bleach can be used as a disinfectant; in an emergency, you can use it to treat water by using 16 drops of regular household liquid bleach per 1 gallon of water (do not use scented or color safe bleaches or bleaches with added cleaners)
- Fire extinguisher
- Matches in a waterproof container
- Feminine supplies and personal hygiene items
- Mess kits, paper cups, plates and plastic utensils, paper towels
- Paper and pencil
- Entertainment—including games and books, favorite dolls, and stuffed animals for small children
- Kitchen accessories—a manual can opener; utility knife; sugar and salt; aluminum foil and plastic wrap; resealable plastic bags
- Sanitation and hygiene items—shampoo, deodorant, toothpaste, toothbrushes, comb and brush, lip balm, sunscreen, contact lenses and supplies, any medications regularly used, toilet paper, towelettes, soap, hand sanitizer, liquid detergent, plastic garbage bags (heavy-duty) and ties (for personal sanitation uses), medium-sized plastic bucket with tight lid, disinfectant, household chlorine bleach.

- Other essential items—paper, pencil, needles, thread, small A-B-C-type fire extinguisher, medicine dropper, whistle, emergency preparedness manual
- A map of the area marked with places you could go and their telephone numbers
- An extra set of keys and identification—including keys for cars and any properties owned and copies of driver's licenses, passports, and work identification badges; copies of credit cards
- Copies of medical prescriptions
- A small tent, compass, and shovel

Pack the items in easy-to-carry containers, label the containers clearly and store them where they would be easily accessible. Duffle bags, backpacks, and covered trash receptacles are good candidates for containers. In a disaster situation, you may need access to your disaster supplies kit quickly—whether you are sheltering at home or evacuating. After a disaster, having the right supplies can help your household endure home confinement or evacuation.

Make sure the needs of everyone who would use the kit are covered, including infants, seniors and pets. It is a good idea to involve whoever is going to use the kit, including children, in assembling it.

FIGURE 11-4   Food Kit

- Store *at least* a 3-day supply of nonperishable food.
- Select foods that require no refrigeration, preparation, or cooking and little or no water.
- Pack a manual can opener and eating utensils.
- Avoid salty foods because they will make you thirsty.
- Choose foods your family will eat.
  - Ready-to-eat canned meats, fruits, and vegetables
  - Protein or fruit bars
  - Dry cereal or granola
  - Peanut butter

- Dried fruit
- Nuts
- Crackers
- Canned juices
- Nonperishable pasteurized milk
- High-energy foods
- Vitamins
- Food for infants
- Comfort/stress foods

(Adapted from FEMA: *Ready America* [www.ready.gov] and the Centers for Disease Control and Prevention: *Emergency preparedness and response* [www.bt.cdc.gov/planning].)

Mass Casualty Incident Management

Mass casualty incidents are events that cause casualties in numbers large enough to overwhelm the available medical and public health services of the affected community. The severity and diversity of injuries and illness, in addition to the number of victims, will be major factors in determining whether an MCI requires resources and assistance from outside the impacted community.

Today's complex disasters, especially those involving terrorism and weapons of mass destruction (chemical, biological, or nuclear), may result in an austere environment. An *austere environment* is a setting in which resources, supplies, equip-

---

FIGURE 11-5   First Aid Kit

In any emergency, you or a family member may be cut, burned, or suffer other injuries.

THINGS YOU SHOULD HAVE
- Two pairs of Latex, or other **sterile gloves** (if you are allergic to Latex)
- **Sterile dressings** to stop bleeding
- **Cleansing agent**/soap and antibiotic towelettes to disinfect
- **Antibiotic ointment** to prevent infection
- **Burn ointment** to prevent infection
- **Adhesive bandages** in a variety of sizes
- **Eye wash solution** to flush the eyes or as general decontaminant
- **Thermometer**
- **Prescription medications** you take every day, such as insulin, heart medicine, and asthma inhalers;

periodically rotate medicines to account for expiration dates
- **Prescribed medical supplies** such as glucose and blood pressure monitoring equipment and supplies

THINGS IT MAY BE GOOD TO HAVE
- Cell phone
- Scissors
- Tweezers
- Tube of petroleum jelly or other lubricant

NONPRESCRIPTION DRUGS
- Aspirin or nonaspirin pain reliever
- Antidiarrheal medication
- Antacid (for upset stomach)
- Laxative

(Adapted from FEMA: *Ready America* [www.ready.gov] and the Centers for Disease Control and Prevention: *Emergency preparedness and response* [www.bt.cdc.gov/planning].)

---

ment, personnel, transportation, and other aspects of the physical, political, social, and economic environments are limited. As a result of these limitations, severe constraints on the availability and adequacy of immediate care for the population in need will be imposed. Prehospital providers must anticipate the reality that, in such situations, the level of care provided to the sick and injured will be altered and interventions normally offered to all patients may be provided only to those individuals who meet specific criteria and who are likely to survive.[9]

Medical concerns related to MCIs include the following four elements:

- *Search and rescue*—the process of systematically looking for those individuals who have been impacted by an event and rescuing them from the hazardous situation. This often requires the use of specially trained teams, particularly when extrication issues are involved.
- *Triage and initial stabilization*—the process of systematically evaluating and categorizing each victim as to the seriousness of their injury or illness and providing initial medical care to address immediate life- or limb-threatening problems.
- *Definitive medical care*—the provision of the specific care needed to treat the patient's specific injuries. This care will usually be provided at hospitals; however, alternate care facilities may be used in major events when hospitals are overwhelmed with casualties or when hospitals have been directly impacted and damaged by the incident.
- *Evacuation*—the process of transporting disaster victims and injured patients away from the disaster site, either to a safe location or to a definitive care facility.

Public health concerns related to MCIs include the following:

- Water (ensuring a safe supply of potable water)
- Food (ideally nonperishable and needing no refrigeration or cooking)
- Shelter (a place for cover, protection, refuge)
- Sanitation (protection from contact with human and animal feces, solid waste, and wastewater)
- Security and safety
- Transportation
- Communication (includes information about communicable diseases)
- Endemic and epidemic diseases (endemic diseases are ones that are always present in a given area or population but that usually occur with low frequency, whereas an epidemic disease is one that develops and spread rapidly to the population at risk)

Failing to address the public health issues associated with a disaster may further exacerbate the medical needs during a major event.

Both medical and public health disaster response activities are coordinated through one organizational structure, the incident command system.

Incident Command System

Many different organizations participate in the response to a disaster. The incident command system (ICS) was created to allow different types of agencies and multiple jurisdictions of similar agencies (fire, police, Emergency Medical Services [EMS]) to work together effectively using a common organizational structure and language in response to a disaster (Figure 11-6; also see Chapter 3).

The incident command system recognizes that, regardless of the specific nature of the incident (police, fire, or medical), a number of functions must always happen. The ICS is organized around these necessary functions. The components of the ICS are:

1. Command
2. Planning
3. Logistics
4. Operations
5. Finance

These functions apply to all incidents and are now used in the medical setting to organize the response to a disaster.

From a medical perspective, several important ICS principles will help during an MCI response, as follows:

1. ICS must be started early, preferably upon arrival to the scene, before the incident management gets out of control.
2. Medical and public health responders, often used to working independently, need to implement the ICS management structure and coordinate their response assets to better respond to an MCI.
3. Using ICS will allow for the integration of the medical response into the overall response to the incident.

Detailed information and training about the incident command system is available on the FEMA website at http://training.fema.gov/EMIWeb/IS/ICSResource/index.htm.

Medical Response to Disasters

The effective response to an MCI depends on the initiation of a series of actions that, combined, will help to minimize the mortality and morbidity of victims of the event. Although these actions will be discussed sequentially in this chapter, it is important to remember that during an actual disaster many of these will be occurring simultaneously (Figure 11-7).

Initial Response. The first step is notification and activation of the EMS response system. This is usually performed by witnesses to the event who then call the local emergency dispatch center seeking response by appropriate police, fire, and emergency medical agencies.

The first medical responders to arrive at the scene have a number of important functions to fulfill that will set the stage for the entire medical response to the incident. Most importantly, these actions do *not* include finding and treating the most critically injured patients, as would be the case in most non-MCI situations. This can be paraphrased as "Don't just do something, stand there." Before beginning the process of providing medical assistance, the first medical personnel should take the time to perform an overall scene assessment. The goals of this assessment are to evaluate any potential hazards, estimate the potential number of casualties, determine what additional medical resources will be needed at the scene, and evaluate whether any specialized equipment or personnel, such as search and rescue teams, will be required.

Once this assessment is complete, the next step is to communicate the overall assessment to the dispatch center, where the process of acquiring and dispatching the needed resources can be performed. After this, the medical personnel should identify appropriate locations to perform triage; collect casualties; and stage incoming ambulances, personnel, and supplies so as not to impede rapid ingress and egress when necessary or expose responding assets to potential hazards from the event.

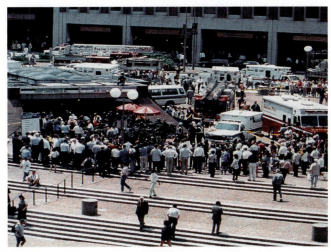

FIGURE 11-6 Incident command system (ICS) allows integration of fire, police, and EMS assets at a disaster scene.

FIGURE 11-7   The Basic Steps in Medical Response to Disasters

Initial response
Notification and activation of EMS
EMS response to the scene
Assess the situation
    Cause
    Number of casualties
    Additional resources
        Medical
        Other
    Communicate the situation and needs
Activation of the medical community
    Notify receiving facilities
Search and rescue
    Triage (treat airway and hemorrhage life-threats)
    Casualty collection
    Treatment
    Transport
    Retriage

In addition to providing for the medical response to the disaster scene, it is essential that the responding EMS agency notify the likely receiving hospitals in the community so that they can activate their disaster plans to prepare to receive casualties. EMS agencies must remember that the field component of the disaster response is the first link in the overall chain of medical care for a disaster patient and that they are responsible for notifying and activating the other components of the healthcare system.

Search and Rescue. At this point, the on-scene process of initiating patient care can begin. Generally, this will start with a search and rescue effort to identify and evacuate casualties from the impacted site to a safer location. The local population near a disaster site as well as survivors themselves, if they are able, are often the immediate search and rescue resource and may have already begun to search for victims.[13] Experience has demonstrated that the local community will respond to a disaster site and begin the process of aiding victims. In addition, many countries and communities have developed formal, specialized search and rescue teams as an integral part of their national and local disaster response plans. Members of these teams receive specialized training in "confined-space environments" and are activated as needed for a particular event. These search and rescue units generally include the following:

- A cadre of medical specialists
- Technical specialists knowledgeable in hazardous materials, structural engineering, heavy equipment operation, and technical search and rescue methods (e.g., listening equipment, remote cameras)
- Trained canines and their handlers

Local construction companies may provide valuable search and rescue assets by providing equipment, tools, and wooden planks that can be used at the disaster site to assist in moving heavy debris.

Triage. As patients are identified and evacuated, they are brought to the triage site, where they can be assessed and a triage category assigned (Figure 11-8). *Triage* is a French word that means "to sort." From a medical perspective, triage means sorting casualties based on the severity of their injuries. This further serves to prioritize the patient's need for medical care and transportation to the hospital.

Triage is one of the most important missions of any disaster medical response. As noted previously, the objective of conventional triage in the nondisaster setting is to do the greatest good for the individual patient. This usually means finding and treating the sickest patient. The objective of mass casualty triage is to do the greatest good for the greatest number of people. Mass casualty triage in the field must be overseen by a trained triage officer. A *triage officer* should have a wide breadth of clinical experience in the assessment and management

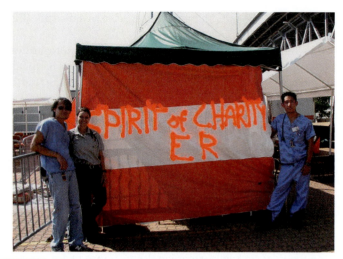

FIGURE 11-8 Triage and initial stabilization at a makeshift medical treatment facility, Hurricane Katrina, Louisiana, 2005.

ment of field injuries because potentially difficult decisions may have to be made about patients who will be deemed critical versus those who will be classified as mortally wounded with little chance of survival. A paramedic with significant field experience usually meets this requirement. A trained physician with experience in the field may also function in this capacity.[4,5]

A number of different methodologies exist for evaluating and assigning the triage category.[11] One common method is to evaluate the anatomic injuries and assign the priority for medical care and transport based on the severity of the injury and the likelihood of need for surgical intervention. Another method involves a rapid physiologic and mental status evaluation. This triage process is referred to as the "START" triage algorithm (**s**imple **t**riage **a**nd **r**apid **t**reatment). This system evaluates the respiratory status, perfusion status, and mental status of the patient in making a prioritization for initial transfer to definitive care facilities[5,6] (see Chapter 3). In addition, other triage systems include MASS (*m*ove, *a*ssess, *s*ort, *s*end) and the Sacco triage method.

In an effort to provide national guidance and bring uniformity to the triage process, the U.S. Centers for Disease Control and Prevention convened a multidisciplinary group of experts to develop a consensus-based triage system, now known as SALT.[11] This triage system involves **s**orting the patients based on their ability to move, **a**ssessing the patient for the need for **l**ife-saving interventions, performing those interventions, and **t**reatment and **t**ransport.

Regardless of the exact triage method used, all of these systems ultimately classify patients into one of (usually) four injury severity categories. Highest priority patients are those who are identified as having critical, but likely survivable, injuries and are usually categorized as *critical* and color-coded *red*. Patients with moderate injuries who can potentially tolerate a short delay in care are categorized as *delayed* patients and color-coded *yellow.* Patients with relatively minor injuries, often referred to as the "walking wounded," are classified as *minimal* victims and color-coded *green.* Patients who have expired on the scene or whose injuries are so severe that death is imminent or is likely are categorized as "dead" or "expectant," respectively, and color-coded *black.* Of note, some triage systems, particularly SALT, specifically separate those patients classified as mortally wounded from those who are dead and color code the expectant as *gray.* All these color codes refer to "disaster tags," which are attached to patients once they have been triaged at disaster scenes. The color code provides an immediate visual reference to their triage category. Some triage systems also use a classification system in which critical, delayed, minimal and the dead or expectant patients are referred to as class I, class II, class III, and class IV, respectively.

It is important that all triage personnel keep in mind that they must avoid the temptation to stop performing triage in favor of treating a critically injured patient that they encounter. As mentioned earlier, the primary principle involved in dealing with an MCI is to do the most good for the most people. During this initial triage phase, medical interventions are limited to those actions that are performed easily and rapidly, and that are not labor intensive. Generally, this means performing only procedures such as manual airway opening and external hemorrhage control. Interventions such as bag-mask ventilation and closed chest compression involve the use of significant personnel and are not performed.

Once patients have been triaged, they are collected together at casualty collection points according to their triage priority. Specifically, all the "red" category or critical patients are grouped, as are the delayed ("yellow") and minimal ("green") patients. Casualty collection sites should be located close enough to the disaster site to easily carry the victim to and offer rapid treatment but far enough away from the impact site to be safe. Important features include the following:

- Proximity to the disaster site
- Safety from hazards and uphill and upwind from contaminated environments
- Protection from climatic conditions (when possible)
- Easy visibility for disaster victims and assigned personnel
- Convenient exit routes for air and land evacuation

As additional medical staff and resources arrive and become available on-scene, medical care and interventions are provided at the casualty collection points according to the triage priority. These are appropriate locations to which physicians responding to the scene may be assigned to further evaluate and treat injured patients.

Finally, as transportation resources become available, patients are then transported for definitive care according,

once again, to their triage priority (Figure 11-9). Critical patients are not held on scene for the provision of further medical care if transport is available. Needed medical interventions should be conducted during transport to the definitive care facility (Figure 11-10).

Because of visible, critical injuries, emergency personnel often have a tendency to move individual patients forward for immediate treatment and transport and to bypass the triage process. This must be avoided so that all victims can be evaluated, the most life-threatening casualties can be treated first, and the best care can be provided for the majority of victims. However, bypassing the triage process is indicated in certain situations. These conditions include (1) risk, as in bad weather; (2) potential impending darkness without the capabilities of lighting resources; (3) the continued risk of injury as a result of natural or intentional events; (4) no triage facility or triage officer immediately available; and (5) any tactical situation in a law enforcement scenario where the victims are

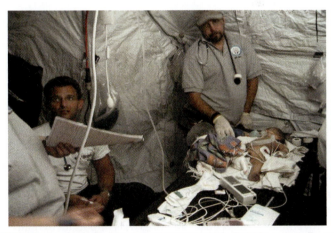

FIGURE 11-9 Definitive medical care, U.S. field hospital, Bam, Iran earthquake, 2005.

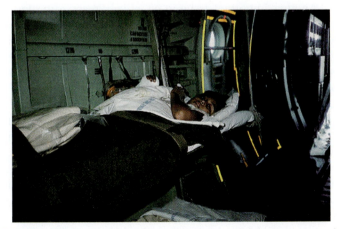

FIGURE 11-10 Interior of a military transport plane converted for medical evacuation with patient litters.

rapidly moved from the impact site to the collection point for transportation.[6,7]

Lastly, triage is not a static process, meaning that once a patient is evaluated and categorized, the patient carries that triage category for the remainder of their care. Instead, it is dynamic and ongoing. As a patient's condition changes, the triage category may change as well. For example, a patient with a major extremity wound and hemorrhage may initially be categorized as an "immediate" patient; however, after pressure is applied to the wound and the bleeding is controlled, the patient may be retriaged as "delayed." Alternatively, a patient initially categorized as "immediate" could deteriorate and subsequently be retriaged as "expectant."

Retriage should occur on the scene while patients are waiting for transport resources. In addition, patients will undergo retriage upon arrival at the receiving destination and again as they are prioritized for surgery.

Treatment

Because the number of casualties will initially exceed the available resources, treatment on the scene is generally limited to manually opening the airway and external hemorrhage control. Only when adequate resources have arrived on scene, or during transport to the hospital, will additional interventions be provided.

Transport

The transport of patients from a mass casualty incident to the receiving hospitals involves a coordinated effort using a variety of transport vehicles. Critically injured or ill patients will be taken to the hospital in ambulances or helicopters (if available and conditions permit). Those incidents that result in huge numbers of casualties, particularly casualties in the *minimal* category, may require the use of nontraditional transport vehicles such as buses and vans. It is important to remember, however, that when such alternate transport mechanisms are used, medical personnel with adequate supplies and equipment must be assigned to accompany the casualties in that vehicle.

Another important issue in effectively responding to an MCI relates to the decision-making process for patient destination once transport is initiated.[12] Recent events have demonstrated that casualties with non–life-threatening injuries will often depart the disaster site using any available means of transportation and make their own way to the hospital.[13] Often this results in large numbers of "walking wounded" arriving at the hospital closest to the disaster site. In fact, approximately 70% to 80% of casualties will get to a hospital without EMS ambulance transport.

Prehospital providers must therefore understand that the hospital closest to a disaster scene may be overwhelmed with casualties even before the arrival of the first transporting ambulance. Before taking a patient to the closest hospital, contact should be made to ascertain the status of the emergency department (ED) and the capability to accept and treat

victims being transported by ambulance. If the closest hospital is overwhelmed, the EMS system should transport patients to more distant facilities, when possible. Although the transport time will be longer, the patient's care will not be complicated by the presence of numerous other casualties. Dispersal of casualties to multiple institutions will ultimately better preserve the ability of all the receiving hospitals to optimize the patient care they provide.

Even if the closest medical facility is not overwhelmed with self-transported patients, it is imperative that prehospital providers themselves not overwhelm the nearest hospital with patients transported by ambulance. Often, the natural desire is to transport a patient to the closest hospital so that the ambulance and its crew can quickly return to the disaster scene to pick up and transport another patient. Transferring the mass casualty incident from the disaster site to the closest hospital will negatively impact the ability of medical facilities to provide the "most good for the most patients." However, in those communities that have limited numbers of hospitals, EMS will have no option other than to transport patients to the nearest hospital.

Medical Assistance Teams

If the disaster is of significant proportion that additional on-scene resources are needed, some hospitals have developed disaster response teams to help augment the EMS field response and provide on-site care, thus allowing prehospital providers to be freed from the task of providing medical care at casualty collection points and instead perform patient transport. If outside resources are needed through the state or federal government, other medical response teams are available in many municipalities (Figure 11-11). As a result of the Metropolitan Medical Response System (MMRS) in the United States, MMRS task forces or strike teams have been created in many cities. These response assets comprise medical personnel from emergency medicine, trauma surgery, surgical subspecialties and nursing. These teams can respond with resources that have been purchased through state and

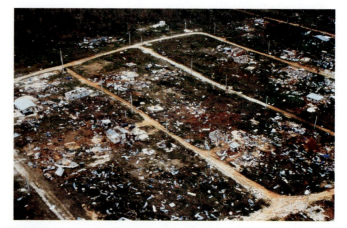

FIGURE 11-11 Aerial view of devastation caused by Supertyphoon Pongsona, Guam, 2002.

federal funds and can be used to augment medical facilities or to staff mobile medical facilities that are established to provide surge capacity and medical care to victims.

On a larger scale, the U.S. government has capabilities through the National Disaster Medical System to mobilize Disaster Medical Assistance Teams (DMATs). These teams are able to provide field care as well as create mobile medical facilities, some of which have the capability to perform surgical interventions and meet the critical care needs of the victims. A request for these teams must come through the appropriate channels via the state emergency management authority and the governor's office through the federal government to the Department of Health and Human Services (DHHS), which houses the National Disaster Medical System's response program.

Threat of Terrorism and Weapons of Mass Destruction

Terrorism may present one of the most challenging MCIs for emergency responders. The spectrum of terrorist threats is limitless, ranging from suicide bombers, conventional explosives, and military weapons to weapons of mass destruction (nuclear, biologic, or chemical WMDs). Terrorist events have the greatest potential of all manmade disasters to generate large numbers of casualties and fatalities.

Terrorists have demonstrated their ingenuity and capacity to not be limited by conventional technology or weaponry. During the terrorist attacks on September 11, 2001, the terrorists used passenger jets full of fuel as "flying bombs," generating massive destruction of life and property.

One of the unique features of a terrorist threat, especially involving WMDs, is that psychogenic casualties usually predominate. Terrorists do not need to kill a large number of people to achieve their goals; they only need to create a climate of fear and panic to overwhelm the medical infrastructure. In the March 1995 sarin attacks in Tokyo, 5000 casualties presented to hospitals. Of these, fewer than 1000 had physical effects from the sarin gas; the remaining presented with psychological stress. The recent anthrax incidents in the United States also dramatically increased the number of individuals presenting to EDs with nonspecific respiratory symptoms that ultimately did not result from actual anthrax infection.

Explosions and bombings continue to be the most frequent cause of mass casualties in terrorism-related disasters. The majority of these bombings consist of relatively small explosives that produce low mortality rates. However, when strategically placed in buildings, pipelines, or moving vehicles, their impact can be much greater (Figure 11-12). The high morbidity and mortality is related not only to the intensity of the blast but also to the subsequent structural damage that leads to collapse of the targeted buildings. A greater threat will be disasters caused by conventional explosives in combination with a chemical, biologic, or radiologic agent,

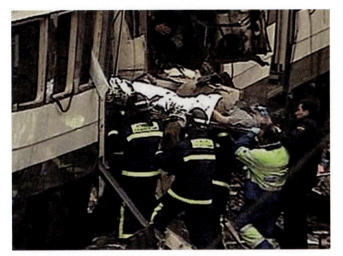

FIGURE 11-12   Madrid terrorist bombing, 2004.

such as a "dirty bomb" that combines a conventional explosive with radioactive material.

WMDs creating "contaminated environments" may prove to be the greatest disaster challenge. Emergency responders will not be able to bring victims into hospitals because of the risk of contaminating medical facilities. Medical responders must be prepared and equipped to perform triage not only to determine the extent of the injuries but also to assess the potential for contamination and need for decontamination and initial stabilization. At the same time, prehospital care providers need to take appropriate steps to protect themselves from potential contamination.

Decontamination

Decontamination is an important consideration for all disasters involving hazardous materials (hazmat) and WMDs (Figure 11-13). Terrorist events, with their larger number of patients, unknown substances, and large numbers of "wor-

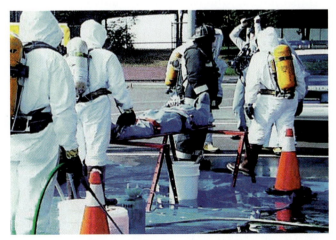

FIGURE 11-13   Decontamination of casualties in the "warm zone" by personnel in level B personal protective equipment (PPE).

ried well," significantly increase the possibility of contaminated or potentially contaminated casualties (see part 2 of the chapter, page 316 for additional information).

Treatment Area

When responding to a disaster involving hazmat and WMDs, it is critical that the triage and treatment areas be at least 300 yards upwind and uphill of the contaminated area.

Psychological Response to Disasters

Psychological trauma and other adverse psychological sequelae are common side effects of events such as natural disasters and unintentional disasters caused by humans.[10] In contrast, one of the objectives of terrorism is to inflict psychological pain, trauma, and disequilibrium.

Characteristics of Disasters That Affect Mental Health

Not all disasters have the same level of psychological impact. Disaster characteristics that seem to have the most significant mental health impact include the following:

- Little or no warning
- Serious threat to personal safety
- Potential unknown health effects
- Uncertain duration of the event
- Human error or malicious intent
- Symbolism related to the terrorist target

Factors Impacting Psychological Response

Everyone who experiences a disaster, whether as a victim or as a responder, is affected by it in some fashion. Fortunately, this does not mean that most individuals will develop a mental health disorder. It does mean, however, that all affected individuals will have some type of psychological or emotional response to the event.

Similarly, there are both individual and collective reactions that interact with each other as individuals and communities recover from these extraordinary events.

Factors affecting individual response to disasters include the following:

- Physical and psychological proximity to the event
- Exposure to gruesome or grotesque situations
- Diminished health status before or because of the disaster
- Magnitude of loss
- Trauma history

Factors impacting collective response to trauma are as follows:

- Degree of community disruption
- Pre-disaster family and community stability
- Community leadership
- Cultural sensitivity of recovery efforts

Psychological Sequelae of Disasters

Post-disaster psychological responses are wide ranging, from mild stress responses to full-blown post-traumatic stress disorder (PTSD), major depression, or acute stress disorder.[8] Although many people may exhibit signs of psychological stress, relatively few (typically 15%–25%) of those most directly impacted will subsequently develop a diagnosable mental disorder.

Interventions

The following interventions can be helpful in managing the psychological sequelae of disasters:

1. Return to normal activities as soon as possible.[8]
2. In persons with no diagnosed mental disorder, it is helpful to provide educational materials that help people understand what they and their families are experiencing.
3. Brief crisis counseling should be provided, followed by referral when treatment is indicated.
4. When a mental disorder is diagnosed, therapeutic interventions can be helpful, including cognitive behavioral therapy and psychiatric medications.

Worker Stress

Disaster workers can also become secondary victims of stress and other psychological sequelae. This can adversely affect their functioning during and after an event. It can also adversely impact their personal well-being as well as their family and work relationships. Supervisory personnel and colleagues should be alert for the development or manifestations of stress and psychological distress in those individuals who were involved in the incident response.

A number of intervention strategies are often used in an effort to help prevent and manage stress after an incident. These include debriefing, defusing, and grief management sessions. Collectively these processes have been referred to as critical incident stress management (CISM). It is important to note that some aspects of CISM, particularly mandatory debriefing sessions, have become controversial, with some researchers questioning the effectiveness of this process. Regardless of the final results of ongoing investigations into the value of specific components of CISM, psychological support, and in some cases treatment, of providers who are having difficulty in dealing with the aftermath of the event is crucial.

Signs of Stress in Workers. Some common signs of stress in workers include physiologic, emotional, cognitive, and behavioral elements.

Physiologic Signs
- Fatigue, even after rest
- Nausea
- Fine motor tremors

- Tics
- Paresthesias
- Dizziness
- Gastrointestinal upset
- Heart palpitations
- Choking or smothering sensations

Emotional Signs
- Anxiety
- Irritability
- Feeling overwhelmed
- Unrealistic anticipation of harm to self or others

Cognitive Signs
- Memory loss
- Decision-making difficulties
- Anomia (inability to name common objects or familiar people)
- Concentration problems or distractibility
- Reduced attention span
- Calculation difficulties

Behavioral Signs
- Insomnia
- Hypervigilance
- Crying easily
- Inappropriate humor
- Ritualistic behavior

Managing Worker Stress On-Site

The following on-site interventions can assist in reducing worker stress:

- Limited exposure to traumatic stimuli
- Reasonable hours
- Adequate rest and sleep (Figure 11-14)
- Reasonable diet
- Regular exercise program
- Private time

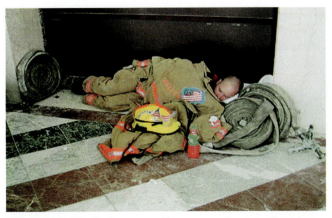

FIGURE 11-14 Fatigue contributes greatly to worker stress.

- Talking to somebody who understands
- Monitoring signs of stress
- Identifiable endpoint for involvement

Disaster Education and Training

The development and implementation of a formal educational and training program will improve the prehospital care provider's ability to respond efficiently to an MCI. The prehospital provider may well fulfill a variety of roles in disaster and mass casualty management, including mitigation and preparedness, search and rescue, triage, acute medical care, transport, and post-event recovery. Preparedness with regard to education and learning can be accomplished in various structured as well as unstructured learning environments. Each has its individual advantages and disadvantages, as measured by educational impact and comparative cost. For optimal learning from educational exercises, it is imperative that interdisciplinary training events be conducted often to include all the appropriate agencies and participants in a disaster response.

Independent learning is the foundation of disaster preparedness. A multitude of resources are available through printed literature as well as via the internet. The Centers for Disease Control and Prevention (CDC), public health agencies, Federal Emergency Management Agency (FEMA), and the military all have internet-based learning opportunities and resources that are available to individuals. Courses can be completed on an independent basis on a time-flexible schedule. The limitation of this modality of learning is that it does not allow for an interactive learning experience.

Group training is directed at specific response teams with regard to disaster response. Training programs are broadly available and include understanding command structure and WMD preparedness. Numerous professional and paraprofessional organizations have developed training programs and modules specific to their scope of professional practice, including public health, emergency medicine, critical care, and surgical and medical specialties, as well as all levels of prehospital care providers.

Simulations provide a training opportunity that brings together many individuals from varied and different backgrounds who are essential to the implementation of a disaster response. As mentioned earlier, these exercises come in two specific forms: a tabletop exercise and a fully active, field training exercise. *Tabletop exercises* are cost-effective and highly useful methods to test and evaluate a disaster response. A starting point with focused incident goals and accomplishments and order for completion of the exercise are usually established in advance. Tabletop exercises can allow for real-time communications and interaction between multidisciplinary agencies. These activities require direction in the form of a facilitator guiding the participants through the objective and critical evaluation of the results at the conclusion.

Field exercises are the most realistic training events, involving the actual execution and performance of the community disaster response plan. The field exercise allows for a real-time assessment of the physical capacity to meet the objectives as defined in writing. Ideally, the exercises will involve moving victims from the point of impact and injury through the EMS response system and into definitive care at medical facilities. These events, however, are labor intensive, long, and have significant cost.

Common Pitfalls of Disaster Response

Numerous studies performed after significant MCIs have identified several consistent shortcomings in the medical response to these events. Identification of these deficiencies has resulted from subsequent evaluations of the response to these incidents as well as from communities that have performed risk, vulnerability, and needs assessments mandated by the U.S. government in order to receive funding resources to enhance the disaster response infrastructure.

Preparedness

As responders in a community, prehospital care providers prepare for the devastation that can occur in a mass casualty event and plan for such events in a variety of ways. Although one method of preparing is the tabletop drill, it does not truly test the ability of the provider to perform the necessary duties as well as the ability of the EMS agency to bring resources and assets to the site in a timely and efficient manner. Realistic functional disaster drills during which victims are triaged, evaluated, "treated," and transported through the medical response system into a hospital facility in a realistic fashion better test the emergency medical response that will be required. The ability to provide for "surge capacity" and for supplying the large number of staff, ambulances, and other equipment needed for victims must be appropriately addressed by the medical response community.

Unfortunately, few agencies have actually tested a surge-capacity response in real time and instead have relied on tabletop drills as a measure of their ability to respond. Only through community-wide drills that involve multiple EMS agencies and ambulance services can the true level of preparedness to respond to an MCI as a community be assessed.

Communications

Many events have demonstrated that the lack of a unified communication system significantly hinders the ability to mount a coordinated response to an MCI. Individual communication systems are effective, but relying on a single system for communication is doomed to failure. The use of cellular phones became impossible when the central communication center located in the World Trade Center was no longer in existence. Also, the failure of the police, fire, and EMS agencies to be able to communicate with each other because of different radio technologies or frequencies is a serious defi-

ciency that significantly reduces the ability to respond to MCIs effectively. Redundancy in the system is of paramount importance, regardless of the chosen source for primary communications. Landlines, hardwired phone systems, cellular phone systems, satellite phone systems, VHF radios, and 800- to 900-MHz frequency systems all have some degree of vulnerability. The following two principles are essential:

1. A unified communication system to which all pertinent responders in the community have access.
2. System redundancy such that if one modality of communication fails or is disabled, another source can be used efficiently as an appropriate backup.
3. Another common problem is the use of "codes" as a form of communication short-hand. Unfortunately, there is no single, agreed-upon set of codes for all agencies to use; thus, a response agency may find itself at a scene with other agencies, all of whom are using codes that have the same terminology but different meanings. It is for this reason that ICS and the National Incident Management System recommend the use of plain English during an incident to avoid any confusion in meaning.

Scene Security

Scene security has become an ever-increasing problem in MCIs. Scene security is important for the following reasons:

1. To protect the response teams from a second strike resulting in further casualties
2. To provide for the ingress and egress of rescue workers and victims unencumbered by onlookers to the disaster
3. To protect and assist in securing the scene and physical evidence

Scene security becomes a significant challenge during a disaster event because, by definition, all resources are being stretched to the maximum of their capabilities and limits. Coordination with local law enforcement leaders is essential for the prehospital and medical community to ensure that security will be available.

Self-Dispatched Assistance

In many MCIs, public safety and EMS agencies (as well as medical responders of all other types) from adjacent and even distant communities have responded to the scene without any formal request for assistance from the impacted jurisdiction.[13] These self-dispatched responders, although well intentioned, often serve only to further complicate and confuse an already chaotic situation. Interagency communications issues are often made more difficult by noncompatible radio systems. Coordinated rescue efforts are often impossible because of the lack of participation in the incident command structure. Ideally, public safety and EMS agencies should respond to a disaster site only if they have been specifically requested to do so by the responsible jurisdiction and incident commander.[14] In addition, it is extremely helpful if access to the scene is controlled and a staging area is set up as soon as possible to which all responding units and volunteers can be directed to better incorporate them into the incident response.

Supply and Equipment Resources

Most municipalities have plans for the routine utilization of supplies and have purchased supplies based on this demand. Events of large magnitude will rapidly exhaust these resources. Having a seamless plan for the reconstitution of supplies is essential for the ongoing mission of treating victims. Supplies must be available in a timely fashion, and appropriate mechanisms must be in place for distribution, which cannot include the care providers in the field, who will already be utilized to their fullest availabilities. In those communities that have been designated to receive Metropolitan Medical Response System (MMRS) funds, community stockpiles have been or are being purchased in preparation for such events.

Failure To Notify Hospitals

In the confusion of responding to and assessing a mass casualty incident as well as performing the numerous tasks that must be accomplished in initiating the medical response to such an event, it is often easy for EMS providers to overlook the need to contact hospitals and have them activate their internal disaster plans. Numerous actual events have demonstrated that unless hospital notification and activation are integral parts of the EMS agency's MCI plan, hospitals may be left on their own to discover that an incident has occurred, either when patients self-transport and report the event or when the first ambulance arrives to an unprepared facility. It is essential that EMS agencies include hospital notification as part of their plan so that a coordinated seamless transition from field care to hospital care can occur.

In addition, ongoing communication from the field (or emergency operations center) to the hospital and from the hospital to the field are important for monitoring the status of the event and the patient load at hospitals.

Media

The media are often seen as a detriment to the physical and operational process of a disaster response. However, communities are encouraged to partner with the media because these outlets can be an asset during a disaster response. The media can provide for the dissemination of appropriate and accurate information to the general population, giving them directions as to how to respond to maintain personal safety and where to report to obtain information or to reunite with family members, as well as communicating other needed information. It is inevitable that the media will broadcast information to the public, and as responders, prehospital care providers have the responsibility to partner with the media to ensure that the information provided is accurate as well as helpful to the response process.

SUMMARY

- Disasters result from natural climactic or geologic events; however, they may also result from intentional or unintentional acts of man.
- Although disasters may be unpredictable, adequate preparation can turn an unthinkable event into a manageable situation.
- Appropriate disaster response involves much more than the medical component.
- Implementation of the Incident Command System allows multiple agencies to collaborate in the disaster response.

- Despite the fact that disasters occur in varying sizes and result from many different causes, common pitfalls have been identified that hinder management of such an event.
- Disaster response may take a heavy psychological toll on those involved, both victims and rescuers.
- The best outcomes in response to MCIs result from the creation of a well-devised disaster plan that has been rehearsed, tested, and critiqued to identify and improve problem areas.

SCENARIO 1 SOLUTION

After the blast event, precautionary measures are taken to evaluate the risk potential for collapse of the damaged structure as well as an ongoing gas leak and the potential for a second explosion. Appropriate personal protective equipment and Standard Precautions are used when treating patients.

Crowd control is of the utmost importance after such an event to prevent well-meaning bystanders from entering the building to search for victims and help with rescue. The ICS should be used to manage the resources required to deal with this event. A staging area for responding units should be designated. Patients are triaged using whatever triage system the EMS provider has in place. Casualty collection points are set up and located in strategic areas to allow for rapid loading and evacuation of victims.

In addition to patient care needs, remember that rescue workers will have hydration, nutrition, and sanitary needs throughout the rescue effort. ■

Weapons of Mass Destruction

SCENARIO 2

You are dispatched to the scene of a reported explosion at an outdoor fair. The number of victims is unknown. Other public safety agencies have been dispatched to the location.

On arrival at the location, you note that you are the first EMS responder on scene. No incident command has yet been established. Dozens of people are running about the scene. Many are screaming for you to assist victims who are obviously bleeding. Others patients are lying on the ground and at least one of the victims appears to be having a seizure.

What will you do first?

What are your priorities as you determine your course of action?

How will you care for so many people?

Preparing to manage a WMD event challenges EMS systems every day. Recent history has demonstrated that these events can occur at any time and in any location. The 1993 World Trade Center bombing resulted in only 6 deaths, but yielded 548 casualties, with more than 1000 victims being assisted by EMS. Responders became casualties as well, with 105 firefighters reporting injuries. The 1995 explosion at the Murrah Federal Building in Oklahoma City resulted in 168 deaths, with 700 injuries. One third of the patients brought to one Oklahoma City hospital came by EMS, and they were the sickest, with 64% requiring admission to the hospital, whereas only 6% of those who self-referred to the emergency department needed admission. The 2001 World Trade Center attacks resulted in more than 1100 injured survivors, with almost a third of those patients arriving at the hospital by EMS. Rescue workers accounted for 29% of the injured victims.

Although conventional high explosives are the most commonly used and most likely form of WMD event, EMS systems have also been challenged by chemical and biohazard events. The 1994 sarin gas attack in Matsumoto, Japan, killed 7, and injured more than 300. The more widely known 1995 sarin gas attack in the Tokyo subway system killed 12, but more than 5000 victims sought medical attention. The Tokyo Fire Department sent 1364 firefighters to the 16 affected subway sites; 135 responders (10%) were affected by direct or indirect exposure to the nerve agent.

No life-threatening bioterrorism assault in the United States has yielded a large number of casualties, but this does not mean that EMS systems have not been challenged to prepare for bioterrorism threats. During 1998 and 1999, almost 6000 persons across the United States were affected by a series of anthrax-related hoaxes in more than 200 incidents. The anthrax letters delivered in the fall of 2001 resulted in only 22 cases of clinical anthrax but generated countless calls for EMS to respond to suspicious packages and powders. Also, although not a bioterrorist event, a naturally occurring biohazard, severe acute respiratory syndrome (SARS), seriously challenged the Toronto EMS system. During the epidemic, 526 of their paramedics had to be quarantined, the vast majority secondary to potential unprotected exposure to the virus, seriously straining that EMS system's ability to mitigate the crisis.

The threat that EMS may one day have to respond to a radiologic WMD event grows, with increasing speculation that terrorists may detonate a radiologic dispersal device ("dirty bomb") that will generate injuries and panic about radioactive contamination.

General Considerations

Scene Assessment and Incident Command System

The ability of the prehospital care provider to assess the scene properly and recognize the use of a WMD will be crucial to ensuring the provider's safety and that of other responders and will ensure the best delivery of service to the patient. WMD events pose significant threats to responding emergency services. In the case of a high-explosives detonation, there may be fire, spilled hazardous materials, power line hazards, and risk of falling debris or subsidence. A rescue worker was killed by falling debris in response to the Oklahoma City bombing,[15] and many more were killed in the 2001 World Trade Center attack. Chemical attacks potentially expose the emergency responder to the offending agent not only from its primary source, the weapon, but also from con-

tamination of victims' skin, clothing, and personal belongings. Biohazards, depending on the form of their delivery, pose a risk of illness from the offending agent (e.g., aerosolized anthrax spores) or from transmission of a communicable disease (e.g., plague or smallpox). A further risk to emergency responders and patients alike is the possibility of a secondary device, for example, a second bomb placed at the scene of the incident, set to explode after arrival of emergency responders, with the intention of increasing not only injury, but also confusion and panic.

Because many of the WMDs pose an inhalation risk, particularly the chemical and biologic agents, responding units from all involved agencies must take care to approach the scene from an upwind direction to minimize the potential for inadvertent exposure. In addition, any incident that involves the release of liquid chemical mandates that responders stage uphill from the spill.

Access to and egress from the potentially contaminated site must be controlled. Concerned bystanders and volunteers must not be allowed to enter the scene because they may contribute to the casualty count if they expose themselves to the agent. Victims of the incident must also be contained as they seek to evacuate the scene, because self-transport may only serve to further disseminate a dangerous chemical or substance to unsuspecting contacts. Just as would occur at a hazardous materials incident, scene control zones (hot, warm, cold) should be established with controlled access points and transit corridors to prevent spread of the contaminants, inadvertent exposure, and safe areas for patient evaluation and treatment (Figure 11-15). The zones are further described in the following section on Personal Protective Equipment.

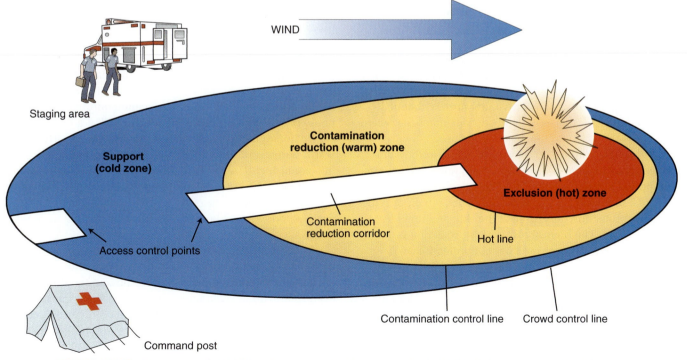

WIND

Staging area

Support (cold zone)

Contamination reduction (warm) zone

Exclusion (hot) zone

Access control points

Contamination reduction corridor

Hot line

Command post

Contamination control line   Crowd control line

FIGURE 11-15 The scene of a WMD or hazmat incident is generally divided into hot, warm, and cold zones. (Modified from Chapleau W: *Emergency first responder,* St Louis, 2004, Mosby.)

All of these factors must be taken into consideration when evaluating a scene and their significance comprehended before taking action. In addition, a critical evaluation, from a safe distance, of how patients are presenting must be included as part of the scene assessment, with particular attention to the clues suggesting a possible chemical or biologic agent release. Prehospital providers also need to communicate their observations through the chain of command so that proper steps can be taken to mount an appropriate response, increasing the safety of the responders and the delivery of care to patients. The incident command system (ICS) defines the chain of command through which this communication takes place.

ICS offers a management structure that coordinates all available resources to ensure an effective response. All incidents, regardless of size or complexity, will have a designated incident commander, who may be the first responding prehospital provider until relieved by some other competent authority. It is essential that prehospital providers be familiar with and have the opportunity to practice implementation of the ICS.

Personal Protective Equipment

When responding to WMD events, the wearing of proper personal protective equipment needs to be considered. PPE requirements may range from the standard daily uniform to a fully encapsulated suit with self-contained breathing apparatus (SCBA), depending on the specific agent involved and the specific role assigned to the responder. PPE is designed to protect the prehospital provider from exposure to offending agents by providing defined levels of protection of the respiratory tract, skin, and other mucous membranes. Civilian PPE has generally been described in terms of the following levels (Figure 11-16):

- *Level A.* This level offers the highest respiratory and skin protection. The respiratory tract is protected by a SCBA or supplied air respirator (SAR) delivering air to the prehospital provider with positive pressure. A chemical-resistant barrier that completely encapsulates the wearer protects the skin and mucous membranes.
- *Level B.* The respiratory tract is protected in the same manner as in level A protection, with positive-pressure–supplied air. Nonencapsulated chemical-resistant garments, including suit, gloves, and boots, which provide splash protection only, protect the skin and mucous membranes. The highest respiratory protection is afforded, with a lower level of skin protection.
- *Level C.* The respiratory tract is protected by an air-purifying respirator (APR). This may be a powered air-purifying respirator (PAPR), which draws ambient air through a filter canister and delivers it under positive pressure to a facemask or hood, or a non-powered APR, which relies on the wearer to draw ambient air through a filter canister by breathing through a properly fitted mask. The skin protection is the same as for level B.
- *Level D.* This represents standard work clothes (i.e., uniform for prehospital care provider) and may also include a gown, gloves, and surgical mask. This level provides minimal respiratory protection and minimal skin protection.

PPE is selected based on the known (or suspected) hazards of the environment and proximity to the threat. Proximity to the threat has often been described in terms of the following zones:

- The *hot zone* is the area where there is immediate threat to health and life. This includes an environment contaminated with a hazardous gas, vapor, aerosol, liquid, or powder. PPE adequate to protect the prehospital care provider is determined based on potential routes of exposure to the substance and the likely agent. Level A protection is most often used in the hot zone.
- The *warm zone* is characterized as an area where the concentration of the offending agent is limited. In the case of a WMD scene, this is the area to which victims are brought from the hot zone and where decontamination is taking place. The prehospital care provider is still at risk for hazmat exposure in this area because the agent is carried from the hot zone on victims, responders, and equipment. PPE is recommended based on potential routes of exposure to the substance.
- The *cold zone* is the area outside the hot and warm zones that is not contaminated, where there is no risk of hazmat exposure, and thus no specific level of PPE is required beyond standard Universal Precautions.

It is important to note that it is often difficult to define these hazard zones and that they are often dynamic and not static. Factors that contribute to the dynamics of the zones include the activity of the victims and responders and ambient conditions. Unless completely incapacitated, contaminated victims might walk toward prehospital care providers in the "cold zone" or leave the scene completely, either in panic or with the intention of seeking aid at a nearby medical treatment facility or their personal physician. By design, warm zones and cold zones are designated upwind of the hot zone, but if wind direction changes, prehospital care providers would be at risk of hazmat exposure if unable to don personal PPE or to retreat. These contingencies must be anticipated when planning for or responding to a WMD event.

It might be concluded that the best protective posture for a prehospital care provider is always to respond in the highest level of protection, level A, regardless of the threat. However, this is not a reasonable response. Level A protection is cumbersome, often making manual tasks difficult to perform. Significant training and experience are required when using an SCBA. Level A protection puts the wearer at risk for heat stress and physical exhaustion. It can make communication between responders and victims difficult. Appropriate PPE

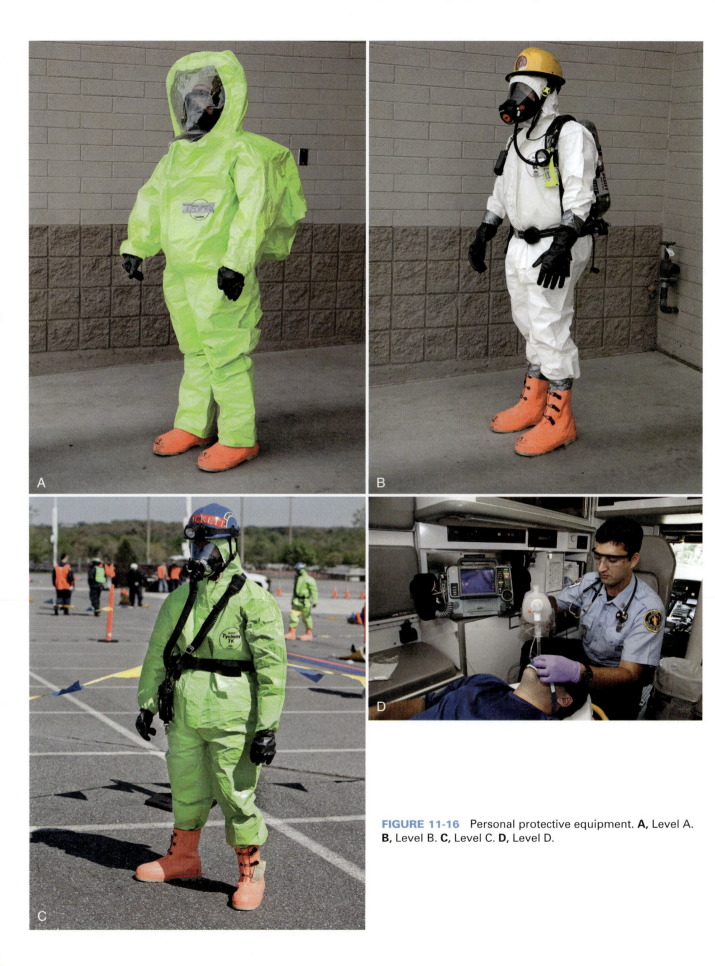

FIGURE 11-16 Personal protective equipment. **A,** Level A. **B,** Level B. **C,** Level C. **D,** Level D.

must be selected based on the threat and the operational responsibilities of the prehospital care provider.

Patient Triage

Prehospital care providers will potentially face a large and overwhelming number of victims who will require evaluation and treatment after a WMD event. Every EMS system should identify and rehearse a mechanism for rapidly triaging victims. The objective of patient triage in a WMD incident is to do the greatest good for the greatest number of victims.

Whatever patient triage system is utilized, it must be employed in routine EMS operations to promote familiarity and to ensure recognition among emergency service providers at all levels of care, including the medical treatment facility.

Principles of Decontamination

Patients and prehospital care providers alike may require decontamination after exposure to adherent solids or liquids that may pose a risk to the patient or other health care personnel. These individuals should have decontamination procedures performed in the field in a designated decontamination area. Decontamination areas are typically upwind and uphill of the affected area when conditions allow. Known exposure to only vapor or gases does not require decontamination to prevent secondary contamination, although the victim's clothing should be removed.

Decontamination is a two-step process that first involves removal of all clothing, jewelry, and shoes, which are bagged and tagged for later identification. The simple act of removing clothing achieves removal of 70% to 90% of contamination. Any solid contaminant should be carefully brushed away from the patient, and any liquid contamination should be blotted off. The second step involves washing the skin surfaces with water or water and a mild detergent to ensure removal of all substances from the patient's skin. Avoid using harsh detergents or bleach solutions on skin as well as vigorous scrubbing. Chemically or physically aggravating the skin may contribute to increased absorption of the offending agent. When washing, skin folds, axillae, groin, buttocks, and feet must receive special attention because contaminants can collect in these areas and may be overlooked by patients in their cleansing efforts.

Decontamination should be performed in a systematic manner to avoid missing areas of contaminated skin. For the eyes, contact lenses should be removed and mucous membranes irrigated with copious amounts of water or saline, especially if the patient is symptomatic. Ambulatory patients should be able to perform their own decontamination under instruction from prehospital care providers. Nonambulatory patients will require the assistance of individuals properly outfitted with PPE to decontaminate litter patients. Expeditious decontamination may be warranted in the effort to decrease exposure time to various life-threatening substances. All prehospital care providers need to be familiar with a hasty

decontamination procedure that may be executed even before arrival of the formal hazmat/decontamination team, to minimize exposure time for both patients and responders.

Issues to consider include (1) offering privacy for males and females required to disrobe, (2) having warm water available for irrigation and showering, (3) providing a suitable substitute for clothing at the completion of decontamination, (4) assuring victims that their personal belongings will be secure until a final disposition is made regarding their return or necessary disposal, and (5) collection of effluent, if practical.

Specific Threats

Explosions and Explosives

Understanding injury from explosives is essential for all providers of emergency care in both civilian and military settings. A study of the 36,110 U.S. bombing incidents reported by the Bureau of Alcohol, Tobacco, and Firearms (ATF) between 1983 and 2002 concluded, "The US experience reveals that materials used for bombings are readily available [and] healthcare providers... need to be prepared."[46]

Explosions occur in homes (primarily due to gas leaks or fires) and are an occupational hazard of many industries, including mining and those involved in demolition, chemical manufacture, or handling fuel or dust-producing substances such as grain. Industrial explosions result from chemical spills, fires, faulty equipment maintenance, or electrical/machinery malfunctions and may produce toxic fumes, building collapse, secondary explosions, falling debris, and large numbers of casualties. Another common cause of explosion is the rupture of a pressurized containment vessel, such as a boiler, when the internal pressure exceeds the capability of the container to withstand the elevated pressure.

As a whole, however, unintentional explosions are responsible for relatively few injuries and deaths (e.g., 150 in the United States in 2004[47]) compared with the large numbers of injuries and deaths produced by explosives used by terrorists and military adversaries.

Terrorists worldwide are increasingly using bombs, especially improvised explosive devices (IEDs), against civilian targets. This is because these devices are inexpensive, made from easily obtained materials, and result in the devastating havoc that focuses international exposure on their cause. An emergency provider is thousands of times more likely to encounter injury from conventional explosives than from a chemical, biological, or nuclear attack. Because both civilian and military responders may be called upon during a bomb attack on civilian populations, all healthcare providers need to be familiar with their roles during these increasingly frequent occurrences.

Review of the U.S. State Department's historical data on terrorist incidents worldwide between 1961 and 2003 reveals a significant increase beginning in 1996 and an exponential increase after the attacks of September 11, 2001.[48] In past decades, there has been a shift from bomb attacks occurring largely in certain "trouble spots," such as Northern Ireland

(1970s) or Paris (1980s), to incidents occurring in all regions of the world, from Atlanta to Jerusalem to Nairobi. In recent years, however, a primary trouble spot has been Iraq, where 60% of the fatalities (a total of 13,606) caused by terrorist attacks occurred in 2007.[49]

At present, although the United States is not typically exposed to as many bomb attacks as other countries, bomb attacks reported in 2007 totaled 445 (more than one per day) and other explosive-related incidents occurred, including theft/recovery of explosives, accidental explosions, and so on (Figure 11-17).[46]

Worldwide, a total of 14,499 terrorist attacks were reported in 2007, which resulted in 44,310 injuries and 22,685 deaths, a 20% to 30% increase over 2006.[46,52] A majority (approximately 70%) were civilians.[46] Continuing the trend from the previous year of "the transition from expeditionary to guerilla terrorism,"[46] most attacks in 2007 were carried out by terrorists using bombs and small arms. This large increase is in part attributed to the increase in suicide bomb attacks.[52] Also in 2007, terrorists continued to coordinate secondary attacks to target first responders and intensified their enhancement of IEDs with chlorine gas to create clouds of toxic fumes.[52] More

recently, however, the number of terror attacks and their associated injuries and deaths declined, by 18%, 30%, and 23%, respectively (Figure 11-18).[49]

Categories of Explosives

Clinicians need to consider the type of explosive device and its location when evaluating casualties of terrorist blast incidents.[16] Explosives fall into one of two categories based on the velocity of detonation: low explosives and high explosives.

High explosives react almost instantaneously. Because they are designed to detonate and release their energy very quickly, HEs are capable of producing a shock wave, or *overpressure phenomenon,* which can result in primary blast injury. The initial explosion creates an instantaneous rise in pressure, creating a shock wave that travels outward at supersonic speed (1400–9000 meters per second [m/sec]).[28] The *shock wave* is the leading front and an integral component of the *blast wave,* which is created upon the rapid release of enormous amounts of energy, with subsequent propulsion of fragments, generation of environmental debris, and often intense thermal radiation.

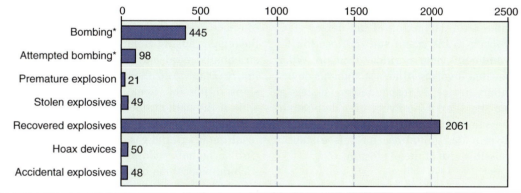

FIGURE 11-17   Explosion-related incidents, United States, 2007.

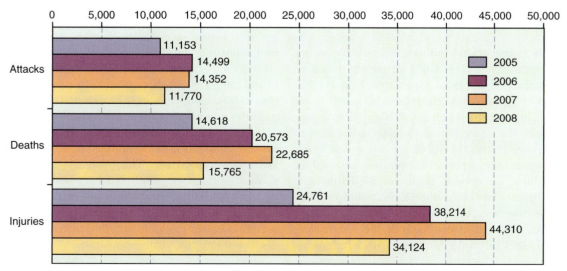

FIGURE 11-18   Terrorist attacks worldwide, with associated injuries and deaths: 2005–2008.

Common examples of high explosives are 2,4,6-trinitrotoluene (TNT), nitroglycerin, dynamite, ammonium nitrate/fuel oil, and the more recent polymer-bonded explosives that have 1.5 times the power of TNT, such as Gelignite and the ubiquitous plastic explosive, Semtex. High explosives have a sharp, shattering effect *(brisance)* that can pulverize bone and soft tissue, create blast overpressure injuries *(barotrauma)*, and propel debris at ballistic speeds *(fragmentation)*. It is also important to note that a high explosive may result in a low order explosion, particularly if the explosive has deteriorated as a result of age (Semtex) or in some cases become wet (dynamite). The reverse, however, is not true—a low explosive cannot produce a high-order explosion.

Low explosives (e.g., gunpowder), when activated, change relatively slowly from a solid to a gaseous state (in an action more characteristic of burning than of detonation), generally creating a blast wave that moves less than 2000 m/sec. Examples of LE include pipe bombs, gunpowder, and pure-petroleum–based bombs such as Molotov cocktails.[19] Explosions resulting from container rupture and ignition of volatile compounds fall into this category as well. Because they release their energy much more slowly, LE are not capable of producing this overpressure.

The type and amount of explosive will determine the size of the blast associated with detonation of the device. This fact makes the approach to the scene and the location for staging responders and equipment a critical decision. When responding to a scene that involves either a suspicious device or a potential secondary device, all responders must stage at a safe distance from the site in the event of a detonation. (refer to Scene Assessment in Chapter 3 for more information). Figure 11-19 provides guidelines for safe distances depending on the possible size of the explosion.

Mechanisms of Injury

Traumatic injury after explosions has generally been divided into three categories: primary, secondary, and tertiary blast injury.[20] In addition to the injuries that result directly from the blast, additional categories of injuries classified as quaternary and quinary have been described and result from complications or toxic effects that are related to the explosive or contaminants. Although these are described separately, they may occur in combination in victims of explosions. Figure 11-20 shows the effects of explosions on the human body.

Primary blast injury (PBI) results from high-order explosive detonation and the interaction of the blast over-pressure wave with the body or tissue to produce stress and shear waves. *Stress waves* are supersonic pressure waves that (1) create high local forces with small, rapid distortions; (2) produce microvascular injury; and (3) are reinforced and reflected at tissue interfaces, thereby enhancing injury potential, especially in gas-filled organs such as the lungs, ears, and intestines. This is not to be confused with wind generated by a blast; a *shock or blast wave* is significantly increased atmospheric pressure produced by the almost instantaneous

detonation of HE. Overpressures from these detonations can exceed 4 million pounds per square inch (psi), compared with 14.7 psi ambient pressure. The shock wave or pressure wave then propagates from the point of origin, gradually dissipating as the distance from the point of combustion increases. Depending on the proximity of the victim to the blast, as well as shielding or augmentation of the wave secondary to detonations in a closed space, a victim may suffer PBI.

Injuries from the stress waves are caused by (1) pressure differentials across delicate structures such as the alveoli, (2) rapid compression of and subsequent re-expansion of gas-filled structures, and (3) reflection of the *tension wave* (a component of the compressive stress wave) at the tissue–gas interface. *Shear waves* are waves with a lower velocity and longer duration that cause asynchronous movement of tissues. The degree of damage depends on the extent to which the asynchronous motions overcome inherent tissue elasticity, resulting in tearing of tissue and possible disruption of attachments. However, muscle, bone, and solid-organ injury are much more likely to result from the tertiary and quaternary effects of the blast than from the blast wave alone.[44,45]

PBI occurs in gas-filled organs such as the lung, bowel, and middle ear. The injury to the tissue occurs at the gas–fluid interface, presumably from a rapid compression of the gas in the organ, causing violent collapse of that organ, followed by an equally rapid and violent expansion, resulting in tissue injury. Damage to the lung manifests as pulmonary contusions, or possibly hemopneumothoraces, resulting in hypoxemia if the patient does not immediately succumb from the injuries (Figure 11-21). Alveoli can also become disrupted, resulting in arterial gas emboli, which may cause cerebral or cardiac embolic complications. Damage to the bowel may include petecchiae or hematomas of the bowel wall or even perforation of the bowel. Tympanic membrane rupture or disruption of the middle ear ossicles also may occur.

Evidence of PBI to the lung is more often found in patients who die minutes after the explosion from associated injuries; however, pulmonary PBI has been noted more frequently among surviving victims of confined-space explosions.[32–34] It has also been associated with other severe injuries and is indicative of increased mortality in survivors. After an open-air explosion in Beirut, only 0.6% of survivors had evidence of PBI, and 11% of those died.[21] In a confined-space explosion in Jerusalem, 38% of survivors had evidence of PBI, with a similar mortality rate of approximately 9%.[22] Similarly, two of the three bombs that were detonated in the London subway system exploded in wide tunnels, resulting in six and seven fatalities, respectively. The third device detonated in the subway system was exploded in a narrow tunnel, causing 26 fatalities. This difference in mortality between open- and closed-space bombing results from the reflection of the blast wave back onto the victims rather than the blast wave being dispersed into the surrounding area.

Secondary blast injury is caused by flying debris and bomb fragments. Fragment (fragmentation) injury, or second-

Improvised Explosive Device (IED) Safe Standoff Distance Cheat Sheet

	Threat Description	Explosives Mass[1] (TNT equivalent)	Building Evacuation Distance[2]	Outdoor Evacuation Distance[3]
High Explosives (TNT Equivalent)	Pipe Bomb	5 lbs 2.3 kg	70 ft 21 m	850 ft 259 m
	Suicide Belt	10 lbs 4.5 kg	90 ft 27 m	1,080 ft 330 m
	Suicide Vest	20 lbs 9 kg	110 ft 34 m	1,360 ft 415 m
	Briefcase/Suitcase Bomb	50 lbs 23 kg	150 ft 46 m	1,850 ft 564 m
	Compact Sedan	500 lbs 227 kg	320 ft 98 m	1,500 ft 457 m
	Sedan	1,000 lbs 454 kg	400 ft 122 m	1,750 ft 534 m
	Passenger/Cargo Van	4,000 lbs 1,814 kg	640 ft 195 m	2,750 ft 838 m
	Small Moving Van/ Delivery Truck	10,000 lbs 4,536 kg	860 ft 263 m	3,750 ft 1,143 m
	Moving Van/Water Truck	30,000 lbs 13,608 kg	1,240 ft 375 m	6,500 ft 1,982 m
	Semitrailer	60,000 lbs 27,216 kg	1,570 ft 475 m	7,000 ft 2,134 m

	Threat Description	LPG Mass/Volume[1]	Fireball Diameter[4]	Safe Distance[5]
Liquefied Petroleum Gas (LPG - Butane or Propane)	Small LPG Tank	20 lbs/5 gal 9 kg/19 l	40 ft 12 m	160 ft 48 m
	Large LPG Tank	100 lbs/25 gal 45 kg/95 l	69 ft 21 m	276 ft 84 m
	Commercial/Residential LPG Tank	2,000 lbs/500 gal 907 kg/1,893 l	184 ft 56 m	736 ft 224 m
	Small LPG Truck	8,000 lbs/2,000 gal 3,630 kg/7,570 l	292 ft 89 m	1,168 ft 356 m
	Semitanker LPG	40,000 lbs/10,000 gal 18,144 kg/37,850 l	499 ft 152 m	1,996 ft 608 m

UNCLASSIFIED

FIGURE 11-19 Explosives safe distance stand-off chart.
(Courtesy National Ground Intelligence Center, United States Army—unclassified.)

[1] Based on the maximum amount of material that could reasonably fit into a container or vehicle. Variations possible.
[2] Governed by the ability of an unreinforced building to withstand severe damage or collapse.
[3] Governed by the greater of fragment throw distance or glass breakage/falling glass hazard distance. These distances can be reduced for personnel wearing ballistic protection. Note that the pipe bomb, suicide belt/vest, and briefcase/suitcase bomb are assumed to have a fragmentation characteristic that requires greater standoff distances than an equal amount of explosives in a vehicle.
[4] Assuming efficient mixing of the flammable gas with ambient air.
[5] Determined by U.S. firefighting practices wherein safe distances are approximately 4 times the flame height. Note that an LPG tank filled with high explosives would require a significantly greater standoff distance than if it were filled with LPG.

FIGURE 11-20   Blast Injury Categories

Effects	Impact	Mechanism of injury	Typical Injuries
Primary	Direct blast effects (over- and under-pressurization)	■ Produced by contact of blast shockwave with body ■ Stress and shear waves occur in tissues ■ Waves reinforced/reflected at tissue density interfaces ■ Gas-filled organs (lungs, ears, etc.) at particular risk	Tympanic membrane rupture Blast lung Eye injuries Concussion

Secondary	Projectiles propelled by explosion	■ Ballistic wounds produced by:
		  Primary fragments (pieces of exploding weapon)
		  Secondary fragments (environmental fragments, e.g., glass)
			Penetrating injuries
			Traumatic amputations
			Lacerations
			Concussion

Tertiary	Propulsion of body onto hard surface or object, or propulsion of objects onto individuals	■ Whole body translocation ■ Crush injuries caused by structural damage and building collapse	Blunt injuries Crush syndrome Compartment syndrome Concussion
Quaternary	Heat and/or combustion fumes	■ Burns and toxidromes from fuel, metals ■ Septic syndromes from soil and environmental contamination	Burns Inhalation injury Asphyxiation

Quinary	Additives such as radiation or chemicals (e.g., dirty bombs)	■ Contamination of tissue from:
		  Bacteria, radiation, or chemical agents
		  Allogenic bone fragments
			Variety of health effects, depending on agent

(From Department of Defense Directive: *Medical research for prevention, mitigation, and treatment of blast injuries,* Number 6025.21E, July 5, 2006, Defense Technical Information Center. Available at www.dtic.mil/whs/directives/corres/html/602521.htm. Accessed November 21, 2008.)

ary injury, is the most common category of injury in terrorist bombings and low-order explosions. These projectiles may be components of the bomb itself, as from military weapons designed to fragment, or from improvised bombs augmented with nails, screws, and bolts. Secondary blast injury is also caused by debris that is carried by the blast wind. Blast winds associated with the force required to create enough overpressure to rupture 50% of exposed eardrums (approximately 5 psi) can briefly generate winds of 145 mph. Winds associated with the force necessary to create an overpressure resulting in significant PBI may exceed 831 mph.[20] Although brief in duration, these winds can propel debris with great force and for great distances, causing both penetrating and blunt trauma.

Tertiary blast injury is caused by the victim's body being thrown by the blast wind, resulting in tumbling and collision with stationary objects. This can result in the whole spectrum of injuries associated with blunt trauma and even penetrating trauma, such as impalement.

Following the blast itself, *quaternary effects* may be seen.[19] These injuries include burns and toxicities from fuel, metals, trauma from structural collapse, infection from soil, and environmental contamination. The increasing threat of radiation-enhanced explosives (i.e., "dirty bombs") has given rise to a fifth *(quinary)* category of effects, which includes injuries caused by radiation, chemicals, or biologic agents and material.[29,30]

Injury Patterns

The prehospital care provider will be confronted with a combination of familiar penetrating, blunt, and thermal injuries and possibly survivors with PBI.[31] The numbers and types of injury will depend on multiple factors, including explosion magnitude, composition, environment, and location and number of potential victims at risk.

Various mortality rates have been associated with different types of bombing. One study that examined 29 terrorist bombings showed that 1 of 4 victims died immediately after structural-collapse bombings, 1 of 12 died immediately in closed-space bombings, and 1 of 25 died immediately after open-space bombings.[16] Additional studies have documented the finding that mortality is higher when an explosion occurs in an enclosed space.[17,18] Soft tissue injuries, orthopedic trauma, and traumatic brain injury (TBI) are predominant among survivors. For example, of 592 survivors of the Oklahoma City bombing,[22] 85% had soft tissue injuries (lacerations, puncture wounds, abrasions, contusions), 25% had sprains, 14% had head injuries, 10% had fractures/dislocations, 10% had ocular injuries (nine with ruptured globes), and 2% had burns. The most common location for soft tissue injury was the extremities (74%), followed by head and neck (48%), face (45%), and chest (35%). Eighteen survivors had severe soft tissue injuries, including carotid artery and jugular vein lacerations, facial and popliteal artery lacerations, and severed nerves, tendons, and ligaments. Seventeen survivors had serious internal organ injury, including partial

FIGURE 11-21	**Blast Lung Injury: What Prehospital Providers Need To Know**

Current patterns in worldwide terrorist activity have increased the potential for casualties related to explosions, yet few civilian Emergency Medical Services (EMS) providers in the United States have experience treating patients with explosion-related injuries. Blast lung injury (BLI) presents unique triage, diagnostic, and management challenges and is a direct consequence of the blast wave from high-explosive detonations upon the body. Persons in enclosed space explosions or those in close proximity to the explosion are at a higher risk. BLI is a clinical diagnosis characterized by respiratory difficulty and hypoxia. BLI can occur, although rarely, without obvious external injury to the chest.

CLINICAL PRESENTATION

- Symptoms may include dyspnea, hemoptysis, cough, and chest pain.
- Signs may include tachypnea, hypoxia, cyanosis, apnea, wheezing, decreased breath sounds, and hemodynamic instability.
- Victims with greater than 10% BSA burns, skull fractures, and penetrating torso or head injuries may be more likely to have BLI.
- Hemothoraces or pneumothoraces may occur.
- Due to tearing of the pulmonary and vascular tree, air may enter the arterial circulation ("air emboli") and result in embolic events involving the central nervous system, retinal arteries, or coronary arteries.
- Clinical evidence of blast lung injury is typically present at the time of initial evaluation; however, it has been reported to occur over the course of 24 to 48 hours after an explosion.
- Other injuries are often present.

PREHOSPITAL MANAGEMENT CONSIDERATIONS

- Initial triage, trauma resuscitation, and transport of patients should follow standard protocols for multiple injured patients or mass casualties.
- Note the patient's location and the surrounding environment. Explosions in a confined space result in a higher incidence of primary blast injury, including lung injury.
- All patients with suspected or confirmed BLI should receive supplemental high-flow oxygen sufficient to prevent hypoxemia.
- Impending airway compromise requires immediate intervention.
- If ventilatory failure is imminent or occurs, patients should have their airways managed; however, prehospital providers must realize that mechanical ventilation and positive pressure may increase the risk of alveolar rupture, pneumothorax, and air embolism in BLI patients.
- High-flow oxygen should be administered if air embolism is suspected, and the patient should be placed in a prone, semi–left lateral, or left lateral position.
- Clinical evidence of, or suspicion for, a hemothorax or pneumothorax warrants close observation. Chest decompression should be performed for patients clinically presenting with a tension pneumothorax. Close observation is warranted for any patient with suspicion of BLI who is transported by air.
- Fluids should be administered judiciously, as overzealous fluid administration in the patient with BLI may result in volume overload and the worsening of pulmonary status.
- Patients with BLI should be transported rapidly to the nearest, appropriate facility, in accordance with community response plans for mass casualty events.

(From Centers for Disease Control and Prevention, Atlanta.)

bowel transection, lacerated kidney and spleen, and liver, pneumothorax, and pulmonary contusion. Of patients with fractures, 37% had multiple fractures. Of those diagnosed with a head injury, 44% required admission to the hospital.[23]

Evaluation and Management

The general evaluation and management of trauma patients (secondary and tertiary blast injury) is applicable to the WMD victim and is addressed in other chapters. Unique to this patient population, however, is the possibility of PBI. Primary blast injuries might increase the likelihood that prehospital care providers will encounter patients with bloody sputum (hemoptysis) and pulmonary contusions, pneumothorax or tension pneumothorax, or even arterial gas embolism. Among survivors of primary blast injury, clinical manifestations may be present immediately[56,57] or may have a delayed onset of 24 to 48 hours.[26] Hemorrhage into the lung tissue and focal

alveolar swelling result in frothy bloody secretions and lead to difficulty breathing. Hypoxia results with increased work of breathing, pathophysiologically similar to pulmonary contusions induced by other mechanisms of nonpenetrating thoracic trauma.[27]

Primary blast injuries are not immediately apparent; therefore, care at the scene should include (1) monitoring for frothy secretions and respiratory distress and (2) provision of oxygen.

The likelihood of multisystem trauma is increased in bomb victims.[35] Management principles are similar to those for trauma from other mechanisms.

Transportation Considerations

Patients requiring transport must be brought to an appropriate medical treatment facility for further evaluation and management. These patients will often require the services of a designated trauma center. Prehospital providers should be aware of the epidemiology of patient transport after these events. Patient arrival at hospitals is usually bimodal, with ambulatory patients arriving first and more critically ill patients arriving later by ambulance. This was demonstrated in the Oklahoma City bombing. Patients began to arrive in the EDs 5 to 30 minutes after the bombing, with patients requiring admission taking longer to arrive by ambulance. Also, the geographically closest hospitals in Oklahoma City received the majority of victims, as seen with other disasters. Nearby hospitals that are overwhelmed by the first wave of self-transported patients may experience some difficulty managing the critically ill patients that arrive by ambulance in the second wave. In Oklahoma City the aggregate peak arrival rate of patients to EDs was 220 per hour at 60 to 90 minutes; 64% of patients visited EDs within a 1.5-mile radius of the event. Prehospital care providers should consider this latter fact when determining the destination of patients from the bomb scene.[15]

Incendiary Agents

Incendiary agents are typically encountered in the military and are used to burn equipment, vehicles, and structures. The three incendiaries recognized most often are magnesium, thermite, and white phosphorus. All three are highly flammable compounds that burn at extremely high temperatures.

Thermite is powdered aluminum and iron oxide that burns furiously at 3600° F and scatters molten iron.[36] Its primary mechanism of injury is partial-thickness or full-thickness burns. The primary and secondary assessment is performed with intervention directed at treating burns. Thermite wounds can be irrigated with copious amounts of water and any residual particles or material subsequently removed.

Magnesium is also a metal in powdered or solid form that burns furiously hot. In addition to its ability to cause second-degree and third-degree burns, magnesium can react with tissue fluid and cause alkali burns. The same chemical reaction produces hydrogen gas, which can cause the wound to bubble. Inhalation of magnesium dust can produce respiratory symptoms, including cough, tachypnea, hypoxia, wheeze, pneumonitis, and airway burns. Residual magnesium particles in a wound will react with water, so irrigation is discouraged until the wounds can be debrided and the particulate removed. If irrigation is required for other reasons, such as decontamination of another suspected material, care should be taken to ensure flushing or removal of magnesium particles from the wound.[36]

White phosphorus (WP) is a solid that spontaneously ignites when exposed to air, causing a yellow flame and white smoke. WP that comes in contact with skin can quickly result in second-degree and third-degree burns. WP can become embedded in the skin, propelled by the blast of WP munitions. The substance will continue to burn in the skin if exposed to air. Prehospital care providers can decrease the likelihood of combustion in the skin by immersing the affected areas in water or applying saline-soaked dressings to the area. Oily or greasy dressings are avoided in these patients because

WP will dissolve in fats and application of these dressings may increase the likelihood of systemic toxicity.

Chemical Agents

Many scenarios could expose the prehospital care provider to chemical agents, including an industrial complex accident, a spilled tanker truck, unearthed military ordnance, or a terrorist attack. The 1984 Union Carbide industrial accident in Bhopal, India, and the sarin gas attack in Tokyo in 1995 are examples of such incidents.

Classification of Chemical Agents. Chemical agents can be classified as follows:

1. Cyanides:
   Hydrogen cyanide, cyanogen chloride
2. Nerve agents:
   Tabun (GA), sarin (GB), soman (GD), GF, VX
3. Lung toxicants (choking agents):
   Chlorine, phosgene, diphosgene, ammonia
4. Vesicants (blistering agents):
   Mustard, lewisite
5. Incapacitating agents:
   3-quinuclidinyl benzilate (BZ)
6. Lacrimating agents (riot control agents):
   Tear gas (CN, CS)
7. Vomiting agents:
   Adamsite

Physical Properties of Hazardous Materials

The physical properties of a substance are affected by its chemical structure, the environmental temperature, and ambient pressure. These factors will determine whether a substance exists as a solid, liquid, or gas. Understanding the physical state of a material is important for the prehospital care provider because it gives clues as to the likely route of exposure and the potential for transmission and contamination.

Primary contamination is defined as exposure to the hazardous substance at its point of release. For example, primary contamination occurs, by definition, in the "hot zone." Gases (vapors), liquids, solids, and aerosols can all play a role in primary contamination. Secondary contamination is defined as exposure to the hazardous substance after it has been carried away from the point of origin by a victim, a responder, or a piece of equipment. Secondary contamination generally occurs in the "warm zone," although it may happen at more remote locations if the exposed victim is able to self-evacuate. Solids and liquids (and sometimes aerosols) generally contribute to secondary contamination. Gases (vapors), which cause injury by inhalation of the substance, do not deposit on skin and therefore do not typically play a role in secondary contamination, although vapors can become trapped in clothing and long hair.

Volatility plays a significant role in risk of secondary contamination. More volatile substances are considered "less persistent," meaning that because they vaporize, the likelihood of long-lasting physical contamination is very low. These agents will readily disperse and be carried away by the wind. Less volatile substances are considered "more persistent." These substances do not vaporize, or do so at a very slow rate, thereby remaining on exposed surfaces for a long time, increasing the risk of secondary contamination. For example, the nerve agent sarin is a nonpersistent agent, whereas the nerve agent VX is a persistent agent.[37]

Personal Protective Equipment

PPE is selected based on the threat of exposure to the hazardous substance. Level A provides respiratory and skin protection from gases (vapors), solids, liquids, and aerosols. This level of protection is appropriate for rescuers entering into the primary contaminated site. Because it also has supplied air, level A PPE is suitable for oxygen-deprived environments. Level B provides the same respiratory protection as level A but only provides skin and splash protection suitable for solids and liquids. Level C provides respiratory protection from selected vapors and aerosols and skin and splash protection from solids and liquids. Level D provides no particular respiratory or skin protection from chemical hazards.

Evaluation and Management

After ensuring the safety of the scene, the prehospital provider will first confirm that victims are undergoing decontamination. Patients with likely skin exposure to the liquid form of a chemical will require decontamination with water. If available, soap may be used as well, but showering with copious amounts of water will generally suffice. Exposure to a gas only does not mandate decontamination but rather removal from any ongoing exposure as well as removal of any clothing that may have trapped residual vapors.

Once the victim has been properly decontaminated, the prehospital care provider will likely encounter patients with signs and symptoms of exposure to a hazardous substance that has not yet been specifically identified. Victims of chemical agents can manifest signs and symptoms of exposure that affect (1) the respiratory system, affecting oxygenation and ventilation; (2) the mucous membranes, causing eye and upper airway injury; (3) the nervous system, resulting in seizures or coma; (4) the gastrointestinal (GI) tract, causing vomiting or diarrhea; and (5) the skin, causing burning and blistering. It is important to evaluate the presenting signs and symptoms and whether or not they are improving or progressing. Patients with worsening clinical findings likely had incomplete cleansing of the contaminant and should undergo repeat decontamination to assure complete removal.

Patients will require a primary survey to determine what lifesaving intervention may be immediately required. A secondary survey may then assist in the identification of symptom constellations that might indicate the nature of the hazardous substance and suggest a specific antidote. This constellation of signs and symptoms has been called a *toxidrome*. A toxidrome is a collection of clinical signs and symptoms that suggest exposure to a certain class of chemical or toxin.[38]

The *irritant gas toxidrome* will include burning of the eyes, nose, and mouth and inflammation, coughing, and difficulty breathing. Agents responsible might include chlorine, phosgene, or ammonia.

The *asphyxiant toxidrome* is caused by lack of oxygen in cells. This can result from inadequate oxygen availability, as in an oxygen-poor atmosphere; inadequate oxygen delivery to the cells, as in carbon monoxide poisoning; or inability to utilize oxygen at the cellular level, as in cyanide poisoning. Signs and symptoms include shortness of breath, chest pain, cardiac dysrhythmias, syncope, seizures, coma, and death.

The *cholinergic toxidrome* is characterized by runny nose (rhinorrhea), respiratory secretions, difficulty breathing, nausea, vomiting, diarrhea, profuse sweating, pinpoint pupils and possible altered mental status, seizures, and coma. Pesticides and nerve agents can cause these cholinergic signs and symptoms.

Most often, prehospital care providers will initiate supportive therapy without knowing the specific cause of the injury. If the offending agent is properly identified, or if its identity is suggested by the toxidrome or clinical presentation, therapy specific to the agent may be delivered by advanced level providers. Cyanide and nerve agent victims are examples of patients who can benefit from agent-specific antidote therapy.

Transportation Considerations

Patients must be brought to an appropriate medical treatment facility for further evaluation and management. Communities may identify preferred hospitals for the management of chemical casualties. These facilities may be more capable of managing these patients by virtue of specialized training or availability of critical care services and specific antidotes. Also, considerations similar to those previously noted for explosive incidents, regarding transport epidemiology, also apply to these patients. Nearby EDs may become overwhelmed by ambulatory, self-evacuated, self-transported patients. Of 640 patients presenting to one hospital in Tokyo after the sarin incident, 541 arrived without EMS assistance.[15] Hospitals closest to the event will likely receive the largest number of ambulatory patients. These factors should be considered in determining the destination of casualties transported via ambulance.

Selected Specific Agents[37,39,40]

Cyanides. Most commonly, prehospital care providers might encounter cyanides when responding to a fire in which certain plastics are burning or in certain industrial complexes, where it can found in large quantities and is used in chemical syntheses, electroplating, mineral extraction, dyeing, printing, photography, and agriculture, and in the manufacture of paper, textiles, and plastics. However, cyanide has been inventoried in military stockpiles and some terrorist websites have provided the instructions for making a cyanide dispersal device.

Hydrogen cyanide is a highly volatile liquid and thus will most often be encountered as a vapor or gas. It therefore has greater potential for mass casualties in a confined space with poor ventilation than if released outdoors. Although a smell of bitter almonds has been associated with this agent, this is not a reliable indicator of hydrogen cyanide exposure. It is estimated that as much as 40% to 50% of the general population is incapable of detecting the odor of cyanide.

Cyanide's mechanism of action is to prevent the use of oxygen at the cellular level, quickly resulting in cell death. Victims of cyanide poisoning actually are able to inhale and absorb oxygen into the blood but are unable to use it at the cellular level.

The organs most affected are the central nervous system (CNS) and the heart. Symptoms of mild cyanide poisoning include headache, dizziness, drowsiness, nausea, vomiting, and mucosal irritation. Severe cyanide poisoning includes alteration of consciousness, dysrhythmias, hypotension, seizures, and death. Death can occur within a few minutes after inhalation of high levels of cyanide gas.

Supportive therapy is important, including high-concentration oxygen delivery. Cyanide antidote kits are available for patients with known or suspected cyanide poisoning. These antidotes may be administered by advanced life support providers at the scene or once the victim is transported to the receiving hospital.

Nerve Agents. Nerve agents were originally developed as insecticides, but once their effects on humans were recognized, numerous different types were developed in the early and mid-1900s as weapons. These deadly chemicals can be found in the military stockpiles of many nations. Nerve agents have also been produced by terrorist organizations, the most notorious releases occurring in Matsumoto (1994) and Tokyo (1995), Japan. Commonly available pesticides (e.g., malathion, Sevin) and common therapeutic drugs (e.g., physostigmine, pyridostigmine) share properties with nerve agents, causing similar clinical effects.

Nerve agents are usually liquids at room temperature. *Sarin* is the most volatile of the group. *VX* is the least volatile and is found as an oily liquid. The main routes of intoxication are through inhalation of the vapor and absorption through the skin. Nerve agents can injure or kill at very low doses. A single, small drop of VX, the most potent nerve agent, if evenly distributed, could kill 1000 victims. Because nerve agents are liquids, they pose a risk for secondary contamination from contact with contaminated clothes, skin, and other objects.

The mechanism of action of nerve agents is to prevent the enzyme acetylcholinesterase from inactivating acetylcholine which is a neurotransmitter that stimulates cholinergic receptors. These receptors are found in smooth muscles, skeletal muscles, the CNS, and most exocrine (secretory) glands.

The mnemonics *DUMBELS* (**d**iarrhea, **u**rination, **m**iosis, **b**radycardia, bronchorrhea, bronchospasm, **e**mesis, **l**acrimation, **s**alivation, sweating) and *MTWHF* (**m**ydriasis [rarely seen], **t**achycardia, **w**eakness, **h**ypertension, hyperglycemia, **f**asciculations) represent the constellation of symptoms associated with nerve agent toxicity. The CNS effects include confusion, convulsions, and coma.

The clinical effects depend on the dose and route of nerve agent exposure (inhalation or dermal). Small amounts of vapor exposure primarily cause irritation to eyes, nose, and airways. Large amounts of vapor exposure can quickly lead to loss of consciousness, seizures, respiratory arrest, and muscular flaccidity. Miosis (constricted pupils) is the most sensitive marker of exposure to vapor. Symptoms of dermal exposure also vary according to dose, as does time of onset. Small doses may not result in symptoms for up to 18 hours. Underlying muscle fasciculations and local sweating at the site of the skin exposure may occur, followed by GI symptoms, nausea, vomiting, and diarrhea. Large dermal doses will result in onset of symptoms in minutes, with effects similar to a large vapor exposure.

Clinical symptoms of the nerve agents include rhinorrhea (runny nose), chest tightness, miosis (pupil is pinpoint, and patient complains of blurry or dim vision), shortness of breath, excessive salivation and sweating, nausea, vomiting, abdominal cramps, involuntary urination and defecation, muscle fasciculations, confusion, seizures, flaccid paralysis, coma, respiratory failure, and death.

Management of nerve agent poisoning includes decontamination, a primary survey, administration of antidotes, and supportive therapy. Ventilation and oxygenation of the patient may be difficult because of bronchoconstriction and copious secretions. The patient will likely require frequent suctioning. These symptoms improve after the antidote is administered by advanced level providers.

Lung Toxicants. Lung toxicants, including chlorine, phosgene, ammonia, sulfur dioxide, and nitrogen dioxide, are present in numerous industrial manufacturing applications. *Phosgene* has been stockpiled for military applications and was the most lethal chemical warfare agent used in World War I.

Chemical pulmonary agents may be gases (vapors) or aerosolized liquids or solids. Ammonia and sulfur dioxide cause irritation and injury to the eyes, mucous membranes, and upper airways. Phosgene and nitrogen oxides tend to cause less immediate irritation and injury to the eyes, mucous membranes, and upper airways, thus providing little warning to the victim and allowing for prolonged exposure to these agents. Prolonged exposure makes it more likely that the alveoli will be injured, resulting not only in upper airway injury but also in alveolar collapse and noncardiogenic pulmonary edema. Chlorine can cause both upper airway and alveolar irritation.

The mechanisms of injury vary among the lung toxicants. Ammonia, for example, combines with the water in the mucous membranes to form a strong base, ammonium hydroxide. Chlorine and phosgene, when combined with water, produce hydrochloric acid, causing injury to the tissues.

These agents cause burning of the eyes, nose, and mouth. Tearing, rhinorrhea, coughing, dyspnea, and respiratory distress secondary to glottic irritation or laryngospasm are possible. Bronchospasm can result in coughing, wheezing, and dyspnea. Agents causing injury to the alveoli can immediately injure the alveolar epithelium in the case of a large exposure, leading to death from acute respiratory failure, or with less massive exposure can result in a delayed onset (24–48 hours) of respiratory distress secondary to development of mild non-cardiogenic pulmonary edema or to fulminant acute respiratory distress syndrome (ARDS), depending on the dose.

Management of lung toxicants includes removal of the patient from the offending agent, decontamination with copious irrigation (if solid, liquid, or aerosol exposure, especially for ammonia), primary survey, and supportive therapy, which will likely require interventions to maximize ventilation and oxygenation. Eye irritation can be managed with copious irrigation using normal saline. Contact lenses should be removed. Expect to manage copious airway secretions, which will require suctioning. Hypoxia will require correction with high-flow oxygen. All exposed patients should be taken to a hospital for evaluation and observation for the delayed onset of symptoms.

Vesicant Agents. The vesicants, or blister agents, include sulfur mustard, nitrogen mustards, and lewisite. These agents have been stockpiled for military operations by many countries. Sulfur mustard was first introduced to the battlefield in World War I. It was reportedly used by Iraq against its Kurdish population and also in its conflict with Iran (1980). It is relatively easy and inexpensive to manufacture.

Sulfur mustard is an oily, clear to yellow-brown liquid that can be aerosolized by a bomb blast or a sprayer. Its volatility is low, allowing it to persist on surfaces for a week or more. This allows for easy secondary contamination. The agent is absorbed through the skin and mucous membranes, resulting in direct cellular damage within minutes of the exposure, although clinical symptoms make take 1 to 12 hours (usually 4–6 hours) after exposure to develop. The delayed onset of symptoms often makes it difficult for the victim to recognize that the exposure occurred and therefore increases the potential for secondary contamination. Warm, moist skin increases the likelihood of skin absorption, making the groin and axillary regions are particularly susceptible. The eyes, skin, and upper airways can develop a range of findings, from erythema and edema to vesicle development and necrosis. Upper airway involvement can result in cough and bronchospasm. High-dose exposures can result in nausea and vomiting, as well as bone marrow suppression.

Treatment involves decontamination, primary survey, and supportive therapy; no antidote exists for the effects of mustard agents. Eyes and skin should be decontaminated with copious amounts of water as soon as exposure is recognized,

to minimize further absorption of the agent and prevent secondary contamination. Absorbed agent cannot be decontaminated and will result in cellular injury. The fluid in resulting vesicles and blisters is not a source of secondary contamination. Skin wounds should be treated as burns, with regard to local wound care.

Biologic Agents

Biologic agents in the form of contagious disease represent a threat to prehospital care providers on a daily basis. Proper infection control procedures must be in place to prevent the contraction or transmission of tuberculosis, influenza, human immunodeficiency virus (HIV), methicillin-resistant staphylococci (MRSA), SARS, and myriad other organisms.

Preparing for bioterrorist events increases the complexity of EMS system preparation. An intentional terrorist act might include delivery of a hazardous agent with the potential to cause disease or illness, such as aerosolized spores, aerosolized live organisms, or an aerosolized biologic toxin. Patients with pathogens not typically seen by EMS personnel, such as plague, anthrax, and smallpox, might be encountered, requiring appropriate PPE and precautions. Familiar infection control procedures will be effective in the safe management of these potentially contagious patients. If the prehospital care provider is responding to an overt event, appropriate precautions regarding decontamination of victims and PPE are required, similar to other hazmat events.

Classification of Biologic Agents
Biologic agents can be classified as follows:

- Bacterial agents
  - Anthrax
  - Brucellosis
  - Glanders
  - Plague
  - Q fever
  - Tularemia
- Viral agents
  - Smallpox
  - Venezuelan equine encephalitis
  - Viral hemorrhagic fevers
- Biologic toxins
  - Botulinum
  - Ricin
  - Staphylococcal enterotoxin B
  - T-2 mycotoxins

Biohazard Agent versus Infected Patient. Prehospital care providers can experience bioterrorism in two forms. The first scenario involves the overt release of a material that is either identified as or thought to be a biologic agent. In this situation, the provider will encounter an environment or a patient contaminated with a suspicious substance. EMS services may be summoned to suspicious activity, such as a device delivering an unknown aerosol agent. The nature of the threat at these events is usually unknown, and precautions for personal safety should always be paramount. These events must be respected as hazmat events until characterized otherwise. If the suspicious substance is in fact a concentrated aerosol of an infectious organism or toxin, PPE appropriate for the hazard and decontamination are required. The anthrax hoaxes of 1998 and 1999 and the anthrax letters of 2001 are good examples. Prehospital providers responded on countless occasions to individuals covered in "white powder" or suspected anthrax.

In this situation, prehospital care providers will not be caring for patients with the clinical disease, but rather, victims contaminated with suspected biologic agent on their skin or clothing. Any person coming in direct physical contact with a substance alleged to be a biologic should remove articles of clothing and perform a thorough washing of exposed skin with soap and water.[19] Clinically significant reaerosolization of material from victims' skin or clothing is unlikely, and the risk to the provider is negligible.[42] As a matter of routine prac-

tice, however, clothing normally removed by pulling over the face and head should instead be cut off to minimize any risk of inadvertent inhalation of contaminant. Decontamination may then proceed using water or soap and water. Consultation with appropriate public health and law enforcement officials will then determine the need for antibiotic prophylaxis.

The second scenario involves a response to a patient who has been a victim of a remote, covert bioterrorist event. Perhaps an individual inhaled anthrax spores after a covert attack at work and now, several days later, is manifesting signs of pulmonary anthrax. Perhaps a terrorist has inoculated himself or herself with smallpox, and you are summoned to assist the victim with a suspicious rash. In these cases, personal and public safety can be ensured by knowledge of proper infection control procedures and the proper donning and removal of PPE appropriate for the biohazard (Figures 11-22 and 11-23). Decontamination of the patient in

---

FIGURE 11-22 Sequence for Donning Personal Protective Equipment (PPE)

The type of PPE used will vary based on the level of precautions required (e.g., Standard Precautions and contact, droplet, or airborne infection isolation).

1. GOWN
- Fully cover torso from neck to knees, arms to end of wrists, and wrap around the back
- Fasten in back of neck and waist

2. MASK OR RESPIRATOR
- Secure ties or elastic bands at middle of head and neck
- Fit flexible band to nose bridge
- Fit snug to face and below chin
- Fit-check respirator

3. GOGGLES OR FACE SHIELD
- Place over face and eyes and adjust to fit

4. GLOVES
- Extend to cover wrist of isolation gown

  Use safe work practices to protect yourself and limit the spread of contamination:

- Keep hands away from face
- Limit surfaces touched
- Change gloves when torn or heavily contaminated
- Perform hand hygiene

(From Centers for Disease Control and Prevention, Atlanta.)

FIGURE 11-23 Sequence for Removing Personal Protective Equipment (PPE)

Except for the respirator, remove PPE at doorway or in an anteroom. Remove respirator after leaving patient room and closing door.

1. GLOVES
- *Outside of glove is contaminated*
- Grasp outside of glove with opposite gloved hand; peel off
- Hold removed glove in gloved hand
- Slide fingers of ungloved hand under remaining glove at wrist
- Peel glove off over first glove
- Discard gloves in waste container

2. GOGGLES
- *Outside of goggles or face shield is contaminated*
- To remove, handle by headband or earpieces
- Place in designated receptacle for reprocessing or in waste container

3. GOWN
- *Gown front and sleeves are contaminated*
- Unfasten gown ties
- Pull away from neck and shoulders, touching inside of gown only
- Turn gown inside out
- Fold or roll into a bundle and discard

4. MASK OR RESPIRATOR
- *Front of mask/respirator is contaminated—do not touch*
- Grasp bottom, then top ties or elastics, and remove
- Discard in waste container

(From Centers for Disease Control and Prevention, Atlanta.)

this scenario is not necessary because the exposure occurred several days in the past.

PPE for infection control purposes should be familiar to all prehospital care providers. Different types of PPE are recommended, depending on the potential for transmission and the likely route of transmission. Transmission-based PPE is used in addition to the Standard Precautions, which are used in the care of all patients. These include contact, droplet, and aerosol precautions.

Contact Precautions. This level of protection is recommended to reduce the likelihood of transmission of microorganisms by direct or indirect contact. Contact precautions include the use of gloves and a gown. Commonly encountered organisms that require contact precautions include viral conjunctivitis, methicillin-resistant staphylococci, scabies, and herpes simplex or zoster virus. Organisms that might be encountered as a result of bioterrorism include bubonic plague or the viral hemorrhagic fevers, such as Marburg or Ebola, as long as the patient does not have pulmonary symptoms or profuse vomiting and diarrhea.

Droplet Precautions. This level of protection is recommended to reduce the likelihood of transmission of microorganisms that are known to be transmitted by large droplets expelled by an infected person in the course of talking, sneezing, or coughing or during routine procedures such as suctioning. These droplets infect the susceptible individual by landing on the exposed mucous membranes of the eye and mouth. Because the droplets are large, they do not remain suspended in air, and therefore contact must be in close proximity, usually defined as 3 feet or less. Droplet precautions include the gloves and gown of contact precautions, but also add eye protection and a surgical mask. Because the droplets do not remain suspended in air, no additional respiratory protection or air filtration is required. Typically encountered organisms in this category include influenza, *Mycoplasma* pneumonia, and invasive *Haemophilus influenzae* or *Neisseria meningitidis* causing sepsis or meningitis. Pneumonic plague is an example of a possible agent encountered as a result of a bioterrorist event.

Aerosol Precautions. This level of protection is recommended to reduce the likelihood of transmission of microorganisms by the airborne route. Some organisms can become suspended in the air attached to small droplets or attached to dust particles. In this case, microorganisms can become widely dispersed by air currents immediately around the source or far from the source, depending on conditions. These patients are kept in isolation rooms in which the exhaust ventilation can be filtered. Aerosol precautions include gloves, gown, eye protection, and a fit-tested high-efficiency particulate air (HEPA) filter mask, such as the N-95. Examples of illnesses typically encountered include tuberculosis, measles, chickenpox, and SARS. Smallpox and viral hemorrhagic fever with pulmonary symptoms are examples that could possibly be related to a bioterrorist event.

Note that many illnesses associated with bioterrorist events require no additional protection beyond Standard Precautions, provided there is no risk of exposure to a concentrated agent. Examples include patients with inhalational anthrax or a biologic toxin such as botulinum. However, in most cases, the specific biologic agent will likely not be identified for several days. Although some, such as anthrax, are not spread from person to person, providers must assume the worst—that the agent is contagious—and therefore use all available precautions, including standard and aerosol precautions.

Radiologic Disasters

Since the terrorist attacks of September 11, 2001, new consideration has been given to the likelihood of EMS systems needing to manage a radiologic emergency. Historically, planning has focused on civil defense preparation for a strategic exchange of military nuclear weapons or the rare occurrence of a nuclear power plant accident. Currently, however, there is increasing awareness of the possibility that terrorists could deploy an improvised nuclear detonation device, or perhaps more likely a radiologic dispersal device, that uses conventional explosives to disseminate radioactive material into the environment.

Although radiologic accidents are rare, there have been 243 radiation accidents since 1944 in the United States with 1342 casualties that met criteria for significant exposure. Worldwide, 403 accidents have occurred, with 133,617 victims, 2965 with significant exposure, and 120 fatalities. The Chernobyl disaster was responsible for 116,500 to 125,000 exposed casualties and close to 50 deaths as of 2005, although it is estimated that the total number of deaths could reach as many as 4,000 as additional cancer victims succumb.[43,54]

Radiation disasters have the potential to generate fear and confusion in both victims and responders. Familiarization with the hazard and management principles will help to ensure an appropriate response and help to reduce panic and disorder (Figure 11-24).

Exposure to ionizing radiation and radioactive contamination may result from several different scenarios: (1) detonation of a nuclear weapon, whether high grade or an improvised low-yield device; (2) detonation of a "dirty bomb" or radiation dispersion device (RDD), in which there is no nuclear detonation, but rather conventional explosives are detonated to disperse a radionuclide; (3) sabotage or accident at a nuclear reactor site; and (4) mishandled nuclear waste.

Medical Effects of Radiation Catastrophes

The injuries and risks associated with a radiologic catastrophe will be multifactorial. In the case of a nuclear detonation, casualties will be produced by the explosion, resulting in primary, secondary, and tertiary blast injuries, thermal injury (burns), and structural collapse. Victims may be further subject to radiation injury from irradiation; from external radioactive contamination, which can be deposited on skin and clothing; or from internal radiation through radioactive par-

1. Assess the scene for safety.
2. All patients should be medically stabilized from their traumatic injuries before radiation injuries are considered. Patients are then evaluated for their external radiation exposure and contamination.
3. An external source of radiation, if great enough, can cause tissue injury, but it does not make the patient radioactive. Patients with even lethal exposures to external radiation are not a threat to medical staff.
4. Patients can become contaminated with radioactive material deposited on their skin or clothing. More than 90% of surface contamination can be removed by removal of clothing. The remainder can be washed off with soap and water.
5. Protect yourself from radioactive contamination by observing, at a minimum, Standard Precautions, including protective clothing, gloves, and a mask.
6. Patients who develop nausea, vomiting, or skin erythema within 4 hours of exposure have likely received a high external radiation exposure.
7. Radioactive contamination in wounds should be treated as dirt and irrigated as soon as possible. Avoid handling any metallic foreign body.
8. Potassium iodine (KI) is only of value if there has been a release of radioactive iodine. KI is not a general radiation antidote.
9. The concept of time/distance/shielding is key in the prevention of untoward effects from radiation exposure. Radiation exposure is minimized by *decreasing time* in the affected area, *increasing distance* from a radiation source, and using metal or concrete *shielding*.

(Modified from Department of Homeland Security, Working Group on Radiological Dispersion Device Preparedness/Medical Preparedness and Response Subgroup: *Radiologic medical countermeasures,* 2004. Available at www1.va.gov/emshg/docs/Radiologic_Medical_Countermeasures_051403.pdf.)

ticulate contamination, which victims may inhale, ingest, or have deposited in wounds.

Accidents at nuclear reactors can generate large doses of ionizing radiation without a nuclear detonation, especially under circumstances in which the reactor reaches a point of "criticality." Explosions, fire, and gas release can also result in radioactive gas or particulate matter, which may expose responders to risk of exposure to contamination with radioactive particles.

RDDs typically would not deliver enough radiation to cause immediate injury. However, RDDs would complicate management for prehospital care responders by distributing radioactive particulates that could contaminate victims and responders and make it difficult to manage the injuries caused by the conventional explosive. RDDs could cause confusion and panic among responders concerned about radioactivity, hindering efforts to assist victims.

Ionizing radiation causes injury to cells by interacting with atoms and depositing energy. This exposure results in *ionization,* which can either damage the cell nucleus directly, causing cell death or malfunction, or indirectly, damaging cell components by interacting with water in the body and resulting in toxic molecules. Acute exposure to large doses of penetrating ionizing radiation (irradiation with gamma rays and neutrons) in a short time can result in acute radiation illness. Types of ionizing radiation include alpha particles, beta particles, gamma rays, and neutrons.

Alpha particles are relatively large and cannot penetrate even a few layers of skin. Intact skin or a uniform offers adequate protection from external contamination emitting alpha particles. Ionizing radiation from alpha particles is a concern only if it is internalized by inhaling or ingesting alpha-particle emitters. When internalized, alpha-particle radiation can cause significant local cellular injury to adjacent cells.

Beta particles are small charged particles that can penetrate more deeply than alpha particles and can affect deeper layers of the skin, having the ability to injure the base of the skin, causing a "beta burn." Beta-particle radiation is found most frequently in nuclear fallout. Beta particles also result in local radiation injury.

Gamma rays are similar to x-rays and have the ability to easily penetrate tissue. Gamma rays are emitted with a nuclear detonation and with fallout. They can also be emitted from some radionuclides that might be present in an RDD. Gamma radiation can result in *whole-body exposure,* which can lead to acute radiation illness (Figures 11-25, 11-26, and 11-27).

Neutrons can penetrate tissue easily, with 20 times the destructive energy of gamma rays, disrupting the atomic structure of cells. Neutrons are released during a nuclear detonation but are not a fallout risk. Neutrons also contribute to whole-body radiation exposure and can result in acute radiation illness. Neutrons have the ability to convert stable metals into radioactive isotopes. This has significance in patients with metal hardware or those in possession of metal objects at the time of exposure.

Acute radiation illness generally follows a defined progression that first manifests in a prodromal phase characterized by malaise, nausea, and vomiting. This is followed by a latent phase, in which the patient is essentially asymptomatic. The length of the latent phase depends on the total absorbed dose of radiation. The greater the dose of radiation, the shorter the latent phase. The latent phase is followed by the subsequent illness, as manifested by the organ system that has been injured. Damage to the bone marrow results in decreasing levels of white blood cells and decreasing resistance to infection over several days to weeks. Decreased platelets can result in easy bruising and bleeding. Decreased red blood cells will result in anemia. As the dose of radiation increases, the GI tract will also be affected, resulting in diarrhea, volume loss,

---

FIGURE 11-25   **Terrorism with Ionizing Radiation: General Guide**

DIAGNOSIS
Be alert to the following:

1. The acute radiation syndrome follows a predictable pattern after substantial exposure or catastrophic events (Figure 11-26).
2. Individuals may become ill from contaminated sources in the community and may be identified over much longer periods based on specific syndromes (Figure 11-27).
3. Specific syndromes of concern, especially with a 2- to 3-week prior history of nausea and vomiting, are:
    - Thermal burnlike skin effects without documented thermal exposure
    - Immunologic dysfunction with secondary infections
    - Tendency to bleed (epistaxis, gingival bleeding, petecchiae)
    - Marrow suppression (neutropenia, lymphopenia, and thrombocytopenia)
    - Epilation (hair loss)

UNDERSTANDING EXPOSURE
Exposure may be known and recognized or clandestine through:

1. Large recognized exposures, such as a nuclear bomb or damage to a nuclear power station
2. Small radiation source emitting continuous gamma radiation, producing group or individual chronic intermittent exposures (e.g., radiologic sources from medical treatment devices, environmental water or food pollution)
3. Internal radiation from absorbed, inhaled, or ingested radioactive material (internal contamination)

(Modified from Department of Veterans Affairs pocket guide produced by Employee Education System for Office of Public Health and Environmental Hazards. This information is not meant to be complete, but to be a quick guide; please consult other references and expert opinion.)

---

and hematochezia (bloody stools). With extremely high doses, the patient will manifest symptoms of the neurovascular syndrome, experiencing the prodromal phase of nausea and vomiting, a short latent phase lasting only a few hours, followed by a rapid deterioration of mental status, coma, and death, sometimes accompanied by hemodynamic instability. Doses this high can occur after a nuclear detonation, but the victim will most likely have been killed by injuries associated with the blast. Victims could also be exposed to these high doses at a nuclear power facility where no blast has occurred but a reactor core has reached criticality.[44]

Not all radiation accidents or terrorist events will result in high-dose radiation exposure. Low-dose radiation exposure, as would most likely occur after an RDD detonation, probably would not produce acute injury secondary to radiation. Dependent on dose, the patient may have an increased future risk of developing cancer. The acute effects of RDD detonation, besides the effects of the detonation of the conventional explosive, will likely be psychological, including stress reactions, fear, acute depression, and psychosomatic complaints, which will significantly strain the EMS agencies and medical infrastructure.

Patients can become contaminated with material that emits alpha, beta, and even gamma radiation. Patients can easily be decontaminated by clothing removal and washing with water or soap and water. It is impossible for a patient to be so contaminated as to be a radiologic hazard to health care providers caring for the individual, so management of traumatic life-threatening injury is an immediate priority and should not be delayed pending decontamination.[44]

As described, radioactive particles can be inhaled, ingested, or absorbed through the skin or contaminated wounds. This type of exposure to radiation will not result in acute effects of radiation exposure but can result in delayed effects. Any victims, or responding personnel who operate in an area at risk for airborne radioactive particles, without the benefit of respiratory protection will require subsequent evaluation to identify internal contamination, which may require medical intervention to dilute or block the effects of the radionuclide.

Personal Protective Equipment

Prehospital care providers will be operating in an environment with risk of exposure to ionizing radiation after a radiologic disaster. The radiation risk will depend greatly on the type of radiologic event.

PPE available to prehospital care providers for use in chemical and biologic hazards will offer some protection from radioactive particulate contamination. It will not provide protection from high-energy radiation sources, however, such as a damaged reactor or nuclear blast at ground zero.

Radioactivity can be present in gases, aerosols, solids, or liquids. If radioactive gases are present, SCBA will offer the highest protection. If aerosols are present, an APR may be adequate to prevent internal contamination caused by inhalation of contaminated particles. An N-95 mask will offer some protection from inhaled particulates. Wearing a standard splash-resistant suit will protect against particulates that emit alpha radiation and will offer some protection from beta radiation but will provide no protection from gamma radiation or neutrons. This type of barrier protection will assist in the decontamination of particulate matter from an individual, but it does not protect against the risks of acute radiation illness when the person is exposed to high-energy sources of external radiation. None of the typical PPE carried by prehospital providers protects from a high-energy point source of radiation.

FIGURE 11-26   **Acute Radiation Syndrome**

Feature	Effects of Whole-Body Irradiation, from External Radiation or Internal Absorption, by Dose Range in rad (1 rad = 1 cGy; 100 rad = 1 Gy)					
	0–100	100–200	200–600	600–800	800–3000	>3000
PRODROMAL PHASE OF SYNDROME						
Nausea, vomiting	None	5%–50%	50%–100%	75%–100%	90%–100%	100%
Time of onset		3–6 hr	2–4 hr	1–2 hr	<1 hr	Minutes
Duration		<24 hr	<24 hr	<48 hr	48 hr	N/A
Lymphocyte count	Unaffected	Minimally decreased	<1000 at 24 hr	<500 at 24 hr	Decreases within hours	Decreases within hours
Central nervous system (CNS) function	No impairment	No impairment	Routine task performance Cognitive impairment for 6–20 hr	Simple, routine task performance Cognitive impairment for >24 hr	Rapid incapacitation May have a lucid interval of several hours	
LATENT PHASE OF SYNDROME						
No symptoms	>2 wk	7–15 days	0–7 days	0–2 days	None	None
MANIFEST ILLNESS						
Signs/ symptoms	None	Moderate leukopenia	Severe leukopenia, purpura, hemorrhage, pneumonia, hair loss after 300 rad		Diarrhea, fever, electrolyte disturbance	Convulsions, ataxia, tremor, lethargy
Time of onset		>2 wk	2 days–4 wk	2 days–4 wk	1–3 days	1–3 days
Critical period		None	4–6 wk; greatest potential for effective medical intervention		2–14 days	1–46 hr
Organ system	None		Hematopoietic; respiratory (mucosal) systems		Gastrointestinal tract Mucosal systems	CNS
Hospitalization duration	0%	<5% 45–60 days	90% 60–90 days	100% 100+ days	100% Weeks to months	100% Days to weeks
Mortality	None	Minimal	Low with aggressive therapy	High	Very high; significant neurologic symptoms indicate lethal dose	

(Modified from Armed Forces Radiobiology Institute: *Medical management of radiological casualties*, Bethesda, Md, 2003, U.S. Army Publications.)

FIGURE 11-27   **Symptom Clusters As Delayed Effects After Radiation**

1	2	3	4
Headache Fatigue Weakness	Anorexia Nausea Vomiting Diarrhea	Partial-thickness and full-thickness skin damage Epilation (hair loss) Ulceration	Lymphopenia Neutropenia Thrombocytopenia Purpura Opportunistic infections

(Modified from Armed Forces Radiobiology Institute: *Medical management of radiological casualties*, Bethesda, Md, 2003, U.S. Army Publications.)

Unlike a chemical hazmat, the inhalation, ingestion, or skin absorption of radiation-emitting gas or particulate will not immediately incapacitate a prehospital care provider or victim. All prehospital providers who have operated in an environment potentially contaminated with radioactive material will have to undergo a radiation survey to determine if internal contamination has occurred and undergo active management if warranted.

Dose rate meters or alarms should be worn if available. Standards exist for acceptable doses of ionizing radiation in the occupational environment under normal and emergency conditions.[45] Dose rates of ionizing radiation can be measured to prevent responders from putting themselves at risk for acute radiation illness or an unacceptably higher incidence of cancer. The incident commander should be approached for guidance on radiation exposure readings and limits.

Evaluation and Treatment

Patients who have been injured in a radiologic catastrophe should receive primary and secondary surveys as dictated by the mechanism of injury. Prehospital care providers can expect to evaluate patients who have sustained blast injury and thermal injury in the case of a nuclear detonation, or from the conventional HE detonation of an RDD (Figure 11-28). Decontamination of the victim is recommended to eliminate radioactive particulate contamination but should not delay care of patients requiring immediate intervention for their injuries. Treatment of traumatic, life-threatening injuries always takes priority over decontamination for radiologic exposure. If the patient does not show signs of serious injury requiring immediate intervention, the patient can be decontaminated first.

Transportation Considerations

Patients should be transported to the nearest appropriate medical center that is capable of managing trauma and radiation injuries. All hospitals are required to have a plan for management of a radiologic emergency, but communities may have identified institutions that have decontamination facilities, are capable of managing trauma, and have staff trained to deal effectively with possible external or internal radioactive contamination, as well as the complications of whole-body exposure to ionizing radiation.

FIGURE 11-28 Treatment and Decontamination Considerations for Radiation Exposure

TREATMENT CONSIDERATIONS
- If trauma is present, treat
- If external radioactive contaminants are present, decontaminate
- If radioiodine (e.g., reactor accident) is present, consider giving prophylactic potassium iodide (Lugol's solution) within first 24 hours only (ineffective later)

(See www.afrri.usuhs.mil or www.orau.gov/reacts/guidance.htm)

DECONTAMINATION CONSIDERATIONS
- Exposure without contamination requires no decontamination
- Exposure with contamination requires Standard (Universal) Precautions, removal of patient clothing, and decontamination with water
- Internal contamination will be determined at the hospital
- Treating contaminated patients before decontamination may contaminate the facility; plan for decontamination before arrival
- Patient with life-threatening condition: treat, then decontaminate
- Patient with non–life-threatening condition: decontaminate, then treat

(Modified from Armed Forces Radiobiology Institute, *Medical management of radiological casualties,* Bethesda, Md, 2003, U.S. Army Publications.)

SUMMARY

- Weapons of mass destruction manufactured by terrorist regimes pose a significant threat to civilized society.
- Prehospital care providers may also come in contact with explosions and chemical and radiologic material as the result of industrial mishaps.
- The safety of providers is paramount, and they should possess a working knowledge of levels of personal protective equipment and the fundamentals of decontamination.
- Explosive agents have predominated in recent terrorist attacks. High-order explosives produce primary blast injuries in survivors who are in close proximity to the blast, and secondary injuries result from flying debris.

- Chemical agents may injure the skin and pulmonary system but may also result in systemic illness, manifesting as a specific toxidrome that yields clues to the agent. Antidotes are used for some of these agents.
- Biologic agents can be highly virulent bacteria or viruses or can be toxins produced by living organisms. The types of protective precautions used by providers vary with the specific agents.
- Several types of radiation exist. Exposure to these agents may result in acute radiation sickness, which is typically a function of the type of radiation and the length of exposure.

SCENARIO 2 SOLUTION

The first priority is safety. Assess the scene. Look also for obvious evidence of a secondary device that may pose a threat to responders. Are there other hazards? Look for hanging debris, downed or exposed power lines, or hazmat spills. Briefly observe the crowd for evidence of a toxidrome. Is there an unusually high proportion of respiratory difficulty? Are victims vomiting and seizing? Is there evidence of agent dispersal in addition to the explosive blast? Don PPE appropriate for the scenario.

Communicate with your chain of command. As the first EMS responder, the communications center will be relying on you for information. Describe pertinent details of the scene, observed hazards, numbers of victims, and likely number of resources required to manage the scene and victims. Based on your observations, the communications center and the on-duty supervisor can apprise other units and agencies of your situation and dispatch the necessary resources. A predefined disaster response plan may be activated.

Once the personal safety of the team has been assured and information has been communicated to the chain of command, prepare to serve as the incident commander until relieved by another competent authority. As soon as is feasible, approach the victims with the intention of triaging them for treatment and transport using the START algorithm. Without engaging in the medical management of victims initially, sort the victims into immediate, urgent, delayed, and expectant categories. As other assistance arrives, direct personnel to assume roles of the incident command system, until supervisory personnel arrive to assume command and control functions. ■

References

1. Noji EK: *The public health consequences of disasters,* New York, 1997, Oxford University Press.

2. Noji EK, Siverston KT: Injury prevention in natural disasters: a theoretical framework. *Disasters* 11:290, 1987.

3. Cuny SC: Introduction to disaster management. Lesson 5. Technologies of disaster management. *Prehosp Disaster Med* 6:372, 1993.

4. Burkle FM, editor: *Disaster medicine: application for the immediate management and triage of civilian and military disaster victims,* New Hyde Park, NY, 1984, Medication Examination Publishing.

5. Burkle FM, Hogan DE, Burstein JL: *Disaster medicine,* Philadelphia, 2002, Lippincott Williams & Wilkins.

6. *Super-G START: A triage training module,* Newport Beach, Calif, 1984, Hoag Memorial Hospital Presbyterian.

7. Burkle FM, Newland C, Orebaugh S, et al: Emergency medicine in the Persian Gulf. Part II. Triage methodology lessons learned. *Ann Emerg Med* 23:748, 1994.

8. West H: Addressing the traumatic impact of disasters on individuals, families, and communities (White Paper). Available at www.nh.gov/safety/divisions/bem/behavhealth/documents/atc_white_paper.PDF. Accessed September 1, 2008.

9. Agency for Healthcare Research and Quality: *Mass medical care with scarce resources: A community planning guide* (AHRQ Publication No. 07-0001), Rockville, Md, 2007, Agency for Healthcare Research and Quality. Available at www.ahrq.gov/research/mce/. Accessed September 1, 2008.

10. Hick JL, Ho JD, Heegaard WG, et al: Emergency medical services response to a major freeway bridge collapse. *Disaster Med Public Health Preparedness* 2(Suppl 1):S17–S24, 2008.

11. Lerner EB, Schwartz RB, Coule PL, et al: Mass casualty triage: An evaluation of the data and development of a proposed national guideline. *Disaster Med Public Health Preparedness* 2 (Suppl 1): S25–S34, 2008.

12. Bloch YH, Schwartz D, Pinkert M, et al: Distribution of casualties in a mass-casualty incident with three local hospitals in the periphery of a densely populated area: lessons learned from the medical management of a terrorist attack. *Prehosp Disast Med* 22:186–192, 2007.

13. Auf der Heide E: The importance of evidence-based disaster planning. *Ann Emerg Med* 47:34–49, 2006.

14. Asaeda G, Cherson A, Richmond N, et al: Unsolicited medical personnel volunteering at disaster scenes. A joint position paper from the National Association of EMS Physicians and the American College of Emergency Physicians. *Prehosp Emerg Care* 7:147–148, 2003.

15. Hogan DE, Waeckerle JF, Dire DJ, et al: Emergency department impact of the Oklahoma City terrorist bombing. *Ann Emerg Med* 34:160, 1999.

16. Arnold J, Halpern P, Tsai M: Mass casualty terrorist bombings: a comparison of outcomes by bombing type. *Ann Emerg Med* 43:263, 2004.

17. Arnold JL, Tsai MC, Halpern P, et al: Mass-casualty, terrorist bombings: epidemiological outcomes, resource utilization, and time course of emergency needs (Part I). *Prehosp Disaster Med* 18(3):220–234, 2003.

18. Halpern P, Tsai MC, Arnold JL, et al: Mass-casualty, terrorist bombings: implications for emergency department and hospital emergency response (Part II). *Prehosp Disaster Med* 18(3):235–241, 2003.

19. Centers for Disease Control and Prevention: *Explosions and blast injuries: a primer for clinicians.* Available at www.bt.cdc.gov/masstrauma/explosions.asp. Accessed August 2004.

20. Wightman JM, Gladish JL: Explosions and blast injuries. *Ann Emerg Med* 37:664, 2001.

21. Frykberg ER, Tepas JJ, Alexander RH: The 1983 Beirut Airport terrorist bombing: injury patterns and implications for disaster management. *Am Surg* 55:134, 1989.

22. Katz E, Ofek B, Adler J, et al: Primary blast injury after a bomb explosion in a civilian bus, *Ann Surg* 209:484, 1989.
23. Mallonee S, Shariat S, Stennies G, et al: Physical injuries and fatalities resulting from the Oklahoma City bombing, *JAMA* 276:382, 1996.
24. Caseby NG, Porter MF: Blast injury to the lungs: clinical presentation, management and course. *Injury* 8:1, 1976.
25. Leibovici D, Gofrit ON, Shapira SC: Eardrum perforation in explosion survivors: is it a marker of pulmonary blast injury? *Ann Emerg Med* 34:168, 1999.
26. Coppel DL: Blast injuries of the lungs. *Br J Surg* 63:735, 1976.
27. Cohn SM: Pulmonary contusion: review of the clinical entity. *J Trauma* 42:973, 1997.
28. DePalma RG, Burris DG, Champion HR, et al: Blast injuries. *N Engl J Med* 352(13):1335–1342, 2005.
29. Kluger Y, Nimrod A, Biderman P, et al: Case report: the quinary pattern of blast injury. *J Emerg Manage* 4(1):51–55, 2006.
30. Sorkine P, Nimrod A, Biderman P, et al: The quinary (Vth) injury pattern of blast (Abstract). *J Trauma* 56(1):232, 2007.
31. Nelson TJ, Wall DB, Stedje-Larsen ET, et al: Predictors of mortality in close proximity blast injuries during Operation Iraqi Freedom. *J Am Coll Surg* 202(3):418–422, 2006.
32. Almogy G, Mintz Y, Zamir G, et al: Suicide bombing attacks: can external signs predict internal injuries? *Ann Surg* 243(4):541–546, 2006.
33. Garner MJ, Brett SJ: Mechanisms of injury by explosive devices. *Anesthesiol Clin* 25(1):147–160, 2007
34. Avidan V, Hersch M, Armon Y, et al: Blast lung injury: clinical manifestations, treatment, and outcome. *Am J Surg* 190(6):927–931, 2005.
35. Peleg K, Limor A, Stein M, et al: Gunshot and explosion injuries: characteristics, outcomes, and implications for care of terror-related injuries in Israel. *Ann Surg* 239(3):311, 2004.
36. Burstein JL: CBRNE. Incendiary agents: magnesium and thermite. Available at www.emedicine.com/emerg/topic917.htm. Accessed October 2004.
37. Sidell FR, Takafuji ET, Franz DR, editors: *Medical aspects of chemical and biological warfare.* TMM series, Part 1: Warfare, weaponry and the casualty, Washington, DC, 1997, Office of the Surgeon General, TMM Publications.
38. Walter FG, editor: *Advanced HAZMAT life support,* ed 2, Tucson, 2000, Arizona Board of Regents.
39. U.S. Army, Medical Research Institute of Chemical Defense: *Medical management of chemical casualties handbook,* ed 3, 2000, Aberdeen Proving Ground, Md, U.S. Army Publications.
40. Greenfield RA, Brown BR, Hutchins JB, et al: Microbiological, biological and chemical weapons of warfare and terrorism. *Am J Med Sci* 323(6):326, 2002.
41. Ingelsby TV, Henderson DA, Bartlett JG, et al: Anthrax as a biological weapon: medical and public health management. *JAMA* 281(18):1735, 1999.
42. Keim M, Kaufmann AF: Principles for emergency response to bioterrorism. *Ann Emerg Med* 34(2):177, 1999.
43. Hogan DE, Kellison T: Nuclear terrorism. *Am J Med Sci* 323(6):341, 2002.
44. Armed Forces Radiobiology Institute: *Medical management of radiological casualties,* Bethesda, Md, 2003, U.S. Army Publications.
45. Department of Homeland Security, Working Group on Radiological Dispersion Device Preparedness/Medical Preparedness and Response Subgroup: *Radiologic medical countermeasures.* Available at www1.va.gov/emshg/docs/Radiologic_Medical_Countermeasures_051403.pdf. Accessed September 2004.
46. Kapur GB, Hutson HR, Davis MA, Rice PL: The United States twenty-year experience with bombing incidents: implications for terrorism preparedness and medical response. *J Trauma* 2005;59:1436–1444.
47. Hall JR Jr: Deaths due to unintentional injury from explosions. Quincy, MA: National Fire Protection Association, Fire Analysis and Research Division, March 2008. Available at www.arfireprevention.org/pdf/Deaths_Due_to_Unintentional_Injury_from_Explosions.pdf. Accessed December 17, 2008.
48. Office of the Historian, Bureau of Public Affairs, U.S. Department of State: *Significant terrorist incidents, 1961–2003: a brief chronology,* Washington, DC, 2004. Available at www.state.gov/r/pa/ho/pubs/fs/5902.htm. Accessed October 2004.
49. National Counterterrorism Center: *2007 report on terrorism,* April 30, 2008. Available at www.terrorisminfo.mipt.org/GetDoc.asp?id=6051&type=d. Accessed December 15, 2008.
50. United States Bomb Data Center: Explosive incidents, 2007. In *2007 USBDC explosives statistics.* Available at www.atf.gov/aexis2/statistics.htm. Accessed December 15, 2008.
51. National Counterterrorism Center: *Report on terrorist incidents—2006,* April 30, 2007. Available at www.wits.nctc.gov/reports/crot2006nctcannexfinal.pdf. Accessed December 15, 2008.
52. U.S. Department of State: *Country reports on terrorism, 2007,* April 2008. Available at www.state.gov/s/ct/rls/crt/2007/index.htm. Accessed December 15, 2008.
53. National Counterterrorism Center: *2008 report on terrorism,* April 30, 2009. Available at http://wits.nctc.gov/ReportPDF.do?f=crt2008nctcannexfinal.pdf. Accessed May 25, 2009.
54. World Health Organization, International Atomic Energy Agency, United Nations Development Programme. Chernobyl: the true scale of the event. Accessed August 27, 2010. http://www.who.int/mediacentre/news/releases/2005/pr38/en/index.html.
55. Caseby NG, Porter MF: Blast injury to the lungs: clinical presentation, management and course, *Injury* 8:1,1976.
56. Leibovici D, Gofrit ON, Shapira SC: Eardrum perforation in explosion survivors: is it a marker of pulmonary blast injury? *Am Emerg Med* 34:168,1999.

Additional Resources

Centers for Disease Control and Prevention Emergency Preparedness and Response Site www.bt.cdc.gov/

U.S. Army Center for Health Promotion and Preventive Medicine http://phc.amedd.army.mil/home/

U.S. Army Medical Research Institute of Infectious Diseases www.usamriid.army.mil/

U.S. Army Soldier and Biological Chemical Command (SBCCOM) http://hld.sbccom.army.mil/

Suggested Reading

Briggs SM, Brinsfield KH: *Advanced disaster medical response: manual for providers,* Boston, 2003, Harvard Medical International.

De Boer J, Dubouloz M: *Handbook of disaster medicine, emergency medicine in mass casualty situations,* National Society of Disaster Medicine, Netherlands, 2000, Van der Wees.

De Boer J, Rutherford WH: Definition and quantification of disaster: introduction of a disaster severity scale. *J Emerg Med* 8:602, 1990.

Eachempati SR, Flomenbaum N, Barie PS: Biological warfare: current concerns for the health care provider. *J Trauma* 52:179, 2002.

Emerg Med Clin North Am 14(2), 1996 [entire issue].

Feliciano DV, et al: Management of casualties from the bombing at the centennial Olympics. *Am J Surg* 176(6):538, 1998.

Hirshberg A, Holcomb JB, Mattox KL: Hospital trauma care in multiple-casualty incidents: a critical view. *Ann Emerg Med* 37(6):647, 2001.

Rutherford WH, De Boer J: The definition and quantification of disaster. *Injury* 15:1, 1983.

Slater MS, Trunkey DD: Terrorism in America: an evolving threat. *Arch Surg* 132(10):1059, 1997.

Stein M, Hirshberg A: Medical consequences of terrorism: the conventional weapon threat. *Surg Clin North Am* 79(6):1537, 1999.

CHAPTER 12

Golden Principles of Prehospital Trauma Care

CHAPTER OBJECTIVES

At the completion of this chapter, the reader will be able to do the following:

✓ Understand the importance of the "golden period."

✓ Discuss why trauma patients die.

✓ Understand and discuss the 14 "Golden Principles" of prehospital trauma care.

In the late 1960s, R Adams Cowley, MD, conceived the idea of a crucial time period during which it was important to begin definitive patient care for a critically injured trauma patient. In an interview he said, "There is a 'golden hour' between life and death. If you are critically injured, you have less than 60 minutes to survive. You might not die right then—it may be 3 days or 2 weeks later—but something has happened in your body that is irreparable."

Is there a basis for this concept? The answer is definitely *yes*. However, an important realization is that a patient does not always have the luxury of a "Golden Hour." A patient with a penetrating wound of the heart may have only a few minutes to reach definitive care before the shock caused by the injury becomes irreversible. At the other end of the spectrum is a patient with slow, ongoing internal hemorrhage from an isolated femur fracture. Such a patient may have several hours to reach definitive care and resuscitation. Because the Golden *Hour* is not a strict 60-minute time frame and varies from patient to patient based on the injuries, the more appropriate term is the Golden *Period*. If a critically injured patient is able to obtain definitive care—that is, hemorrhage control and resuscitation—within that particular patient's Golden Period, the chance of survival is greatly improved.[1]

No call, scene, or patient is the same. Each requires flexibility by the healthcare team members to act and react to situations as they develop. The management of prehospital trauma must reflect these contingencies. The goals, however, have not changed: (1) gain access to the patient, (2) identify and treat life-threatening injuries, and (3) package and transport to the closest appropriate facility, all in the least amount of time. The majority of the techniques and principles discussed are not new, and most are taught in an initial education program. This text is different in the following ways:

1. It provides current, evidence-based practices of management for the trauma patient.
2. It provides a systematic approach for establishing priorities of patient care for trauma patients who have sustained injury to multiple body systems.
3. It provides an organizational scheme for interventions.

The Prehospital Trauma Life Support (PHTLS) program teaches that the prehospital care provider can make correct judgments leading toward a good outcome only if the provider is supplied with a good base of knowledge. The foundation of the PHTLS program is that patient care should be *judgment* driven, not protocol driven; thus, the medical detail provided in this course. This chapter addresses the key aspects of prehospital trauma care and "brings it all together."

Why Trauma Patients Die

Studies that analyze the causes of death in trauma patients have several common themes. A study from Russia of trauma deaths found that most patients who rapidly succumbed to their injuries fell into one of three categories: massive acute blood loss (36%), severe injury to vital organs such as the brain (30%), and airway obstruction and acute ventilatory failure (25%).[2] In an analysis of trauma patients who died of their injuries at a level I trauma center, 51% of trauma patients died from severe trauma to the central nervous system (CNS, e.g., traumatic brain injury), 21% from irreversible shock, 25% from both severe CNS trauma and irreversible shock, and 3% from multiple organ failure.

But what is happening to these patients on a cellular level? The metabolic processes of the human body are driven by energy, similar to any other machine. As with machines, the human body generates its own energy but must have fuel to do this. Fuel for the body is oxygen and glucose. The body can store glucose as complex carbohydrates (glycogen) and fat to use at a later time. However, oxygen cannot be stored. It must be constantly supplied to the cells of the body. Atmospheric air, containing oxygen, is drawn into the lungs by the action of the diaphragm and intercostal muscles. Oxygen then diffuses across the alveolar and capillary walls in the lungs, where it binds to the hemoglobin in the red blood cells (RBCs) and is transported to the body's tissues by the circulatory system. In the presence of oxygen, the cells of the tissues then "burn" glucose though a complex series of metabolic processes to produce the energy needed for all body functions. Without sufficient energy, essential metabolic activities cannot function normally and organs begin to fail.

Shock is viewed as a failure of energy production in the body. The sensitivity of the cells to a lack of oxygen varies from organ to organ (Figure 12-1). The cells within an organ can be fatally damaged but can continue to function for a time. This delayed death of cells, leading to organ failure, is what Dr. Cowley referred to in his statement quoted earlier. The condition he described, shock, resulted in death if a patient was not treated promptly. His definition included transporting the patient to the operating room for control of internal hemorrhage. The American College of Surgeons (ACS) Committee on Trauma has used this concept of a Golden Period to emphasize the importance of transporting a patient to a facility where expert trauma care is immediately available.

The Golden Period represents a time interval during which shock is worsening, but this condition is almost always **reversible** if proper care is received. Failure to initiate appropriate interventions aimed at improving oxygenation and controlling hemorrhage allows shock to progress, becoming **irreversible.** For trauma patients to have the best chance of survival, interventions should start in the field with prehospital care provid-

---

FIGURE 12-1   Shock

When the heart is deprived of oxygen, the myocardial cells cannot produce enough energy to pump blood to the other tissues. For example, a patient has lost a significant number of red blood cells and blood volume from a gunshot wound to the aorta. The heart continues to beat for several minutes before failing. Refilling the vascular system, after the heart has been without oxygen for several minutes, will not restore the function of the injured cells of the heart. This process is called irreversible shock. The specific condition in the heart is known as pulseless electrical activity (PEA). Cellular function is still present; however, it is not sufficient to pump blood to the body's cells. The patient has a rhythm on electrocardiogram (ECG) but not enough contractile power to force blood out of the heart to the rest of the body.

Another example of this same process but with a less severe outcome is congestive heart failure. Many of the cells of the heart have been damaged by ischemia secondary to coronary artery disease, but some are not. The damage is not complete, so enough functioning cells are left for the pumping process to continue.

Although ischemia, as seen in severe shock, may damage virtually all tissues, the damage to the organs does not become apparent at the same time. In the lungs, acute respiratory distress syndrome (ARDS) often develops within 48 hours after an ischemic insult, whereas acute renal failure and hepatic failure typically occur several days later. Although all body tissues are affected by insufficient oxygen, some tissues are more sensitive to ischemia. For example, a patient who has sustained a traumatic brain injury may develop cerebral edema (swelling) that results in permanent brain damage. Although the brain cells cease to function and die, the rest of the body may survive for years.

---

systems. Although this text presents the body systems individually, most severely injured patients have injury to more than one body system; thus, the name *multisystem trauma patient* (also known as *polytrauma*). A prehospital care provider needs to recognize and prioritize the treatment of patients with multiple injuries, following the "Golden Principles of Prehospital Trauma Care" described next.

1. Ensure the Safety of the Prehospital Care Providers and the Patient.

Prehospital care providers need to ensure that scene safety remains their highest priority (Figure 12-2). This includes not only the safety of the patient, but their own safety as well. Based on information provided by dispatch, potential threats can often be anticipated before arrival at the scene. For a motor vehicle crash (MVC), threats may include traffic, hazardous materials, fires, and downed power lines; for a shooting victim, providers need to be aware that the perpetrator may still be in the area. When a violent crime is involved, law enforcement personnel should first enter the scene and secure the area. A prehospital care provider who takes needless risk may also become a victim; in doing so, the provider is no longer of help to the original trauma patient. Except in the most unusual circumstances, only those with proper training should attempt rescues.

Another fundamental aspect of safety involves the use of Standard Precautions. Blood and other body fluids can transmit infections, such as human immunodeficiency virus (HIV) and hepatitis B virus (HBV). Protective gear should always be worn, especially when caring for trauma patients in the presence of blood.

The safety of the patient and possible hazardous situations should also be identified. Even if a patient involved in

ers and then continue in the emergency department (ED), the operating room (OR), and the intensive care unit (ICU). Trauma is a "team sport." The patient "wins" when all members of the trauma team—from those in the field to those in the trauma center—work together to care for the individual patient.

The Golden Principles of Prehospital Trauma Care

The preceding chapters discuss the assessment and management of patients who have sustained injury to specific body

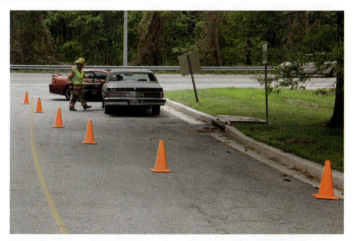

FIGURE 12-2 Ensure the safety of the prehospital care providers and the patient.

an MVC has no life-threatening conditions identified in the primary survey, rapid extrication is appropriate if threats to patient safety are noted, such as a significant potential for fire or a precarious vehicle position.

2. Assess the Scene Situation to Determine the Need for Additional Resources.

During the response to the scene and immediately on arrival, a quick assessment is performed to determine the need for additional or specialized resources. Examples include additional Emergency Medical Services (EMS) units to accommodate the number of patients, fire suppression equipment, special rescue teams, power company personnel, medical helicopters, and physicians to aid in the triage of a large number of patients. The need for these resources should be anticipated and requested as soon as possible.

3. Recognize the Kinematics That Produced the Injuries.

Chapter 2 provides the reader with a foundation of how kinetic energy can translate into injury to the trauma patient. As the scene and the patient are approached, the kinematics of the situation are noted (Figure 12-3). Understanding the principles of kinematics leads to better patient assessment. Knowledge of specific injury patterns aids in predicting injuries and knowing where to examine. Consideration of the kinematics should not delay the initiation of patient assessment and care but can be included in the global scene assessment and in the questions directed to the patient and bystanders. The kinematics may also play a key role in determining the destination facility for a given trauma patient (mechanism of injury criteria for triage to trauma centers). The key aspects of the kinematics noted at the scene should also be relayed to the physicians at the receiving facility.

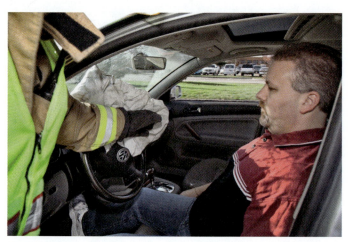

FIGURE 12-3 Recognize the kinematics that produced the injuries.

4. Use the Primary Survey Approach to Identify Life-Threatening Conditions.

The central concept in the PHTLS program is the emphasis on the primary survey. This brief survey allows vital functions to be rapidly assessed and life-threatening conditions to be identified through systematic evaluation of the ABCDEs: airway, breathing, circulation, disability, and expose/environment. On initial approach to the scene and as field care is provided, the prehospital care provider receives input from several senses (sight, hearing, smell, touch) that must be sorted, placed in a priority scheme of life-threatening or limb-threatening injuries, and used to develop a plan for correct management (Figure 12-4).

The primary survey involves a "treat as you go" philosophy. As life-threatening problems are identified, care is initiated at the earliest possible time. Although taught in a step-wise fashion, many aspects of the primary survey can be

---

FIGURE 12-4 **Critical or Potentially Critical Trauma Patient: Scene Time of 10 Minutes or Less**

Presence of any of the following life-threatening conditions:
1. Inadequate or threatened airway
2. Impaired ventilation as demonstrated by the following:
   - Abnormally fast or slow ventilatory rate
   - Hypoxia
   - Dyspnea (shortness of breath)
   - Open pneumothorax or flail chest
   - Suspected pneumothorax
3. Significant external hemorrhage or suspected internal hemorrhage
4. Shock, even if compensated
5. Abnormal neurologic status
   - GCS score = 13
   - Seizure activity
   - Sensory or motor deficit
6. Penetrating trauma to the head, neck, or torso, or proximal to the elbow and knee in the extremities
7. Amputation or near-amputation proximal to the fingers or toes
8. Any trauma in the presence of the following:
   - History of serious medical conditions (e.g., coronary artery disease, chronic obstructive pulmonary disease, bleeding disorder)
   - Age > 55 years
   - Hypothermia
   - Burns
   - Pregnancy

performed simultaneously. During transport, the primary survey should be reassessed at reasonable intervals so that the effectiveness of the interventions can be evaluated and new concerns addressed.

In children, pregnant patients, and elderly persons, injuries should be considered (1) to be more serious than their outward appearance, (2) to have a more profound systemic influence, and (3) to have a greater potential for producing rapid decompensation. In pregnant patients, there are at least two patients to care for—the mother and the fetus—both of whom may have sustained injury. Compensatory mechanisms differ from younger adults and may not reveal abnormalities until the patient is profoundly compromised.

The primary survey also provides a framework to establish management priorities when faced with numerous patients. At a multiple casualty incident, for example, patients who have serious problems identified with their airway, ventilation, or perfusion are managed and transported before patients with only altered levels of consciousness.

5. Provide Appropriate Airway Management While Maintaining Cervical Spine Stabilization.

Management of the airway remains the highest priority in the treatment of critically injured patients. This should be accomplished while maintaining the head and neck in a neutral inline position, if indicated by the mechanism of injury. All prehospital care providers must be able to perform the "essential skills" of airway management with ease: manual clearing of the airway, manual maneuvers to open the airway (trauma jaw thrust and trauma chin lift), suctioning, and the use of oropharyngeal and nasopharyngeal airways.

6. Support Ventilation and Deliver Oxygen.

Assessment and management of ventilation is another key aspect in the management of the critically injured patient. The normal ventilatory rate in the adult patient is 12 to 20 ventilations per minute. A rate slower than this often significantly interferes with the body's ability to oxygenate the RBCs passing through the pulmonary capillaries and to remove the carbon dioxide (CO_2) produced by the tissues. These bradypneic patients require assisted or total ventilatory support with a bag-mask device connected to supplemental oxygen. When patients are tachypneic (adult rate > 20 breaths/minute), ventilations should be assisted with a bag-mask device connected to supplemental oxygen.

Supplemental oxygen is administered to any trauma patient with obvious or suspected life-threatening conditions. Oxygen can be administered through a non-rebreathing mask to the spontaneously breathing patient or with a bag-mask device connected to supplemental oxygen for those patients receiving assisted or total ventilatory support.

7. Control Any Significant External Hemorrhage.

In the trauma patient, significant external hemorrhage is a finding that requires immediate attention. Because blood is not available for administration in the prehospital setting, hemorrhage control becomes a paramount concern for prehospital care providers in order to maintain a sufficient number of circulating RBCs; *every RBC counts*. Extremity injuries and scalp wounds, such as lacerations and partial avulsions, may be associated with life-threatening blood loss.

Most external hemorrhage is readily controlled by the application of direct pressure at the bleeding site or, if resources are limited, by the use of a pressure dressing created with gauze 4×4 pads and an elastic bandage. If direct pressure or a pressure dressing fails to control external hemorrhage from an extremity, the prehospital care provider may consider applying a tourniquet. Although taught for many years in first-aid and basic emergency care courses, evidence shows that elevation of an extremity or applying pressure over a pressure point adds little to direct pressure or a pressure dressing.[3] Tourniquets are routinely used in surgical procedures, with an excellent safety record, and may be lifesaving in the prehospital setting. When faced with a patient who has external hemorrhage that is difficult to control and not amenable to application of a tourniquet, the provider may consider application of a topical hemostatic agent.

Control of external hemorrhage and recognition of suspected internal hemorrhage, combined with prompt transport to the closest appropriate facility, represent opportunities in which prehospital care providers can make significant impact and save many lives.

8. Provide Basic Shock Therapy, Including Appropriately Splinting Musculoskeletal Injuries and Restoring and Maintaining Normal Body Temperature.

At the end of the primary survey, the patient's body is exposed so that the prehospital care provider can quickly scan for additional life-threatening injuries. Once this is completed, the patient should be covered again because hypothermia can be fatal to a critically injured trauma patient. The patient in shock is already handicapped by a marked decrease in energy production resulting from widespread inadequate tissue perfusion. If the patient's body temperature is not maintained, severe hypothermia can ensue. Hypothermia drastically impairs the ability of the body's blood clotting system to achieve hemostasis. Blood coagulates (clots) as the result of a complex series of enzymatic reactions leading to the formation of a fibrin matrix that traps RBCs and stems bleeding. These enzymes function in a very narrow temperature range. A drop in body temperature below 95° F (35° C) may significantly contribute to the development of a *coagulopathy* (decreased ability for blood clotting to occur). Therefore, it is important to maintain and restore body heat through the use of blankets and a warmed environment inside the ambulance.

When fracture of a long bone occurs, surrounding muscle and connective tissue are often torn. This tissue damage, along with bleeding from the ends of the broken bones, can result in significant internal hemorrhage. This blood loss can range from about 500 mL from a humerus fracture up to 1 to 2 L from a single femur fracture. Rough handling of a fractured extremity can worsen the tissue damage and aggravate bleeding. Splinting assists in reducing the loss of additional blood into surrounding tissues, thus helping to preserve circulating RBCs for oxygen transport. For this reason, as well as for pain management, fractured extremities are splinted.

With a critically injured trauma patient, there is no time to splint each individual fracture. Instead, immobilizing the patient to a long backboard will splint virtually all fractures in an anatomic position and diminish internal hemorrhage. The one possible exception to this is a mid-shaft fracture of the femur. Because of the spasm of the very strong muscles in the thigh, the muscles contract, causing the bone ends to override one another, thereby damaging additional tissue. These types of fractures are best managed by use of a traction splint if time allows its application during transport. For the vast majority of trauma calls, when no life-threatening conditions are identified in the primary survey, each suspected extremity injury can be appropriately splinted.

9. Maintain Manual Spinal Stabilization Until the Patient Is Immobilized on a Long Backboard.

When contact with a trauma patient is made, manual stabilization of the cervical spine should be provided and maintained until the patient is either (a) immobilized on a long backboard, or (b) deemed not to meet indications for spinal immobilization (see Indications for Spinal Immobilization Algorithm, Figure 6-23, p. 156) (Figure 12-5). Satisfactory spinal immobilization involves immobilization from the head to the pelvis. Immobilization should not interfere with the patient's ability to open the mouth and should not impair ventilatory function.

For the victim of penetrating trauma, spinal immobilization is performed only if the patient has spine-related neurologic complaint or if a motor or sensory deficit is noted on physical examination. In a patient with blunt trauma, spinal immobilization is indicated if the patient has an altered level of consciousness (Glasgow Coma Scale [GCS] score < 15) or a neurologic complaint, or if spinal tenderness, an anatomic abnormality, or a motor or sensory deficit is identified on physical examination. If the patient has sustained a mechanism of injury that causes concern, spinal immobilization is indicated if the patient has evidence of alcohol or drug intoxi-

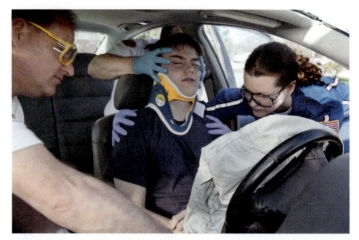

FIGURE 12-5   Maintain manual spinal immobilization until the patient is immobilized on a long backboard.

cation, a significant distracting injury, or an inability to communicate because of an age or language barrier.

10. For Critically Injured Trauma Patients, Initiate Transport to the Closest Appropriate Facility within 10 Minutes of Arrival on Scene.

Numerous studies have demonstrated that delays in transporting trauma patients to appropriate receiving facilities lead to increases in mortality rates (Figure 12-6). Although prehospital care providers have become proficient at airway management, ventilatory support, and circulatory support, most critically injured trauma patients are in hemorrhagic shock and are in need of two things that cannot be provided in the prehospital setting: blood and control of internal hemorrhage. Because human blood is a perishable product, it is

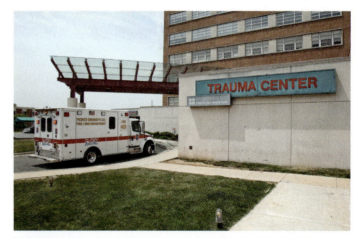

FIGURE 12-6   For critically injured trauma patients, initiate transport to the closest appropriate facility within 10 minutes of arrival on scene.

impractical for administration in the field under most circumstances. Control of internal hemorrhage almost always requires emergent surgical intervention best performed in an operating room. Resuscitation can never be achieved in the patient with ongoing internal hemorrhage. Therefore, the goal of the prehospital care provider is to spend as little time on scene as possible.

This concern for limiting scene time should not be construed as a "scoop and run" mentality in which no attempts are made to address key problems before initiating transport. Instead, the PHTLS program advocates a philosophy of "limited scene intervention," focusing on a rapid assessment aimed at identifying threats to life and performing interventions that are *believed* to improve outcome. Examples include airway and ventilatory management, control of external hemorrhage, and spinal immobilization. Precious time should not be wasted on procedures that can be instituted en route to the receiving facility. Patients who are critically injured (see Figure 12-4) should be transported within 10 minutes of the arrival of EMS on the scene whenever possible—the "Platinum 10 Minutes" of the Golden Period. Reasonable exceptions to the Platinum 10 Minutes include situations that require extensive extrication or time needed to secure an unsafe scene, such as law enforcement ensuring that a perpetrator is no longer present.

The *closest* hospital may not be the *most appropriate* receiving facility for many trauma patients. Those patients who meet certain physiologic, anatomic, or mechanism of injury criteria benefit from being taken to a trauma center—a facility that has special expertise and resources for managing trauma. Ideally, patients who meet physiologic, anatomic, or mechanism of injury criteria, and those with special circumstances, should be transported directly to a trauma center if one is within a reasonable distance (i.e., 30 minutes driving time). Air medical helicopters can also be utilized to transport patients from the scene directly to trauma centers, provided the delay in transport related to awaiting arrival of the helicopter does not exceed the time of ground transport to the closest hospital when a trauma center is not readily available. Thus, each community, through a consensus of surgeons, emergency physicians, and prehospital care providers, must decide where these types of trauma patients should be transported. These decisions should be incorporated into protocols that designate the best destination facility—the closest *appropriate* facility. In some situations, it is appropriate to bypass non-trauma centers to reach a trauma center. Even if this causes a moderate increase in the transport time, the overall time to definitive care will be shorter. Ideally, in the urban setting, a critically injured patient arrives at a trauma center within 25 to 30 minutes of being injured. The hospital also must work equally efficiently to continue resuscitation and, if necessary, transport the patient quickly to the operating room (all within the Golden Period) to control hemorrhage.

11. Ascertain the Patient's Medical History and Perform a Secondary Survey when Life-Threatening Problems Have Been Satisfactorily Managed or Have Been Ruled Out.

If life-threatening conditions are found in the primary survey, key interventions should be performed and the patient prepared for transport within the Platinum 10 Minutes. Conversely, if life-threatening conditions are not identified, a secondary survey is performed. The secondary survey is a systematic, head-to-toe physical examination that serves to identify all injuries. At this time a SAMPLE history (**s**ymptoms, **a**llergies, **m**edications, **p**ast medical history, **l**ast meal, **e**vents preceding the injury) is also obtained. For critically injured trauma patients, a secondary survey is performed only if time permits and once life-threatening conditions have been appropriately managed. In some situations where the patient is located close to an appropriate receiving facility, a secondary survey may never be completed. This approach ensures that the prehospital care provider's attention is focused on the most serious problems—those that may result in death if not properly managed—and not on lower-priority injuries. The patient should be reassessed frequently because patients who initially present without life-threatening injuries may subsequently develop them.

12. Provide Thorough and Accurate Communication Regarding the Patient and the Circumstances of the Injury to the Receiving Facility.

Communication about a trauma patient involves three components: (1) prearrival warning, (2) verbal report upon arrival, and (3) written documentation of the encounter in the patient care report (PCR). Care of the trauma patient depends on a team effort. The response to a critical patient begins with the prehospital provider and continues in the hospital. Thus, providing information from the prehospital setting to the receiving hospital allows for notification and mobilization of appropriate hospital resources to ensure optimal reception of the patient in the receiving institution, Then, upon arrival at the receiving facility—ideally a trauma center for the most critically injured—the prehospital care provider relates a verbal report to those who are assuming the care of the trauma patient. This report should be succinct, accurate, and serve to inform receiving personnel of the patient's presenting condition, kinematics of the injury, assessment findings, interventions, and response to interventions. Because of their ability to interview family members and bystanders, and because a patient's mental status may deteriorate during transport, prehospital care providers may have key information essential to assessment and management of the patient that the in-hospital personnel may not be able to ascertain. Direct communication from provider to provider during patient hand-on ensures continuity of care.

Upon completion of patient care duties, the prehospital care provider carefully and accurately completes a patient care report (PCR). Like other medical records, this document serves as a organized report of the encounter with this patient. A PCR includes all important information from the patient and family or bystanders, as well as findings identified in the physical examination. Additionally, interventions performed are listed, as well as any changes in the patient's condition noted during ongoing assessment. Although several different options exist for documentation, this record should "paint a picture" to the reader of the patient's appearance and provide chronology of interventions. PCRs should be accurate because they are a medicolegal document and also provide crucial information that is included in hospital trauma registries and may be utilized for research.

13. Above All, Do No Further Harm.

The medical principle that states "Above all, do no further harm" dates back to the ancient Greek physician Hippocrates. Applied to the prehospital care of the trauma patient, this principle can take many forms: developing a backup plan for airway management, protecting a patient from flying debris during extrication from a damaged vehicle, or using methods for controlling significant external hemorrhage. Recent experience has shown that prehospital care providers can safely perform many of the lifesaving skills that can be delivered in a trauma center. However, the issue in the prehospital setting is not, "What *can* providers do for critically injured trauma patients?" but rather, "What *should* providers do for critically injured trauma patients?"

When caring for a critically injured patient, prehospital care providers need to ask themselves if their actions at the scene and during transport will reasonably benefit the patient. If the answer to this question is either *no* or *uncertain,* those actions should be withheld and emphasis placed on transporting the trauma patient to the closest appropriate facility. Interventions should be limited to those that prevent or treat physiologic deterioration. Trauma care must follow a given set of priorities that establish an efficient and effective plan of action, based on available time frames and any dangers present at the scene, if the patient is to survive (Figure 12-7). Appropriate intervention and stabilization should be integrated and coordinated between the field, the ED, and the OR. It is essential that every provider at every level of care and at every stage of treatment be in harmony with the rest of the team.

Another important component to the principle of "above all, do no further harm" relates to the issue of secondary injury. It has become clear that injury occurs not only from the initial traumatic event, but also from the physiologic consequences that result from the direct trauma. Specifically,

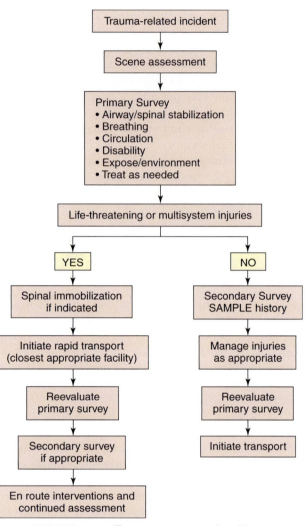

FIGURE 12-7 Trauma response algorithm.

hypoxia, hypotension, and hypothermia all produce additional injury, over and above the primary insult. Failure to recognize that these problems are present, allowing them to develop during the course of treatment, or failure to correct them in a timely fashion offers an opportunity for added complications and greater morbidity and mortality.

In discussing the issue of "do no further harm," the concept of financial harm should be considered in addition to the common thought of physical harm. Specifically, on a regular basis, manufacturers introduce new medications and devices designed to replace or improve existing modalities of treatment. It is important to consider a number of issues before implementing new treatments, including the following:

- What is the medical evidence supporting the efficacy of the new treatment?
- Is the new intervention as good as or better than existing interventions?
- How does the cost of providing the new intervention compare to the existing intervention?

As a general principle, there should be convincing medical evidence that demonstrates that a new intervention is at least as good as, and preferably better than, existing treatments before it is formally accepted and implemented. Because the cost of a new intervention often exceeds that of an existing intervention, the absence of evidence indicating superiority of the new intervention leads to added charges to the patient, resulting in financial harm.

Critically injured trauma patients arriving at a trauma center can have a worse outcome when transported by EMS rather than private vehicle. A significant factor that probably accounts for the increased mortality rate is the actions of well-intentioned prehospital care providers who fail to understand that trauma is a *surgical* disease; most critically injured patients require immediate surgery to save their lives. Anything that delays surgical intervention translates into more hemorrhage, more shock, and ultimately death.

Even with the best planned and executed resuscitation, not all trauma patients can be saved. However, with attention focused on the reasons for early traumatic death, a much larger percentage of patients may survive, with a lower residual morbidity rate than would otherwise result without the benefit of correct and expedient field management. ***The fundamental principles taught in PHTLS—rapid assessment, key field interventions, and rapid transport to the closest appropriate facility—have been shown to improve outcomes in critically injured trauma patients.***

SUMMARY

The following are the Golden Principles of Prehospital Trauma Care:

- Ensure the safety of the prehospital care providers and the patient.
- Assess the scene situation to determine the need for additional resources.
- Recognize the kinematics that produced the injuries.
- Use the primary survey approach to identify life-threatening conditions.
- Provide appropriate airway management while maintaining cervical spine stabilization.
- Support ventilation and deliver oxygen.
- Control any significant external hemorrhage.
- Provide basic shock therapy, including restoring and maintaining normal body temperature and appropriately splinting musculoskeletal injuries.
- Maintain manual spinal stabilization until the patient is immobilized on a long backboard.
- For critically injured trauma patients, initiate transport to the closest appropriate facility within 10 minutes of arrival on scene.
- Ascertain the patient's medical history and perform a secondary survey when life-threatening conditions have been satisfactorily managed or have been ruled out.
- Provide thorough and accurate communication regarding the patient and the circumstances of the injury to the receiving facility.
- ***Above all, do no further harm.***

References

1. Lerner EB, Moscati RM: The Golden Hour: scientific fact or medical "urban legend"? *Acad Emerg Med* 8:758, 2001.
2. Tsybuliak GN, Pavlenko EP: Cause of death in the early posttraumatic period. *Vestn Khir Im I I Grek* 114(5):75, 1975.
3. 2005 International Consensus on Cardiopulmonary Resuscitation (CPR) and Emergency Cardiovascular Care (ECC) Science with Treatment Recommendations. Part 10. First aid. *Circulation* 112(suppl I):III–115, 2005.

Glossary

accelerated motion A sudden surge or increase in motion, e.g., from the transferring of energy in a rear-impact collision; occurs as a slower moving or stationary object is struck from behind.

acetabulum The cup-shaped hip socket on the lateral surface of the pelvis that holds the head of the femur.

acidosis Accumulation of acids and decreased pH of the blood.

acute radiation syndrome The physiologic consequences of whole-body radiation.

acute respiratory distress syndrome (ARDS) Respiratory insufficiency as a result of damage to the lining of the capillaries and alveoli in the lung, leading to the leakage of fluid into the interstitial spaces and alveoli.

acute tubular necrosis (ATN) Acute damage to the renal tubules, usually due to ischemia associated with shock.

adolescent A child with the body size and physical development normally found in children between 13 and 16 years of age.

adult A person (generally 16 years of age or older) whose body has reached maturity and has finished its progression through the phases of pediatric growth and development.

aerobic metabolism Oxygen-based metabolism that is the body's principal combustion process; most efficient process for the production of cellular energy.

aerosol Solid particles and liquid particles that are suspended in air.

afterload The pressure against which the left ventricle must pump out (eject) blood with each beat.

air bags Bags that automatically inflate in front of the driver or passenger upon collision to cushion the impact. The bags absorb the energy slowly by increasing the body's stopping distance. These bags are only designed to cushion forward motion on the initial impact.

alveoli The terminal air sacs of the respiratory tract where the respiratory system meets the circulatory system and gas exchange occurs.

Alzheimer's disease A form of brain disease commonly associated with premature senile dementia.

amnesia A loss of memory.

amputation A severed part or a part that is surgically totally separated (removed) from the rest of the body.

anaerobic metabolism Metabolism not using oxygen, an inefficient process for the production of cellular energy.

analgesia The relief of pain.

anatomical splinting "Splinting" the body on a long backboard, in a supine position and securing the patient to the board.

angina (angina pectoris) A cramping, crushing midsternal chest pain caused by myocardial anoxia. It often radiates to either arm, most commonly the left, or the jaw and is associated with a feeling of suffocation and impending death.

anhidrosis The absence of sweating.

anisocoria Inequality of pupil size.

anterior cord syndrome Damage to the anterior portion of the spinal cord, usually as a result of bony fragments or pressure on spinal arteries.

anterocaudad Forward and toward the feet.

anterograde amnesia Amnesia for events occurring after the precipitating trauma; inability to form new memories.

anticoagulant A substance or drug that prevents or delays coagulation or the forming of blood clots.

antihypertensive A drug that reduces high blood pressure (hypertension).

aortic tear Complete or partial tear of one or more layers of tissue of the aorta.

apnea An absence of spontaneous breathing.

arachnoid mater (arachnoid membrane) Spiderweb-like transparent membrane between the dura mater and the pia mater; the middle of the three meningeal membranes surrounding the brain.

ARDS See *acute respiratory distress syndrome*.

ascending nerve tracts Nerve pathways in the spinal cord that carry sensory impulses from body parts up to the brain.

ataxic breathing Erratic breathing with no rhythm. Commonly associated with head injury and increased intracranial pressure.

atelectasis Collapse of alveoli or part of the lung.

atherosclerosis A narrowing of the blood vessels; a condition in which the inner layer of the artery wall thickens while fatty deposits build up within the artery.

atlas First cervical vertebra (C1); the skull perches upon it.

austere environment A setting in which resources, supplies, equipment, personnel, transportation, and other aspects of the physical, political, social, and economic environments are extremely limited.

autonomic nervous system The part of the central nervous system that directs and controls the involuntary functions of the body.

avulsion The ripping or tearing away of a part; a flap or partially separated tissue or part.

axial unloading Taking the weight of the head off the cervical spine.

axis Second cervical vertebra (C2); its shape allows for the wide possible range of rotation of the head. Also, an imaginary line that passes through the center of the body.

bag-mask device Mechanical ventilation device consisting of a self-inflating bag made of plastic or rubber and several one-way valves; squeezing the bag results in positive-pressure ventilation through a mask or endotracheal tube. May be used with or without supplementary oxygen.

baroreceptor A sensory nerve ending that is stimulated by changes in blood pressure. Baroreceptors are found in the walls of the atria of the heart, vena cava, aortic arch, and carotid sinus.

basal metabolic rate The number of calories the body burns while at rest, resulting in heat production as a byproduct of metabolism.

basilar skull fracture Fracture of the floor of the cranium.

Battle's sign Discoloration posterior and slightly inferior to the outer ears due to bleeding into the subcutaneous tissue caused by an occipital basilar skull fracture.

birdshot Small metal pellets loaded into shotgun shells.

blunt trauma Nonpenetrating trauma caused by a rapidly moving object that impacts the body.

body surface area (BSA) Outer surface of the body covered by the skin; percentage of the body's total surface area represented by any body part. Used as one factor in determining size of a burn.

bradycardia Heart rate less than 60 beats per minute.

brain stem The stem-like part of the brain that connects the cerebral hemispheres with the spinal cord.

bronchioles The smaller divisions of the bronchial tubes.

Broselow Resuscitation Tape A commercially available system for estimating pediatric medication dosing and equipment sizing based on patient length.

Brown-Séquard syndrome Caused by penetrating injury and involves hemitransection of the spinal cord involving only one side of the cord.

buckshot Large metal pellets loaded into shotgun shells.

capillaries The smallest blood vessels. Minute blood vessels that are only one cell wide, allowing for diffusion and osmosis of oxygen and nutrients through the capillary walls.

capnography (end-tidal carbon dioxide) The method of monitoring the partial pressure of carbon dioxide in a sample of gas. It can correlate very closely to the arterial partial pressure of carbon dioxide ($PaCO_2$).

cardiac output The volume of blood pumped by the heart at each contraction (reported in liters per minute).

cardioaccelerator center The brain center that activates the sympathetic response that increases the rate of the heart.

cardiogenic shock Shock that results from failure of the heart's pumping activity; causes can be categorized as either intrinsic, a result of direct damage to the heart itself, or extrinsic, related to a problem outside the heart.

cardioinhibitory center A part of the medulla that slows or inhibits the heart's activity.

cardiovascular Referring to the combination of the heart and blood vessels.

cataract Milky lens that blocks and distorts light entering the eye and blurs vision.

catecholamines Group of chemicals produced by the body that work as important nerve transmitters. The main catecholamines made by the body are dopamine, epinephrine (also called adrenalin), and norepinephrine. They are part of the body's sympathetic defense mechanism used in preparing the body to act.

caudad Toward the tail (coccyx).

cavitation Forcing tissues of the body out of their normal position; to cause a temporary or permanent cavity (e.g., when the body is struck by a bullet, the acceleration of particles of tissue away from the missile produces an area of injury in which a large temporary cavity occurs).

cellular respiration The use of oxygen by the cells to produce energy.

central cord syndrome Damage to the central portion of the spinal cord that usually occurs with hyperextension of the cervical area.

central neurogenic hyperventilation Pathologic rapid and shallow ventilatory pattern associated with head injury and increased intracranial pressure.

cephalad Toward the head.

cerebellum A portion of the brain that lies beneath the cerebrum and behind the medulla oblongata and is concerned with coordination of movement.

cerebral perfusion pressure The amount of pressure needed to maintain cerebral blood flow; calculated as the difference between the mean arterial pressure (MAP) and the intracranial pressure (ICP).

cerebrospinal fluid (CSF) A fluid found in the subarachnoid space and dural sheath; acts as a shock absorber, protecting the brain and spinal cord from jarring impact.

cerebrum The largest part of the brain; responsible for the control of specific intellectual, sensory, and motor functions.

cervical flexion Bending the head forward or downward, causing bending of the neck.

cervical spine The neck area of the spinal column containing seven vertebrae (C1–C7).

chemical burn Burn that occurs when skin comes into contact with various caustic agents.

chemical energy The energy, usually in the form of heat, that results from the interaction of a chemical with other chemicals or human tissue.

chemoreceptor cells Cells that stimulate nerve impulses by reacting to chemical stimuli. Certain chemoreceptor cells control the ventilatory rate.

chemoreceptor A sensory nerve ending that is stimulated by and reacts to certain chemical stimuli; located outside of the central nervous system. Chemoreceptors are found in the large arteries of the thorax and neck, the taste buds, and the olfactory cells of the nose.

Cheyne-Stokes breathing Pathologic ventilatory pattern with periods of shallow, slow breathing increasing to rapid, deep breathing and then returning to shallow, slow breathing followed by a short apneic period. Commonly associated with traumatic brain injury and increased intracranial pressure.

chin lift A way to open the airway of a patient with suspected cervical spine injury; adaptation of chin lift airway maneuver that includes manual immobilization of the head in a neutral in-line position.

cilia Hair-like processes of cells that propel foreign particles and mucus from the bronchi.

cingulate herniation The cingulate gyrus along the medial surface of the cerebral hemispheres is forced under the falx, usually as a result of hemorrhage or edema, causing injury to the medial cerebral hemispheres and the midbrain.

closed fracture A fracture of a bone in which the skin is not interrupted.

coagulopathy Impairment in the normal blood-clotting capabilities.

coagulative necrosis The type of tissue damage that results from acid exposure; the damaged tissue forms a barrier that prevents deeper penetration of the acid.

coccygeal spine The most caudad part of the spinal column; contains the three to five vertebrae that form the coccyx.

cold zone A geographic area that is free from contamination from a hazardous material.

Colles' fracture Fracture of the wrist. If the victim falls forward onto outstretched hands to break a fall, this may result in a silver fork deformity.

compartment syndrome The clinical findings noted from ischemia and compromised circulation that can occur from vascular injury causing hypoxia of muscles in an extremity compartment. The cellular edema produces increased pressure in a closed facial or bony compartment.

compensated shock Inadequate peripheral perfusion as evidenced by signs of decreased organ perfusion but with normal blood pressure.

complacency A feeling of safety or security in the unacknowledged face of potential danger.

complete cord transection Complete damage and severing of the spinal cord; all spinal tracts are interrupted, and all cord functions distal the site are lost.

complication An added difficulty that occurs secondary to an injury, disease, or treatment. Also, disease or incident superimposed upon another without being specifically related yet affecting or modifying the prognosis of the original disease.

compressibility Ability to be deformed by the transfer of energy.

compression injuries Injuries caused by severe crushing and squeezing forces; may occur to the external structure of the body or to the internal organs.

compression Type of force involved in impacts resulting in a tissue, organ, or other body part being squeezed between two or more objects or body parts.

concussion A temporary alteration in neurologic function, most commonly a loss of consciousness, and no intracranial abnormality is identified by computed tomography (CT) scan.

conduction The transfer of heat between two objects in direct contact with each other.

consensual reflex The reflexive constriction of one pupil when a strong light is introduced into the other eye. A lack of consensual reflex is considered a positive sign of brain injury or eye injury.

contact wounds The type of wound that occurs when the muzzle of a gun touches the patient at the time of discharge, resulting in a circular entrance wound, often associated with visible burns, soot, or the imprint of the muzzle.

contraindication Any sign, symptom, clinical impression, condition, or circumstance indicating that a given treatment or course of treatment is inappropriate. Relative contraindication is usually considered as a contraindication but under special circumstances may be overruled by a physician as an accepted medical practice on a case-by-case basis.

contralateral On the opposite side.

contrecoup injury An injury to parts of the brain located on the side opposite that of the primary injury.

contusion A bruise or bruising.

convection The transfer of heat from the movement or circulation of a gas or liquid, such as the heating of water or air in contact with a body, removing that air (such as wind) or water, and then having to heat the new air or water that replaces what left.

cord compression Pressure on the spinal cord caused by swelling, which may result in tissue ischemia and, in some cases, may require decompression to prevent a permanent loss of function.

cord concussion The temporary disruption of the spinal cord functions distal to the site of a spinal cord injury.

cord contusion Bruising or bleeding into the tissue of the spinal cord, which may also result in a temporary loss of cord functions distal to the injury.

cord laceration Occurs when spinal cord tissue is torn or cut.

coup injury An injury to the brain located on the same side as the point of impact.

cranial vault The space within the skull or cranium.

crash Energy is exchanged between a moving object and the tissue of the human body or between the moving human body and a stationary object.

crepitus Crackling sound made by bone ends grating together.

cricothyroid membrane The thin, tough layer of tissue that is located between the thyroid and the cricoid cartilages, the site where a surgical opening is created during a cricothyrotomy.

crush syndrome The physiologic consequences that occur from severe muscle trauma after part of the body is crushed under a heavy weight, manifested by renal failure and death.

Cullen's sign Ecchymosis around the umbilicus.

Cushing's phenomenon The combination of increased arterial blood pressure and the resultant bradycardia that can occur with increased ICP.

cyanosis Blue coloring of skin, mucous membranes, or nail beds indicating unoxygenated hemoglobin and a lack of adequate oxygen levels in the blood; usually secondary to inadequate ventilation or decreased perfusion.

dead space The amount of space that contains air that never reaches the alveoli to participate in the critical gas exchange process.

decerebrate posturing Characteristic posture that occurs when a painful stimulus is introduced, the extremities are stiff and extended and the head is retracted. One of the forms of pathologic posturing (response) commonly associated with increased intracranial pressure.

decontamination Reduction or removal of hazardous chemical, biologic, or radiologic agents.

decorticate posturing A characteristic pathologic posture of a patient with increased intracranial pressure; when a painful stimulus is introduced, the patient is rigidly still with the back and lower extremities extended while the arms are flexed and fists clenched.

definitive care Care that resolves the patient's illness or injury after a definitive diagnosis has been established. Clear and final care that is without question what the particular patient needs for his or her individual problem.

density The number of particles in each given area of tissue.

dermatome The sensory area on the body for which a nerve root is responsible. Collectively, they allow the body areas to be mapped out for each spinal level and to help locate a spinal cord injury.

dermis Layer of skin just under the epidermis made up of a framework of connective tissues containing blood vessels, nerve endings, sebaceous glands, and sweat glands.

diaphragm The dome-shaped muscle that divides the chest and abdomen and which functions as part of the breathing process.

diaphragmatic rupture (diaphragmatic herniation) A tearing or cutting of the diaphragm so that the abdominal and thoracic cavities are no longer separated, allowing abdominal contents to enter the thoracic cavity. Usually a result of increased intra-abdominal pressure producing a tear in the diaphragm.

diaphyseal Part of or affecting the shaft of a long bone.

diastole Ventricular relaxation (ventricular filling).

diastolic blood pressure The resting pressure between ventricular contractions, measured in millimeters of mercury (mm Hg).

diffusion The movement of solutes (substances dissolved in water) across a membrane.

distraction The pulling apart of two structures; i.e., pulling apart the fractured components of a bone or part of the spine.

distributive shock Shock that occurs when the vascular container enlarges without a proportional increase in fluid volume.

Don Juan syndrome The pattern of injury that often occurs when victims fall or jump from a height and land on their feet. Bilateral calcaneus (heel bone) fractures are often associated with this syndrome. After the feet land and stop moving, the body is forced into flexion as the weight of the still-moving head, torso, and pelvis come to bear. This can cause compression fractures of the spinal column in the thoracic and lumbar areas.

dorsal root The spinal nerve root responsible for sensory impulses.

down-and-under pathway When a vehicle ceases its forward motion, the occupant usually continues to travel downward into the seat and forward into the dashboard or steering column.

dura mater The outer membrane covering the spinal cord and brain; the outer of the three meningeal layers. Literally means "tough mother."

dural sheath A fibrous membrane that covers the brain and continues down to the second sacral vertebra.

dysarthria Difficulty speaking.

dysbarism The changes that result physiologically as a result of changes in ambient environmental pressure.

dysrhythmia (cardiac) Abnormal, disordered, or disturbed rhythm of the heart.

ecchymosis A bluish or purple irregularly formed spot or area resulting from a hemorrhagic area below the skin.

eclampsia A syndrome in pregnant women that includes hypertension, peripheral edema and seizures; also called Toxemia of pregnancy.

edema A local or generalized condition in which some of the body tissues contain an excessive amount of fluid; generally includes swelling of the tissue.

edentulism The absence of teeth.

electrical energy The result of movement of electrons between two points.

electrolytes Substances that separate into charged ions when dissolved in solution.

empyema Collection of pus in the pleural space.

endotracheal intubation Insertion of a large tube into the trachea for direct ventilation from outside of the body.

epidermis The outermost layer of the skin, which is made up entirely of dead epithelial cells with no blood vessels.

epidural hematoma Arterial bleeding that collects between the skull and dura mater.

epidural space Potential space between the dura mater surrounding the brain and the cranium. Contains the meningeal arteries.

epiglottis Leaf-shaped structure that acts as a gate or flapper valve and directs air into the trachea and solids and liquids into the esophagus.

epinephrine Chemical released from the adrenal glands, it stimulates the heart to increase cardiac output by increasing the strength and rate of contractions.

epiphyseal The end of the long bone.

escharotomy Incision made to allow the tissues underlying the tough, leathery damaged skin created by severe burns to expand as they swell.

eucapnia Normal blood carbon dioxide level.

euhydration The physiologic state of normal body water balance.

euvolemia Normal circulating blood volume.

evaporation Change from liquid to vapor.

event phase The moment of the actual trauma.

evisceration When a portion of the intestine or other abdominal organ is displaced through an open wound and protrudes externally outside the abdominal cavity.

expiration The forcing of air out of the lungs from the relaxation of the intercostal muscles and diaphragm, resulting in the return of the ribs and diaphragm to their resting positions.

explosion Physical, chemical, or nuclear reactions that result in the almost instantaneous release of large amounts of energy in the form of heat and rapidly expanding, highly compressed gas, capable of projecting fragments at extremely high velocity.

exsanguination Total loss of blood volume, producing death.

external respiration The transfer of oxygen molecules from the atmosphere to the blood.

extraluminal pressure Pressure in the tissue surrounding the vessel.

extreme altitude Elevations higher than 18,045 feet.

fight-or-flight response A defense response that the sympathetic nervous system produces that simultaneously causes the heart to beat faster and stronger, constricts the arteries to raise blood pressure, and increases the ventilatory rate.

FiO$_2$ Fraction of oxygen in inspired air stated as a decimal. An FiO$_2$ of 0.85 means that 85 hundredths or 85% of the inspired air is oxygen.

flail chest A chest with an unstable segment produced by multiple ribs fractured in two or more places or including a fractured sternum.

flat bones Thin, flat, and compact bones, such as the sternum, ribs, and scapulae.

flexion A bending movement around a joint that decreases the angle between the bones at the joint. In the cervical region, it is a forward bending motion of the head, bringing the chin nearer to the sternum.

foot-pounds of force A measure of mechanical force brought to bear. Force = Mass × Deceleration or Acceleration.

foramen magnum The opening at the base of the skull through which the medulla oblongata passes.

foramina Small opening.

fourth-degree burn Burn injury that involves all layers of the skin, as well as the underlying fat, muscles, bone, or internal organs.

fracture A broken bone. A simple fracture is closed without a tear or opening in the skin. An open fracture is one in which the initial injury or bone end has produced an open wound at or near the fracture site. A comminuted fracture has one or more free-floating segments of disconnected bone.

fragmentation When an object breaks up to produce multiple parts or rubble, and, therefore, creates more drag and more energy exchange.

frostbite The actual freezing of body tissue as a result of exposure to freezing or below-freezing temperatures.

full-thickness (third-degree) burns Burn to the epidermis, dermis, and subcutaneous tissue (possibly deeper). Skin may look charred or leathery and may be bleeding.

G-force (gravitational force) Measured force of acceleration or deceleration or of centrifugal force.

gastric ventilation Air undesirably forced down the esophagus and into the stomach rather than into the lungs.

geriatric Dealing with aging and the diagnosis and treatment of injuries and diseases affecting the elderly.

Glasgow Coma Scale A scale for evaluating and quantifying level of consciousness or unconsciousness by determining the best responses of which the patient is capable to standardized stimuli, including eye-opening, verbal, and motor responses.

global overview The simultaneous 15- to 30-second overview of the patient's condition. The global overview focuses on the patient's immediate ventilatory, circulatory, and neurologic status.

glycogen Glucose molecules strung together, used for carbohydrate storage purposes.

Golden Period The period of time a patient has to reach definitive care to achieve the best possible outcome.

Grey Turner's sign Ecchymosis involving the flanks.

heat cramps Acute painful spasms of the voluntary muscles after hard physical work in a hot environment, especially when not acclimated to the temperature.

heat exhaustion Results from excessive fluid and electrolyte loss through sweating and lack of adequate fluid replacement when the patient is exposed to high environmental temperatures for a sustained period of time, usually several days.

heat stress index The combination of ambient temperature and relative humidity.

heat stroke An acute and dangerous reaction to heat exposure characterized by high body temperature and altered mental status.

hematocrit A measure of the packed cell volume of red blood cells in the total blood volume.

hemianesthesia Loss of sensation on one side of the body.

hemiparesis Weakness limited to one side of the body.

hemiplegia Paralysis on one side of the body.

hemoglobin The molecule found in red blood cells that carry oxygen.

hemopericardium Blood accumulation inside the pericardial space that can lead to pericardial tamponade.

hemoptysis Coughing up blood.

hemorrhage Bleeding. Also, a loss of a large amount of blood in a short period of time, either outside or inside the body.

hemorrhagic shock Hypovolemic shock resulting from blood loss.

hemothorax Blood in the pleural space.

high altitude An elevation above 5,000 to 11,480 feet.

homeostasis A constant, stable internal environment. Balance necessary for healthy life processes.

homeotherm Warm-blooded animal.

hot zone The geographic area of highest contamination from a hazardous material; only specially trained and equipped workers may enter this area.

hypercarbia Increased level of carbon dioxide in the body.

hyperchloremia Increase in the blood chloride level.

hyperextension Extreme or abnormal extension of a joint; a position of maximum extension. Hyperextension of the neck is produced when the head is extended posterior to a neutral position and can result in a fracture or dislocation of the vertebrae or in spinal cord damage in a patient with an unstable spine.

hyperflexion Extreme or abnormal flexion of a joint. A position of maximum flexion. Increased flexion of the neck can result in a fracture or dislocation of the vertebrae or in spinal cord damage in a patient with an unstable spine.

hyperglycemia Elevated blood glucose.

hyperhydration Over-consumption of water.

hyperkalemia Increased blood potassium.

hyperrotation Excessive rotation.

hypertension Having a blood pressure greater than the upper limits of the normal range; generally considered to exist if the patient's systolic pressure is greater than 140 mm Hg.

hypertensive crisis A sudden severe increase in blood pressure with signs of organ damage, such as renal failure or cardiac compromise.

hyperthermia Body temperature much higher than normal range.

hypertonic Osmotic pressure greater than serum or plasma.

hypochlorite solutions Solutions used in the production of household bleaches and industrial cleaners.

hypoglycemia Decreased blood glucose.

hypoperfusion Inadequate blood flow to cells with properly oxygenated blood.

hypopharynx The lower portion of the pharynx that opens into the larynx anteriorly and the esophagus posteriorly.

hypotension Blood pressure below normal acceptable range.

hypothalamus The area of the brain that functions as the thermoregulatory center and the body's thermostat to control neurologic and hormonal regulation of body temperature.

hypothenar eminence Fleshy part of the palm along the ulnar margin.

hypothermia Subnormal core body temperature below normal range, usually between 78° and 90° F (26° and 32° C).

hypotonic A solution of lower osmotic pressure than another. Also, having a lower osmotic pressure than normal serum or plasma.

hypoventilation Inadequate ventilation when minute volume falls below normal.

hypovolemia Inadequate (below normal range) fluid or blood volume.

hypovolemic shock Shock caused by loss of blood or fluid.

hypoxia (hypoxemia) Deficiency of oxygen; inadequate available oxygen. Lack of adequate oxygenation of the lungs due to inadequate minute volume (air exchange in the lungs) or a decreased concentration of oxygen in the inspired air. Cellular hypoxia is inadequate oxygen available to the cells.

immune system A related group of responses by various body organs and cells that protects the body from disease organisms, other foreign bodies, and cancers. The main components of the immune response system are the bone marrow, thymus, lymphoid tissues, spleen, and liver.

incident command system A system that defines the chain of command and organization of the various resources that respond during a disaster.

incisura (tentorial incisura) Opening in the tentorium cerebelli at the junction of the midbrain and the cerebrum. The brain stem is inferior to the incisura.

incomplete cord transection Partial transection of the spinal cord in which some tracts and motor/sensory functions remain intact.

infant A child between 7 weeks and 1 year of age.

inhalation The process of drawing air into the lungs.

injury A harmful event that arises from the release of specific forms of physical energy or barriers to normal flow of energy.

intentional injury Injury associated with an act of interpersonal or self-directed violence.

intercostal muscles The muscles located between and that connect the ribs to one another.

internal respiration The movement or diffusion of oxygen molecules from the red blood cells into the tissue cells.

interstitial fluid The extracellular fluid located between the cell wall and the capillary wall.

intervertebral disc Cartilage-like discs that lie between the body of each vertebra and act as shock absorbers.

intervertebral foramina A notch through which nerves pass in the inferior lateral side of the vertebra.

intracellular fluid Fluid within the cells.

intracranial hypertension Increased intracranial pressure.

intraosseous Within the bone substance.

intubation Passing a tube into a body aperture. Endotracheal intubation is the insertion of a breathing tube through the mouth or nose into the trachea to provide an airway for oxygen or an anesthetic gas.

involuntary guarding Rigidity or spasm of the abdominal wall muscles in response to peritonitis.

ipsilateral On the same side.

ischemia Local deficiency of blood supply due to obstruction of circulation to a body part or tissue.

ischemic sensitivity The sensitivity of the cells of a tissue to the lack of oxygen before cell death occurs.

jaw thrust A maneuver that enables the airway of a trauma patient to be opened while the head and cervical spine are manually maintained in a neutral in-line position.

jugular vein distention (JVD) Backup of pressure on the right side of the heart resulting in venous pooling and neck vein distention (engorgement) due to decreased filling of the left heart and reduced left heart output.

keraunoparalysis Transient paralysis that results from a lightning strike.

kinematics The process of looking at the mechanism of injury of an incident to determine what injuries are likely to have resulted from the forces and motion and changes in motion involved; the science of motion.

kinetic energy (KE) Energy available from movement. Function of the weight of an item and its speed. $KE = \frac{1}{2}$ of the mass $\times$ the velocity squared.

kyphosis A forward, humplike curvature of the spine commonly associated with the aging process. Kyphosis may be caused by aging, rickets, or tuberculosis of the spine.

larynx The structure located just above the trachea that contains the vocal cords and the muscles that make them work.

laws of motion Scientific laws relating to motion. Newton's first law of motion: A body at rest will remain at rest and a body in motion will remain in motion unless acted upon by some outside force.

ligament A band of tough, fibrous tissue connecting bone to bone.

ligamentum arteriosum A remnant of fetal circulation and point of fixation at the arch of the aorta.

limbus Junction of the cornea and the sclera.

liquefaction necrosis The type of tissue injury that occurs when alkali damages human tissue; the base liquefies the tissue which allows for deeper penetration of the chemical.

logroll A way to turn a person with a possible spine injury from one side to the other or completely over while manually protecting the spine from excessive, dangerous movement. Used to place patients with a suspected unstable spine injury onto a longboard.

long bones Femur, humerus, ulna, radious, tibia, and fibula.

lumbar vertebrae The five spine vertebrae located below the thoracic vertebrae, these are the most massive, and allow for movement in several directions.

lucid interval Period of normal mental functioning between periods of disorientation, unconsciousness, or mental illness.

lumbar spine Part of the spinal column found at the lower back inferior to the thoracic spine, containing the five lumbar vertebrae (L1–L5).

lymphedema Obstruction of lymph channels, leading to edema.

mass (multiple) casualty incident (MCI) An incident (such as a plane crash, building collapse, or fire) that produces a large number of victims from one mechanism, at one place, and at the same time.

mass The victim's weight.

mean arterial pressure The average pressure in the vascular system, estimated by adding one third of the pulse pressure to the diastolic pressure.

mechanical energy The energy that an object contains when it is in motion.

mediastinum The middle of the thoracic cavity containing the heart, great vessels, trachea, mainstem bronchi, and esophagus.

medulla (medulla oblongata) Part of the brain stem. The medulla is the primary regulatory center of autonomic control of the cardiovascular system.

meninges Three membranes that cover the brain tissue and the spinal cord.

metabolic acidosis Acidosis resulting from increase in acids produced by impaired or abnormal metabolic processes.

metabolism The sum of all physical and chemical changes that take place within an organism; all energy and material transformations that occur within living cells.

minute volume The amount of air exchanged each minute; calculated by multiplying the volume of each breath (tidal volume) by the number of breaths per minute (rate).

miosis Constricted pupil, the patient often complains of blurry or dim vision.

multisystem trauma patient Having injury to more than one body system.

myocardial contusion A bruising of the heart or the heart muscle.

myocardial hypertrophy An increase in the heart's muscle mass and size.

myocardium The middle and thickest layer of the heart wall; composed of cardiac muscle, often used as a general term to refer to all muscle in the heart.

myoglobin A protein found in muscle that is responsible for giving muscle its characteristic red color.

myoglobinuria The release of myoglobin into the bloodstream in considerable amounts, causing a reddish or tea-colored urine, toxicity to the kidneys, and kidney failure.

nares (singular naris) The openings in the nose that allow passage of the air from the outside to the throat. The anterior nares are the nostrils. The posterior nares are a pair of openings in the back of the nasal cavity where it connects with the upper throat.

nasopharyngeal airway An airway that is placed in the nostril and follows the floor of the nasal cavity directly posterior to the nasopharynx. This airway is commonly tolerated by patients with a gag reflex.

nasopharynx The upper portion of the airway, situated above the soft palate.

neural arches Two curved sides of the vertebrae.

neurogenic shock Shock that occurs when a cervical spine injury damages the spinal cord above where the nerves of the sympathetic nervous system exit, thus interfering with the normal vasoconstriction and leading to decreased blood pressure.

newborn A child from birth to 6 weeks of age.

Newton's first law of motion A body at rest will remain at rest and a body in motion will remain in motion unless acted on by an outside force.

norepinephrine Chemical released by the sympathetic nervous system, it triggers constriction of the blood vessels to reduce the size of the container and bring it more into proportion with the volume of the remaining fluid.

nonpatent airway An obstructed airway.

nonrebreather reservoir mask (NRB) An oxygen mask with a reservoir bag and nonrebreather valves that allow the exiting of exhaled air. It delivers high oxygen concentrations of between 85% and 100% to the patient when attached to a high-liter-flow oxygen source.

obtundation Diminished mental capacity, usually as a result of trauma or disease.

occipital condyles The two rounded knuckle-like bumps on either side of the occipital bone at the back of the head.

oculomotor nerve The third cranial nerve; controls pupillary constriction and certain eye movements.

odontoid process The toothlike protrusion on the upper surface of the second vertebra (axis) around which the first cervical vertebra (atlas) turns, allowing the head to rotate through approximately 180 degrees.

off-line medical direction Written protocols that can direct most prehospital care.

oncotic pressure Pressure that determines the amount of fluid within the vascular space.

online medical direction Medical direction that allows the prehospital care provider to discuss patient care over the radio or phone while in the field.

open fracture A fracture of a bone in which the skin is broken.

open pneumothorax (sucking chest wound) A penetrating wound to the chest causes the chest wall to be opened, producing a preferential pathway for air moving from the outside environment into the thorax.

oropharyngeal airway An airway that, when placed in the oropharynx superior to the tongue, holds the tongue forward to assist in maintaining an open airway. It is only used in patients with no gag reflex.

oropharynx The central portion of the pharynx lying between the soft palate and the upper portion of the epiglottis.

orthostatic hypotension Decrease in blood pressure when attempting to stand or sit after lying down, often manifested by lightheadedness, dizziness, or syncope.

osmosis The movement of water (or other solvent) across a membrane from an area that is hypotonic to an area that is hypertonic.

osteomyelitis Bone infection.

osteophysis Calcification of bone.

osteoporosis A loss of normal bone density with thinning of bone tissue and the growth of small holes in the bone. The disorder may cause pain (especially in the lower back), frequent broken bones, loss of body height, and various poorly formed parts of the body. Commonly a part of the normal aging process.

overtriage The problem of minimally or noninjured patients being taken to trauma centers.

oxygen consumption The volume of oxygen consumed by the body in 1 minute.

oxygen delivery The process of oxygen transfer from the atmosphere to the RBC during ventilation and the transportation of these RBCs to the tissues via the cardiovascular system.

palpation Process of physically examining a patient by application of the hands or fingers to the external surface of the body to detect evidence of disease, abnormalities, or underlying injury.

paradoxical motion The motion caused by the combination of the lower pressure in the chest and the higher atmospheric pressure outside the chest that causes a flail segment to move inward, rather than outward, during inspiration.

paradoxical pulse Condition in which the patient's systolic blood pressure drops more than 10 to 15 mm Hg during each inspiration, usually due to the effect of increased intrathoracic pressure such as would occur with tension pneumothorax or from pericardial tamponade.

para-anesthesia Loss of sensation in the lower extremities.

paraplegia Paralysis of the lower extremities.

parasympathetic acute stress reaction Slows bodily functions and may result in syncope.

parasympathetic nervous system The division of the nervous system that maintains normal body functions.

paresis Localized weakness or partial (less than total) paralysis related in some cases to nerve inflammation or injury.

parietal pleura A thin membrane that lines the inner side of the thoracic cavity.

Parkland formula Formula for fluid replacement in the burned patient.

partial-thickness (second-degree) burns Burns that involve both the epidermis and dermis. Skin presents with reddened areas; blisters; or open, weeping wounds.

patent airway An open unobstructed airway of sufficient size to allow for normal volumes of air exchange.

pathophysiology The study of how normal physiologic processes are altered by disease or injury.

PEARRL Pupils equal and round, reactive to light; the term used when checking the patient's eyes to determine if they are round, appear normal, and appropriately react to light by constricting, or whether they are abnormal and unresponsive. Generally the presence of consensual reflex is included in this examination term.

pediatric trauma score (PTS) A clinical scoring system based on clinical information that is predictive of severity of injury and can be used for triage decision making.

pediatric Dealing with children; dealing with injuries and diseases affecting children (birth to 16 years of age).

penetrating trauma Trauma that results when an object penetrates the skin and injures underlying structures. Generally produces both permanent and temporary cavities.

percutaneous transtracheal ventilation (PTV) A procedure in which a 16-gauge or larger needle through which the patient is ventilated is inserted directly into the lumen of the trachea through the cricothyroid membrane, or directly through the tracheal wall.

perfusion Blood passing through an organ or a part of the body.

pericardial space The space existing between the heart muscle (myocardium) and the pericardium.

pericardial tamponade Compression of the heart by blood collecting in the pericardial sac, which surrounds the heart muscle (myocardium); also sometimes called cardiac tamponade.

pericardiocentesis A procedure to remove accumulated blood or fluid inside the pericardial space.

pericardium A tough, fibrous, flexible but inelastic membrane that surrounds the heart.

peristalsis The propulsive, muscular movements of the intestines.

peritoneal space Space in the anterior abdominal cavity that contains the bowel, spleen, liver, stomach, and gallbladder. The peritoneal space is lined with the peritoneum.

peritoneum Lining of the abdominal cavity.

peritonitis Inflammation of the peritoneum.

phantom pain The experience of sensation in the missing part or limb after amputation.

pharynx The throat; a tubelike structure that is a passage for both the breathing and digestive tracts. Oropharynx area of the pharynx posterior to the mouth; nasopharynx area of the pharynx beyond the posterior nares of the nose.

photophobia Light sensitivity.

pia mater A thin vascular membrane closely adhering to the brain and spinal cord and proximal portions of the nerves; the innermost of the three meningeal membranes that cover the brain.

pleura A thin membrane that lines the inner side of the thoracic cavity and the lungs. The part that lines the thoracic cavity is called the parietal pleura; the fold covering the lung is called the visceral pleura.

pleural fluid Fluid that creates surface tension between the two pleural membranes and causes them to cling together.

pneumatic antishock garment (PASG) A garment designed to put pressure on the lower portion of the body and prevent pooling of blood in the abdomen and pelvis. Also called military or medical antishock trousers (MAST).

pneumothorax Injury that results in air in the pleural space; commonly producing a collapsed lung. A pneumothorax can be open with an opening through the chest wall to the outside or closed resulting from blunt trauma or a spontaneous collapse.

polytrauma See *multisystem trauma patient*.

post-event phase This phase begins as soon as the energy from the crash is absorbed and the patient is traumatized; the phase of prehospital care that includes response time, "golden period," and critique of a call.

pre-event/precrash phase This phase includes all of the events that precede an incident (e.g., ingestion of drugs and alcohol) and conditions that predate the incident (e.g., acute or pre-existing medical conditions). This phase includes injury prevention and preparedness.

preload The volume and pressure of the blood coming into the heart from the systemic circulatory system (venous return).

premature ventricular contraction A premature, irregular, extra contraction of the ventricles due to an ectopic stimulus, causing a contraction rather than the normal stimuli from the normal pacing node. Second most common abnormal rhythm of the heart.

presbycusis Gradual decline in hearing.

presbyopia Farsightedness.

preschooler A child with the body size and physical development normally found between 2 and 6 years of age.

priapism Prolonged erection. It may be caused by a urinary stone, sickle cell disease, or an injury to the lower spinal column.

primary brain injury Direct trauma to the brain and associated vascular injuries.

primary contamination Exposure to a hazardous substance at its point of release.

primary hypothermia Decrease in body temperature that occurs when healthy individuals are unprepared for overwhelming acute or chronic cold exposure.

primary injuries of blasts Injuries that are caused by the pressure wave of the blast (e.g., pulmonary bleeding, pneumothorax, perforation of the gastrointestinal tract).

primary survey The initial assessment of airway, breathing, circulation, disability, and environment/exposure to identify and manage any life-threatening injuries.

pruritus Severe itching.

psychogenic shock A temporary neurogenic shock as a result of psychological stress (fainting).

pulmonary contusion A bruising of the lungs. This can be secondary to blunt or penetrating trauma.

pulmonary diffusion Movement of oxygen from the alveoli across the alveolar capillary membrane and into the red blood cells or the plasma.

pulmonary function Controlled patent airway, ventilation, diffusion, and perfusion, resulting in arterial blood that contains adequate oxygen for aerobic metabolism and a proper level of carbon dioxide to maintain tissue acid-base balance.

pulse oximeter A machine that provides measurement of arterial oxyhemoglobin saturation. It is determined by measuring the absorption ratio of red and infrared light passed through the tissue.

pulse pressure The increase in pressure (surge) that is created as each new bolus of blood leaves the left ventricle with each contraction. Also, the difference between the systolic and diastolic blood pressures (systolic pressure minus diastolic pressure equals pulse pressure).

quadriplegia Paralysis of all four extremities.

quaternary effects Injuries from a blast or explosion that include burns and toxicities from fuel, metals, trauma from structural collapse, septic syndromes from soil, and environmental contamination.

raccoon eyes (periorbital ecchymosis) Ecchymotic area around each eye, limited by the orbital margins.

radiation The direct transfer of energy from a warm object to a cooler one by infrared radiation.

radiation energy Any electromagnetic wave that travels in rays and has no physical mass to it.

rapid sequence intubation A method of patient intubation that includes pharmacologic adjuncts for sedation and muscle relaxation.

rebound tenderness A physical examination finding that occurs by pressing deeply on the abdomen and then quickly releasing the pressure causing more severe pain when the abdominal pressure is suddenly released.

residual volume Air that remains trapped in the alveoli and bronchi that cannot be forcibly exhaled.

respiration The total ventilatory and circulatory processes involved in the exchange of oxygen and carbon dioxide between the outside atmosphere and the cells of the body. Sometimes in medicine limited to meaning breathing and the steps in ventilation.

respiratory tract The pathway for air movement between the outside air and the alveoli; includes the nasal cavity, oral cavity, pharynx, larynx, trachea, bronchi, and lungs.

response time The time interval from the time an incident occurs until arrival of emergency medical services on scene.

retrograde amnesia Loss of memory for events and situations just preceding the time (immediate preinsult period) of the patient's injury or illness. Also, loss of memory for past events.

retroperitoneal space Space in the posterior abdominal cavity that contains the kidneys, ureters, bladder, reproductive organs, inferior vena cava, abdominal aorta, pancreas, a portion of the duodenum, colon, and rectum.

revised trauma score A method for scoring and quantifying the severity of trauma in patients.

rotational impact When one vehicle strikes the front or rear side of another, causing it to rotate away from the point of impact. Also, when one corner of the vehicle strikes an immovable object or one moving slower or in the opposite direction of the vehicle, resulting in it rotating.

rule of nines A topographic breakdown (mostly of 9% and 18% portions) of the body in order to estimate the amount of body surface covered by burns.

sacral spine (sacrum) Part of the spinal column below the lumbar spine containing the five sacral vertebrae (S1–S5), which are connected by immovable joints to form the sacrum. The sacrum is the weight-bearing base of the spinal column and is also a part of the pelvic girdle.

safety Evaluation of all possible dangers and ensuring that no unreasonable threats or risks still exist.

SAMPLE History A mnemonic to remember the components of the history of symptoms, allergies, medication, past medical and surgical history, last meal, and events leading up to the injury.

SAR Search and rescue.

scalp The outermost covering of the head.

scene Environment to be evaluated in which an injury occurred. In a motor vehicle crash, this includes evaluation of the number of vehicles, the forces that acted upon each, and the degree and type of damage to each.

school-age child A child with the body size and physical development normally found between about 6 and 12 years of age.

seat-belt sign Ecchymosis or abrasion across the chest or abdomen resulting from compression of the trunk against the shoulder harness or lap belt.

secondary brain injury An extension of the magnitude of the primary brain injury by factors such as hypoxia and hypertension that result in a larger, more permanent neurologic deficit.

secondary contamination Exposure to a hazardous substance after it has been carried away from the point of origin by a victim, a responder, or a piece of equipment.

secondary hypothermia Decrease in body temperature as a consequence of a patient's systemic disorder, including hypothyroidism, hypoadrenalism, trauma, carcinoma, and sepsis.

secondary injuries of blasts Injuries that occur when the victim is struck by flying glass, falling mortar, or other debris from the blast.

secondary survey Head-to-toe evaluation of the trauma patient. This assessment is only done after the primary survey is complete and there are no immediate life-threatening problems; usually done en route in urgent patients.

semipermeable membrane Membrane that will allow fluids (solvents) but not the dissolved substance to pass through it.

senescence The process of aging.

sensory examination A gross examination of sensory capability and response to determine the presence or absence of loss of sensation in each of the four extremities.

sepsis Infection that has spread to involve the entire body.

septic shock Shock resulting from locally active hormones due to widespread systemic infection, causing damage to the walls of blood vessels, producing both peripheral vasodilation and a leakage of fluid from the capillaries into the interstitial space.

sesamoid bones Bones, usually small and round, located within tendons.

shear Change-of-speed force resulting in a cutting or tearing of body parts.

shock A widespread lack of tissue perfusion with oxygenated red blood cells that leads to anaerobic metabolism and decreased energy production.

short bones Metacarpals, metatarsals, phalanges.

simple pneumothorax The presence of air within the pleural space.

sinoatrial node Node at junction of superior vena cava with right cardiac atrium; regarded as the pacing or starting point of the heartbeat. In healthy patients, pacing from this node causes atrial contraction and then results in contraction of the ventricles.

situation Events, relationships, and roles of those parties who, with the patient, were involved in a call. The situation (e.g., domestic dispute, single vehicle crash without an apparent reason, elderly person living alone, a shooting) is important in scene assessment.

skull (cranium) Several bones that fuse into a single structure during childhood to house and protect the brain.

slugs A single metallic missile; bullet.

sniffing position A slightly superior anterior position of the head and neck to optimize ventilation as well as the view during endotracheal intubation.

spinal shock A term that refers to an injury to the spinal cord that results in a temporary loss of sensory and motor function.

spinal stenosis Narrowing of the spinal canal.

spinous process Tail-like structure on the posterior region of the vertebrae.

sprain An injury in which ligaments are stretched or even partially torn.

stellate wound Star-shaped wound.

strain A soft tissue injury that occurs around a joint when the muscles or tendons are stretched or torn anywhere in the musculature.

stroke volume The volume of blood pumped out by each contraction (stroke) of the left ventricle.

subarachnoid hemorrhage Bleeding into the cerebrospinal fluid-filled space beneath the arachnoid membrane.

subarachnoid space Space between the pia mater proper and arachnoid membrane; contains cerebrospinal fluid and meningeal veins. The subarachnoid space is a common site of subdural hematomas.

subcutaneous layer Layer of skin just under the dermis that is a combination of elastic and fibrous tissue as well as fat deposits.

subdural hematoma A collection of blood between the dura mater and the arachnoid membrane.

sublimation When solids emit vapors, bypassing the liquid state.

superficial (first-degree) burns Burns to the epidermis only; red, inflamed, and painful skin.

supine hypotension syndrome Decrease in blood pressure caused by compression of the vena cava by the pregnant uterus.

surgical cricothyrotomy A procedure to open a patient's airway that is accomplished by cutting a slit into the cricothyroid membrane in the neck to open the airway into the trachea.

surveillance The process of collecting data within a community, usually for infectious diseases.

sutural bones The flat bones that make up the skull.

sympathetic acute stress reaction The "fight-or-flight" response in which bodily functions increase and pain masking occurs from a release of epinephrine and norepinephrine.

sympathetic nervous system Division of the nervous system that produces the fight-or-flight response.

syncope Fainting.

synovial fluid Fluid found inside joints.

systemic vascular resistance The amount of resistance to the flow of blood through the vessels. It increases as the vessel constricts. Any change in lumen diameter or vessel elasticity can influence the amount of resistance.

systole Ventricular contraction.

systolic blood pressure Peak blood pressure produced by the force of the contraction (systole) of the ventricles of the heart.

tachycardia Abnormally fast rate of heartbeats; defined as a rate over 100 beats per minute in an adult.

tachypnea Increased breathing rate.

tendon A band of tough, inelastic, fibrous tissue that connects a muscle to bone.

tension pneumothorax Condition when the air pressure in the pleural space exceeds the outside atmospheric pressure and cannot escape. The affected side becomes hyperinflated, compressing the lung on the involved side and shifting the mediastinum to partially collapse the other lung. A tension pneumothorax is usually progressive and is an imminently life-threatening condition.

tentorial herniation The process by which part of the brain is pushed down through the incisura as a result of increased intracranial pressure, tentorial herniation occurs.

tentorium cerebelli (tentorium) An infolding of the dura that forms a covering over the cerebellum. The tentorium is a part of the floor of the upper skull just below the brain (cerebrum).

tertiary injuries of blasts The injuries that occur from an explosion when the victim becomes a missile and is thrown against some object. These injuries are similar to those sustained in ejections from vehicles, in falls from significant heights, or when the victim is thrown against an object by the force wave resulting from an explosion. Tertiary injuries are usually blunt injuries.

tetany Muscle contraction or spasms that are sustained in duration.

thermal energy Energy associated with increased temperature and heat.

thoracic spine The part of the spinal column between the cervical spine (superiorly) and the lumbar spine (inferiorly) containing the 12 thoracic vertebrae (T1–T12). The 12 pairs of ribs connect to the thoracic vertebrae.

thorax (thoracic cavity) Hollow cylinder supported by 12 pairs of ribs that articulate posteriorly with the thoracic spine and 10 pairs that articulate anteriorly with the sternum. The 2 lowest pairs are only fastened posteriorly (to the vertebrae) and are called floating ribs. The thoracic cavity is defined and separated inferiorly by the diaphragm.

tidal volume Normal volume of air exchanged with each ventilation. About 500 ml of air is exchanged between the lungs and the atmosphere with each breath in a healthy adult at rest.

toddler A child with the body size and physical development normally found between about 1 and 2 years of age.

tonsil-tip catheter Rigid suction catheter designed for rapid removal of large amounts of fluid, vomitus, blood, and debris from the mouth and pharynx to avoid aspiration.

tonsillar herniation The process by which the brain is pushed down toward the foramen magnum and pushes the cerebellum and medulla ahead of it, causing damage and, ultimately, death.

total lung capacity The total volume of air in the lungs after a forced inhalation.

transmural pressure Difference between the pressure inside a blood vessel and the pressure outside the vessel.

transverse process Protuberances at each side of a vertebra near the lateral margins.

trauma chin lift This maneuver is used to relieve a variety of anatomic airway obstructions in patients who are breathing spontaneously. It is accomplished by grasping the chin and lower incisors and then lifting to pull the mandible forward.

trauma jaw thrust This maneuver allows an open airway with little or no movement of the head and cervical spine. The mandible is thrust forward by placing the thumbs on each zygomatic arch and placing the index and long fingers under the mandible and at the same angle, thrusting the mandible forward.

traumatic aneurysm An abnormal dilation, bursting, or tearing of a major blood vessel (usually an artery) caused by or related to an injury.

traumatic asphyxia Blunt and crushing injuries to the chest and abdomen with marked increase of intravascular pressure, producing rupture of the capillaries.

traumatic rhabdomyolysis See *crush syndrome.*

Trendelenburg position Simultaneous lowering of the patient's head while elevating the patient's legs. Usually done by raising the foot end of a flat bed or longboard higher than the head end. In this position (with the abdomen higher than the thorax), the weight of the abdominal contents presses on the diaphragm, producing some ventilatory difficulty. A modified Trendelenburg position with the head and torso horizontal and only the legs elevated will minimize ventilatory problems.

triage French word meaning "to sort;" a process in which a group of patients is sorted according to their priority of need for care. When only several patients are involved, triage involves assessing each patient, meeting all of the patients' highest priority needs first, and then moving to lower priority items. In a mass casualty incident with a large number of patients involved, triage is done by determining both urgency and potential for survival.

tumble End-over-end motion. Bullets commonly tumble when resistance is met by the leading edge of the missile.

uncal herniation The process by which an expanding mass (usually hemorrhage or swelling) along the convexity of the brain pushes the medial portion of the temporal lobe downward through the tentorium that supports the cerebrum, causing damage to the brainstem.

uncus The medial portion of the temporal lobe.

undertriage The problem that arises when seriously injured patients are not recognized as such and are mistakenly taken to nontrauma centers.

unified command The process by which the incident commanders of all of the various agencies responding to an event work together to manage the incident.

up-and-over pathway The pathway in a motor vehicle crash in which the body's forward motion carries it up-and-over the steering wheel; the chest or abdomen commonly impacts the steering wheel and the head strikes the windshield. In the semisitting position common in passenger vehicles, once the down-and-under motion has ended as the knees are stopped by the dashboard, the body then continues in an up-and-over movement. In some trucks, in which the driver is sitting fully upright with his feet stopped by the pedals, the up-and-over movement may occur initially.

vagal Dealing with stimulation of the vagus (tenth cranial) nerve; the parasympathetic system's response that slows the heart rate and reduces the force of contractions, keeping the body within workable limits. This response can normally override the sympathetic nervous system's chemical release, keeping the heart rate in an acceptable range. Accidental vagal stimulation, however, can result in producing an undesirable bradycardia, further reducing the patient's cardiac output and circulation.

vagus nerve The tenth cranial nerve; when stimulated, slows the heart rate regardless of levels of catecholamines. It contains motor and sensory functions and a wider distribution than any of the other cranial nerves.

vapor A solid or liquid in a gaseous state, usually visible as a fine cloud or mist.

velocity Speed, as in the speed of a moving mass, and the direction of movement.

ventilation Movement of air into and out of the lungs through the normal breathing process; the mechanical process by which air moves from the atmosphere outside the body through the mouth, nose, pharynx, trachea, bronchi, and bronchioles, and into and out of the alveoli. To ventilate a patient is to provide positive-pressure inspirations with a ventilating device, such as a bag-mask device, and then alternately allowing time for passive exhalation to occur; used in patients who are apneic or who cannot provide adequate ventilation for themselves.

ventral root The spinal nerve root responsible for motor impulses.

vertebra Any of the 33 bony segments of the spinal column.

vertebral body The part of the vertebrae that bears most of the weight of the spine.

vertebral foramen Holes in the bony structure of the vertebrae through which blood vessels and nerves pass.

vertebral foramina Openings in the vertebral body.

very high altitude Elevation levels between 11,480–18,045 ft.

vestibular folds The false vocal cords that direct airflow through the vocal cords.

visceral pleura A thin membrane that covers the outer surface of each lung.

volatility The likelihood that solids or liquids vaporizes into a gaseous form at room temperature.

voluntary guarding When palpating a tender area of the abdomen, the patient tenses up the abdominal muscles in that area.

warm zone A geographic area of diminished contamination from a hazardous material and the location for the contamination reduction corridor where exposed patients are decontaminated by the hazmat team.

whistle-stop catheter (whistle-tip catheter) A soft catheter used for suctioning the nasal passage, deep oropharynx, or endotracheal tube; allows for controlled intermittent suction. Its name is derived from the opening (whistle-stop) found in the side of the proximal end of the catheter. Suction is not produced at the distal tip until this hole or port is covered with one of the operator's fingers, producing a closed system to the opening at the distal tip.

white phosphorus An incendiary agent used in the production of munitions.

zygomatic arches The bones that form the superior area of the cheeks of the face. Laterally, superior to the molars, these extend more anteriorly than the maxilla, giving the individual some of his or her unique facial structure; commonly called the cheekbones.

Index

Page numbers followed by f indicate figures.